# PUBLIC HEALTH ADMINISTRATION IN THE UNITED STATES

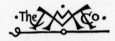

THE MACMILLAN COMPANY
NEW YORK · BOSTON · CHICAGO · DALLAS
ATLANTA · SAN FRANCISCO

MACMILLAN AND CO., Limited
LONDON · BOMBAY · CALCUTTA · MADRAS
MELBOURNE

THE MACMILLAN COMPANY
OF CANADA, Limited
TORONTO

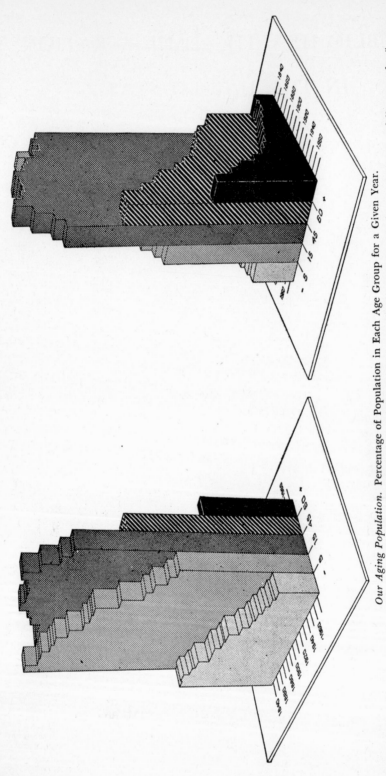

*Our Aging Population.* Percentage of Population in Each Age Group for a Given Year.

The graph gives the percentage of the population in various age groups by decades, from 1840 to 1980. The age groups are as follows: under 5 years; 6 to 15 years; 16 to 45 years; 46 to 60 years; over 60 years. The greatest proportional decline occurs in young children, and the greatest increase in the aged. The productive age group—15 to 45 years—remains quite constant. These changes in our population will require a complete reorientation of health and welfare activities. Old-age insurance was instituted just in time, but other social and economic readjustments remain to be made.

# PUBLIC HEALTH ADMINISTRATION

# IN THE UNITED STATES

*by*

## WILSON G. SMILLIE

A.B., M.D., Dr.P.H., Sc.D. (Hon.)

PROFESSOR OF PUBLIC HEALTH AND PREVENTIVE MEDICINE
CORNELL UNIVERSITY MEDICAL COLLEGE
NEW YORK CITY

*THIRD EDITION*

NEW YORK
THE MACMILLAN COMPANY
1951

Fifth Printing, 1951.

This book is dedicated to the
Pioneers of the Modern Public Health Movement
in the United States,
who in 1872
founded the American Public Health Association
and at that first meeting
laid the foundation stones on which
Public Health Administration in the United States
has been built.

"No subject is more intimately connected with the happiness and prosperity of a people than the degree of public health that they enjoy."

LEMUEL SHATTUCK

"A Census of the City of Boston"

1845

# PREFACE TO THE SECOND EDITION

FIVE years ago, when this text was introduced with the statement that public health was in the developmental stage in the United States, we had no conception of the rapid growth and expansion of public health administration that were about to occur.

These developments have not been of a revolutionary nature, for the basic principles have remained unchanged. But the work has been more effective. Increased knowledge of the epidemiology of disease has made it possible to carry out more precise control measures. We have learned to apply in a more well-defined way the scientific knowledge that has accumulated in relation to communicable disease control. Thus, it becomes necessary to revise our administrative procedures in the control of scarlet fever, typhoid fever, measles, whooping cough, tuberculosis, influenza, syphilis, gonorrhea, and pneumonia, as well as in many other diseases of lesser import.

We have greatly increased our knowledge concerning the importance of nutrition to individual and community welfare, and have discovered the useful part that the health department may play in improving the general nutritional state of the people within its jurisdiction.

All these matters have been discussed in this revised edition.

The extraordinary change that has occurred during the past few years has been the growth of public interest in national health affairs. The Social Security Act of 1935 is concrete evidence of this interest. This Act revolutionized the United States Public Health Service and the Children's Bureau, and made possible a true national health program. Immediately after the passage of this Act there began a tremendous movement, which in real estate terms would be called a "boom," in public health. This phenomenal growth in public health occurred under competent national leadership, and relatively few serious mistakes were made.

In retrospect, it becomes clear that the nation was ready for this expansion. All the years of careful planning and experimentation in administrative technics, largely under sponsorship of voluntary health agencies, had prepared the soil and fitted the personnel for successful cultivation of this fertile field. The United States Congress provided the funds, and the United States Public Health Service and the Children's Bureau, with the assistance of experienced state health officers and other experts who volunteered their services, provided the leadership. As a result, during the past five years, more extensive and substantial advances have been made in public health administration than occurred during the previous quarter of a century. Full time local health departments have increased fourfold, state health departments have been placed on an effective basis, child health activities have been developed in an adequate manner, increased facilities have been provided for the technical training of all types of public health personnel—all within the period from 1935 to 1940.

We have attempted to review these developments of the national health program, to indicate how the present gains may be consolidated, and to anticipate what may unfold in the immediate future.

The field of the health administrator is expanding; more and more responsibility is being placed on his shoulders. It is our modest hope that these pages may be of some assistance to those who desire to inform themselves concerning our present knowledge of the administration of public health affairs.

We wish to thank all those who have given us criticisms and suggestions in relation to the first edition of this book. These corrections and additions have been incorporated in the new text.

I take this opportunity to express my sincere thanks to Miss Lina Garland Odom for her unflagging interest in the tedious editorial detail work of this manuscript.

W. G. S.

# PREFACE TO THE THIRD EDITION

THE author understood, when he first began to write this text (about 1930), that public health in the United States was in the developmental stages, with little crystallization of ideas concerning those public health procedures that were most profitable and worth while.

But little did he realize, at that time, the rapid developments that would occur in the field of public health during the following twenty years. The changes in our social organization have been so abrupt and so profound that it has become necessary to revise completely the original book, so that it has become only a skeleton upon which to frame a new text.

The major events that transpired during these past years were: a nation-wide economic depression, followed by a world-wide war. As a direct result, there occurred all the social upheavals that such catastrophes entail. Even from great disasters, some benefits to society usually accrue. As an example, there is an extraordinary phenomenon that has always been observed in American history, namely, that every war in which the nation has participated, has brought with it, as a by-product, a resurgence in medical science, and a great advancement in the public health. World War II was no exception to this rule.

One striking change during and following this war was the advance that was made in our knowledge of the epidemiology of a great many important diseases. This knowledge was acquired as a direct result of war exigencies and war efforts. Since control of communicable disease rests on epidemiologic knowledge, it has become necessary to change our concepts and adapt our control methods to meet these new ideas. Thus important changes are found in this third edition in the control methods for scarlet fever and all the streptococcoces, in the pneumonias, in tuberculosis, and particularly in the control of syphilis, together with the other venereal diseases. Newer knowledge has been acquired in malaria control, in tetanus, in epidemic cerebrospinal meningitis, in influenza, and in fact the whole range of the acute infectious diseases.

The war efforts also brought about new information and new control procedures in the whole field of environmental sanitation. The new concepts of housing, the development of effective insecticides, the revolutionary methods that have been initiated in the control of air-borne infection through aerosols, and many other sanitary procedures, are notable. The discovery of a host of new antibiotics changed our concepts and procedures entirely, in relation to such devastating infections as plague, lobar pneumonia, and the bacillary dysenteries, as well as many other diseases.

New laboratory procedures for the detection of carriers of a great many diseases, new technics for rapid cultivation of the tubercle bacillus, and for isolation and cultivation of viruses, represent a great resurgence of scientific interest and accretion of knowledge in the whole field of communicable disease control.

The nation-wide depression caused an acute interest in the economic aspects of nutrition. This was followed by food scarcities due to the war. The result was an increased interest in the development of research in the whole field of nutrition. This was a subject that was seized avidly by the general public, and was exploited by commercial interests. Concomitantly there developed an awakened interest of the general population in the whole field of personal hygiene, as well as in all other matters relating to the health promotion of the individual and the community. Health educators emerged to meet this need, and the role of a health educator in the administration of a health service began to be apparent.

During this period we became aware that we were an *aging population*. Furthermore, the great scarcity of labor during the war years led to an appreciation of the importance to the community of the health and welfare of the individual. Labor scarcity also led to a greater appreciation of the necessity for conservation of the health of the worker. It became obvious that health departments must take more interest in the prevention of the diseases of middle life, and must attempt to postpone the advent of the degenerative diseases.

Industrial health services developed rapidly, the word *geriatrics* was coined, and the community began to be more conscious of the need for a co-ordination of health services for *all the people*.

Out of these concepts grew the idea that provision of comprehensive medical care for all the people was a community function, and that a community-wide plan of this sort must encompass preventive services, as well as curative and rehabilitation facilities. These would then become a single function, and responsibility of government.

This great ferment of ideology, and the development of new social theories in relation to public health administration, obviously cannot be discussed adequately in a text of this sort.

We have simply attempted to present the newer knowledge that has been gained, and to point out the trends in social thinking. This, as has been noted above, has resulted in an almost complete revision of the text.

It will be observed that detailed budgets have, for the most part, been omitted from the text. The reason is that fluctuations in the cost of living, together with variations in the standards of living in different parts of the country, have caused our readers some confusion when details of budgets have been presented.

Pertinent references to a specific subject have been placed as footnotes on the same page with the quotations. At the end of each chapter will be found a list of *general references,* which are intended to guide the student in further reading. An extensive general bibliography of public health subjects is not given, since it soon becomes antiquated. The public health worker is referred to the "Bibliography on Public Health and Allied Subjects" that is published annually by the Book Service of the American Public Health Association, 1790 Broadway, New York City. Most valuable of all is the list on *Basic Books for Public Health Workers.*

In the appendix will be found the standard minimum qualifications that have been set by the Committee on Professional Education of the American Public Health Association. We have published the qualifications for key personnel only. Qualifications for other types of public health personnel can be obtained from this committee of the American Public Health Association. It is important to remember that these standards are minimum, and that they are revised every few years by the Committee.

The author wishes to thank most sincerely all those who aided him in the revision of this third edition. We are particularly indebted to Dr. George A. Denison for his suggestions on rabies control, to Dr. Gaylord Anderson for his assistance in communicable disease control, and in the section of field training of public health personnel. Dr. John W. Smillie gave valuable suggestions in the chapter on nutrition, and Dr. Leona Baumgartner in the chapter on child health.

To Miss May McKean, for her tireless and loyal assistance in the editorial work of this third edition, I wish to express my special gratitude.

W. G. S.

# INTRODUCTION

PUBLIC health administration in the United States is in the developmental stage. Many of our present practices have not had sufficient opportunity to demonstrate their real worth; our ideas in regard to them have not crystallized to a degree that will warrant a comprehensive summary, with formal, clear-cut conclusions. However, many individuals who have spent the best part of their lives in the pioneer phases of public health organization in the United States believe that the public health movement has now passed its initial developmental stages, and that many practices that were undertaken more or less in an experimental way have firmly established themselves and proved their worth. If this is so, then we should begin to consolidate the ground that has been gained and extend the worth-while methods and practices of preventive medicine to the whole people.

Everyone who has been interested in public health administration has recognized that it would be a valiant, though perhaps foolhardy, undertaking if the attempt were made to gather together all the diverse and multiform public health practices of all the various official and voluntary agencies of the United States, to analyze them, weigh and measure their value, and to set forth, in a single volume, a digest of these practices with suggestions as to the most fruitful methods of procedure and the probable trend of future developments in the public health field.

With a feeling which the fool must have had when he rushed in where the angel feared to tread, the author has endeavored to summarize our present information as to the most suitable methods of public health administration in the United States, and, to some degree at least, to indicate possible developments of this type of work in the future.

It is undoubtedly true that there is real need for a book of this type. There is no single place where the student of public health can turn for ready information concerning the various phases of public health administration as now practiced in the United States. There are excellent texts on the general subject of the administration of government. Municipal health administration, and, to a lesser degree, rural health administration, have been treated comprehensively, and this material is readily available. Many detailed studies have been made upon special subjects relating to public health administration, such as hospitalization for tuberculosis, promotion of infant and child hygiene, public health programs for nurses, industrial hygiene programs, etc.

In this text we have not made a comprehensive analysis of all these various subjects, but have compiled the material that is available concerning the administrative aspects of public health organization and procedure. We have attempted to correlate one activity with another, and fit each into its proportionate place; to present an analysis of present practices, and to suggest probable future developments.

The limitations of such an attempt are obvious and almost insurmountable. No person can possibly possess the knowledge and experience that would be required to encompass so broad a field in an adequate manner. We are an enormous nation, consisting of some forty-eight sovereign and very different governmental bodies. Each state has its own peculiar problems, with great variation in historical development, racial constitution and climate, and with widely varying types of industrial life. The people of the several states possess different traditions and customs,—even different modes of thought. It is not possible to devise a single plan or even a general type of public health organization that will prove adequate or suitable for all the forty-eight states.

Organization of a local health department service is even more difficult. Total population and area influence profoundly the public health machinery in any governmental unit. Our municipalities vary in size from a few hundred persons to many millions. Some rural populations are compact and homogeneous; others are widely scattered. Some communities are very poor; others well-to-do. Some local governments have an advanced social development; others have remained almost unchanged for over a hundred years. We cannot evade these difficulties, neither can we adjust them to fit some simple, uniform formula.

Another important defect of a textbook is that once a general principle is elaborated and placed within the pages of a book, the subject tends to become static. There is a real danger that the book will be referred to as an authority rather than simply be taken as a guide.

If public health administration is to assume a real place in the scientific application of knowledge, it must be based on the principles of preventive medicine. These principles are changing constantly with the accretion of new knowledge. Thus public health must be dynamic, not static. The health officer should be free to try out new methods, and, more important still, to discard old practices that are unfruitful. He must be constantly changing emphasis, activities, type of personnel, and point of view. Stability is an important asset, but it must not degenerate into stagnation.

The author of a textbook is under obligation to set forth a concrete, more or less didactic, statement of his opinion upon the subject under discussion; but if this opinion is to be taken as the last word that may be said on the subject, it had better not be written.

Understanding all these difficulties and responsibilities, the author has attempted the compilation of a book on the administration of public health in the United States. Its purpose is to select those public health administrative methods that have been employed by competent, experienced men and that have the merit of successful application.

No attempt has been made to describe in detail the technic of any special type of activity. The student of public health will find elsewhere much more adequate treatment of the technical details of the school health program, the functions of the public health nurse, the exacting and varied duties of the sanitary inspector, the procedures to be followed in an epidemiological investigation, or the intricate technic of health education.

We have considered first the basic, essential public health functions of any government as we now conceive them. Each has been discussed, irrespective of the relation of this function to any special division or unit of government.

The various divisions of government that are common to our political life in the United States—the federal, state and local units—have then been considered. We have attempted to show just what part each governmental unit must play in a properly correlated, unified plan of health promotion and protection. The relation of the various voluntary agencies to the official program is given consideration, as well as the functions of various professional groups,—particularly the relation of the practicing physician to the general public health program.

Certain suggestions have been made as to suitable personnel and budgets for different types of work. Many health authorities will feel that the estimates are too low, and that the plans suggested do not represent adequate service. This point is granted willingly. We will grant also that health protection and promotion are paramount obligations of society and must be given proper emphasis by government. One must realize, however, that governmental funds are limited, that other governmental services are considered by students of government to be equally essential. All make a demand upon the public treasury. Thus every proposed item of expenditure for public health purposes must be scrutinized and weighed in the light of its importance in relation to other necessary governmental expenditures. Our enthusiasm and interest in our own subject must not blind us to the fact that public health protection and promotion are an integral but, in truth, relatively small part of a complete political structure. The fact that the health officer deals with matters of life and death more directly and intimately perhaps than any other governmental agency does not entitle him to the special privilege of departing from the sound rules of good administrative practice. One must be courageous in insisting upon suitable consideration of essential public health activities, but we cannot reasonably expect that other equally essential public needs shall be neglected in order to achieve our own ends.

The author wishes to acknowledge his gratitude to those who have given him aid and counsel in the compilation of this book, and for the many helpful suggestions that have been received. Sincere thanks are extended to the following public health specialists for their reviews of certain chapters:

Dr. M. J. Rosenau and Dr. Mazyck P. Ravenel, the chapter on The Development of Public Health in the United States.

Dr. L. R. Thompson, the chapter on Federal Health Administration.

Dr. W. Lloyd Aycock, the chapter on Poliomyelitis and Cerebrospinal Meningitis.

Dr. Gaylord W. Anderson, the chapter on the Communicable Diseases of Childhood.

Dr. Leon C. Havens, the chapter on Public Health Laboratories.

Miss Sophie C. Nelson, the chapter on Public Health Nursing.

Mr. Philip Drinker, the chapter on Industrial Hygiene.

Dr. W. Frank Walker, the chapter on Appraisal of Health Activities.

Dr. R. G. Hoskins, the chapter on Mental Hygiene.

Mr. Geddes Smith, the chapter on Budgets and Budget Making.

Dr. Clarence L. Scamman, for his encouragement during the laborious compilation of all parts of the text and for his many helpful suggestions and corrections.

Particularly, I wish to express my gratitude to my secretary, Mrs. Margaret E. Codrington, for her tireless efforts in the preparation and revision of the manuscript of the first edition.

W. G. S.

# CONTENTS

## PART IV

## ORGANIZATION OF PUBLIC HEALTH PROGRAMS

# LIST OF ILLUSTRATIONS

# PART I

# CHAPTER I

## FUNCTIONS OF A HEALTH ORGANIZATION

PUBLIC health has been defined as "the art and science of preventing disease, prolonging life and promoting physical and mental efficiency *through organized community effort."* (C.-E. A. Winslow.)

Public health administration is the application of public health principles and technics for the benefit of the community, by official or unofficial organizations.

In order to determine the obligations of a community in relation to the organization of services for the protection of the health of the individual and the mass, it is essential that we set forth the desirable minimum functions of government that are required to attain proper health protection.

Let us consider briefly the major public health functions of government as they are recognized and, to a great degree, accepted by the public health leaders and students of government of the present day.

### SANITATION

One of the fundamental obligations of a community is the protection of the health of its people through sanitation of the environment.

**Safe and Adequate Water Supply.** Water is a universal human requirement. It may readily become a source of infection which will result in community disaster. The health department must provide safeguards for all water supplies, both public and private, commercial and household, so that a pure, safe, and adequate water supply may be available for dietary, cleansing, and recreational use.

**Suitable Disposal of Human Waste.** The method employed in sewage disposal by any community is a fairly accurate index of the degree of civilization of the people. The Eskimo, representing one of the lowest degrees of communal culture, lives in a common household with his families and his dogs, and the feces of human beings and dogs are scattered indiscriminately about the huts. The nomadic Indian has a higher state of culture and will not pollute his environment. Feces are always deposited on the downstream side of the camp and water obtained on the upstream side. Still to be found in the United States are isolated rural communities that possess only the most rudimentary facilities for feces disposal. In fact, one of the major activities of many rural health organ-

3

izations at the present time is education of the people concerning the importance of proper disposal of human wastes and the necessity for installation of suitable toilet facilities.

By contrast, most of our large cities possess elaborate and highly effective systems of sewage disposal, with ramifications extending into every household.

It is the obligation of the health department to promote proper systems for disposal of all human wastes in any community, large or small, to supervise their installation and keep a constant check on their effectiveness.

**Safe and Adequate Food Supply.** The complexities of modern civilization have resulted in a great modification in methods for distribution of food. One need only cite as an example the elaborate machinery that has been developed to provide an adequate and safe milk supply for the large municipalities.

Refrigeration and other methods of food preservation and storage have made a complete change in the dietary habits of the whole nation. The old standard dietary of meat, potatoes, bread and coffee, with fruits and vegetables available during a short season only, has changed to such a degree that even the most humble home may now procure a variety of fresh fruits and vegetables at any season of the year. The promotion of this desirable state of affairs, and the safeguarding of this food supply from contamination, is one of the primary functions of a good health service.

**Disposal of Garbage and Refuse.** Disposal of garbage and refuse was formerly considered a public health function. This was due to the fact that disease was thought to be propagated by decaying vegetable and animal matter. We now realize that suitable garbage and refuse disposal is a matter of community cleanliness, and bears little relationship to the prevalence of disease, or the prevention of illness. Thus it becomes a function of the department of public works, rather than of the health department. In most cities the health department no longer has the responsibility for garbage and refuse disposal. It should not do so, for it is not a public health function.

**Cleanliness of the Environment.** Under this general title one may include such functions as the cleaning of the streets, the prevention of dust, the abatement of the smoke nuisance, the abatement of nuisances in general, and many other activities. Indirectly, these situations may represent a health hazard, and some of the activities toward amelioration of these conditions have been incorporated by various municipalities as health department functions. They are, more properly, functions of the public works department. In some cities, abatement of nuisances is logically assigned to the police department.

**Housing regulations and city planning,** as well as recreational parks and playgrounds, bear a direct relationship to the promotion of health and the prevention of disease; but these activities are usually assigned to some other governmental department than that of public health. Advantages to health are effected by:

a. Prevention of overcrowding.
b. Provision for adequate sunlight.
c. Ventilation of buildings, particularly schoolhouses and public places of congregation, etc.

**Safeguards for protecting human life against accident,** and particularly industrial safeguards and promotion of methods that may be utilized for the prevention of disease due to industrial processes, all come within the field of interest of the health officer, though he may have no direct administrative responsibility in relation to these activities.

**The control of the intermediate sources of disease transmission** is, in some areas, a very important public health function. As examples, we may cite the methods employed for the control of breeding of anopheles mosquitoes, in order to prevent malaria; the control of house fly breeding; the control of rat propagation in prevention of plague and typhus fever, and many other similar activities.

All the functions of a health department that have been enumerated above pertain to the general field of sanitation of the environment. They represent the earliest types of health activities that were undertaken by government in this country, and are still matters of primary importance in every official health service.

## CONTROL OF COMMUNICABLE DISEASE

Spasmodic attempts were made toward control of a few of the important epidemic diseases in early colonial times. Not until about 1870, however, were serious, continuous efforts made by health departments to prevent the spread of communicable disease in the community. Great disasters in the form of epidemics of disease have been potent stimuli to the organization of health departments in the United States, and many of the activities of official health organizations at the present time are related, directly or indirectly, to communicable disease control. In the mind of the average man on the street, the sole reasons for existence of the health department are:

a. To control communicable disease.
b. To abate nuisances.

**Public Health Laboratory Service.** Laboratory service has become one of the increasingly important functions of a health department. The diagnostic laboratory is an essential part of communicable disease control and is a normal outgrowth of this function. But public health laboratory service now includes many additional activities, particularly those concerned with chemical and bacteriological analyses of water and sewage, of milk and other foods.

The public health laboratory is organized usually as a separate division of health service, though it clearly is not a separate function, but is an accessory to other primary health activities.

**Vital Statistics.** Apparently it never occurred to those who first kept a record of the births, deaths and marriages that this activity was a public health function, or even a governmental function. For generations it was considered a semi-religious function, and the records were kept by the local parish priests as part of the church archives. In the Province of Quebec, Canada, to-day the local registrar in many of the townships is still the parish priest.

We now realize fully that mortality statistics give us an important, though gross, index of the success or failure of public health programs. The recording and analysis of vital statistics are now generally recognized as public health functions.

Morbidity statistics are, by far, our most delicate measure of the control of communicable disease. If a satisfactory system has been worked out for reporting communicable disease promptly, one can determine the course of an epidemic and check its spread. Every one will grant, therefore, that a comprehensive system for the collection of morbidity statistics, particularly those pertaining to communicable disease, is an important function of public health departments, and a special adjunct to a communicable disease control system.

## PUBLIC HEALTH EDUCATION

The education of the individuals of a community in personal and community hygiene is a primary public health function. Mass education in regard to specific procedures has become, in fact, one of the most important phases of public health work. It is axiomatic that any piece of public health work which requires the co-operation of masses of people can be successful only if carried out with full approval and understanding of the program by the community. The people must be thoroughly convinced that the project is for their benefit and best interest. Lack of foresight in this one essential has been a major mistake in many public health undertakings. Public health education is a slow process. Often progress is greatly retarded because it must await the gathering force of public opinion. Health officers have been slow to understand and loath to accept the principle that they should not proceed with a program until they have secured a fully informed public. It is worth noting that this principle was thoroughly appreciated from the very first by public health leaders of the nation. Elisha Harris, at the initial meeting of the American Public Health Association, in 1873, said: "In the United States, the permanent value and success of any method or system of sanitary government will depend upon the degree in which the people are generally enlightened, concerned, and made responsible in regard to sanitary duties."

Modern public health practice has shown how to prevent a large proportion of sickness and premature death. It is the responsibility of the health department to make this knowledge available to the average man in a form which he can understand and can incorporate into his daily life.

## INDIVIDUAL HEALTH PROTECTION AND PROMOTION

Some authorities believe that the activities of the health department should be limited to the first three functions that we have already considered. In recent years a fourth function has been included by most communities as a fundamental health department activity, namely, the organization through community effort of a medical and nursing service for the early diagnosis of disease in the individual and for the prevention of permanent defects.

Beginning about 1900, communities began to interest themselves in a purposeful way in providing facilities for the promotion of the health of the individual. The initial activities were undertaken almost entirely by voluntary, and not by official, health agencies. In some communities at the present time the organized medical profession does not yet sanction the assumption of this function by public health officials.

Is this function one which should be promoted by organized official community effort, or should it be a matter of private enterprise and individual initiative? The whole question is still a matter of debate and has aroused a great deal of acrimonious controversy. In general, it may be stated that certain definite and quite successful steps have been taken, through organized community effort, in relation to the hygiene of maternity and infancy and the promotion of health of children of the preschool age. The plans for promotion of the health of school children have been the most successful of all the activities of this type. All the above efforts may be grouped under the general title of child hygiene.

In addition to those medical, dental and nursing activities which are intended primarily for the prevention of disease and the promotion of the health of the mother and child, there have been organized, under public auspices, diagnostic clinics, nursing service and hospitalization for tuberculosis; diagnostic and treatment clinics for venereal disease; as well as other special diagnostic medical services and nursing care. The most noteworthy of these have been concerned with cancer, heart disease, poliomyelitis, lobar pneumonia, and nutritional disturbance, such as pellagra. In a few instances health departments have offered as a public health measure a medical service for systematic physical check-up of normal adults.

There is no clear-cut crystallized opinion in the United States at the present time as to the exact line of demarcation between public health functions and private initiative. In general, it may be said that the consensus of foresighted public health leaders is that the health department should not assume permanently the clinical functions that rightly belong to, and are best carried out by, well trained private practitioners of medicine. It is the obligation of the health department to demonstrate effective methods and to stimulate the public interest to strive for such medical, dental and nursing services as may be necessary for promotion of health of the individual. In addition, the health department should arrange for suitable care, by clinics or otherwise, for those individuals in the community who are too poor to pay for essential preventive services. We must recognize, however, that measures for the prevention of disease and promotion of health of the individual are essentially the function of the practitioner of medicine, and health departments should do everything in their power to develop a satisfactory system whereby this ideal condition can be achieved.

## RESEARCH IN DISEASE PREVENTION

The health department must not be content to be simply an agency for the application of well-proved methods for prevention of disease. In order to maintain health service at a high level, the whole subject must be approached with an inquiring and critical mind. Only with such a point of view can we hope to achieve improvement in technic, as well as in administrative procedure.

Some portion of the time and attention of the personnel of each of the major divisions of the health department should be devoted to research and inquiry. If this policy is followed, organized public health service will become a source of new and accurate knowledge concerning the principles and the application of methods in public health promotion. Furthermore, this policy will tend to attract the best type of intelligent, enthusiastic young men to the public health field.

## THE DEVELOPMENT OF A NATION–WIDE PROGRAM OF ADEQUATE COMPREHENSIVE MEDICAL CARE

It is now generally agreed, in theory at least, that this sixth basic function is, or will soon become, a governmental function. Will the initiative and momentum that will be required to bring about this result come from the medical and public health personnel of the United States, or from those whose interests are more closely related to the field of sociology? Will the administrative duties and the necessary funds be assigned to the official department of public health, the department of public welfare, or to some other governmental agency?

No one had given this matter very much thought until the financial crisis which began in 1929. A standard of living had been built up which was more than adequate for proper maintenance of health of individuals, and for the community as a whole. Suddenly the foundation seemed to slip out from under society. There was an abundance of food to supply all the necessary caloric and vitamin requirements of the nation, yet people were going hungry. There were ample facilities for the production of adequate clothing, but children were without enough clothes to keep them warm. There were plenty of physicians and dentists and nurses, and, for the large cities at least, adequate hospital facilities, but many people suffered from lack of adequate medical care, and particularly from lack of preventive service. At first there was a good deal of confusion and wasted effort. Gradually, methods were evolved through organized community effort, governmental and otherwise, to meet the requirements of the situation. Most of these activities were centralized in newly formed governmental agencies and not assigned to existing agencies, such as the health and welfare departments; but in many areas, particularly in rural sections, it was found that the local full-time health personnel were the best available groups to carry out the necessary plans. Health officers found themselves carrying out activities that they had always considered as public welfare and not public health functions. They found not only that their departments were equipped to do the work well, but also that the work supplemented many of their previous activities and made it possible for them to accomplish results toward which they had been striving for years. In retrospect, we realize that when public health officials first began—about 1900—to take an interest in the promotion of the health of the individual, they took the first steps toward a nation-wide program for the provision of adequate medical, nursing, and hospital care of all the people in each of the communities of the nation.

These ideas developed slowly, and met with great opposition. Every one agreed as to the desirability of the objectives; the controversy related to such matters as how the plan should be developed, and who should administer it.

In general, organized medicine has felt that the responsibility should be local—an individual community enterprise, with local autonomy. Other strong groups have felt that the plan should be developed under Federal auspices, with heavy subsidy from the National Government. Some have believed that a single governmental agency should be established, and that the health officer should be trained to administer all matters relating to community-supported medical care. Others believed that the health department should limit its activity strictly to the established public health procedures. A fairly definite national policy of Federal Government subsidy to states and local communities for the purpose of developing adequate public health services was established in 1935 by the Social Security Act. Future leadership in the development of a national health program will undoubtedly be provided on a nation-wide basis. Time and the experimental method will determine which mode of organization and procedure will prove most efficient in promoting the national health program.

## SUMMARY

In the above discussion we have simply attempted to outline in a general way the desirable minimum functions of a community health service and have considered briefly the present trends which indicate the direction that future developments will take. In the subsequent pages we shall discuss in detail the administration of the basic divisions of a health service. We shall then discuss the special public health functions and the suitable, more or less accepted and established, administrative procedures of the national government, the state government and the local health department. We shall consider as well the relationship of unofficial organizations and private physicians to official public health activities, and attempt to outline procedures whereby public health methods can be applied successfully for the greatest benefit of the individual, and the community.

# CHAPTER II

## DEVELOPMENT OF PUBLIC HEALTH ADMINISTRATION IN THE UNITED STATES

THE story of the development of public health administration in the United States from its beginning is a fascinating one, and teaches some very practical lessons. It shows us why some of the residual activities, now obsolete, are still carried on because of the momentum of tradition and precedent. We learn how difficult it is to give up established practices, and how important to consider very carefully the introduction of new and untried measures. The eager, intelligent health officer who has met stupid and unreasoning opposition to well-thought-out programs learns forbearance, patience, and tolerance when he discovers that his predecessors had even greater difficulty than he has had in spanning the chasm between new scientific discoveries in preventive medicine and the actual application of these principles in current public health procedure.

A mere fragmentary outline of major events will serve to pay incomplete tribute to the "giants that walked the land" in those pioneer days, and illustrate the fact that many practices, now well accepted and established, are a direct outgrowth of seed planted long ago.

Our forefathers were much more interested in the preservation of human souls than human bodies, and the promotion of spiritual rather than physical welfare. Disease, at first considered as a visitation of Providence, was later believed to be propagated and spread by decomposing animal and vegetable matter and other unfavorable environmental influences. Public health organization as such was practically non-existent. The chief public health acts were measures relating to promotion of municipal cleanliness as a means of protecting the public health. The Massachusetts Bay Colony statutes are illustrative. In 1647 the Colonial Legislature first passed regulations for prevention of pollution of Boston Harbor. During the period from 1692 to 1708 Boston, Salem and Charlestown passed acts concerning nuisances and also relating to trades offensive or dangerous to public health. The drainage act was passed in 1709. The city did not assume direct control of sewers until 1824. The drains were used for collection of ground and surface water. Not until 1833 was permission given to discharge fecal matter from privy vaults into the city drains. Isolation and quarantine regulations concerning smallpox were first passed in 1701. Ship quarantine laws were initiated in 1700, and a ship quarantine hospital was authorized in 1736.

In 1797 the act authorizing the first local *Boards of Health* was passed, and Boston, in 1799, by a special act of legislature, formed a Board of Health with the ubiquitous and many-talented Paul Revere as its chairman. The chief powers of these local boards of health related to abatement of nuisances. It is worth noting that the organization, functions, and non-medical type of personnel of these local boards of health in Massachusetts have remained fundamentally unchanged up to the present day.

The entire attention of sanitarians in the early days of the nation was concerned with control of the environment, and slight attention was paid to control of the individual as a means of protecting him from infection, or, when he became infected, preventing him from spreading disease. Some attempts were made to control smallpox by isolation, quarantine and immunization, and sporadic attempts were made to control yellow fever by isolation, quarantine and disinfection. Port quarantine against yellow fever was attempted many times, particularly when the disease was prevalent in the West Indies.

The earliest immunization procedures were initiated by Zabdiel Boylston in Boston. He introduced attenuated smallpox inoculation in 1721, but the method did not make much progress, and was abandoned when Benjamin Waterhouse obtained threads of cowpox vaccine from Jenner, and introduced cowpox vaccination in Cambridge, Massachusetts, in 1800.

Disinfection was employed from the earliest colonial times. Boston regulations in 1628 mention the use of sulphur, coal tar and sunlight.

Public health measures were not carried out by permanent governmental bodies as a rule, but by temporary appointment of commissions and by grants of funds to meet emergencies.

As an index of public health opinion and practices at the turn of the eighteenth century, we may select New York City, with a population of some 75,000. Vital statistics were compiled on the basis of sextons' returns for interments. The public health committee appointed in 1806 was concerned with:

1. Pure water supplies.
2. Construction of common sewers.
3. Drainage of lowland marshes.
4. Interment of the dead.
5. Construction of a masonry wall along the water front.
6. Planting of trees and healthy vegetables.
7. Habitation in damp cellars.

The period from 1800 to 1850 was marked by rapid expansion of the country, but little growth in public health knowledge or administration. Epidemic after epidemic swept the land. The overtones were smallpox, yellow fever and typhus fever. But in 1850 scarlet fever was second in the list of causes of death from "zymotic" diseases, and tuberculosis caused the death of three thousand people in Massachusetts in that year,—a rate of over 300 per 100,000 population. By 1845 New York City had grown to nearly 300,000 population. A city inspector system was in vogue. The division was a branch of the municipal police. There was one chief inspector and one assistant. These men concerned themselves with attempts at control of outbreaks of yellow fever and smallpox. Public health measures related chiefly to overcrowding, uncleanliness of streets, regulation of slaughter houses, public baths and pig sties.

In 1845 Lemuel Shattuck of Boston wrote a "Census of the City of Boston," "embracing collateral facts and statistical research illustrating the history and condition of the population and their means of progress and prosperity." This census dealt with many factors that influenced public welfare, public health, religion, education, crime and poverty. Shattuck was the first in the United States to apply the statistical method as an interpretation of public health procedure. The principal source of his information was the "Abstracts from the Bills of Mortality" prepared by the superintendent of burying grounds. He analyzed the available data concerning causes of death in Boston from 1810 on, and pointed out the prevalence of certain epidemic and contagious diseases, stressing the importance of scarlet fever, measles and smallpox.

Lemuel Shattuck in 1850 wrote a still more extraordinary book,—a "Report of the Sanitary Commission of Massachusetts." He was not a physician, but had a wonderful insight in relation to the public health needs of the state and nation. This report recommended the establishment of a State Board of Health, with powers to appoint a suitable, competent, well-paid, full-time secretary. Many other important recommendations were proposed that are quite in line with modern practice, including recommendations for the establishment of nurses' training schools, the teaching of sanitary science in medical schools, the incorporation of preventive medicine in clinical practice, the establishment of competent local boards of health, the inclusion of vital statistics as a function of the health department, and many others.

Shattuck's recommendations were far ahead of the times, but, as a direct result of his work and recommendations, the first State Board of Health was finally organized in Massachusetts in 1869.

The nation was half through the century and no single state had, as yet, organized a state board of health. Twenty-one cities had more or less active health organizations. Some of the smaller towns, due to serious emergencies, had been the first to organize boards of health. Toner, at the first meeting of the American Public Health Association, gave a summary of the organization of city health departments. The dates are not well established, but are given for what they are worth.

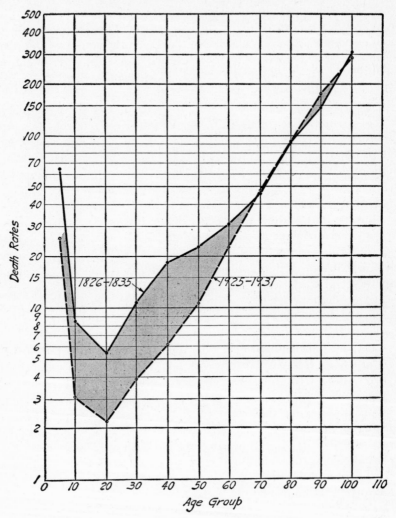

AVERAGE DEATHRATES PER 1,000 POPULATION
IN BOSTON, MASSACHUSETTS.

FIG. 1. *Conservation of Life during a 100-year Period.* Average death rates per 1,000 population from all causes at specified ages in Boston, Massachusetts. 1830 compared with 1930. Sources: Lemuel Shattuck 1845, from Bills of Mortality 1810–1849. Mass. Vital Statistics 1929, 1930, 1931. The semilogarithmic graphic representation indicates that the proportionate conservation of life has been as great in the second, third, and fourth decades as in the first 10-year period.

*Organized* [1]

| | |
|---|---|
| Petersburg, Virginia | 1780 |
| Baltimore, Maryland | 1798 |
| Stoughton, Connecticut | 1801 |
| Alexandria, Virginia | 1804 |
| Charleston, S. Carolina | 1815 |
| Philadelphia, Pennsylvania | 1818 |
| Pensacola, Florida | 1822 |

Baltimore was the first of the large cities to organize a health department (1798); the others were slow to follow.

*Organized*

| | |
|---|---|
| Baltimore, Maryland | 1798 |
| Philadelphia, Pennsylvania | 1818 |
| Providence, Rhode Island | 1832 |
| Cambridge, Massachusetts | 1846 |
| New York City | 1866 |
| Chicago, Illinois | 1867 |
| Louisville, Kentucky | 1870 |
| Indianapolis, Indiana | 1872 |
| Boston, Massachusetts | 1873 |

The first state board of health was organized in Massachusetts in 1869.[2] By 1875 the following states had established boards of health (J. M. Toner. "Report of the American Public Health Association." Vol. I):

*Organized*

| | |
|---|---|
| Massachusetts | 1869 |
| California | 1870 |
| District of Columbia | 1871 |
| Virginia | 1872 |
| Minnesota | 1873 |
| Michigan | 1873 |
| Maryland | 1874 |
| Alabama | 1875 |

A Bureau of Vital Statistics was established apart from the Bureau of Sanitary Inspection in New York City in 1854. Stephen Smith[3] made a very important sanitary survey of New York City in 1864. This survey resulted in legislation for the formation of the Metropolitan Health Board. Its chief concerns and achievements, according to Dr. Smith, were:

[1] There is a good deal of uncertainty as to the exact dates of organization of local boards of health, and the criteria used by Toner are not clear. New York City, for example, had a board of health in 1796 and Boston in 1799. These boards were tenuous affairs at best with part-time personnel, functioning sporadically, and with little or no funds.

[2] Louisiana had developed a quarantine board in conjunction with the City of New Orleans in 1855.

[3] See Chapter I, "History of Public Health" by Stephen Smith in *A Half Century of Public Health*, edited by M. P. Ravenel.

1. Underdrainage of the soil.
2. Removal of cellar populations to homes in open air and sunlight.
3. Removal of offensive industries.
4. Enforcement of rigid sanitary regulations.

## THE AMERICAN PUBLIC HEALTH ASSOCIATION

By 1870, a considerable number of talented men had become vitally interested in public health affairs. These men formed the American Public Health Association in 1872, and Stephen Smith was elected as its

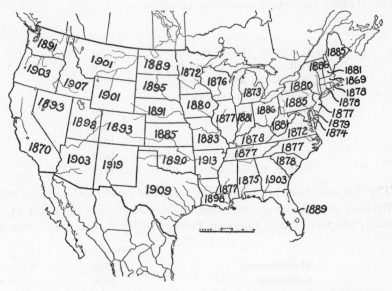

FIG. 2. *The Date of Creation of Each State Board of Health for the Purpose of Promoting State-wide Public Health Work.* From Health Departments of the United States and Canada. U.S.P.H. Service Bulletin #184. 1932, p. 8.

first president. National Sanitary Conventions had been called in Philadelphia in 1857, in Baltimore in 1858, in New York in 1859 and in Boston in 1860. These ceased with the advent of the Civil War, and no further attempt was made to organize a public health association until Stephen Smith called a preliminary committee together in his office in 1872.

Ravenel, in "A Half Century of Public Health," has said, "No more opportune time could have been chosen for the formation of the American Public Health Association. The art of medicine was becoming the science of medicine; modern preventive medicine was being born. The discoveries of Pasteur had substituted the bed rock of science as a foundation on which has been erected the wonderful structure of medicine as it exists today."

The first volumes of the Proceedings of the American Public Health Association are a mine of information, for they indicate the vital matters that concerned the leaders of that day. Many of the principles that were presented in the very first report have become the foundation stones on which public health in America has been built.

The broad viewpoint and scope of interests of these pioneers may be indicated by the subjects that were discussed at the first meeting. Among others one notes:

1. Public health education, which was considered even at that time to be of primary importance in public health affairs.

2. Vital statistics—race and nationality, rural and urban factors in relation to mortality.

3. The germ theory of disease.

4. The epidemiology of typhoid fever and particularly the relationship of water supplies to this disease.

5. Control of specific diseases, particularly smallpox, yellow fever and cholera.

6. Quarantine and disinfection.

7. Water purification, street cleaning and scavenging.

8. Organization of state, local and national boards of health, and many other topics.

Elisha Harris, secretary of the Association (Vol. I, p. 472), stated certain broad principles of public health administration that are applicable to the present day.

1. He advocated state boards of health for all states, with the framing of general laws for giving enlightened and systematic direction to sanitary administration.

2. He believed local administration to be the form of public health government best designed to enlist popular support, and recommended avoidance of unnecessary assumption by the state of local duties, or interference with local health officers.

3. He recommended a statute requiring every township or county to organize a local board of health.

4. He recognized the county as the most acceptable unit of local sanitary administration. Towns and villages should organize and administer their own activities in connection with, often as parts of, the county system.

5. He clearly understood that the chief purpose of state administration was to promote local efficiency.

6. He emphasized the point that compilation of vital statistics should be supervised by the state board of health in order to secure uniformity of practice and comparable results.

7. He recommended that the state board of health attempt to establish a general sanitary system which is adapted to local needs. "The faithfulness, efficiency, good influence and permanency of local boards of health cannot be secured without central (state) influence and certain kinds of authority."

What a splendid far-sighted administrative platform for public health! How long a period will be required for its complete realization? Yet there were only two state boards of health in existence at the time.

The discussion by Dr. C. C. Cox upon the subject, "The Necessity for a National Sanitary Bureau" (Vol. I, p. 522), is equally well marked by clear thinking and real vision.

As Ravenel truly says, modern public health practice may be said to have been born at that first meeting of the American Public Health Association in 1872.

Local boards of health began to require reporting of the more important contagious diseases about 1870. Environmental sanitation became a secondary activity of the health department, and control of communicable disease a major function. Providence established the first diagnostic laboratory in 1888. New York City followed in 1894. Tuberculosis began to be recognized as a communicable disease and not a family taint, and was made reportable by health departments about 1895. Diphtheria antitoxin was introduced in 1894 and was adopted almost at once, with relatively little of the controversy that harasses so many of the important medical discoveries before they become incorporated in public health procedure.

Thus from 1875 on through the next 50 years, the chief activity of sanitarians related to attempts toward the control of communicable disease. In many instances success was astounding; other attempts met with complete failure. The cause of typhoid fever was discovered, its mode of spread determined and control measures were instituted. Tuberculosis, malaria, diphtheria, smallpox all declined as causes of death. The respiratory infections, particularly influenza and pneumonia, were not affected by any public health measures that were employed, and the infant death rate remained high. Formaldehyde fumigation came and went. Communicable disease hospitals were built. Scarlet fever became less virulent. At the turn of the nineteenth century many of the hitherto important communicable diseases were on the wane.

A National Board of Health was organized in 1879, but had a short life. It was sponsored in great part by the men who formed the American Public Health Association. Its organization was poorly conceived, and it was doomed to failure almost from the start. The Army, the Navy, and the Marine Hospital Service all were anxious to gain control of the National Board of Health, but it was set up as a separate body, with twelve members. Dr. J. L. Cabell, a fine southern gentleman, was President throughout its existence. The struggle to maintain this first attempt to develop a national health program is buried in the reports of the Board. Its final destruction is generally attributed to Dr. J. H. Hamilton, but in reality it failed because of its own inherent weakness, and because the country as a whole was not yet ready for a nation-wide health promotion service.

A new phase of public health began about 1900, namely, a trend toward improving the health of individuals. Infant hygiene, school health work, industrial hygiene, public health nursing and health education are all outgrowths of this period of research in public health administrative method.

About 1900 the voluntary agencies began to interest themselves in public health affairs. The visiting nursing associations had been concerned chiefly with the home care of the sick poor, but the leaders in this field realized the importance and value of the preventive methods. Public health nursing was slowly evolving. The Anti-tuberculosis League and the Red Cross entered the field of public health.

Formal attempts at public health education were undertaken. The old school books on hygiene, which were concerned primarily with anatomy and physiology, were discarded, and new programs were instituted. School medical inspection was initiated. Vaughan's report of the shocking sanitary conditions of the concentration camps of Florida in the Spanish-American War of 1898 educated the whole people as to the mode of spread of typhoid fever through careless disposal of human excreta. It emphasized also the menace of the house fly that existed in myriads in every home.

One event tumbled over another in adding new information and new control methods, by means of which the community might protect itself against disease. Information outran action. Application lagged far behind the acquisition of new knowledge because of antiquated health machinery, untrained personnel, and lack of public understanding and support. Gradually, the more enlightened health officers consolidated the information that had become available. They discarded ineffective procedures, such as the notorious "swat the fly" campaigns; and sloughed off ancient activities, such as garbage collection and cleaning of the streets, that bore no further relationship to disease prevention.

Biggs was State Health Commissioner of New York, Sternberg was Surgeon General of the United States Army, Sedgwick was firing the imagination of a brilliant group of students at the Massachusetts Institute of Technology, and Whipple was beginning his eventful career at Harvard. Park was developing public health laboratory procedures in New York City. Chapin, in Providence, with his analytic and forceful intelligence, was founding the basic principles of municipal health procedures. Evans introduced compulsory pasteurization of milk in Chicago in 1908. In 1909 under the aegis of President Eliot, the first department of Preventive Medicine in a medical college was established in the Harvard Medical School and Dr. M. J. Rosenau was selected to head the department. A short time afterward Rosenau's "Preventive Medicine and Hygiene" was published. There can be no doubt that this one book did as much to advance public health as any single factor.

These stirring events called for men, well trained, who were interested in social advancement and were willing to devote their lives at any sacrifice to the welfare of mankind. In 1913 Sedgwick, Whipple, and Rosenau formed a School of Public Health for the training of such men, utilizing the joint facilities of Massachusetts Institute of Technology and Harvard University. As a direct outgrowth of this pioneer effort, Schools of Public Health were established in Johns Hopkins, Harvard, and Toronto Universities that were equipped to train medical health officers for positions of responsibility. Several other universities, notably Yale, the Universities of Michigan and California, and Massachusetts Institute of Technology, developed courses of training in the special technics of public health.

Another factor which has had a tremendous influence upon public health administration was the establishment during the first quarter of the century of the private foundations. With their immense resources they have interested themselves in public health affairs and stimulated the development of new administrative methods. Their funds have made possible the development of the experimental method in public health administration, and have enabled state and local health officials to promote preventive measures far more rapidly and effectively than could have occurred if the health officials had been entirely dependent upon public funds.

Public health administration in the United States, both in local and state government, is at present in the developmental stage. Much of the present methodology may be discarded in the future; new methods will undoubtedly be introduced when they are shown to be more efficient than present ones.

The next fifty years will undoubtedly see a more comprehensive development in public health procedure in the United States than has occurred during the past one hundred years. Within a single generation it is more than probable that our whole conception of the functions of government in relation to protection and promotion of the public health will be radically modified and an entirely new philosophy will be developed concerning the proper place of public health in the organization and administration of government.

## REFERENCES

1. Ravenel, M. P. *A Half Century of Public Health.* Amer. Pub. Health Assn. 1921.
   Note particularly special chapters on:
   *History of State and Municipal Control of Disease.* Chas. V. Chapin. P. 133.
   *The History of Public Health 1871–1921.* Stephen Smith. P. 1.
2. Shattuck, Lemuel. *A Census of Boston.* 1845. (Out of print.)
3. Shattuck, Lemuel. *A Sanitary Survey of Massachusetts.* 1850. (Out of print.)
4. *Reports of Proceedings of the American Public Health Association.*
   Note particularly Vol. I.

a. *Germ Theory of Disease and Its Relation to Hygiene.* F. A. P. Barnard, President of Columbia University. Vol. I, p. 70.

b. *Relation of Water to Propagation of Fever.* Austin Flint. Vol. I, p. 164.

c. *Boards of Health in the United States.* J. M. Toner. Vol. I, p. 499.

d. *General Health Laws and Local Ordinances Considered with Reference to State and Local Sanitary Organization.* Elisha Harris. Vol. I, p. 472.

e. *A Report on the Necessity for a National Sanitary Bureau.* C. C. Cox. Vol. I, p. 522.

5. Annual Reports of the National Board of Health. 1879, 1880, 1881, 1882.

# PART II

ADMINISTRATIVE CONTROL OF COMMUNICABLE
DISEASES

# CHAPTER III

## ADMINISTRATIVE PRINCIPLES OF COMMUNICABLE DISEASE CONTROL

THE administrative methods that may be employed in the attempt to prevent the spread of a given communicable disease depend in great part upon the epidemiological characteristics of that disease. Since no two communicable diseases present the same epidemiological features, no uniform method can be adopted which will be effective for the control of every disease. Certain general principles may be developed, which represent essentials; the details will vary for each disease, and these details will be considered when each specific disease is discussed. The common measures that are taken to prevent the spread of communicable disease may be described briefly:

**Notification.** The reporting system must be simple. The law usually requires a report to the health department in writing and within a limited period of time by the attending physician. In case there is no physician in attendance, the householder is commonly required by law to report communicable disease to the health department. Though excellent in theory, this plan does not work well in practice. The simplest method is an informal report by telephone from the physician in charge of the case, and this type of reporting is now generally acceptable to local health departments. The essentials of the report are:

*a.* The patient's name.
*b.* His residence.
*c.* His age.
*d.* The disease.
*e.* The physician's name.
*f.* The date of the report.

What diseases should be reported to the health department? The list is long,—thirty to forty diseases in most states; but many of the diseases on the list are encountered rarely, as for example, yellow fever, plague, and cholera. The tendency is to shorten the list of notifiable diseases. Chapin's dictum is an excellent one; namely, that we should not require reporting of a communicable disease unless some specific action will be taken immediately by the health department on receipt of the report. If this rule were followed, it would greatly increase the degree of completeness of reporting by physicians, and also result in more effective control work.

Geiger [1] has divided the list of reportable diseases into three groups:

"1. Diseases which, because of relatively little risk of infection by contact, or because cases may be handled in accordance with conditions of the moment, may be listed as reportable only, include:

| | | |
|---|---|---|
| Anthrax | Glanders | Rocky Mountain spotted |
| Beriberi | Hookworm | fever |
| Botulism | Jaundice (infectious) | Septic sore throat |
| Coccidioidal granuloma | Malaria | Tetanus |
| Dengue | Pellagra | Trichinosis |
| Fluke infection | Pneumonia (lobar) | Tularemia |
| Food poisoning | Relapsing fever | Vincent's infection |

"2. Diseases in which *isolation* of the case or carrier is practiced:

| | | |
|---|---|---|
| Chickenpox | Influenza | Rabies (human) |
| Dysentery (amebic) | Measles | Syphilis |
| Dysentery (bacillary) | Mumps | Trachoma |
| Erysipelas | Ophthalmia neonatorum | Tuberculosis |
| German measles | Psittacosis | Whooping cough |
| Gonococcus infection | Rabies (animal) | |

"3. Diseases in which *quarantine* is applied. This list is selected on the basis of a marked degree of infectiousness of the case itself, and also implies a degree of likelihood of indirect transmission or transmission by carrier:

| | |
|---|---|
| Cholera | Plague |
| Diphtheria | Scarlet Fever |
| Encephalitis (epidemic) | Smallpox |
| Leprosy | Typhoid and paratyphoid fevers |
| Meningitis (epidemic) | Typhus fever |
| Poliomyelitis (acute anterior) | Yellow fever" |

Geiger's division of reportable diseases is a useful one to the administrator. He recognizes fully, of course, that local conditions or increasing epidemiological knowledge may require the transfer of a given disease from one classification to another, or perhaps an inclusion in or exclusion from the lists.

Physicians are lax in reporting communicable disease to the health department when they believe that no action will be taken and no service rendered to the patient or the community. Under present conditions, poliomyelitis and typhoid fever are reported more completely than other diseases on the list. Measles and whooping cough are reported inadequately in most communities.

**Investigation.** The health department should make an immediate investigation of reported cases of communicable disease. Otherwise the

[1] Geiger, J. C.: *Health Officers' Manual.* W. B. Saunders Company. Philadelphia. 1939.

whole value of prompt notification is nullified. The purpose of this pre-liminary investigation is:

a. To detect the source of the original infection.
b. To discover other possible cases of the disease.
c. To prevent spread of the disease from the discovered source.
d. To do whatever possible to minimize the effects of the disease in persons already infected.

Health departments should furnish laboratory and other diagnostic aids to practicing physicians in order that the earliest possible diagnosis of suspicious cases may be made. The essential epidemiological data should be obtained on the first visit to the case. These essential data are:

a. Names of all members of the household.
b. Their ages.
c. Occupation or school.
d. Previous attacks of the disease.
e. Source of the milk supply.
f. Exposure to other cases of the disease.

This simple information should be recorded in the home.

The data concerning this case, together with those of related cases, should be assembled and the source of infection determined at once, if possible. Often the determination of the original source of infection is of great aid in preventing further spread of the outbreak. An example of the value of a simple epidemiological report which may be compiled from a summary of data obtained by careful investigation of cases of communicable disease that are reported to the health department is the following, from the Westchester County Health Department.[2]

### DIPHTHERIA IN THE HEALTH DISTRICT

Within the past few weeks twelve cases of diphtheria have been reported in the health district. Two of them resulted fatally. A twenty months old child of Croton-on-Hudson succumbed to a laryngeal infection and an adult male of Millwood died of a virulent nasal diphtheria. Other single cases occurred in Harrison, Rye and Tarrytown.

The only concentration of the disease has been in Elmsford where there have been seven cases, six of them in two families. The accompanying chart explains the spread of the disease. C. M., a colored boy 12 years of age, who had received toxin-antitoxin some years ago, had a sore throat beginning September 12. Subsequent examination revealed the fact that he was a carrier of virulent diphtheria bacilli. His brother, age 9, immunized at the same time, was also found to be a carrier of virulent organisms. The latter sat at the same table in the same classroom at school with G. S. and R. R. who evidently started the disease in their respective families. Both of these boys had sore throats, one on September 17

[2] Report from the Westchester County, New York, Department of Health. Nov. 5. 1934.

and the other on October 8. The former is a virulent carrier; the virulence test has not been completed for the latter. In addition to the six cases in the S and R families, one isolated case has appeared in the village. This child, M. B., is 4 years of age and lives in an entirely different section of the community. It has

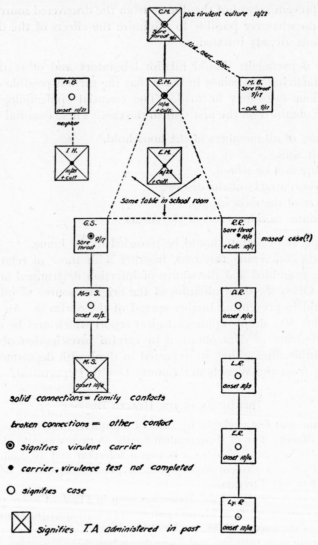

FIG. 3. *An Outbreak of Diphtheria in Elmsford, N. Y.* A routine communicable disease report. From Westchester County Health Bulletin. 1934.

recently been found that I. H., age 9, a neighbor who has been in contact with M. B., is a carrier but a virulence test has not been completed. Although this child is a classmate of C. M., G. S., and R. R., apparently she was not the cause of infection of M. B. When investigation of the Elmsford cases began, cultures were made of all children in this particular class and at that time examinations of both nose and throat secretions of I. H. were negative. It was not until after M. B. became ill that positive cultures were secured from I. H. Aside from the remote possibility of error in laboratory technique in the early examination of I. H. all efforts to connect M. B. with the main outbreak have been unsuccessful.

It is of interest to note that of the seven cases in Elmsford only one had ever had toxin-antitoxin. As a corollary, it is an equally interesting fact that of five children who had at some time had toxin-antitoxin or toxoid, four became carriers, thus demonstrating their immunity to the infection.

Although surveys made recently indicate that the percentage of presumably immunized children is large enough to prevent any widespread epidemic of diphtheria in the health district, this does not protect the unimmunized child against the disease if he comes in contact with a carrier.

**Isolation.** Once the diagnosis of communicable disease has been made, suitable steps must be taken toward isolation of the patient. The health officer, after consultation with the attending physician and the family, must determine whether the patient may be isolated at home or in the hospital. Isolation at home has limited value. England's experience with fever hospitals demonstrates clearly that hospital isolation of communicable disease has little or no effect in preventing the march of an epidemic through a community. Hospitalization has real value in promoting the welfare of the infected person, and does aid in prevention of household infection with scarlet fever and diphtheria, particularly in the very young children in the family.

Hospitalization for communicable disease is a fairly widespread practice in the United States, particularly in the larger municipalities. No one questions the value of the procedure in typhoid fever, meningitis, poliomyelitis, lobar pneumonia and tuberculosis. Complete hospitalization of other communicable diseases is a very expensive procedure because of the irregularity of the load. The plan would be more feasible if communicable disease hospitalization could be administered as part of a general hospitalization program. This has been accomplished in a few cities, but there are many objections to it, and the plan has not been accepted generally. The general standards for communicable disease hospitalization are twenty to thirty beds (exclusive of beds for tuberculosis) for each 100,000 of the population. During epidemics, this small number of beds is entirely inadequate; but in interepidemic periods, most of the beds are empty.

It seems quite probable that in the future diminishing emphasis will be placed upon the importance of separate isolation hospitals for communicable disease. We must recognize that hospitalization has not proved to be an effective method for the prevention of spread of communicable diseases in the community, and that the chief benefits of hospitalization are derived from the better care that the patients receive in a well conducted hospital.

Since official funds allotted to control of communicable disease are usually quite limited, the general trend of health department practice is to expend the available monies for items which will yield the greatest return in *community* benefit. The result has been and probably will continue to be a curtailment by health departments of expenditures for extensive communicable disease hospitalization.

**Quarantine.** Quarantine is instituted for those individuals who have been exposed to infection, and thus may be in the incubation period of the disease. Specific regulations in regard to both isolation and quarantine have been formulated for each communicable disease. These regulations are arbitrary; and in general are determined so as to allow a margin of safety to the community. Details concerning these matters will be given in the discussion of the various specific diseases. The report of the Sub-Committee on Communicable Disease Control of the American Public Health Association [3] gives complete data and recommendations concerning all the common communicable diseases.

Individualization of isolation and quarantine is obviously the next logical step in communicable disease control. It is successful in diphtheria, where release may be permitted after two successive negative nose and throat cultures. This plan of individualization has real disadvantages, and is often misinterpreted by the public, which feels that everyone with a given disease should be subjected to the same regulations. Gordon has pointed out the value of individualization in scarlet fever. In the summer time, for example, he recommends release of children from isolation after three weeks and adults in two weeks, if the patients have had no complications.

In many instances at present quarantine is instituted on an individual, rather than a purely arbitrary basis. For example, the health officer may quarantine only the particularly susceptible persons in a household, or quarantine persons on the basis of occupation. Thus, food handlers who may have been exposed to typhoid fever, or a school teacher exposed to scarlet fever, would receive special consideration.

The health officer must always use his own judgment also in relation to quarantine of immediate and general contacts. He must depend upon his knowledge of the epidemiology of the disease in question, and consider also the particular circumstances of any given situation. Closing of schools, for example, will seldom check an outbreak of disease. Among scattered rural populations, however, the method may be of value. Popular demand frequently requires the closing of schools during an epidemic of poliomyelitis, but under average conditions the children are in no greater danger of exposure in school than out of school.

The public demands both isolation and quarantine, and this demand should be given due consideration. On the other hand, individuals rebel

3 *The Control of Communicable Diseases.* American Public Health Association, 1945.

against rigid regulations of this type, and should not be unfairly penalized.

In the last analysis it must be confessed that isolation and quarantine have not proved to be highly successful methods for control of communicable disease, nor can we expect more favorable results in the future. The reasons why the methods do not meet with success are obvious.

a. The health department is seldom successful in finding every case of the disease.
b. The plan presupposes that every case of the disease is readily recognizable. This is seldom true.
c. Healthy carriers of disease are often hard to detect.
d. Many of the communicable diseases are highly infectious before they become recognizable clinically.

Carefully collected data from Norwegian and other sources suggest that local quarantine and isolation for most communicable diseases is of little value and might well be dispensed with altogether. The findings do not apply to international quarantine, nor does it seem feasible to abandon local quarantine and isolation measures until other, more effective control measures may be substituted.

**Placarding.** Placarding of communicable disease is a device which has a very limited value in communicable disease control. Its principal value is that it does unquestionably aid in effecting better reporting of communicable diseases, particularly measles and whooping cough.

**Disinfection.** Destruction of the infecting organism is a logical step in preventing the spread of disease. Concurrent disinfection is the most important of the disinfection procedures. It simply represents an immediate and proper disposal of all the excretions of the patient. Terminal disinfection is essentially a question of cleanliness, and is brought about by soap, water and sunshine. Terminal gaseous disinfection has been abandoned, except for destruction of insects and vermin.

**Control of Carriers.** The problem of carriers of infection has always been a very difficult one. This is true whether the patient has had the disease and recovered, or has never suffered from symptoms of the infection. The methods commonly used in the prevention of the spread of infection by carriers will be discussed when each specific disease is considered.

**General Measures to Prevent the Spread of Communicable Disease.** In addition to the specific methods that are employed in an attempt to prevent the spread of an infection that has already invaded a community, certain general measures are employed that are of great value in preventing disease from gaining access to the community.

a. Measures are instituted to protect from possible infection the vehicles that may carry the etiological agents of disease. For example, general measures are taken to protect the community water supply from pollution, supplementing this action by water purification methods. Supervision of food supplies, and particularly milk sanitation, with superimposed pasteurization, is essentially a communicable disease control activity.

b. The destruction of intermediate hosts of infection will aid in the control of certain diseases, as, for example, malaria, plague, typhus fever, yellow fever and many others.

**Increasing the Resistance of Individuals in the Community to Specific Diseases.** Some communicable diseases may be checked in a community by increasing the resistance of individuals to these specific diseases. Success depends upon the principle that it is possible to raise the community level of resistance to such a point that the disease will not spread, following an average dosage of infection, even after the community is invaded. These measures are difficult to carry out, since the health officer must appeal to individuals to protect themselves. This procedure is not always easy. It is a truism that any new procedure will meet formidable obstacles when success depends upon the co-operation of large groups of people. Fortunately, every single individual need not be immunized in order to protect the community completely. When a sufficient number are immune, the disease cannot spread, even though complete immunity of all individuals has not been attained.

Resistance may be increased by passive immunization, active immunization without actually producing the disease, or by producing a modified form of the disease. An example of the last method is the production of modified measles through the use of convalescent serum.

**Minimizing the Ill Effects of Disease.** The last line of defense in communicable disease control is an effort to minimize the ill effects of the disease after it has invaded the community. This is a confession of failure of previous efforts. We must readily admit, however, that we frequently fail to prevent the spread of disease, and simply do our best to lessen its ravages. Examples of this method are:

a. Distribution of diphtheria antitoxin as a therapeutic measure.
b. After care of poliomyelitis to prevent the serious effects of paralysis.
c. Nursing and medical care in measles to prevent sequelae.

ORGANIZATION OF A COMMUNICABLE DISEASE CONTROL SERVICE

All health departments, whether large or small, must furnish some measure of communicable disease control service. Communicable disease control is one function that the health department should not delegate to any unofficial body. Partial exceptions may be made even in this instance, as, for example, home nursing visits in tuberculosis by visiting nurses' associations.

At least five types of service and personnel are required to carry out a communicable disease control program:

a. Expert diagnostic and consultation service requiring medical personnel.
b. Epidemiological investigations.
c. Home nursing instruction.
d. Clerical personnel to obtain, record and analyze morbidity data.
e. Hospitalization service.

Communicable disease control is usually organized as a separate division, even in small health departments. The director of this work should be a physician, trained in epidemiology and skilled in the diagnosis and methods of treatment of the common communicable diseases. The public health nurse is a very important factor in the communicable disease control program. She explains the purpose of isolation and quarantine, and gives detailed instruction in the necessary procedures that must be carried out. In usual practice, all visits to cases of communicable disease, except for the purposes of diagnosis and epidemiological study, are made by the nurse. The number of nurses required for an adequate public health program will be discussed at the appropriate time. (See Chapter XXI.)

Activities relating to tuberculosis and venereal disease control should logically be incorporated in the division of communicable disease. Because of numerous personnel and extensive budgets required for these activities in large health departments, divisions of tuberculosis control and of venereal disease control are sometimes organized as separate divisions, each with its own full-time director.

Hospitalization is a tremendous item of expense in the communicable disease control program and may overshadow all other activities of the health department. Often the appropriation for hospitalization of tuberculosis exceeds all the other combined official public health expenditures. It is highly advisable to budget all expenditures for hospitalization of communicable disease as separate items rather than incorporate these items in the general budget.

In a well balanced program the local health department should not spend more than 25 per cent of the total appropriation for communicable disease control (exclusive of tuberculosis hospitalization). Thus, in a city of 100,000 population with an average expenditure for health work of $1.00 per capita, not more than $25,000 should be allocated to communicable disease control.

Diagnostic laboratory service is not included in this item, since laboratory service of the health department is usually organized in a separate Division of Laboratories. In smaller health departments the public health laboratory may be successfully incorporated in the division of communicable disease.

Expenditures and emphasis in relation to communicable disease control will vary greatly in each community depending upon special problems; in fact, the emphasis upon a particular subject will change in the same community from time to time. No item in the budget requires greater flexibility. Some states meet this situation through the provision of an emergency fund, to be used only in case of epidemics.

In the following chapters we shall discuss the administrative procedures in control of communicable disease that are in common use at the present time by health officers practicing in the United States. The epidemiological features of each disease, upon which control measures are founded, are set forth briefly. The diseases selected for discussion are those most commonly encountered in everyday practice by health officers. The student is referred to other texts for a more comprehensive and inclusive discussion, particularly in relation to the rarer diseases.

## REFERENCES

1. Scamman, C. L. *The Administrative Control of Communicable Disease*. Amer. J. Pub. Health. April 1928, p. 429.
2. Holst, P. M. *Isolation in Infectious Disease*. Tidsskr. j. d. Norske Laegeforening. 1933, Vol. 53, p. 479.
3. Geiger, J. C. *Health Officers' Manual*. Philadelphia. W. B. Saunders Company. 1939.
4. *The Control of Communicable Diseases* (6th edition), 1945. Publication of the American Public Health Association.
5. Anderson, G. W. and Arnstein, Margaret. *Communicable Disease Control*. New York, Macmillan Company. 1941.
6. Stimson, P. M. *Common Contagious Diseases*. Philadelphia, Lea and Febiger. 1940.
7. Gage, N. D. and Landon, J. F. *Communicable Diseases* (4th edition). Philadelphia, F. A. Davis. 1944.
8. Top, F. H. *Handbook of Communicable Diseases*. St. Louis. C. V. Mosby Company. 1941.
9. Topley, W. W. C. and Wilson, G. S. *Principles of Bacteriology and Immunity* (3rd edition). Baltimore. Wood. 1946.

# CHAPTER IV

## ADMINISTRATIVE METHODS IN CONTROL OF DIPHTHERIA

THE decrease in diphtheria in recent years is one of the major triumphs of preventive medicine. The last great pandemic occurred in the United States in the years 1872 to 1876. Previous to this time the disease had swept over the United States in irregular waves, penetrating every community and leaving a terrible swath of devastation and death in its wake. No other disease struck such terror into the heart of the parent, for diphtheria was almost inevitable and little could be done to save the suffering or even the life of the child. In some epidemics one fourth of the children who developed the disease died.

The great stages in control of the disease have been:

1. The discovery of the etiological agent of the disease, *Corynebacterium diphtheriae,* by Klebs in 1883. This made possible accurate and rapid diagnosis.

2. The development of specific therapy through the use of antitoxin in 1894.

3. Active immunization of the individual, and later the development of community immunization through the combined use of the *Schick Test* and *toxin-antitoxin* (later toxoid) in 1912.

The results of these successive stages of administrative control of the disease are almost unbelievable. Diphtheria has completely disappeared from many cities, even whole states. (See Figure 4 of cases reported in Connecticut.) A whole year may pass in even a large center of population without a single death from the disease. We have no evidence that the disease has decreased in virulence or power of dispersion. There is every reason to believe that it is just as great a potential source of danger as ever before. The decline in the incidence and in the deaths from diphtheria is due, in great part, to an increased specific immunity of the population.

## EPIDEMIOLOGICAL CONSIDERATIONS THAT AFFECT CONTROL

Diphtheria has certain characteristic epidemiological features that influence the methods of administrative control.

**Etiology.** The etiological agent is *Corynebacterium diphtheriae.* The normal habitat of this organism is the human upper respiratory tract. It may live for some hours outside its host, and also may occasionally pro-

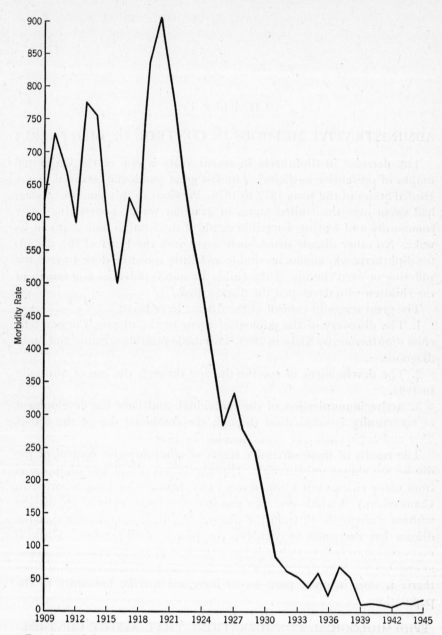

FIG. 4. *Diphtheria Trend in Connecticut, 1909–1945.* Morbidity Rate per 100,000 Children under 15 Years. Data from Connecticut State Department of Health.

duce lesions in other parts of the body, particularly the conjunctiva, the vagina, and, rarely, the skin. The organism is readily recognizable by standard bacteriological technic. Its virulence also may be determined by animal inoculation.

**Prevalence.** The disease has a characteristic seasonal prevalence. It rarely occurs in summer, and is commonest in early winter, particularly December and January.

Diphtheria follows irregular cycles. It may be prevalent in a community for several years, and then decline—to return later with increased virulence.

The disease is more prevalent in the northern than in the southern states, and is believed by some authorities to be less virulent in Negro than in white children.

**Symptomatology.** Diphtheria is very treacherous. Constitutional symptoms are often mild and cause the parents no alarm. Progress is insidious so that many hours of valuable time are lost before a physician is called. Infection is usually localized in the posterior nasopharynx (faucial diphtheria). Laryngeal diphtheria is by far the most dangerous type from the point of view of the patient. The throat culture is sometimes negative in these cases and there may be no obvious membrane. Persons with nasal diphtheria have relatively little absorption of the toxin, and the symptoms are often mild. Sometimes the only suspicious symptom is a slightly bloody nasal discharge. These cases are often missed, and constitute the greatest source of dispersion of the disease. Thus, a child with nasal diphtheria is much more important from a public health point of view than one with any other type. In faucial diphtheria the diagnosis usually is not difficult. The characteristic adherent membrane is seen on the tonsils, and spreading up over the anterior and posterior pillars. Sometimes there is a swelling of the adjacent glands. The diagnosis is readily verified by bacteriological culture, but antitoxin should be given as soon as a presumptive clinical diagnosis has been made.

The differential diagnosis in laryngeal diphtheria is sometimes very difficult, as the chief symptoms are those of laryngeal obstruction. It is always advisable to give diphtheria antitoxin in these cases, if there is a reasonable suspicion that the child has diphtheria.

**Carriers.** Carriers of diphtheria bacilli are common during the winter months (1 to 2 per cent of the total population in northern climates). There is no feasible routine procedure for picking up these carriers in the general population.

**Incubation Period.** The incubation period is 3 to 5 days, but may be several days longer. Usually the organism disappears from the throat of the patient within 2 to 3 weeks.

**Mode of Spread.** Diphtheria is usually spread by direct contact with a case or carrier; sometimes through contact with articles freshly soiled by the patient, and occasionally through infected raw milk. The missed case of mild diphtheria is probably the most important source of dispersion of diphtheria bacilli.

**Therapy.** The use of specific therapy in patients and the passive immunization of contacts with diphtheria antitoxin are very successful methods of controlling the disease in the individual and family. Active immunization by toxoid is a very successful method for the prevention of the disease in the community.

## METHODS OF CONTROL

### THE INDIVIDUAL CASE

**Reporting.** When the family physician has made a presumptive clinical diagnosis of diphtheria, he should report the case immediately to the health department, and should institute preliminary isolation. He should not wait for cultural confirmation of the diagnosis before reporting the case.

**Consultation Service.** The health officer or his representative should be available at all times for consultation in suspected cases of diphtheria. Immediately on making the presumptive diagnosis, the physician should give antitoxin. The dosage depends upon the severity of symptoms and the period that has elapsed since the onset. If seen within 24 to 36 hours, 10,000 to 15,000 units as an initial dose is often sufficient to control the infection. Every hour counts; if seen late in the third day or afterward, a very large dose of even 100,000 units of antitoxin may not save the life of the child. If the family of the patient cannot be kept under constant observation, it may be advisable to give passive immunization (1,000 units) of the antitoxin to all the small children who have been exposed to the patient.

**Isolation.** The disease is readily communicable. The patient should be sent to a hospital, if possible. If he remains at home, he should be isolated in a suitable room with his own attendant. Isolation is continued until two negative cultures from the nose and throat have been obtained on successive days. Usually, the organisms disappear within 15 days.

In some rare instances the throat condition returns to a normal appearance, but the diphtheria bacilli remain for a long period. The virulence of these organisms in chronic carriers may be determined by suitable laboratory tests. Carriers of non-virulent strains may be released from isolation. Persistent carriers of virulent diphtheria bacilli may sometimes be cleared up by treatment with penicillin.

**Quarantine.** If the patient is removed to a hospital, all family contacts should have throat cultures made. If the results are negative, they may be released from quarantine. Some health departments require two successive negative nose and throat cultures, taken not less than 24 hours apart, before releasing contacts. If the patient remains at home, all child contacts, and also all contacts whose occupation involves handling of food or close association with children, should be quarantined during the period of isolation of the patient.

Susceptibility of exposed persons may be determined by the Schick test. The Schick test is performed as follows: 0.1 cc. of solution containing 1/50 M.L.D. of diphtheria toxin is injected *intradermally* in the right forearm. A control of 0.1 cc. of the toxin which has been heated to 75° C. for 1 hour is injected in the left forearm. Readings are made best on the third or fourth day after injection. If the result is positive, there will be a distinct area of induration and redness about the point of injection of the right arm. Certain experience is required before one can distinguish between false and true positive reactions. Active immunization may be given to the susceptibles, but this procedure will not protect a child already exposed to infection. The reason for this is that immunity develops slowly, whereas the incubation period of the disease is short (3 to 7 days). If passive immunization of the exposed susceptibles (1,000 units of antitoxin) has been undertaken, these children should not, of course, be given toxoid concomitantly. A period of at least three weeks should elapse after giving passive immunization, before active immunization can be started.

**Disinfection.** The usual procedures of concurrent disinfection should be followed. Boiling or scalding of all material contaminated by the patient is sufficient. Terminal disinfection is achieved by a thorough cleaning. Terminal fumigation is not necessary.

### COMMUNITY PROGRAM

The community program of diphtheria prevention has two phases:

Measures taken to prevent the disease from gaining a foothold in the community.

Measures to prevent its spread and reduce its ravages, if and when it does invade the community.

**Antitoxin.** A supply of potent diphtheria antitoxin should be made readily available for any emergency. The spectacular dash across the ice by dog team to Nome, Alaska, some years ago to take diphtheria antitoxin to the stricken children of the community aroused great popular enthusiasm and called for supreme heroism of both the men and the dogs. A statue has been erected to commemorate the heroic efforts of the dog which led that team. If this dog had been endowed with human intelligence, one suspects that he would have been exasperated with the lack of human forethought which made that epic effort necessary. Candid truth compels us to admit that a sufficient supply of diphtheria antitoxin should have been available in Nome to meet that emergency.

**Hospital Facilities.** Hospitalization is of great value to the patient with diphtheria and possibly also has some value in preventing the spread of the disease in the community. The great difficulty is that communicable disease hospitals are very expensive to maintain because of the seasonal prevalence and irregular hospital load of this group of diseases. Many cities formerly maintained at least 20 hospital beds per 100,000 population for diphtheria patients. The need for the beds is now rapidly disappearing.

**Laboratory Diagnosis.** The health department must supply adequate facilities for rapid, accurate diagnosis of diphtheria and for release cultures. The laboratory should not be more than six hours by shortest route from any community. In rural communities of large states this is achieved by the establishment of branch laboratories, as the central laboratory may be too far away. The plain cotton swab in a sterile test tube is the best means of sending material to the laboratory for diagnosis of diphtheria.

The laboratory should telegraph or telephone all positive results on cultures sent for diagnosis. Release culture reports may be mailed.

**Epidemiological Investigations.** Epidemiological investigations should be made by the health department in each case of diphtheria, to determine, if possible, the source of the infection. Search should be made for carriers that may have been responsible for the case, and particular efforts should be made to find mild missed cases. The missed cases are usually nasal diphtheria, and many times this source of infection has been only slightly ill and has not been seen by a physician. The health officer must consider that, for all practical purposes, each case of diphtheria has been in recent contact with a case of diphtheria or a carrier of diphtheria bacilli, and that this potential danger probably still exists in the community.

### COMMUNITY IMMUNIZATION

A big step in control of diphtheria has been the development of community immunization programs. The standard immunization technic formerly required three injections of diphtheria toxoid given one week apart. The Havens method of immunization with alum-precipitated toxoid has greatly simplified and improved the process. The optimum spacing and dosage of the alum-precipitated toxoid is a two-dose method, as follows:

First dose                              0.1 to 0.2 cc.
Second dose  (four weeks later)         0.4 to 0.5 cc.

Chesney reports that 1,555 children immunized in this way showed 99.6 per cent negative Schick tests at the end of 8 weeks after the final injection. The Schick test is done about six months after the immunization to determine if the child has really become immune. The most advantageous period to immunize a child is between the sixth and twelfth months of life.

Formerly diphtheria immunization programs were conducted in the schools. Since most cases of diphtheria occur before a child reaches twelve years of age and most deaths occur under six years of age, we now recognize that the immunization program should concentrate on the first year group, with supplementary immunization during the first grade of school life. Godfrey's data prove that a high proportion of the school children in a community may be immunized against diphtheria, with little effect in the control of the disease. But when 35 to 50 per cent of infants and preschool children have been protected, the disease disappears from the community.  (See Fig. 5.)

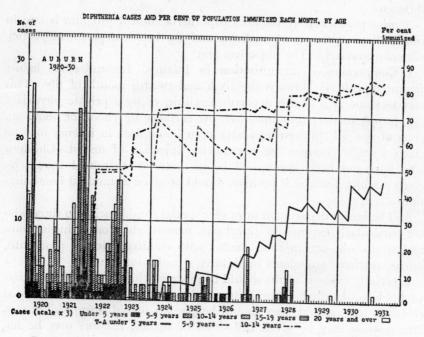

FIG. 5. *Data from Auburn, N. Y.,* which indicate that at least 30 per cent of the children under five years of age must be immunized against diphtheria in order to secure control of the disease. From E. S. Godfrey. Amer. J. Pub. Health. 1932. Vol. 22, p. 242.

Children over twelve years of age usually are not given diphtheria toxoid because most of them are immune. Nurses and attendants constantly exposed to infection should be given a preliminary Schick test, and if positive, should be immunized.

Some health departments recommend a preliminary Schick test for every child before toxoid is given. This greatly increases the cost, with little benefit, as few small children are Schick negative. Since some children are not protected by toxoid, the parents may be advised to have a Schick test done six months or a year after the toxoid administration to determine if the child has become immune or if the immunity has disappeared. Most health officers do not assume responsibility for the final Schick test, since this is an individual rather than a community matter.

The great proportion of health departments have organized diphtheria immunization clinics with their own personnel, and the service has been free to all who apply. Practicing physicians have sometimes felt that the health department was infringing on their province in giving this service free of charge to everyone. The health officer is in a difficult position. He does not desire to encroach upon the clinical practice of medicine, yet he must protect his community against the invasion of diphtheria by immunization of at least 50 per cent of the susceptible preschool age children.

A most practicable community diphtheria control program is one in which all practitioners of medicine and the health department participate co-operatively. The objectives are:

1. Comprehensive immunization in infancy. Immunize all babies against diphtheria between the sixth and twelfth month of life. This may be done at a health department clinic, or by a private physician.

2. Supplementary immunization. At entrance to school, or about six years of age, all children who have been immunized in infancy may be given a single "booster" or re-enforcing injection of toxoid. Children who have not been immunized before entrance to school should be given a Schick test and if positive, should be given a standard immunization.

3. The health department must give special consideration to those who are particularly exposed to diphtheria, namely, children in institutions, and adults who are in close contact with children, such as physicians, nurses, teachers, attendants in children's institutions, etc.

Especially exposed adults should be given a Schick test and if positive, should be immunized. Since adults may have severe local or constitutional reactions from toxoid, they should be given a toxoid susceptibility test. Non-reactors may be given full doses of toxoid; reactors may be immunized by repeated suitably diluted doses of toxoid.

## REFERENCES

1. Wells, D. M., Graham, A. H. and Havens, L. C. *Diphtheria Toxoid Precipitate with Alum.* Amer. J. Pub. Health. 1932, Vol. 22, p. 648.
2. Baker, J. N. and Gill, D. G. *Precipitated Toxoid as an Immunizing Agent against Diphtheria.* Amer. J. Pub. Health. 1934, Vol. 24, p. 22.
3. Monroe, J. D., Volk, V. K. and Park, W. H. *Evaluation of Diphtheria Toxoid Preparations and Methods of Immunizing.* Amer. J. Pub. Health. 1934, Vol. 24, p. 342.
4. Geib, L. O. and Vaughan, H. F. *The Physician as a Health Worker.* J. Amer. Med. Assn. 1931, Vol. 97, p. 367.
5. Anderson, G. W. and Bigelow, G. H. *Diphtheria Immunization and the Private Practitioner.* Amer. J. Pub. Health. 1933, Vol. 23, p. 655.
6. Godfrey, E. S., Jr. *A Study in the Epidemiology of Diphtheria in Relation*

    *to the Active Immunization of Certain Age Groups.* Amer. J. Pub. Health. 1932, Vol. 22, p. 237.

7. Chesney, G. *Diphtheria Immunization: Optimum Spacing of Doses of Alum-Precipitated Toxoid.* Medical Officer. 1939, Vol. 61, p. 127.

8. Zinsser, H., Enders, J. F. and Fothergill, L. D. *Immunity: Principles and Application in Medicine and Public Health.* New York, The Macmillan Company. 1939.

9. Committee of Medical Research, Great Britain Office of Medical Research. *Diphtheria Treatment with Penicillin.* London News Letter 122. Dec. 1944.

10. Kocher, R. A. and Siemsen, W. J. *Diphtheria Carriers Treated with Penicillin.* Ann. Int. Med. May 1946, Vol. 24, p. 883.

11. Ingraham, H. S. and Korns, R. F. *Diphtheria in Upstate New York, 1908–1946.* N. Y. St. Jour. Med. Nov. 1, 1946, p. 2414.

12. Saffron, M. H. *Diphtheria as a Military Problem.* Arch. Dermat. and Syph. 1945, Vol. 51, p. 337.

13. *Changes in the Epidemiology of Diphtheria.* International Medical Digest. 1945, Vol. 47, p. 307.

# CHAPTER V

## ADMINISTRATIVE CONTROL OF STREPTOCOCCAL INFECTION—RESPIRATORY

### SCARLET FEVER, SEPTIC SORE THROAT, AND STREPTOCOCCAL TONSILLITIS

THE epidemiologic exigencies of World War II necessitated extensive studies—clinical, bacteriologic, and immunologic—of the streptococcus infections of the respiratory tract. This new information, taken in conjunction with various additional studies, has demonstrated clearly that one hemolytic streptococcus, Lancefield Group A, is responsible for all of the above infections. It may cause septic sore throat in one person, tonsillitis in another, and in a third person, scarlet fever may be produced.

The clinical picture that is produced by this infectious agent depends upon a number of factors, such as (a) the characteristics of the particular strain that is producing the infection, (b) the portal of entry, (c) the previous history of exposure to streptococcus infection, and many other factors. Thus it is necessary, in discussing the control of these various clinical conditions, to consider them as an entity.

It is now quite clear that the major distinction between scarlet fever and septic sore throat is the appearance of a skin rash. There is ample evidence that the presence or absence of a scarlet fever rash in this type of infection depends largely upon an individual's ability to neutralize the erythrogenic toxin of the infecting hemolytic streptococcus. Thus if two individuals are exposed to the same hemolytic streptococcus, one may develop a sore throat without a rash, because he is immune to the factor that produces the rash, but is susceptible to other factors; whereas the other person, who is not immune to the rash-producing factor, will develop all the symptoms of typical scarlet fever.

It becomes obvious therefore that in planning control measures we cannot, as we have in the past, use clinical distinction to guide us in our control policies, handling scarlet fever in one way, administratively, and tonsillitis or septic sore throat in another.

**Etiology.** Streptococcosis is due to an infection with the beta hemolytic streptococcus Lancefield Group A. This group has been divided into a large number of types. In a family or institutional outbreak, usually one type predominates, but several types are encountered in a community-wide epidemic. Some types elaborate an erythrogenic toxin (the rash-producing factor) ; others do not.

44

**Prevalence.** Infection with this group of organisms is very prevalent, but no actual data of prevalence are available. Scarlet fever, which has been a well recognized clinical entity for generations, has been well reported in some states for years. It has an annual morbidity rate of 500 to 1,000 per 100,000 children under 15 years of age. There has been little or no decline in morbidity over the past fifty years. However, the case fatality rate has declined markedly during this period. From 1830 to 1880 the disease was severe, and community invasion was greatly dreaded. Symptoms were intense, sequelae frequent and severe, and the case fatality rate was high. In some years, twenty per cent of the children who

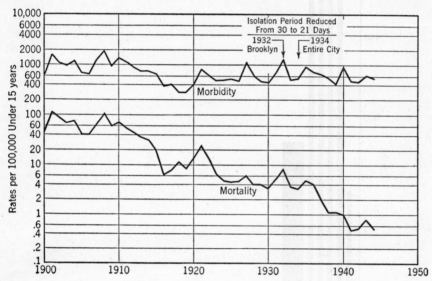

Fig. 6. *Scarlet Fever.* Trends in Morbidity and Mortality Rates, (Cases Reported and Deaths per 100,000 Population under 15 Years of Age), New York City, 1900–1944. Source: New York City Department of Health.

developed the disease died. Beginning about 1885, for some unknown reason, the disease became less severe, and by 1900 the case fatality rate was reduced to two per cent. Complications became less severe and less frequent. This trend has been continued, until at the present time scarlet fever is a relatively unimportant cause of death in childhood. This fact is well illustrated by the records of the New York City Department of Health from 1900 to 1945. (See Fig. 6.)

Scarlet fever is largely a disease of early childhood. It is unusual in infants under one year of age, and is most common in children from 1 to 5 years. Sixty per cent of the cases occur before the sixth year. Almost all the deaths occur in early childhood. (See Fig. 7.)

**Seasonal Prevalence.** Scarlet fever may occur at any season, but is most prevalent in the late winter and early spring, particularly from December to March.

Tonsillitis is prevalent during school age and through adolescence, and adults are frequently infected. The actual community incidence and case fatality rate is not known. Septic sore throat may occur in epidemic form, and is often produced by heavy infection of food, particularly milk and milk products.

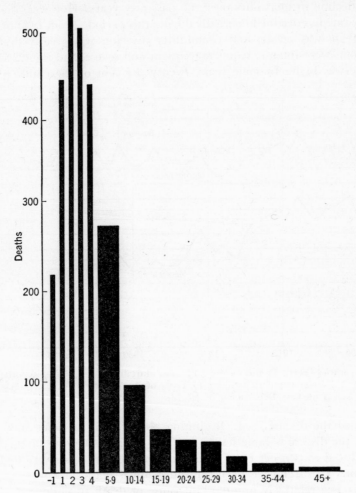

FIG. 7. *Scarlet Fever.* Deaths, by Age Groups, Indiana, 1900–1942. Source: *Indiana State Board of Health Monthly Bulletin,* March 1943.

The disease is much more prevalent in the temperate zones than in the tropics.

**Immunity.** If the infecting strain of streptococcus is erythrogenic, *i.e.,* capable of producing toxin, the individual will build up a strong immunity against the toxin. Thus clinical scarlet fever does not recur. However, no definite bacterial immunity has been demonstrated to streptococcus infections, and thus an individual may have repeated attacks of this type of illness. But he will have scarlet fever only once, even though the subsequent infection is due to an erythrogenic strain of organism.

An individual's susceptibility to the erythrogenic strain may be determined by the Dick test. If positive, the individual has no immunity and will develop scarlet fever.

The Dick test is a standard test dose of Dick toxin, 0.1 cc., which is injected intracutaneously. If positive, an area of erythema of at least 10 mm. in diameter will be present at the site of injection at the end of 24 hours. The test should be read at this time, as it begins to fade in 36 hours.

The incubation period of streptococcus infection is short—usually 3 to 4 days. It is almost never less than 36 hours and no more than 7 days.

The disease is readily transmissible, usually through direct contact with an infected person. As noted above, milk was formerly a very common vehicle of streptococcus infection, but almost universal pasteurization of milk has now minimized this hazard. (See chapter on control of milk-borne infections.) It is important to remember that an epidemic of milk-borne streptococcus infection, if due to an erythrogenic strain of organism, may produce a variety of clinical conditions. Exposed children with a positive Dick test will develop scarlet fever, whereas those immune to the toxic factor will develop septic sore throat, with no rash.

**Carriers.** Healthy carriers of Lancefield Group A hemolytic streptococcus are common. There is a definite seasonal rhythm, the highest carrier rates occurring in the winter, the lowest in the summer. Schwentker, Janney and Gordon,[1] in their Roumanian studies, showed that the carrier rate increased in a village *before the outbreak* of scarlet fever occurred. Schwentker [2] also showed, in a study of an outbreak of scarlet fever in an army camp, that the case incidence of scarlet fever was related to the carrier incidence of the strain (Type 19) that produced the outbreak.

Carriers of hemolytic streptococcus Group A are infrequent in the tropics, and in persons living in isolated communities. It is an organism of civilization. Frequent and close human contact give it the best chance for development.

**Clinical Manifestations of Streptococcus Infection of the Throat.** The disease has a sudden onset, with nausea, vomiting, fever, prostration, and a severe sore throat. The tonsils are markedly engorged, and may be covered with a pseudomembranous exudate. If the streptococcus strain is erythrogenic, and the patient is not immune to the toxin, the characteristic skin rash of clinical scarlet fever will appear on the second or third day. The rash is fine, punctate, and quite characteristic. It begins at

[1] Schwentker, F. F., Janney, J. H. and Gordon, J. E.: *Am. J. Hyg.* 1943, Vol. 38, p. 27.
[2] Schwentker, F. F.: *Am. J. Hyg.* 1943, Vol. 38, p. 207.

the neck and spreads to the trunk and extremities, but does not appear on the face. At times the rash may be confused with other conditions, such as the rash of German measles, various drug rashes, etc. If the diagnosis is in doubt, the Schultz-Charlton reaction may be of value.

**Schultz-Charlton Reaction.** From 0.1 to 0.5 cc. of scarlet fever antitoxin (convalescent serum) is injected intradermally when the rash occurs. A blanching of the injected area within 6 to 36 hours indicates the diagnosis of scarlet fever.

Streptococcus infections of the throat respond readily to therapy with the sulfonamides. Penicillin therapy is also of great value in hemolytic streptococcus infections of the respiratory tract.[3]

In both types of therapy, it is apparent that the drug simply checks further development of the organism, thus giving the body time to build up natural resistance. Symptoms may be relieved immediately following treatment, but if the drug is given over too short a period of time— less than 4 days—relapses are common, and convalescence may be prolonged.

It was hoped that carriers of streptococcus hemolyticus might be cleared up by sulfonamide or penicillin therapy. The results of this method of control have on the whole been quite disappointing.[4]

**Control.** In view of all the new epidemiologic evidence in streptococcus infections of the throat, it becomes apparent that we must revise our methods of control completely. At first it may be difficult, from the administrative point of view, to realize that scarlet fever should not be considered as a separate clinical entity, but must be grouped with other streptococcus infections of the throat. Furthermore, scarlet fever has become so benign, and is so susceptible to clinical control by adequate therapy, that rigorous isolation and quarantine measures are not indicated, as they undoubtedly were 50 years ago. It is a good administrative rule in public health to eliminate procedures that do not give results commensurate with efforts at control that are expended, no matter how firmly grounded are these traditional regulations in the minds of the people of the community.

Our present concepts of a suitable community program for control of this group of infections is as follows:

**Reporting.** Streptococcus infections of the throat should be reported to the health department. Scarlet fever should continue to be reported as a separate clinical entity.

**Isolation.** The uncomplicated case of streptococcus infection of the throat should be carefully isolated until the mucous membranes of the throat regain their normal appearance. This period is never shorter than one week. Two weeks usually covers the period of communicability of the infection.

[3] Plummer, Norman, *et al.*: *J.A.M.A.* 1945, Vol. 127, p. 369.
[4] Rubenstein, A. D. and Foley, G. E.: *New Eng. Jour. Med.* 1945, Vol. 233, p. 315.

The complicated case, with discharging ears or nasal sinus, with mastitis, enlarged or suppurative glands, or with pneumonia, should not be discharged from isolation until complete recovery of the condition occurs. If the complication persists for more than 6 weeks, discharge from isolation may be secured if two successive negative cultures for hemolytic streptococcus, taken not less than 24 hours apart, are obtained from the lesions.

**Disinfection.** Concurrent disinfection of all articles soiled by the patient is a necessary part of control technic, and terminal disinfection of all contaminated objects, including bed clothing, bedroom furniture, floors, and other objects of the sickroom, are indicated.

**Quarantine.** Quarantine of contacts of a case of streptococcus infection of the throat, including scarlet fever, has been abandoned as an ineffective procedure by most health departments. It is a good general rule that the household in which a case of scarlet fever or septic sore throat is present shall not be permitted to sell dairy products or other types of food that may transmit the infection, during the period of isolation of the patient. But the breadwinner of the family need not be excluded from his work, nor the normal children in the family from school.

**Control of Carriers.** Detection of hemolytic streptococcus carriers by use of routine throat cultures is not a practicable procedure. Hamburger [5] suggests that "dangerous" carriers may be detected by nose cultures, and demonstrated that cross infections occurred in a hospital from the nasal carrier.

**Immunization.** A child that is non-immune to the erythrogenic factor may be protected by suitable immunization procedures, and will become Dick negative. Active immunization with Dick toxin is a long and tedious process. Five injections are commonly employed, given at weekly intervals. Reactions sometimes follow the administration of Dick toxin, but they are not severe.

This procedure will protect the child against clinically recognizable scarlet fever, but will not protect against streptococcal infection. It is not a feasible community-wide immunization procedure, but may be employed as clinical judgment indicates by pediatricians in private practice, in institutions for small children, and in various other special conditions.

**Control Measures Employed by the Health Department.** Every practicable effort should be made to prevent the dissemination of hemolytic streptococcus in the community.

Provision should be made for laboratory identification of hemolytic streptococcus and identification of serologic groups. In investigation of an outbreak, the source of infection can frequently be determined by identification of serologic types within Group A. Special attention may be given to the "dangerous," *i.e.* nasal, carriers, but detection and isola-

[5] Hamburger, Morton, *et al.: Jour. Inf. Dis.* 1945, Vol. 77, p. 96.

tion of normal carriers, *i.e.* throat carriers, of streptococcus is not a feasible procedure.

Universal pasteurization of milk is one of the most effective community-wide preventive measures. Persons known to be infected with the hemolytic streptococcus should not be allowed to handle milk or milk products.

Any cows with mastitis should be excluded from the "milking line," and the milk should not be sold until the mastitis has cleared up.

The studies of Robertson [6] and his co-workers of the Surgeon General's Commission on Air-borne Infections indicated that transmission of infection with the streptococcus in soldiers' barracks occurs through the air. If the floor dust is controlled, the danger of infection is lowered, and oiling the blankets greatly decreases the prevalence of organisms in the air. The value of air sterilization by triethylene glycol vapor or other technics may eventually prove to be an important factor in control of this as well as other types of respiratory infection. See chapter on Control of Air-borne Infection.

**Epidemic Control Measures.** When an epidemic of streptococcus infection occurs, the health department should take immediate steps to determine the sources of infection and bring them under control. Children in school should be given a daily morning inspection. All persons exposed or potentially exposed should be observed for 7 days. All suspected food, such as milk or milk products, should be excluded from sale or use, until pasteurized.

Persons who are known to have been definitely exposed to food-borne infection may be protected to some degree by daily administration of small doses of a suitable sulfonamide, given under the direct supervision of a physician.

The reader is referred to the excellent series of studies of streptococcus infections by various members of the Surgeon General's Commission on Air-borne Infections, and to the monograph of Schwentker, Janney and Gordon on "The Epidemiology of Scarlet Fever." [7]

## REFERENCES

1. Plummer, Norman, Duerschner, D. R., Warren, H. D., Rogliano, F. T. and Sloan, R. A. *Penicillin Therapy in Hemolytic Streptococcic Pharyngitis and Tonsillitis.* J.A.M.A. 1945, Vol. 127, p. 369.
2. Hamburger, Morton, Green, M. J. and Hamburger, V. G. *The Problem of the "Dangerous Carrier" of Hemolytic Streptococci. II: Spread of Infection by Individuals with Strongly Positive Nose Cultures Who Expelled Large Numbers of Hemolytic Streptococci.* Jour. Inf. Dis. 1945, Vol. 77, p. 96.

6 Robertson, O. H., *et al.: J.A.M.A.* 1944, Vol. 126, p. 993.
7 Schwentker, F. F., Janney, J. H. and Gordon, J. E.: *Am. Jour. Hyg.* 1943, Vol. 38, p. 27.

3. Rubenstein, A. D. and Foley, G. E. *The Effect of Chemotherapy on the Duration of the Carrier State Following Scarlet Fever.* New Eng. Jour. Med. 1945, Vol. 233, p. 315.

4. Wheeler, S. M. and Foley, G. E. *Serologic Types of Hemolytic Streptococci Isolated from Scarlet Fever in Massachusetts, 1942–1943.* New Eng. Jour. Med. 1944, Vol. 231, p. 287.

5. Foley, G. E., Wheeler, S. M. and Aycock, W. L. *Serological Types of Hemolytic Streptococci Isolated from Multiple Cases of Scarlet Fever in the Same Households.* Am. Jour. Pub. Health. 1944, Vol. 34, p. 1083.

6. Schwentker, F. F. *The Relation between Scarlet Fever Morbidity and Streptococcus Carrier Rates.* Am. Jour. Hyg. 1943, Vol. 38, p. 207.

7. Schwentker, F. F., Janney, J. H. and Gordon, J. E. *The Epidemiology of Scarlet Fever.* Am. Jour. Hyg. 1943, Vol. 38, p. 27.

8. Hare, Ronald. *Haemolytic Streptococci in Normal People and Carriers.* The Lancet. Jan. 18, 1941, p. 85.

9. Hare, Ronald. *The Expulsion of Haemolytic Streptococci by Nasopharyngeal Carriers.* Canadian Pub. Health Jour. Nov. 1940, p. 539.

10. Bormann, F. and Folff, Eisner A. *On the Schultz-Charlton Phenomenon in Scarlet Fever.* Archiv. f. Dermat. u. Syph. 1932, Vol. 164, p. 761.

11. Williams, A. W., Gurley, C. R. *et al. Milk Borne Septic Sore Throat and Scarlet Fever and Their Relation to Beta Hemolytic Streptococci.* J. Bact. 1932, Vol. 23, p. 241.

12. Gordon, J. E. *Epidemiology of Scarlet Fever. A Clinical Approach.* J. Amer. Med. Assn. 1932, Vol. 98, p. 519.

13. Scamman, C. L. *Milk Borne Septic Sore Throat and Scarlet Fever.* Am. Jour. Pub. Health. 1929, Vol. 19, p. 1339.

14. Lombard, H. L. *Septic Sore Throat in Massachusetts. Epidemiology.* J. Prev. Med. 1929, Vol. 3, p. 81.

15. *Epidemic Septic Sore Throat.* Publications Mass. State Dept. of Health. 1929. April Bulletin. See particularly historical review by Dr. Benjamin White, which includes a comprehensive bibliography.

16. Bigelow, G. H. and Forsbeck, F. C. *Milk-borne Disease in Massachusetts, 1927–1929.* Amer. J. Pub. Health. 1930, Vol. XX, p. 104.

17. Henningsen, E. J. and Ernst, J. *Milk Epidemic of Scarlet Fever and Angina Originating from Milkmaid with Scarlatinal Otitis Media.* Jour. of Hyg. 1939, Vol. 39, p. 51 (abstract).

# CHAPTER VI

## OTHER COMMUNICABLE DISEASES OF CHILDHOOD

### MEASLES

MEASLES is the most prevalent of all communicable diseases. As matters now stand, it is almost inevitable that a given individual will develop the disease at some time during his life. There is a very general impression that no procedure yet developed is of much avail in the prevention of measles. We do possess knowledge, however, which enables health officials, family physicians, and parents to prevent many of the serious consequences of measles and to obviate much suffering and disability—even to save many lives.

### EPIDEMIOLOGICAL FEATURES OF MEASLES WHICH MAY AFFECT ITS CONTROL

**Etiology.** Measles is due to a filtrable virus. This virus is present in the secretions of the nose and throat of a patient with measles.

**Transmission.** Measles is transmitted through fairly direct contact with a patient who is passing through the early stages of the disease. All available evidence indicates that there are no carriers of the virus. It is most contagious during the first days of the infection and before the rash appears. Five days, more or less, after the appearance of the rash, the disease is no longer communicable.

**Diagnosis.** This disease is characterized by sudden onset, with fever, malaise and headache, and is accompanied by all the symptoms of an acute upper respiratory infection, including congestion of the conjunctivae and the mucous membranes of the nose and throat, profuse nasal discharge, sneezing and coughing. The typical rash does not appear until the third or fourth day after the initial symptoms appear. Early diagnosis may be made by the appearance of a characteristic eruption on the buccal mucous membranes (Koplik's spots). This eruption is always present in early stages of the disease and has practically disappeared by the time the rash appears on the skin. The average period of incubation of measles is 10 days from exposure to the appearance of initial symptoms, 14 days to the appearance of the rash. The incubation period is very constant. Seldom is it shorter than 10 days, but it may be prolonged up to three weeks, when convalescent serum has been used to modify the symptoms.

**Immunity.** If a mother has had measles, her infants are immune to the disease for three to six months following birth. Otherwise, there is no natural immunity. One attack of measles gives a life-long immunity to subsequent attacks.

**Epidemic Cycles of Measles.** Measles occurs in cycles which happen with sufficient regularity to enable the health officer of a large municipality to predict a pending epidemic with a fair degree of accuracy. The disease is most prevalent in the spring months; its lowest prevalence is in the late summer, but it may occur at any time. In large cities the epidemics tend to occur every three or four years due to the fact that, in a 3 or 4 year interval, enough non-immunes have accumulated by accretion of new births to furnish sufficient inflammable material to produce an epidemic. In smaller communities, the epidemic cycles depend in great part upon proximity to large centers of population and facilities for communication. Epidemics will be less frequent and cycles less constant than in the large cities. In general, children in rural areas contract measles later in life than city dwellers. In sparsely settled areas, many people may escape measles entirely until adult life.

**Fatality Rate.** The case fatality rate in measles varies greatly, depending upon the age of the patients, their physical condition and nutrition, as well as upon the social and economic status of their parents. Healthy children of school age, 6 to 16 years old, practically never die of measles or its complications. Infants (children under 1 year) suffer severely with the disease, with a case fatality rate of 5 to 10 per cent. As the age increases, the type of the disease is rapidly modified. Adults, and particularly aged people, suffer much more severely from measles than children of school age. The severe symptoms which may result from measles are usually due to the invasion of secondary infectious agents, particularly the pneumococci, and hemolytic streptococci. These organisms produce the otitis media, mastoiditis and pneumonia that are frequent sequelae of the disease. In a children's institution such as an orphans' home, where nutrition of the children may be poor, and nursing care insufficient, an epidemic of measles may cause havoc, with a case fatality rate of 25 per cent or higher. In essence, measles is least serious and most prevalent in children between 6 and 16 years of age. In a modern industrial community 85 per cent of the inhabitants will have had measles by the end of their fifteenth year of life.

**Prevention.** Convalescent serum has proved very effective in preventing or modifying the typical course of a case of measles. Four to six cubic centimeters of pooled convalescent serum are injected intramuscularly into the buttock. If given within the first four days after initial exposure a passive immunity is produced which lasts from 4 to 6 weeks. This procedure is not recommended except for infants between 5 and 12 months of age or in children who, for some special reason, must be completely protected from infection. A much more satisfactory procedure is to give the convalescent serum on the fifth or sixth day following initial exposure. In almost every instance, the child will develop a mild, non-complicated form of measles and will become *immune for life.* Some pediatricians now commonly recommend the exposure of normal healthy susceptible children at a suitable time (June or July) to a full-blown case of measles; others recommend the transfer of the virus from the nasal mucous membranes of a case to susceptibles by means of a cotton applicator. Five or six days after inoculation (or exposure) the children are given partial immunization with convalescent serum.

Whole blood from a normal adult who has had measles (such as a parent) may be used if convalescent serum is not available. The dosage is large—25 to 40 cc., and, for many reasons, the method is not so satisfactory or effective as the use of convalescent serum.

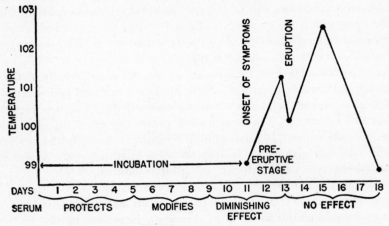

Fig. 8. *Effectiveness of Serum in Prevention and Modification of Measles.* McKhann, C. F. and Coady, H., South Med. J. 1934, Vol. 27, p. 20.

Gamma globulin, a by-product of human blood serum production, has proved even more satisfactory than convalescent serum in prevention of measles. Rake and Shaffer [1] have cultivated measles virus upon chick embryo, and have produced typical measles with this material in rhesus monkeys. Stokes, in co-operation with Rake,[2] inoculated more than 200 susceptible children with chick-embryo-grown measles virus. The disease resembled measles in every way, but was very mild, and in practically all cases produced immunity against subsequent exposure to measles.

Since measles is a universal infection, it seems quite feasible to produce a community-wide immunity against infection, if a living attenuated standardized measles virus can be developed that can be administered at a suitable period in the child's life and which will produce a permanent immunity against subsequent infection.

[1] Rake, G. and Shaffer, M. F.: *J. Immunol.* 1940, Vol. 38, p. 177.
[2] Stokes, J., Jr., *et al.: J. Pediat.* 1943, Vol. 22, p. 1.

ADMINISTRATIVE METHODS IN THE CONTROL OF MEASLES

Obviously, from the discussion of the epidemiology of measles, it becomes quite clear that it is not feasible, perhaps indeed not possible, with our present knowledge, to prevent an individual from contracting measles at some period during his life. In fact, it may not be advisable to postpone infection until adult life, since in some adults the disease will be severe. The chief effort in measles control is to limit the disease to those age groups in which it will do the least harm, and to prevent the development of severe symptoms and sequelae, in so far as it is possible.

**Reporting.** Each case of measles should be reported to the local health department, and each case should be investigated by some member of the health department staff. This work is usually done best by the public health nurse.

**Isolation.** The child should be isolated for his own protection, to avoid, if possible, invasion of secondary organisms which may produce sequelae, and also to avoid transmission of the disease to the young members of the family. Isolation is usually carried out best at home, rather than in a contagious disease hospital, where sequelae to measles tend to be more prevalent. Children under three years of age in the home should be kept from all contact with the patient. Unless concurrent disinfection technic and the usual simple household isolation procedures are followed, infection of the younger members of the family may occur by indirect contact, through an attendant, dishes, clothing, etc. The public health nurse can give proper instructions to the mother in regard to isolation of the infected child. The nurse should also give advice to other mothers in the vicinity who have small children, concerning suitable procedures that they may take to prevent infection of their babies.

**Quarantine.** Quarantine of the family is of little value and discourages reporting. Placarding has largely been discontinued. When a known exposure has occurred, the parents should watch their children carefully and isolate them when the end of the period of incubation draws near. Most school authorities require non-immune children in a family to remain at home during the entire incubation period, but allow the immune children in the household to go to school. A more modern method, practiced chiefly in private schools, is to permit the non-immunes to go to school the first week after known exposure, and then quarantine them at home.

During an epidemic, or where a case of measles has occurred in a school, it is necessary to obtain a census of the non-immunes. These children are observed carefully each morning when they enter school, and those who exhibit initial symptoms of the disease are excluded. The school nurse or the school authorities should inform the parents of a non-immune when an initial case of measles has occurred in their child's room, or when there has been a possibility of contact with a case of measles. If measles occurs in a children's institution, such as a hospital for chronic disease, or an orphanage, the wards containing the infants and young children should be most carefully quarantined against invasion.

**Convalescent Serum.** Measles convalescent serum has not yet been widely adopted as a prophylactic measure. It is certainly a valuable agent in modifying the course of the disease, and if properly given will prevent much suffering and save many lives. It is particularly valuable for the partial immunization of children under three years of age, or in undernourished or otherwise ill children. It is not at all improbable that future health officers and family physicians will recommend the exposure of suitable healthy non-immune children to actual cases of measles at some opportune or convenient time (as in the summer when the disease is milder and sequelae are less prevalent), with the definite intention of producing a modified form of measles through the use of convalescent serum.

This recommendation to the family will probably come through the family physician, but the health department will be called upon to collect, prepare and distribute suitable convalescent serum, and to declare its policy in regard to this matter.

Some municipal contagious disease hospitals now collect convalescent serum, as a routine measure, from measles patients just before they are discharged from the hospital. A few health departments have purchased blood from healthy persons who have recently had measles, and have prepared convalescent serum for emergency use in case of epidemic.

McKhann has utilized to great advantage the antibodies that are found in the human placenta. The placental extracts are pooled, and a highly potent product obtained which may be used in prevention or modification of measles. Gamma globulin is perhaps the most effective and simple preventive agent of all.[3]

**The Syracuse Plan.** Many communities have adopted the plan of measles control that was developed in Syracuse by Dr. George C. Ruhland. It is based on the following premises:

1. Infection with measles is practically inevitable.

2. Children under 4 years of age may suffer severely with measles. The disease is often fatal in very young children: 80 per cent of all deaths from measles occur in children under four years of age.

3. Babies are immune to measles during the first six months of life.

4. Highly susceptible age groups can be *isolated from infection* during the dangerous age periods.

A "measles susceptible" file is kept at all times. It is compiled from birth registration records. A child's name enters the file when he reaches six months of age and remains there until his fourth (or fifth) birthday.

[3] Greenberg, M., Frant, S. and Rutstein, D. D.: *J.A.M.A.* 1944, Vol. 126, p. 944.

When a child has had measles, dies, or leaves the community, his name is removed from the file.

When an epidemic of measles occurs, all nurses of the health department concentrate their efforts upon the special work of saving lives of measles susceptibles. Since 75 per cent of all deaths from measles occur in homes of people of low economic strata, special emphasis is placed on zones of overcrowding and poverty. The simple lessons taught by the nurses in their house-to-house visits are:

1. The dangers to babies under 4 years of exposure to measles.

2. The entry of measles into the home through the school children.

3. The necessity of securing a physician for young children when they develop measles.

4. The methods that may be used to modify measles, if the date of exposure is known.

5. The importance of isolation of the baby with measles, for his own protection against secondary infection.

Under this plan, no city-wide attempt is made to isolate measles, or to check the march of the epidemic through the city. School inspection is utilized chiefly as a means of detecting measles early in older children, and then securing protection of small children in the home from exposure.

This radical modification of the long-established but ineffective standard plan of isolation and quarantine has resulted in a clear-cut reduction in the death rate from measles, wherever the plan has been carried into effect. It does not check an outbreak, but it does save babies' lives.

## GERMAN MEASLES

German measles (rubella) is a very mild, highly contagious disease which presents no real administrative difficulties. Its chief importance lies in the fact that it may be confused with other more serious communicable diseases, such as measles or, more commonly, scarlet fever.

**Incubation Period.** The incubation period in German measles is usually from 2 to 3 weeks, averaging about 15 days. In contrast to measles, the incubation period is not fixed, but may vary greatly. Sometimes it is as short as 8 days.

**Diagnosis.** As in measles, the disease may have a preliminary phase with symptoms resembling coryza. In from 2 to 3 days the skin eruption appears. In many instances there are no obvious prodromal symptoms. The rash covers the entire body, including the face. It may be diffuse or somewhat blotchy on the face and neck, but on the body it appears as a brilliant, pinkish red, discrete macular rash. One important differential diagnostic point is the enlargement of the *posterior auricular glands* that is practically always noted in this disease. The disease is differentiated from a mild case of measles by the characteristic appearance of the rash and the absence of Koplik's spots. It may be difficult at times to differentiate between German measles and a very mild case of scarlet fever.

## Differential points that may be of value are:

| Characteristics of Rash | MILD SCARLET FEVER | GERMAN MEASLES |
|---|---|---|
| 1. Appearance | None on face; appears first on neck, spreading to trunk and then to extremities. | First on face, then on extremities and finally on trunk. |
| 2. Face | A flush with circumoral pallor. | Blotchy, diffuse eruption on face. |
| 3. Body | Punctate. Individual lesions fused, giving generalized eruption. | Discrete lesions, macular in type. |
| 4. Throat | Characteristic eruption on posterior nasopharynx, soft palate and pillars. The throat is sore. | Absence of the symptoms and signs described under scarlet fever. |
| *Glandular Enlargement* | No enlargement of the posterior auricular glands. Usually enlargement of glands draining the nasopharynx. | Posterior auricular glands enlarged. |

The temperature in scarlet fever is usually higher and more prolonged, and usually there is a more marked prostration in scarlet fever than in German measles; but these signs are not of differential diagnostic significance, since scarlet fever may be very mild. It must not be forgotten that desquamation does occur in German measles, but it is fine and branny, as in measles, rather than the coarse desquamation of scarlet fever.

**Transmission.** German measles is transmitted by direct contact with an actual case and is highly communicable, especially during the early stages. This period of communicability lasts about four days after the rash appears and the patient is well within a week. German measles usually occurs in epidemics, mostly in children.

**Immunity.** Natural immunity to the disease probably does not exist. An infant under 3 months may possess immunity, if its mother has had the disease. Some authorities believe that immunity following an attack is slowly lost with age. In any case, physicians and nurses exposed to German measles not infrequently develop the disease.

### ADMINISTRATIVE METHODS IN DEALING WITH GERMAN MEASLES

**Prevalence.** The disease is probably as prevalent as measles, but the data on this point are faulty. The case fatality rate is negligible.

**Reporting.** Because German measles may closely resemble scarlet fever or measles, the disease is reportable in ordinary administrative practice. It is just as important for a representative of the epidemiological division of the health department to investigate a case of German measles as one of measles itself. The differential diagnosis must be made with care.

When the definite diagnosis of German measles has been made, the child should be isolated in the home from other children in the household. Quarantine measures discourage reporting, are of no practical importance, and are not instituted. Placarding is unnecessary.

The infected child should be excluded from school for a week following the appearance of the rash. The school authorities should be informed if a case of German measles has occurred among their pupils, so that the teachers and the school health authorities may be on the alert to detect children with initial symptoms of the disease and exclude them from school.

**Education.** Because of the similarity of the two names, most parents believe that German measles is a modified form of measles and not a distinct disease. The general health information program should stress the fact that German measles is a distinct disease, unrelated to measles, and that an attack does not produce immunity to measles.

Parents should know that the disease may be confused with *mild scarlet fever.* They should be taught the importance of reporting the appearance of all eruptive diseases in childhood in order that the health department may investigate any suspicious case in its very incipiency.

If the people are made to understand that the purpose of reporting disease to the health department is to aid them personally, and incidentally to aid the community in avoiding ill effects of serious disease, and that arduous, troublesome quarantine measures will not be imposed upon them except in case of actual necessity, then the health department will gain in efficiency as well as in popularity.

Recent and rather startling evidence [4] has been introduced, which indicates that German measles in pregnant mothers may be of great potential danger to the unborn child. Congenital defects of various types, including congenital deafness and congenital cataracts, may be due directly to an attack of rubella in the mother during her period of pregnancy. If these observations are substantiated, then we must give much more serious consideration to German measles than has been our custom.

There is strong evidence that nearly 25 per cent of expectant mothers who get German measles during the first three months of pregnancy will give birth to a baby with some defect. In view of this observation, Sycock [5] has made the practical suggestion that all girls should be deliberately exposed to German measles during childhood or early adolescence.

[4] Altmann, F. and Dingmann, A.: "Congenital Deafness and Cataract Following Rubella in the Mother." *Arch. Otolaryng.* 1945, Vol. 42, p. 51.

"Occurrence of Congenital Defects in Children Following Maternal Rubella During Pregnancy." Report of Committee appointed by Director-General of Public Health of New South Wales. *Med. Jour. Australia.* 1945, Vol. 2, p. 122.

[5] Sycock, W. L. and Ingalls, T. H.: *Am. Jour. Med. Sciences.* 1946, Vol. 212, p. 3,366,

## WHOOPING COUGH

Whooping cough is of chief interest to health officials because it is so fatal to young children. Control of the disease has been most troublesome because no definite criteria had been developed to aid in the diagnosis during the early and most communicable stages of the disease. The differential leucocyte count is of some significance during the catarrhal stages of whooping cough, but cannot be considered diagnostic.

Improved techniques have now made it feasible to make an accurate and early diagnosis by the "cough plate" method.

The freshly prepared selective blood agar "cough plates" may be carried in the nurse's or physician's hand bag on daily rounds. The child suspected of having whooping cough is invited to cough, and the open surface of the cough plate is held directly in front of his mouth. If the child has whooping cough, the minute, characteristic, glistening colonies of the *haemophilus pertussis* will grow rapidly on the plate and may be recognized with ease. Calculating the onset of the disease at the first cough, Donald found that 100 per cent of the cases of whooping cough gave positive "cough plates" during the first week of the disease. Practically the same results were obtained during the second and third weeks. At the beginning of the fourth week, positive results fell off rapidly, with only 44 per cent positive plates. In the fifth week, though the children were still whooping strongly, only 2 per cent showed positive plates. These results reveal the practical diagnostic value of the cough plate, and also give us a good indication of the period of communicability.

Saito[6] and his associates recommend a combination of cough plate and a nasal culture. A small nasal swab is inserted through the nostril to the posterior nasopharynx, and the child is induced to cough.

## EPIDEMIOLOGICAL FEATURES OF WHOOPING COUGH WHICH RELATE TO ITS CONTROL

**Etiology.** Whooping cough is due to an infection with *Haemophilus pertussis,* a tiny gram-negative organism that is localized in the larynx, trachea and bronchial tree.

The organisms are discharged in the secretions from the trachea and bronchi. They survive for only a short time outside the human host. Thus whooping cough is always transmitted through direct contact with a case of the disease or through contact with various articles freshly soiled with the discharges from the bronchial tree.

**Incubation Period.** The incubation period of whooping cough is from 7 to 10 days, sometimes a few days longer. The early symptoms resemble those of any acute infection of the larynx and trachea, and the disease is commonly mistaken for an ordinary cold.

6 Saito, T. M., Miller, J. J. and Leach, C. W.: "The Nasopharyngeal Swab in the Diagnosis of Pertussis." *Am. Jour. Pub. Health.* 1942, Vol. 32, p. 471.

**Transmission.** After a week or ten days of the catarrhal stage, the cough becomes paroxysmal and the characteristic "whoop" appears. This paroxysmal cough may persist for weeks, or even to some degree for months, but the period of communicability lasts no longer than four weeks after the "whoop" appears. Thus, in a normal case, the period of greatest communicability begins about a week after exposure, persists during the catarrhal stage, which lasts about a week, diminishes gradually during the period of the spasmodic cough, and disappears between 3 and 4 weeks after the "whoop" began. Formerly we believed that carriers of whooping cough did not exist, but the newer diagnostic methods have demonstrated that temporary carriers are frequently encountered in the family and other close contacts of cases of whooping cough. Furthermore, the disease may run an atypical course. A child who never develops a true "whoop" and perhaps has only a suggestion of spasmodic cough may nevertheless have true whooping cough, and may transmit a severe type of the disease to others.

**Immunity.** Natural immunity to whooping cough probably does not exist, even in early infancy. The disease is highly prevalent and few people in normal community life escape whooping cough during childhood. One attack gives permanent immunity as a rule, but mothers who have undoubtedly had whooping cough in early childhood and who are in intimate contact with their children, nursing them during the disease, not infrequently develop a second attack.

**Prevalence.** Since whooping cough is not highly communicable, it does not occur in explosive outbreaks. The epidemic may linger in a given community for a whole year, without showing great seasonal preference. The greatest mortality from the disease occurs in the spring. Whooping cough tends to spread more rapidly through the larger communities than through the smaller towns. The greatest prevalence at any given period and the highest mortality occur in the congested population districts. Thus, rural children tend to develop the disease later in life than children living under urban conditions.

**Case Fatality.** Children of school age, 6 to 16 years, practically never die of whooping cough or its complications. The disease deserves serious consideration, however, because it may be especially severe in its effects on young children, particularly babies under one year of age. One child in ten who develops whooping cough under 12 months of age will die of the disease. In children from one to two years old the case fatality rate is about 5 per cent. The disease becomes modified in type as the age of a child is increased, so that a child of 5 years or over, unless malnourished or living under very bad hygienic conditions, will be subjected to no great danger from an attack of whooping cough. Children who develop whooping cough suffer much less severely and have fewer complications, if they can be kept in the fresh air and sunshine, and if they can retain their normal appetites and be given a suitable high-vitamin diet.

TABLE 1

Mortality from Whooping Cough by Age Groups

United States, 1941

| Age | Number of Reported Deaths | Per Cent |
|---|---|---|
| Under 1 year | 2,572 | 68.1 |
| 1 year | 714 | 18.8 |
| 2 years | 217 | 5.7 |
| 3 years | 117 | 3.1 |
| 4 years | 48 | 1.2 |
| 5 to 14 years | 98 | 2.6 |
| 15 and over | 19 | 0.5 |
| Total | 3,785 | 100.0 |

Source: Vital Statistics of the United States, 1941, Part I, pp. 106–112.

ADMINISTRATIVE CONTROL OF WHOOPING COUGH

The administrative methods used in the control of whooping cough differ in some respects from those employed in other communicable diseases of childhood. The average patient should not be confined to bed, but should be kept out of doors as much as possible. The period of communicability is long—about four weeks—so that complete isolation from all other children is seldom feasible.

The early diagnosis of the disease is difficult and often a child's contacts have been thoroughly exposed before a definite diagnosis has been made. Almost everyone will contract the disease sooner or later during his life time, so that the health officer's chief concern is to prevent the real harm that may result from the disease, by limiting whooping cough as much as possible to children of school age.

**Reporting and Isolation Procedures.** It is a common practice to require the reporting of whooping cough to the health department. If reporting of the disease is required, then the health department is under obligation to investigate each case. The work is done best by the public health nurse. All children under five years of age, and particularly babies under two years of age, should be protected as carefully as possible from contact with the child who has whooping cough. Since the disease is not highly communicable, this procedure is feasible, even if the patient remains at home. The child with whooping cough is excluded from school and is kept on the home premises for at least 4 weeks after the "whoop" begins, or 5 weeks after the initial symptoms. The "cough plate" technic indicates that this isolation period might be shortened one week without injury to the community. Quarantine discourages reporting and does not aid in the control of the disease. Placarding is unnecessary.

Some health departments use the system of marking a case of whooping cough during the communicable period with a yellow arm band, and permitting the child so marked to play outdoors in his own yard, but not with other children.

When the initial case of whooping cough occurs in a schoolroom, a census of non-immunes should be made. The school health authorities should watch these children carefully and exclude each one from school, if catarrhal symptoms develop, until a definite diagnosis is made.

The public health nurse should keep in close touch with the whole situation in her jurisdiction and should advise the mothers who live in the environs of a case of whooping cough to take special precautions to prevent the infection of their infants and small children.

**Vaccine Therapy.** The vaccines that have been used in the past in the prevention -of, and also in the treatment of, cases of whooping cough have given very disappointing results.

Sauer has insisted that these results have been due to use of an improper antigen. He has reported excellent results in the production of immunity to whooping cough by means of a suitably prepared vaccine. He insists that a very important factor of success is the use of *freshly isolated cultures* for vaccine preparation.

Madsen in 1933 has reported a study from the Faroe Islands which substantiates Sauer's results. The vaccine used was prepared from freshly isolated cultures. Three injections of 0.5, 0.7 and 1.0 cc. were given three or four days apart. Each cubic centimeter contained 10,000 million bacilli. 1,832 children were vaccinated and 446 children were not vaccinated. Of the whole vaccinated group only 458 escaped infection, but practically all the vaccinated children who developed whooping cough had a mild type of the disease, with only one death in the vaccinated group. Only 8 of the 446 controls escaped infection; many were severely ill and 8 died. Thus the case fatality of the unvaccinated group was twenty-five times that of the vaccinated group. Best results were secured when the vaccination had been completed in a community just before the onset of the epidemic. This vaccine is not without its danger. Madsen reports two deaths, probably due to the vaccine, in infants under one month of age. He also points out that the vaccine has been given to a very large number of infants without ill effect, but he does not recommend giving the vaccine to infants under one month of age.

Kendrick and Eldering observed 4,212 children over a period of 44 months, with the following results:

| | Number | Cases Whooping Cough | Annual Attack Rate |
|---|---|---|---|
| Vaccinated | 1,815 | 52 | 2.3 |
| Controls | 2,397 | 348 | 15.1 |

The vaccinated had a less severe disease than the controls.

The vaccine was made with Phase I, ten billion organisms per cc.; a total of 7 cc. was given divided in four weekly doses: 1 cc., 1.5 cc., 1.5 cc., and 3 cc. These authors conclude that there is a statistically significant difference in the pertussis incidence in the test and control groups, and the attacks which did occur in the injected group were milder.

Authorities generally agree that pertussis vaccine as a prophylactic is a useful technic in clinical practice. Many health departments that conduct well baby clinics now give whooping cough immunization to infants just as routinely as diphtheria toxoid, and some state health departments have conducted state-wide immunization programs. Sako [7] and his colleagues recommend the early administration to infants under 3 months of age of alum precipitated pertussis vaccine. His rationale rests on the fact that whooping cough is highly fatal in young babies, and that there is little or no placental transmission of immunity. Local and systemic reactions from this procedure, though infrequent, were troublesome.

Many clinicians give whooping cough vaccine in infancy and follow with a small "booster" dose of 0.1 to 0.5 cc. of the vaccine about the second birthday. Others give a small dose of vaccine as supplementary immunization at yearly intervals until school age.

Anti-pertussis serum prepared from the blood of hyperimmunized rabbits has been found to be seven times more effective than immune human serum. It has been used intensively as a prophylactic in babies that have known exposures to whooping cough, and some clinicians report satisfactory therapeutic results with this serum if given during the early stages of the disease.[8]

Concurrent disinfection of discharges from the throat is an important factor in preventing the infection of others. The simple procedures which are necessary should be explained to the parents by the public health nurse.

**Educational Work.** The educational features of whooping cough control should be part of a general health education program. They may be emphasized during an epidemic with good effect. Parents should understand the simple epidemiological features of the disease. The chief points to be stressed are:

1. Whooping cough in children under two years of age may be serious; in infants it is often fatal.

2. The disease is spread by contact with a case, particularly during the early stages of the infection. The discharges from the trachea and bronchi contain the infectious agent.

3. The catarrhal stage is the most contagious period of the disease, but

---

[7] Sako, W., Treuting, W. L., Witt, D. B. and Nichamin, S. J.: "Early Immunization against Pertussis with Alum Precipitated Vaccine." *J.A.M.A.* 1945, Vol. 127, p. 379.

[8] Bradford, W. L., Scherp, H. W. and Brooks, A. M.: *Proc. Soc. Exper. Biol. and Med.* 1942, Vol. 49, p. 157.

a child may transmit whooping cough as long as 3 or 4 weeks after the "whoop" begins. A child may whoop for three months or more, but will not transmit the disease after one month.

4. Children with whooping cough have less severe symptoms and fewer complications if kept out of doors in the sunshine and fresh air.

5. The public health nurse visits all the cases reported, not for the purpose of enforcing quarantine and isolation, but to aid in the prevention of infection, particularly of little children.

6. With our present knowledge little can be done to lower the absolute morbidity of whooping cough, but the serious consequences of the disease can often be avoided, if suitable precautions are taken.

The general educational measures relating to personal hygiene are of great value in preventing the spread of whooping cough. These include instruction to children in regard to use of individual drinking cups and eating utensils, and the importance of using a handkerchief when coughing, etc.

## MUMPS (INFECTIOUS PAROTITIS)

Mumps is a mild febrile contagious disease of childhood which receives little consideration, either by the parent or the health department. It is practically never fatal and would receive no official recognition by the health department were it not for the fact that the etiological agent sometimes invades secondarily the organs of reproduction, particularly the testes, producing a very painful inflammatory condition which sometimes results in complete sterility. Children are most susceptible to this complication during the period of adolescence.

### EPIDEMIOLOGICAL FEATURES OF THE DISEASE

The etiological agent in mumps is a specific filtrable virus. The disease is characterized by an acute inflammation of the salivary glands, particularly the parotid glands. Usually, one gland first becomes swollen and tender, followed within two days by involvement of the gland on the other side. The disease is transmitted by direct contact with a case. Carriers probably do not occur, but missed cases are common and are important factors in the spread of the disease. The source of infection is the salivary secretions.

The usual period of incubation is 18 to 21 days, though it may be a week shorter or longer. The disease is communicable in its early stages, even before symptoms have appeared, and may be transmitted during the period of enlargement of the glands, 10 to 12 days. Mumps occurs in recurring epidemics and may appear at any season, but is most common in the late winter and spring. There is little or no natural immunity to mumps, but the disease is not as readily communicable as the other acute infectious diseases of childhood. Infection is commonest in the school age period, 6 to 16 years. The actual morbidity of mumps in the United States is not known, but it has been estimated that in a typical industrial municipality, from sixty to seventy per cent of the population contract the disease at some time during life. It is less common in the rural areas, where individuals often reach adult life before contracting the disease. Mumps is practically never fatal. Its effects are most severe in the very young and the aged. It may have serious consequences in young adults, if the glands of reproduction become involved secondarily. Immunity is produced by the disease, but second attacks may sometimes occur.

## ADMINISTRATIVE PROCEDURES IN HANDLING MUMPS

Many health departments take no official recognition of mumps. Where the reporting of the disease is required by the local health department, each case which is reported should be investigated. This procedure is carried out best by the school nurse. The infected child is excluded from school and isolated from contact with susceptible children in the household during the period of communicability. No quarantine measures are required and placarding is unnecessary. There is no known method of preventing secondary invasion of the testes and no method for determining which individuals may become infected. It is assumed that fatigue, overexertion, chilling, or mild injury to the testes predisposes to localization of the infection in these glands.

A viable mumps vaccine, produced from a viable attenuated mumps virus, which has been cultivated serially in chick embryo, produces immunity in animals and offers promise of success in prevention of human mumps.[9]

**Education.** Specific educational methods concerning the prevention of mumps are of limited value. General educational methods are much more important. Since the disease is spread through the salivary secretions, the general hygienic measures that should be instituted in any community are of real value in preventing the spread of mumps. These measures include the installation of proper drinking fountains, abolition of the common drinking utensils, the adoption of individual dishes and other food utensils in schools and eating places, and proper cleansing of all articles that may transmit salivary secretions from one person to another.

## CHICKENPOX (VARICELLA)

Chickenpox is a mild febrile disease usually occurring in children. Its chief importance is that it may closely resemble and be confused with mild smallpox. The disease is usually more severe in adults than children, but the case fatality rate is very low.

---

9 "Improved Mumps Vaccine." Editorial, *J.A.M.A.* 1947, Vol. 133, p. 939.

## EPIDEMIOLOGICAL FEATURES RELATING TO CONTROL
## OF THE DISEASE

Chickenpox is due to a filtrable virus, which is present in the mucous surfaces of the body and in the skin lesions. The disease is transmitted by contact with a case. Carriers do not occur. The incubation period of the disease is from 10 to 18 days. The patient may transmit the disease during the early stages before the skin eruption has appeared, as well as during the eruptive period.

The appearance and distribution of the eruption is fairly characteristic. Lesions are superficial and scattered. Each lesion passes through a development of papular, vesicular and pustular stages, followed by crusting. All stages of development of the lesions may be observed at the same time.

The differential diagnosis between smallpox and chickenpox will be given under the former disease (see page 135).

Natural immunity to chickenpox is rare. One attack usually gives permanent immunity. Practically everyone in the United States develops the disease at one time or another during his life. Over 90 per cent of the population have the disease before the fifteenth birthday.

## ADMINISTRATIVE CONTROL OF CHICKENPOX

**Reporting.** Chickenpox is a reportable disease in general health department practice. The reason for this arduous requirement is that the disease may resemble smallpox very closely. Otherwise, reporting would not be necessary, as the disease itself is very mild and almost never causes death.

**Isolation.** An infected child should be excluded from school for a period of 7 to 10 days after appearance of the eruption and should avoid contacts with other children. No quarantine measures are required and no placarding is necessary.

**Epidemiological Investigations.** A good general rule for the health officer to follow is to investigate all cases of chickenpox in persons over 15 years of age, as well as all reported cases of chickenpox occurring during an epidemic of smallpox. The primary purpose of this investigation is to determine whether or not the patient may have smallpox. A careful history will usually elicit the source of the infection and reveal other cases that have developed from similar exposure. The vaccination history may be very helpful in making the diagnosis. The appearance of the skin lesions usually confirms the diagnosis. If there is any question in the health officer's mind as to the differential diagnosis, the case should be handled as though it were smallpox. In children's institutions, such as orphanages, the small babies may suffer severely from chickenpox and should be protected from contact with a case.

# REFERENCES

## MEASLES

1. *Measles. Report of the Medical Officer of Health and School Medical Officer on the Measles Epidemic, 1931–1932,* Publication of the London County Council. 1933, Published by P. S. King and Son. Ltd., 14 Great Smith St., Westminster.
2. Garrison, H. F., Jr. *Convalescent Serum in the Prevention and Attenuation of Measles.* New Orleans Med. and Surg. J. 1933, Vol. 86, p. 165.
3. Burn, M. *Prevention of Measles Mortality.* J. Roy. San. Inst. 1932, Vol. 53, p. 126.
4. Hunter, T. M. *Prevention of Measles by Convalescent Serum.* Brit. Med. J. 1933, Feb. 11, p. 217.
5. Gunn, G. W. *Convalescent Serum in Prophylaxis of Measles, Chickenpox and Mumps.* Brit. Med. Jour. 1932, Jan. 30, p. 183.
6. McKhann, C. F. and Coady, Harriet, *Immunity in Infants to Infectious Diseases: Placental Antibodies.* Southern Med. J. 1934, Vol. 27, p. 20.
7. Greenberg, M., Frant, S. and Rutstein, D. D. *"Gamma Globulin" and "Placental Globulin"; Comparison of their Effectiveness in Prevention and Modification of Measles.* J.A.M.A. 1944, Vol. 126, p. 944.
8. Rake, G. and Shaffer, M. F. *Studies on Measles; Use of Chorio-allantois of Developing Chicken Embryo.* J. Immunol. 1940, Vol. 38, p. 177.
9. Stokes, J., Jr., *et al. Studies in Measles; Results Following Inoculation of Children with Egg-Passage Measles Virus.* J. Pediat. 1943, Vol. 22, p. 1.
10. Dungal, N. *Convalescent Serum Against Measles.* J.A.M.A. 1944, Vol. 125, p. 20.

## WHOOPING COUGH

1. Sauer, L. W. and Hambrecht, L. *Early Diagnosis of Whooping Cough by the Cough Plate Method.* J. Med. Assn. 1930, Vol. 95, p. 263.
2. Sauer, L. W. *Whooping Cough. A Study in Immunization.* J. Amer. Assn. 1933, Vol. 100, p. 187.
3. Madsen, T. *Vaccination against Whooping Cough.* J. Amer. Med. Assn. 1933, Vol. 101, p. 187.
4. Sauer, L. W. *Immunization with Bacillus Pertussis Vaccine.* J. Amer. Med. Assn. 1933, Vol. 101, p. 1449.
5. Donald, A. B. *Diagnosis of Whooping Cough.* Brit. Med. Jour. 1938, Vol. 2, p. 613.
6. Kendrick, P. and Eldering, G. *A Study in Active Immunization Against Pertussis.* Am. J. Hyg. 1939, Section B, Vol. 29, p. 133.
7. Wheeler, R. E. *Epidemic of Whooping Cough in a Rural Area.* Milbank Memorial Fund Quarterly, 1935, Vol. XIII, No. 4; and 1936, Vol. XIV, Nos. 1 and 2.
8. Saito, T. M., Miller, J. J. and Leach, C. W. *Nasopharyngeal Swab in Diagnosis of Pertussis.* Am. J. Pub. Health. 1942, Vol. 32, p. 471.
9. Kendrick, P. J. and Eldering, G. *Study in Active Immunization Against Pertussis.* Am. J. Hyg. 1939, Vol. 29, p. 133.
10. Cohen, P. and Scadron, S. J. *Placental Transmission of Protective Antibodies*

*Against Whooping Cough by Inoculation of Pregnant Mother.* J.A.M.A. 1943, Vol. 121, p. 656.

11. Bradford, W. L., Scherp, H. W. and Brooks, A. M. *Protective Value of Refined Antipertussis Rabbit Serum.* Proc. Soc. Exper. Biol. and Med. 1942, Vol. 49, p. 157.

12. Dungal, N., Thorroddsen, S. and Agustsson, H. *Vaccination Against Whooping Cough.* J.A.M.A. 1944, Vol. 125, p. 200.

## MUMPS

1. Enders, J. F., Levens, J. H., Stokes, J. Jr., Maris, E. P. and Berenberg, Wm. *Attenuation of Virulence with Retention of Antigenicity of Mumps Virus after Passage in the Embryonated Egg.* J. Immunol. 1946, Vol. 54, p. 283.

Zinsser, H., Enders, J. F. and Fothergill, L. D. *Immunity: Principles and Application in Medicine and Public Health;* should be considered in relation to all the above communicable diseases.

# CHAPTER VII

## ADMINISTRATIVE CONTROL OF TYPHOID FEVER AND ALLIED DISEASES

THE control of typhoid fever and allied diseases is one of the great achievements of health administration in the United States. Only a generation ago this group of diseases was one of those most commonly encountered in the physician's practice. The hospital wards were full of typhoid fever in the autumn season, and the toll of death ranked among the highest of all infectious diseases. Following better health administration and an improvement of the hygienic standards of the people, these diseases have almost disappeared in many states; only the residual typhoid remains,—imported infections, and cases that may chance to be infected by the rapidly disappearing chronic carriers. Most of these carriers had the disease many years ago, when typhoid fever was prevalent. Only a small proportion of cases become permanent carriers so that, as the disease becomes less prevalent, the incidence of typhoid carriers becomes proportionately lower.

The decline in typhoid fever may be illustrated by the records of a single state—North Carolina. The achievement of this state was duplicated in many other states, and the data are typical for the nation as a whole.

Typhoid fever is essentially a disease of rural people. North Carolina began its active rural health program with the promotion of full-time county health services under the state health officer, Dr. Rankin, about 1914. That year there were 8,390 cases of typhoid fever reported in the state, with 839 deaths. In 1943 there were only 117 cases reported, with 19 deaths. The mortality rate per 100,000 population fell from 35.8 to 0.5. The morbidity and mortality data for North Carolina for 30 consecutive years has been plotted on a semilogarithmic graph. (See Fig. 9.) This graph indicates that the reporting of cases was quite satisfactory, since we know from long experience that the case fatality rate in typhoid fever is quite constant, centering around 10 per cent. The data are actual cases and actual deaths, and are not calculated on the basis of cases per 100,000 population. The state has grown in population during the 30 years from 2,350,000 in 1914 to nearly 4,000,000 people in 1946, but most of the growth has been an industrial one, with a centering of the population in large communities, where typhoid fever is more readily controllable.

This reduction in typhoid fever has been accompanied by a similar reduction in other intestinal infections, such as bacillary and amebic dysentery, hookworm disease, and others. Most of the reduction is due to improvement in rural sanitation, with special emphasis on the sanitation of water supplies, proper sewage disposal and milk pasteurization. Extensive typhoid vaccination campaigns have been conducted, with free distribution of typhoid vaccination, and the health education of rural people has been continuous and very effective. Probably the most effective administrative measure in typhoid fever control was the establishment of full-time county health units.

Administrative control of typhoid fever is particularly important to the municipal health officer because the city which he represents may be held financially responsible for any case of typhoid fever that results from improper procedures in supplying water to the people, or from other cause. The epidemic of typhoid fever in Olean, New York, is a good example of the neglect on the part of the city authorities to protect properly the municipal water supply. Following this outbreak, the city had to bond itself for a tremendous indebtedness to pay for the medical and nursing care of the sick, and for the damages incurred to families through loss of life.

## EPIDEMIOLOGICAL PRINCIPLES

The control of typhoid fever depends upon certain general epidemiological principles that characterize this whole group of infections.

1. Typhoid fever is due to a specific organism, *Eberthella typhi*.

2. The incubation period of the disease may vary from 3 to 30 days. In most instances it falls within 7 to 14 days.

3. The disease may occur in either sporadic or epidemic form.

4. The seasonal prevalence is characteristic. In the southern states the first cases of typhoid fever appear in June, the peak is reached in early August, and the disease tends to disappear in September. In the northern states there is a lag of about one month in this seasonal prevalence.

5. One attack of the specific disease gives almost complete immunity.

6. The organisms may live for a considerable period in quiescent state free from the human host.

7. The group of diseases is contracted by mouth, in great part through food and drink. Contact infection may occur; but it is not common.

8. These diseases are spread through the alvine discharges of:

    *a.* The acute case.
    *b.* The carrier.
        The carrier may be temporary or permanent and may or may not have suffered the clinical symptoms of the disease.

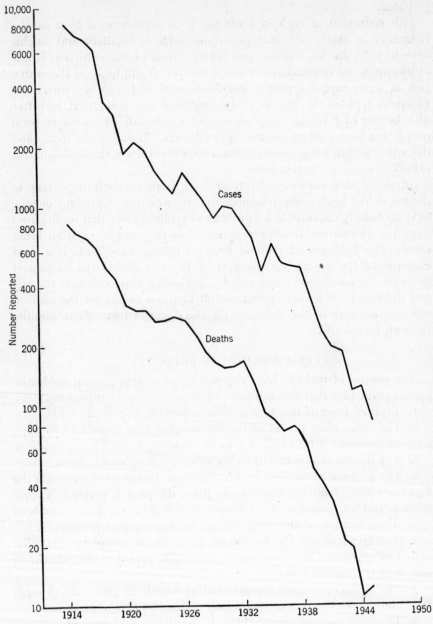

FIG. 9. *Typhoid Fever*. In North Carolina, 1914–1945. Data from North Carolina State Department of Health.

Administrative control of typhoid fever has two phases: (1) The control measures which relate to an actual case of typhoid fever. (2) The general community program.

## CONTROL OF INDIVIDUAL CASE

The control of the disease at its source requires:

**Isolation.** Earliest possible isolation of the case is essential. Thus the physician should report a suspected case of typhoid fever to the health department immediately, preferably by telephone.

Each case should be visited by the epidemiologist of the local health department as soon as the notification is received. It is his duty to aid in confirmation of the diagnosis, to institute suitable protective measures for the family and the community, and to determine, if possible, the source of the infection.

**Diagnosis.** The diagnosis should be verified by the blood culture, if possible. In the first week of the disease, the organisms are found in the blood stream of 95 per cent of the cases; 65 per cent in the second week, and only 40 per cent in the third week. If the blood cultures are negative, feces and urine cultures are of diagnostic value, particularly after the first two weeks of the disease. The Widal test becomes positive late in the disease, and should be used for verification only. It has limited value in differential diagnosis. The Widal test may give a false positive reaction in patients who are suffering from some other infection, and whose positive Widal may be due to a past immunization against typhoid fever. The test is negative in actual cases of typhoid fever until the disease is well advanced. Thus, the Widal test must be interpreted with great care, and cannot be used as an absolute index, as is often done.

**Hospitalization.** The patient should be isolated as soon as typhoid fever is suspected. Hospital treatment is best for the patient, for his family, and for the community. If hospitalization is not possible, then a suitable room in the house should be selected, where the patient may be isolated with his nurse. The patient's nurse should have no additional household duties.

**Concurrent disinfection** should be insisted upon. The public health nurse is the proper person to instruct the family in the technic of bedside prophylaxis. The urine and stools may be disinfected with 4 per cent chlorinated lime. The discharges should be received in a vessel containing a small amount of germicide and an amount then added to make twice the volume of the excretion. The nurse should break up the masses of feces, if necessary, and let stand two hours. The bath water should also be disinfected with chloride of lime solution or bichloride of mercury. The bed linen, clothing, etc., should be soaked in bichloride of mercury 1–1,000 and then boiled. All dishes and utensils entering the room should be boiled after use. All remnants of food should be burned. The room must be screened to keep out flies. Mosquito netting is satisfactory, if wire screens are not available. All these bedside precautions can best be explained by a public health nurse. She should demonstrate the methods to the family, and should make frequent follow-up visits to make sure that all precautions are being followed.

**Epidemiological investigations** should be begun as soon as the diagnosis has been made, in an attempt to determine the source of infection. A case of typhoid fever always means that there is a potential source of danger somewhere in the community. An important part of the epidemiological study is the careful search for missed cases, and for carriers of the typhoid bacillus. The missed case usually has had a very mild attack of the disease and often has not employed a physician. A careful inquiry will usually elicit suspicious symptoms, such as an unexplained fever of a week or more in duration, a diarrhea, perhaps a history of intermittent headache, or a vague malaise and feeling of ill-being. Often the stool examination has become negative at the time the epidemiological investigation is made. A strongly positive Widal test may be the chief indication that the patient has recently suffered from an attack of typhoid fever.

The carrier state is determined by repeated bacteriological examination of the stools and urine of suspected individuals. The Widal test is of some value in searching for typhoid carriers, but should not be relied upon as a definite diagnostic index. Felix has determined that the H and O agglutinations to *B. typhosus* are not reliable guides in the detection of typhoid carriers. He found that 33 of 36 known typhoid carriers did possess $V_1$ antibody in serum dilutions of 1/5 to 1/20. He considered the test to be of practical value in the detection of carriers in two outbreaks, and believes it is the best available technic, though a positive reaction is presumptive and not positive proof of the carrier state. If positive, the Felix $V_1$ test serves as an indication to intensify the bacteriological study of that person. A negative test does not mean that the person is not a carrier. Frequently it is necessary to make three or more bacteriological tests of the stools and urine of a suspected carrier before positive results are obtained. In one classical instance in which all the epidemiological evidence pointed to a single individual as the source of an epidemic of typhoid fever, seven or eight stool examinations were required before the results were positive. These negative results do not represent a failure in bacteriological technic. A few individuals are "intermittent carriers." Their stools remain free from typhoid bacilli for days, with sudden appearance of showers of these organisms. Intermittent carriers are the exception rather than the rule, however. In most cases all the stools of the carriers are positive at all times.

Various types of special selective media have greatly simplified and improved laboratory efficiency in the detection of typhoid carriers. Excellent results are obtained by direct plating with undiluted feces upon these selective media. These new technics enable the laboratory to make a rapid and very accurate diagnosis.

It is not always possible to determine the source of infection of a case of typhoid fever, but persistence and ingenuity will often bring out the hidden danger. Once it has been found, the method of correction and prevention of future infection of others by the carrier is usually apparent.

The family contacts should be protected against typhoid fever by typhoid vaccine. Immunity is produced slowly, so that the administration of vaccine to contacts may be of no avail. If any one of the family contacts is in the incubation stage of the disease when the typhoid vaccine is administered, the disease will not be prevented, though the vaccine will do him no harm.

Some physicians [1] insist that typhoid vaccine should not be given to family contacts, fearing that the "negative phase" of the vaccine may lower the resistance of the exposed individuals to such a degree that typhoid fever may result. There is no justification for the development of this hypothesis. On the contrary, it has been shown conclusively in Ramsey's studies that vaccination of family contacts greatly reduces secondary case incidence.

If the family produces any food for sale, such as milk, butter, cheese, etc., the sale must be discontinued while there is a case of typhoid fever in the house. If the patient goes to a hospital, and if the epidemiological investigation shows clearly that there is no carrier or other source of infection in the family, then sale of food may be recommenced.

Food handlers should not continue at their customary work while living in a household where typhoid fever exists. They have three choices: they may leave the home, leave their work, or send the patient to the hospital. Other members of the family need not be held in strict quarantine. Visitors should not be permitted to the patient, nor to the household.

The public health nurse should make follow-up house visits, to be sure the family understands the precautionary measures, and is carrying them out. The number of visits that should be made to each case by the nurse will vary according to individual conditions, and may be left to the judgment of the nurse.

A patient may be released from isolation following two negative cultures of the stool and urine, taken not less than twenty-four hours apart. This procedure is not an entirely satisfactory indication that an individual with typhoid fever has not become a carrier. However it is not feasible, as a routine, to require more than two laboratory tests. (A few health departments require three negative stools.) A certain proportion of the cases remain temporary carriers for three to six months and then clear up. Only a small proportion remain as permanent carriers, probably less than 3 per cent.

Gray studied 18,500 persons chosen at random in Mississippi to deter-

---

[1] Gerundo: *Kansas Medical Journal.* 1938, Vol. 39, p. 376.

mine the community typhoid carrier rate. He found that 1,547 of these persons had had typhoid fever, and that 3.27 per cent of such individuals were still positive after one year. He estimated (1938) that about 6,000 persons in the State of Mississippi were typhoid carriers. This number will decrease rapidly.

## COMMUNITY PROGRAM

**Sanitation** is the key-note of typhoid fever prevention. It is frequently stated that in order to prevent typhoid fever completely, it is only necessary to prevent human feces and urine from reaching the mouths of human beings. This is not as simple and easy a matter as it would seem, even under modern conditions. The sanitary program of the health department is, in great part, the responsibility of the sanitary engineer, and is divided into several parts:

a. Proper disposal of human urine and feces.
   (1) Community systems of sewage disposal.
   (2) Septic tanks.
   (3) Sanitary privies.
b. Maintenance of a safe community water supply.
   (1) Protection of the watershed from human pollution.
   (2) A suitable water collection and storage system.
   (3) Additional safeguards of filtration, chlorination, etc.
   (4) Protection of individual water systems, such as wells, springs, etc., from pollution.

It is obvious that the water used in making ice should be subjected to the same restriction as the drinking water, as freezing does not destroy typhoid bacilli.

c. Pasteurization of milk and milk products at 140° for 30 minutes, or some equivalent procedure that will destroy typhoid bacilli completely.
d. Disinfection of produce. In areas of heavy endemic infection, vegetables, fruits, and other products eaten raw should be thoroughly washed in a 1–2,000 solution of chlorinated lime.
e. Supervision of shellfish, which should come from officially inspected beds that have met the standard sanitary requirements.

There are, in addition, many minor sanitary activities that aid in the prevention of typhoid fever, such as sanitation of swimming pools and bathing beaches, sanitary supervision of roadside stands and public eating places, etc.

**Carriers.** In many states sanitation has been perfected to such a point that typhoid fever is no longer a serious menace. Connecticut has claimed that not a single case of typhoid fever in the state was traced to water, food, or milk for a period of seven years (1932–1939). New York State reports similar findings. This does not mean that these various sources of infection can be ignored, nor can sanitary vigilance be relaxed. This fact is well illustrated by the extensive and very severe outbreak of typhoid fever that occurred *in a state institution* in Illinois in 1939. The epidemic was traced directly to the improper sewage disposal and water supply system of the hospital.

In great part, however, typhoid fever control in the United States now resolves itself into the control of carriers. They are hard to find.

The New York State Department of Health had 479 chronic typhoid carriers under supervision on January 1, 1946—not including New York City. Twenty-three carriers were added to, and 26 removed from, the register during the year. Since only 71 cases of typhoid fever were reported in the state during the year, it is estimated that only two new carriers resulted from the disease. Since all cases of typhoid fever are due, directly or indirectly, to a carrier, these data clearly indicate that typhoid fever is a disease vanishing slowly but inevitably.

The great proportion of carriers have been discovered in two ways:

(*a*) through epidemiological investigation; and, (*b*) through routine release cultures of persons suffering from the disease.

About two thirds of the carriers are discovered through epidemiological investigations, and less than one third through routine examination of patients who have had typhoid fever and desire to be released from isolation.

Since the typhoid carrier, once he is recognized and properly instructed, rarely is responsible for another case of typhoid fever, it becomes an important part of health department practice to search assiduously for all typhoid carriers in the community. The work of Forsbeck in Michigan proved that discovery and control of typhoid carriers is largely a matter of enthusiastic, tireless, intelligent and continuous effort. It is one of the hardest and most discouraging tasks of a state epidemiologist, but the results obtained warrant the effort that is required. A card index of known carriers should be kept, and each carrier should be visited at least once a year. They should not be permitted to engage in any occupation involving the handling of food.

Some health departments permit modifications of this rigid rule, but any modifications require constant supervision and represent a potential menace because of possible slips in technic.

If an individual has been required to give up an occupation for which he is especially trained, such as cooking or dairy work, because he is a menace to the community, it is only just that he receive some compensation from the state or the local government. This compensation, though it may be small, aids the health department greatly in keeping in touch with carriers.

If the patient is a gall bladder carrier, he may be freed of his organisms in most instances by a suitable surgical operation. Since there are practically always some pathologic changes in the gall bladder of these carriers, the health department is perfectly justified in urging the carrier to have the operation for the sake of his own health. After surgical operation he should not be discharged from observation by the health department as free from typhoid bacilli until at least two specimens of bile that have been obtained by duodenal bucket have been cultured and found negative. These cultures should be made from three to five months after the surgical operation. In Massachusetts, New York State, Michigan, and several other states, the health departments have met the expenses of an operation of this type, if the carrier wishes to have it performed. Operation should not be suggested to the carrier if he is over fifty years of age, as these persons are not good surgical risks.

The adequate control of known typhoid carriers is a serious difficulty to any health department. A dramatic illustration of this fact is the case of Mrs. B, an Italian woman with a large family who lived in a small city. She supplemented the family income by assisting in outside household work, and she also made and sold family food products. A small outbreak of typhoid fever in the city was investigated. She came under suspicion and, although she had never had the disease to her knowledge, she was found to be a typhoid carrier. Though she was a good surgical risk, her father refused to permit a surgical operation. She agreed, however, to give up any activities involving food handling except for her own family. She infected at least three members of her family with typhoid fever at different times, so that eventually it was necessary to keep the non-immune members protected constantly by typhoid vaccination. On two known occasions she violated her agreement with the Board of Health. Once visitors ate at the family table and in due time developed typhoid fever. On another occasion she gave a cake to some neighbors, with the result that typhoid fever developed in several persons who ate this food. Finally, she was placed under strict isolation and under almost constant supervision by the Board of Health. No further cases of typhoid fever were traceable to her for several years. In due time her father died and the family requested the Board of Health that strict isolation be relaxed and that the family be permitted to hold a public funeral. Five of the people who came to the funeral and ate the repast served at that time developed typhoid fever. But now the chief objector to the surgical operation was dead, so that the carrier finally consented to an operation, which was done at the expense of the Board of Health. Thus, after years of effort and many failures, this source of community infection was at last eliminated.

**Food Handlers.** Stool examinations of all food handlers for the typhoid carrier state has been attempted as a routine procedure by some local health departments. The results have not been commensurate with the efforts expended.[2] The procedure is justifiable in large institutions, such as hospitals, hotels, college dining rooms, etc.

Cheese may be an important source of typhoid fever epidemics. The social condition precipitated by World War II resulted in several widespread outbreaks of typhoid fever due to improperly processed cheese

---

[2] A possible exception is dairy workers in the southern states.

made from unpasteurized milk. Notable were the epidemics in northern Indiana and in California.[3]

**Community Immunization.** A general typhoid vaccination program has been developed extensively in some of the rural areas of the southern states and has proved very popular. In order to secure proper protection, the vaccine should be prepared from virulent smooth strains, which possess complete antigenic composition. These campaigns have undoubtedly reduced the incidence of typhoid fever in areas where it was formerly very prevalent. This method of control has many limitations: it is a temporary measure, since the immunity diminishes greatly after three years; the immunity of the individual is not absolute, but relative, depending upon the intensity of exposure. During an epidemic of typhoid fever the results from the vaccine program may be disappointing. The reason for this is that immunity is produced slowly, the maximum being obtained about one week after the last injection. In epidemics the exposure is usually abrupt and of short duration, so that all danger may be passed before vaccination has begun. Vaccine should be given to all household contacts of a case of typhoid fever, for Ramsey has shown that this procedure will reduce the anticipated secondary case rate by at least 75 per cent.

The degree of endemicity of typhoid fever of any given community should determine whether or not an immunization campaign would be fruitful. As a rough index one may state that if the annual typhoid fever morbidity rate is 200 or more per 100,000 population, or the death rate 20 or more per 100,000 population, a typhoid fever vaccination program would be most profitable as a temporary control measure. In areas where the typhoid fever morbidity rate is 10 to 20 per 100,000 or less, a vaccination campaign would probably be unprofitable. Groups of persons that may be subjected to unusual risk, such as soldiers, construction camp workers, etc., should always be immunized against the disease. These vaccination programs should be used as an accessory, rather than a primary method of control. Their chief purpose is to check the spread of the disease until more permanent methods of control have been instituted. Even when typhoid fever is prevalent, vaccination should be selective, rather than a wholesale mass immunization of every person who may apply. For example, children under three years of age and persons over sixty years of age seldom develop typhoid fever and do not require the vaccine.

## BACILLARY DYSENTERY (SHIGELLOSIS) [4]

Bacillary dysentery was the scourge of both Northern and Southern soldiers during the Civil War of 1860—as it has scourged all armies

[3] Meyer, Karl F.: "Cheese-borne Epidemics of Typhoid Fever." *California and Western Medicine.* 1944, Vol. 61, No. 3.

[4] See recommendation of Hardy, A. V. and Watt, James: "The Acute Diarrheal Diseases." *J.A.M.A.* 1944, Vol. 124, p. 1173.

throughout history. In civilian life, during the past centuries, it recurred each summer throughout the land, causing great loss of life in infants, and frequently appeared in institutions for the aged or insane, with disastrous results. Due to the improvements in sanitation and to general public health measures, bacillary dysentery almost disappeared from many parts of the United States by 1940. The importance of the disease was suddenly re-emphasized, with the advent of World War II, particularly in the campaigns in North Africa, Italy, and the South Pacific.

The re-awakened interest lead to intensive studies of the disease, with resultant changes in our knowledge of the epidemiology of this group of infections, and improvements in our methods of diagnosis and control.

Bacillary dysentery is due to a group of organisms called Shigella. In the United States, Sonne is most prevalent and least fatal. Flexner is also frequently encountered. The Shiga strain is highly toxic, and if this type of infection is untreated, 20 per cent of the victims may die. Occasional Shiga outbreaks have been reported in the United States, but they are rare.[5]

The incubation period is very short—4 to 7 days—and susceptibility is general. Children and aged people are much more severely affected by the disease than are young adults. This is in contrast to typhoid fever, which is primarily a disease of young adults. The disease is transmitted through the infected bowel discharges. The acute case is an important factor in transmission, but carriers also may be very important. During an institutional epidemic, the carrier rate of Sonne dysentery may have a ratio of 20 temporary carriers to 1 case. In Flexner dysentery the ratio is about 7 to 1.

Hardy[6] and his colleagues have developed very accurate methods for the cultivation and differentiation of the Shigellas. He and others have shown that sulfadiazine is a very effective drug in the treatment of cases of illness and in the control of carriers.

The disease usually occurs in sharp epidemics. It is most prevalent in early summer. The modes of spread are very similar to those of typhoid fever, but domestic flies are a special and very dangerous factor in the transmission of bacillary dysentery. The disease produces a temporary immunity, which does not persist. Thus subsequent attacks are common. The large state institutions for the insane are particularly vulnerable to epidemics of this disease.

**Control.** The diagnosis is made by direct examination of feces cultures taken by the swab technic. Blood cultures are not of any value.

Control of bacillary dysentery follows the same general rules that are

[5] Caudill, F. W., Teague, R. E. and Duncan, J. T.: "A Rural Shiga Dysentery Epidemic." *J.A.M.A.* 1942, Vol. 119, p. 1402.

[6] Hardy, A. V. and Cummins, S. D.: "Studies of the Acute Diarrheal Diseases." *Pub. Health Reports.* 1943, Vol. 58, p. 693.

See also previous and subsequent series of papers by Hardy on this subject, published serially in *Public Health Reports* in 1941–1945.

utilized in control of typhoid fever. Proper sewage disposal, sanitation of water supplies, and pasteurization of milk are the keystones.

The discovery that sulfadiazine or sulfaguanidine will control these infections has revolutionized our methods of control. Formerly in Shiga dysentery, specific Shiga anti-serum was administered, with life-saving results. Sulfonamide therapy now controls this type of illness.

Carriers can be readily controlled by specific therapy, and if a large group of persons have been exposed to infection—as in a large body of armed troops—the disease may be prevented in all persons by the administration of small doses of sulfonamide daily for from 5 to 7 days.

Routine search for temporary carriers is not a feasible procedure, even during an outbreak.

When an outbreak occurs in a large institution, as for example a state hospital for the insane, all food handlers should be observed with special care. Search for carriers may be indicated, with treatment of all those found positive.

Control of flies is an important factor in prevention of the spread of bacillary dysentery. Concurrent disinfection of the patient's fecal discharges is an essential preventive measure. Immunization against this group of diseases by vaccines has not as yet proved to be a practical procedure.

## SALMONELLOSIS

A variety of organisms of the Salmonella group produce an acute gastrointestinal infection, which is described in some detail under the chapter on food infection and food poisoning. (See page 249.)

The disease is characterized by an acute onset, with prostration, abdominal cramps, nausea, vomiting, and diarrhea.

The disease occurs in sharp, localized outbreaks, and is very common. Individual susceptibility varies, but there is no permanent immunity to the infection, and repeated attacks may occur.

The source of infection is usually from some animal. Infection from human cases or human carriers is rare. Usually human food becomes contaminated with the feces of some animal, as a rat or other rodent, chickens, ducks, or through duck eggs. The meat of animals that may have had the disease may be the source of human infection.

Control of the disease relates almost exclusively to proper handling of food, particularly meat, dairy products, and other protein foods. The human case of illness is not an important source of human infection.

## AMEBIC DYSENTERY

The outbreak of amebic dysentery during the World's Fair in Chicago in 1933 startled public health authorities into a realization of the potential dangers of this infection. Conditions were unusually favorable for the spread of this disease, which extended to 206 known localities in the

United States, with over 900 cases and more than 50 deaths. The secondary case rate was negligible.

The etiological agent of the disease is *E. histolytica*. It is widely distributed throughout the United States: probably 5 per cent of the population are carriers of the cysts. One would anticipate a widespread clinical evidence of the disease, with frequent epidemics, but such is not the case. One reason for this is that the acute case of the disease is not a community menace, as only the cysts are infectious. Apparently massive doses of infectious material are required to produce the disease; thus, simple sanitary precautions should readily control the spread of the infection.

In the Chicago outbreak, gross pollution of the water supply of two large hotels produced the disease. It was not checked at the outset because the infected hotel guests did not remain in the city, but scattered to widely separated parts of the country. Since the water supply was adequately chlorinated, typhoid fever and allied infections did not occur. But the cyst of *E. histolytica* is resistant to ordinary chlorination. Thus, the chlorination masked the water pollution.

**Control of Amebic Dysentery.** The common simple principles of proper community sanitation will control amebic dysentery. Gross pollution of water and food with human feces is now relatively uncommon in the United States. Epidemics of the disease may occur from time to time, due to some chain of fortuitous circumstances, but these should be rare. These epidemics should cause no serious alarm, for they are easily controlled, and the secondary attack rates will be of little import.

The health department must offer the same diagnostic facilities, laboratory service, and public health nursing supervision in these diseases as in typhoid fever.

## PUBLIC HEALTH EDUCATION

Public health education is an important factor in the control of typhoid fever and allied diseases. This includes specific education of the family at the bedside of the patient by the nurse, and general education of all the people by the health department in the interepidemic period, especially in relation to general sanitation. During an epidemic, specific education concerning the prevention of these diseases can be stressed.

## REFERENCES

1. Havens, Leon. *The Control of Typhoid Fever. A Bacteriological Approach.* Commonwealth Fund Publication. 1935.
2. Dean, A. S. *The Olean City Epidemic of Typhoid Fever in 1928.* Amer. J. Pub. Health. 1931, Vol. 21, p. 390.
3. Welch, S. W., Dehler, S. A. and Havens, L. C. *The Prevalence of Typhoid Carriers in a General Population.* J. Amer. Med. Assn. 1925, Vol. 85, p. 1036.
4. Kjellstrand, T. *Chronic Typhoid and Paratyphoid Carriers and Their Treat-*

*ment.* Hygeia. 1933, Vol. 95, p. 295.

5. Bigelow, G. H. and Anderson, G. W. *Cure of Typhoid Carriers.* J. Amer. Med. Assn. 1933, Vol. 101, p. 348.

6. *The Epidemiology of Typhoid Fever.* Mass. State Health Dept. Publications. "The Commonhealth." 1933, Vol. 20, No. 3.

7. Kuttner, A. G. and Zepp, H. D. *Salmonella Suipestifer Infections in Man.* J. Amer. Med. Assn. 1933, Vol. 101, p. 269.

8. Kristensen, M. and Poulsen, K. A. *The Widal Reactions in Chronic Enteric Carriers.* Zeit. f. Bakt. 1933, Vol. 128, p. 450.

9. Jordan, E. O. *Essentials of Typhoid Fever Control To-day.* Amer. J. Pub. Health. 1934, Vol. 24, p. 349.

10. Ramsey, G. H. *What Are the Essentials of Typhoid Fever Control To-day?* Amer. J. Pub. Health. 1934, Vol. 24, p. 355.

11. Felix, A. *Detection of Chronic Typhoid Carriers by Agglutination Tests.* Lancet. 1938, Vol. 2, p. 738.

12. Gray, A. L. *The Probable Typhoid Carrier Incidence in Mississippi.* Amer. J. Pub. Health. 1938, Vol. 28, p. 1415.

13. Ramsey, G. H. *Typhoid Fever among Household Contacts, with Special Reference to Vaccination.* Amer. J. Hyg. 1935, Vol. 21, p. 665.

14. Feemster, R. F. and Anderson, G. W. *Paratyphoid Fever in Massachusetts.* Amer. J. Pub. Health. 1939, Vol. 29, p. 881.

15. Caudill, F. W., Teague, R. E. and Duncan, J. T. *A Rural Shiga Dysentery Epidemic.* J.A.M.A. 1942, Vol. 119, p. 1402.

16. Hardy, A. V., Shapiro, R. L., Chant, H. L. and Siegel, M. *Studies of the Acute Diarrheal Diseases.* IX A. *Shigella Dysenteriae Infections among Institutional Inmates.* Pub. Health Reports. 1942, Vol. 57, p. 1079.

17. Schlesinger, E. R. *Use of Modern Laboratory Aids in the Investigation of a Typhoid Fever Outbreak.* Am. Jour. Pub. Health. 1943, Vol. 33, p. 1257.

18. Hardy, A. V. and DeCapito, T. *Studies of the Acute Diarrheal Diseases.* X A. *Cultural Observations on the Relative Efficacy of Sulfonamides in Shigella Dysenteriae Infections.* Pub. Health Reports. 1943, Vol. 58, p. 689.

19. Hardy, A. V. and Cummins, S. D. *Studies of the Acute Diarrheal Diseases.* X B. *A Preliminary Note on the Clinical Response to Sulfadiazine Therapy.* Pub. Health Reports. 1943, Vol. 58, p. 693.

20. Hardy, A. V., Watt, James and DeCapito, T. *Studies of the Acute Diarrheal Diseases.* XI. *The Typing of Shigella Dysenteriae Flexner.* Pub. Health Reports. 1943, Vol. 58, p. 696.

21. Hardy, A. V. and Watt, James. *The Acute Diarrheal Diseases.* J.A.M.A. 1944, Vol. 124, p. 1173.

22. Meyer, Karl F. *Cheese-borne Epidemics of Typhoid Fever.* California and Western Medicine. Sept. 1944, Vol. 61, no. 3.

23. Watt, James and Hardy, A. V. *Studies of the Acute Diarrheal Diseases.* XIII. *Cultural Surveys of Normal Population Groups.* Pub. Health Reports. 1945, Vol. 60, p. 261.

24. Hardy, A. V. *Studies of the Acute Diarrheal Diseases.* X C. *Further Cultural Observations on the Relative Efficacy of Sulfonamides in Shigella Infections.* Pub. Health Reports. 1945, Vol. 60, p. 1037.

25. Feemster, R. F. and Smith, H. M. *Laboratory Criteria of the Cure of Typhoid Carriers.* Am. Jour. Pub. Health. 1945, Vol. 35, no. 4.

# CHAPTER VIII

## ADMINISTRATIVE METHODS IN CONTROL OF
## TUBERCULOSIS

A TREMENDOUS decline in the death rate from tuberculosis has occurred in the United States in recent years. This decrease has been universal in all groups of society and all parts of the country. The decline has been more rapid in some groups and in some sections than in others, but nowhere has the death rate increased or even remained stationary. This fact is well brought out by Fig. 10, which gives the data for mortality from tuberculosis in the United States Death Registration Area from the period of 1900 to 1945. It will be noted that the trend line descends most rapidly from 1900 to 1925. The deaths continued to decrease, at a lower annual rate, until about 1935, when the curve levels off with a very slow recession during the past ten years. These data for recent years are not at all discouraging. Tuberculosis is a social disease, and the death rate responds to modification in social conditions. The surprising thing is that tuberculosis did not increase from 1930 to 1944. The nation went through a prolonged period of financial depression, only to be followed by the tremendous stress of a world war. Past experience indicated that such devastating nation-wide social disturbances inevitably result in an increase in those diseases that are closely related to social upheaval, notably tuberculosis, typhus fever, venereal disease, and malnutrition. As we shall demonstrate in another chapter, only one of these conditions— the venereal diseases—increased markedly during the years of social distress.

Health educators have stressed the fact that pulmonary tuberculosis is a vanishing disease, and have suggested that if we continue an active program in tuberculosis control, the disease may be practically eliminated from the community by 1960. This would be true if the mortality rate continued to decline during the next generation at the same rate that it had declined during the past 35 years. But unfortunately trend lines almost never assume a straight line, but tend to level off. We have every reason to believe that the tuberculosis death rate will continue to decline, but the incidence of the disease will remain high for many years to come.

**Geographic Distribution.** The death rate for tuberculosis varies enormously in different parts of the nation. (See Fig. 11.) The reasons for this phenomenon, in some instances, are quite clear; in other areas, they are not fully understood. Arizona, which had the highest rate in 1944, has a very large Indian population, and also is a mecca of sufferers from tuberculosis. The southern states, with large Negro populations, formerly all had rates that were above the mean, but the record of South Carolina and Georgia is now superior to Vermont or Connecticut. The heavily industrialized states of New York, New Jersey, Pennsylvania, and Delaware all have rates above the mean, 41.3 per 100,000 population, whereas

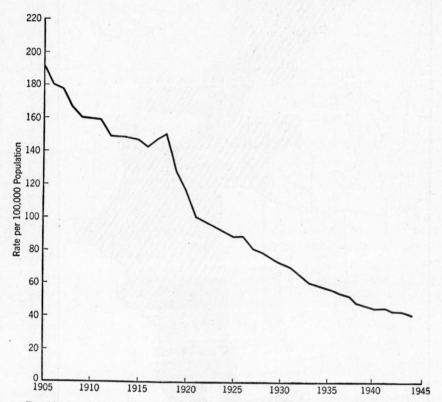

Fig. 10. *Death Rates from Tuberculosis—All Forms.* United States Registration Area, 1905–1945, Total Persons of all Ages. Metropolitan Life Insurance Company.

the midwestern farming and ranching states of Wyoming, Utah, Iowa. North Dakota, and Nebraska all have rates below 18 per 100,000 population. Certain states in the Appalachian chain have always had much higher death rates from tuberculosis than the mean for all states—notably, Tennessee, Kentucky, and West Virginia. The reasons for this are not clear. Massachusetts, New Jersey, New York, and Pennsylvania have conducted active and very intelligent tuberculosis control programs for many years, but the death rates in these states from this disease continue to be much higher than in many states where much less tuberculosis control has been carried on. Some authorities have suggested that tuberculosis

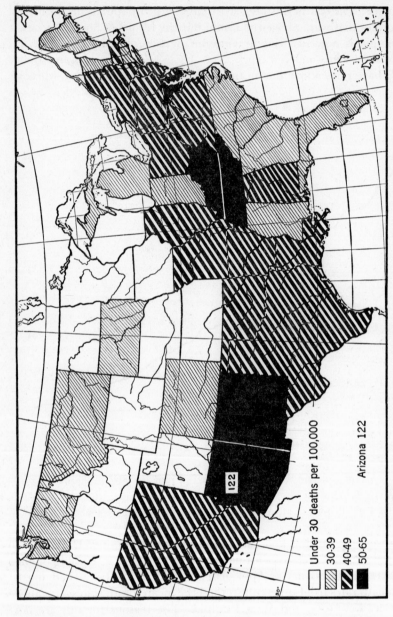

FIG. 11. *Tuberculosis Death Rates per 100,000 Population among Residents of each State, 1944. Death Rate for the United States—41.3.* Source: United States Bureau of the Census.

86

would have declined throughout the nation, even though no active, specific efforts had been undertaken to control the disease. In other words, tuberculosis has declined because of changes in the national economy and social structure, and not because of health department activities. The author believes that a combination of natural control factors and specific epidemiological measures have played an equal and complementary part in the successes that have been achieved in this field.

It is impossible even to guess at the relative importance of the various factors that have produced the enormous saving of life and relief from suffering from tuberculosis. There is a real difference of opinion as to whether or not the activities of health departments or unofficial health agencies have had any material influence on the rate of decline. Hospitalization and sanatorium care have undoubtedly saved many lives, but it is impossible to determine how much this procedure has influenced the incidence of infection or the development of pulmonary disease. How can one measure the relative importance of the numerous factors that have undoubtedly influenced the decrease of this disease, such as better economic conditions, better housing, more abundant supply and utilization of foods, greater and more widespread knowledge of the natural history of the disease, perhaps increase of community immunity, and many other unmeasurable factors? We have evidence that the economic factor is very important, since tuberculosis has almost disappeared in recent years in the more fortunate economic levels of society and has become in great part a disease of poor people. Who knows the importance of the development of better shipping and storage facilities for food, with refrigeration and better marketing? Greater recreational facilities and less overcrowding have influenced the trend of the disease. Most important of all, perhaps, is the better understanding of the disease by the whole population, the general knowledge that tuberculosis is transmitted by contact with infected material, usually by direct contact with an infected individual. The mere knowledge that tubercle bacilli are present in large numbers in the sputum of tuberculous persons has resulted in less promiscuous expectoration, and greatly lowered dispersion of the organism.

Tuberculin testing of cattle and especially the pasteurization of milk have almost eliminated bovine tuberculosis from most communities.

As we have gained knowledge of the disease, we have modified our administrative methods of control more and more to suit the newer knowledge. We have also profited by previous mistakes, and thus rendered our efforts more effective.

**Sources of Infection.** The etiological agent of tuberculosis is *Mycobacterium tuberculosis*. This great discovery by Koch in 1882, together with his proof that the disease is transmitted by contact with an infected individual and is not due to inheritance, unfavorable climate, dampness, fog, miasma, "evil eye" or other environmental phenomena, represents the beginning of, and foundation for, all our attempts toward the development of methods of controlling tuberculosis. Tubercle bacilli are distributed in great part through the sputum of "open cases" of the disease. The infection is usually acquired by direct contact with a person with tuberculosis, but may be acquired through contaminated food, particularly milk, and also by articles soiled with the discharges of the patient.

**Period of Incubation.** There is no method of determining the incubation period in tuberculosis. The period between actual infection and the development of clinical symptoms varies tremendously. The infection is carried by the respiratory system or the circulatory system to the terminal air vesicles in the periphery of the lung. Usually, only a tiny sub-pleural tubercle develops. The lymph channels carry the infection to the lymph glands at the bifurcation of the bronchi, or the trachea. Here tubercles are formed. This is called the *childhood type* of tuberculosis or *hilum* tuberculosis. An infant exposed to a tuberculous mother may develop a generalized tuberculosis from this initial infection and die within a few weeks. In most children the infection never advances beyond the earliest stage. The infected children show no evident clinical symptoms and the only index of infection may be the positive Mantoux test.

The adult type of pulmonary tuberculosis is usually a secondary infection. There may be a new infection from without or re-invasion from the previous lesion. In the adult type of tuberculosis the lung itself is invaded—usually at the apex. If this type of tuberculosis develops in childhood, or, in fact, before the eighteenth year of age, the result is frequently fatal.

**Diagnosis.** It is commonly assumed that every individual living in a modern community inevitably becomes infected with the tubercle bacillus at some time during life—usually before adolescence. Undoubtedly this was true in the past, but the conditions that brought about this situation are rapidly disappearing. Careful tests have shown repeatedly that more than 60 per cent of the young college graduates—all over twenty-one years of age—who enter medical school have a negative tuberculin test. In some of the western universities more than 75 per cent of the students (ages 17–21) have a negative tuberculin test. There is every indication that the tuberculin positive rates of all age groups in practically all parts of the United States are diminishing year by year. As the disease has gradually declined and dispersion of tubercle bacilli has been less wide, it has become an increasingly common occurrence to postpone the age at which the original infection occurs. Furthermore, we have arrived at the stage where exposure to a heavy dosage of infection is less and less frequent.

Formerly, the tuberculin test was considered of limited diagnostic value and useful only in small children. We are rapidly approaching a stage where a negative tuberculin reaction will be the rule in adolescence and early adult life, so that a tuberculin test will be of greater significance as times goes on.

**Mantoux Test.** The procedure commonly used as a routine is as follows: Carefully standardized old tuberculin [1] is used. Freshly prepared dilutions only are employed. The solution is made so that 0.1 cc. of the solution contains 1/100 milligram of tuberculin. The injection (0.1 cc.) is given with a small caliber needle into the skin of the forearm. The reaction is read at the end of 48 hours. Usually, there is no question about the result. A positive test is indicated by a wheal at the site of injection with a surrounding area of redness. In a few instances the reaction is intense with extension of the redness along the lymphatics and with swelling of the axillary glands. This soon disappears. If the reaction is negative or questionable, a second injection of a dilution of the solution of old tuberculin containing 1.0 milligram in 0.1 cc. is given intracutaneously, and the reaction is observed 48 hours later.

The tuberculin test is a very useful method to determine whether or not the individual has been infected with the tubercle bacillus. It does not give information concerning the stage of development of this infection. The method is of particular value in the study of contacts and in determination of sources of infection. It has been used extensively as a screening technic in community-wide surveys.

The second and most important diagnostic aid is the x-ray. It is a simple and exact method for early diagnosis of the disease, and is the most effective technic that we possess for determining the advance or retardation of the infection. Various procedures are employed, depending upon the purpose of the particular investigation. The rapid small film technic is used extensively in pulmonary screening tests, particularly when large numbers of persons are surveyed. The fluoroscope has its place, particularly in the office of the practitioner of medicine. The standard 14- by 17-inch cellulose films are used for accurate verification of the diagnosis, and for study of contacts and search for sources of infection.

The history of the patient is a very valuable aid in diagnosis of early tuberculosis and should be utilized fully.

Physical examination of the patient is an adjunct which has some value in determination of the advance or retardation of the pulmonary process and is a useful aid to the clinician in handling the individual

---

[1] Purified protein derivative—PPD—is preferred to old tuberculin—OT—by some authorities. The technique of administration is the same. Customary doses of PPD are:

| | | |
|---|---|---|
| 1st dose: | 1:50,000 | dilution of 1% PPD |
| 2nd dose: | 1:200 | dilution of 1% PPD |

Seideman believes that the PPD reaction is more specific and more clear-cut. See "A Comparative Study of Old Tuberculin and the Purified Protein Derivative." *American Journal of Hygiene.* 1939, Vol. 30 (section B), page 1.

case. From the public health point of view, a prolonged and detailed examination of the chest by percussion and auscultation has relatively little value or significance, because the early stages of tuberculosis are determined much more readily by other means.

Examination of the sputum is a very important procedure from the point of view of the health officer, and should be utilized to a much greater degree than is the common practice. Dubos' brilliant researches [2] in the cultivation of the tubercle bacillus have revolutionized our cultural methods, and made the cultivation of the tubercle bacillus a relatively simple process.

**Resistance** of the individual depends in the main upon three factors:
1. Racial or familial resistance.
2. Virulence of the invading organisms.
3. Individual resistance.

The latter factor only is subject to some measure of control.

*Racial or Familial Resistance.* The aboriginal races have a low resistance to invasion of the tubercle bacillus. Thus the Negro or Indian will frequently develop a rapidly fulminating case of pulmonary tuberculosis following the initial invasion of the organism. Certain families seem to have a much higher resistance to invasion than others. The Scotch, Irish, and Scandinavian races are highly susceptible to the disease. Those racial or familial groups that are relatively immune probably have not escaped infection. Rather they possess a higher resistance to invasion of their tissues by the organism.

*Virulence of the Invading Organism.* Different strains of tubercle bacilli vary in virulence. This factor undoubtedly plays a real part in the prognosis of any given case of the disease.

*Individual resistance* depends upon many factors, one of the most important of which is the state of general nutrition. All those things which go to make up a healthful life increase resistance to the secondary invasion with resultant pulmonary involvement. This secondary invasion may be initiated by continuous reinfection through frequent exposure to a chronic case, or to undue strain, overwork, poor nutrition, bad living conditions or for other reasons.

Clinical symptoms may develop following some special physiological stress, often appearing at puberty in girls, or in young men when they assume the burden of earning their own living. The breakdown may occur later in life following unusual mental or physical strain.

The factor of resistance to infection, with gradual decrease of community exposure to massive infection, has produced a gradual change in the epidemiological picture of the disease. The incidence of tuberculosis in infants and young children has declined markedly. Between the ages of 6 and 16 years, in all classes of society and all racial groups,

[2] Dubos, R. J.: "Rapid and Submerged Growth of Mycobacteria in Liquid Media." *Proc. Soc. Exp. Biol. and Med.* 1945, Vol. 58, p. 361.

the disease has become of little consequence. Early infection occurs in Negro girls, beginning at about 16 years. From this point on, the incidence of infection increases in all ages and all racial groups. The incidence of infection is probably no higher in Negro than in white persons who live under similar social conditions, but Negroes succumb much more rapidly to tuberculosis than do white people. Thus the death rate from tuberculosis in Negroes who live in American cities is five or six times greater than in the whites.

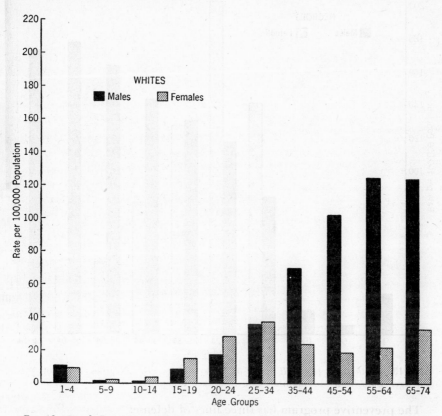

FIG. 12. *Death Rates from All Forms of Tuberculosis—1945.* By Color, Sex and Age. Data from Metropolitan Life Insurance Company.

Furthermore, the disease is much more prolonged in the whites, so that tuberculosis has become in the white race in the United States a disease of past middle life, and the peak of death occurs not in the period of 20 to 30 years, as was the case a generation ago, but rather during the fifth and sixth decade. These data are well illustrated in Fig. 12 and 13.

Since the death rate from tuberculosis is so much higher among the Negroes than in whites, one would anticipate that the disease would be more prevalent in Negro communities. Such is not the case. If a survey is made of two similar communities at the same time, one a community of Negro families and one of white families, the investigators will find more cases of tuberculosis in the white community than in the Negro community.

These matters are discussed in some detail, because they are of importance in making plans for control of the infection.

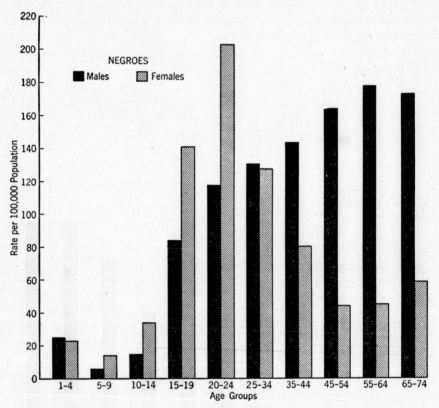

FIG. 13. *Death Rates from All Forms of Tuberculosis—1945*. Negroes, by Color, Sex, and Age. Data from Metropolitan Life Insurance Company.

**The preventive program** has three lines of defense:

1. Prevention of infection.

2. Prevention of development of clinical symptoms in the infected.

3. Prevention of death in those who have developed definite symptoms of disease.

Absolute prevention of infection at some time during life of the individual under modern living conditions is not yet possible, although it is possible to postpone the age at which infection occurs and also to prevent frequent exposure to a heavy dosage of infection. In the past tuberculosis has been, essentially, a disease of youth. Anyone who passed the age of 30 without developing demonstrable tuberculosis could be quite sure that he would never die from that disease. This epidemiological feature of the disease is gradually changing. Prevention of the disease as measured by definite clinical symptoms depends upon a nice balance between invasiveness or virulence of the organisms and resistance of the individual. Prevention of the advance of clinical symptoms and actual death from tuberculosis depends in great part upon suitable, prolonged, expert treatment.

**Period of Communicability.** The disease is communicable until all lesions have been healed. Relapses are common. Following an acute respiratory infection, an individual with quiescent tuberculosis sometimes becomes an "open case," discharging bacilli freely, and is again a menace to his immediate personal contacts. In recent years, the chronic case of tuberculosis, often unrecognized, is probably the most important source of dispersion of tubercle bacilli.

Individuals working in certain trades show a high degree of susceptibility to tuberculosis. The chief factor which produces this increased susceptibility is inhalation of silica dust, and the trades involved are numerous and varied, from granite cutters to zinc miners, and from lens grinders to makers of abrasive soaps.

## METHODS OF CONTROL

Modern methods of control are based on:

1. Early and accurate diagnosis of tuberculosis.

2. Good epidemiological work in determining sources of infection and tracing and examining the contacts of a source of infection that may have been discovered.

3. Good case finding technics.

4. Prevention of dispersion of tubercle bacilli by the open case of tuberculosis. This was attempted in the past by means of partial isolation of the patient in his home, by disinfection of his sputum and by careful education of the patient as to the danger of carelessness. Collapse therapy has greatly simplified the problem of preventing the dispersion of tubercle bacilli. It has proved to be a very valuable public health measure in changing the open case of tuberculosis to a "closed" case.

All the various administrative devices that have been developed in control of tuberculosis—special clinics, sanatoria, visiting nursing service, ambulatory x-ray service, and all the rest have, in their essence, attempted to improve our technic in the four principles mentioned above. Early and accurate diagnosis of the case, determination of contacts, wide search for early active cases, and prevention of further spread from a determined source of infection are basic. As a corollary to this work, every attempt is made to prevent further extension of the pulmonary process in those persons who have already developed the disease, to aid in arrest of the disease of the incipient cases, and to attempt the prolongation of life of those individuals in whom the disease is well advanced.

**Reporting.** All diagnosed cases of tuberculosis should be reported promptly to the local health department by name. Because of former dread and fear of the disease, and the belief that its hereditary character represented a blight on the family name, tuberculosis has often been kept secret as long as possible, and has been reported poorly by physicians. A real index of the standard of education of a people and the effectiveness of a health department is the ratio of cases reported to the health department, to death certificates for tuberculosis that are filed. A good ratio is five cases to one death. In a Negro population the ratio will often be less than one reported case for each annual death.

A card index of all cases of tuberculosis should be kept in a separate file. All "open cases" should be kept in a special file, with a "tickler" system to indicate just when each case should be visited, and a cross index with the "family card" file.

**Laboratory Diagnosis.** The local health department must supply facilities for accurate laboratory diagnosis of sputum. This service should be free, irrespective of the economic status of the patient. The technic is simple and is dependable for diagnostic purposes. It is also a valuable method of determining whether or not the patient is still in the infective stage. Gastric lavage has become a real asset in accurate and early diagnosis of tuberculosis, and should be employed whenever indicated. All large central laboratories should furnish facilities for demonstration of tubercle bacilli by animal inoculation or by cultivation.

**Investigation.** Every case of reported tuberculosis should be investigated by the health department. This work is done best by a skilled, tactful public health nurse, who confers with the family physician and the patient's family to determine if the patient shall remain at home, or be hospitalized. If he remains at home, the nurse should make frequent instructional visits so long as the patient remains infective, and aid the patient in establishing the partial isolation which is so essential in preventing infection of family contacts. The technic of concurrent disinfection should be explained, and, in cases of economic necessity, the health department should furnish the patient with suitable sputum cups and necessary simple antiseptics.

**Isolation and Quarantine.** Compulsory hospitalization is not feasible. Complete isolation of the patient is not necessary. The essential thing is to teach the patient the simple procedures in proper disposal of his discharges, to win his co-operation and persuade him to follow the necessary technic. In rare instances, a criminally careless, recalcitrant patient will refuse to carry out the necessary precautions for protection of his friends and neighbors, and the health officer is compelled to take vigorous measures.

**Hospitalization.** It is generally agreed that the great proportion of cases of tuberculosis require a period of sanatorium care, particularly if the case is active and "open." This procedure is of benefit in saving the life of the patient and in protecting the public. Since treatment is prolonged and expensive, and since most of the cases occur in the lower economic levels of society, the burden of hospitalization falls in great part on the community.

Experience has shown that the average period of hospitalization of a recognized case is one year. The standard recommendations are two available beds for cases of tuberculosis for each actual death. Thus, for a typical city of 100,000 population, with 30 or 40 deaths from tuberculosis each year, from 60 to 80 beds are required. Many communities have provided up to 3 beds per annual death. In view of the continuing decline in tuberculosis incidence in most parts of the United States, it does not seem appropriate to expand the hospitalization program beyond the present standards. The average hospitalization costs per patient per year are at least $1,200, not including initial construction costs and depreciation. These standards represent almost prohibitive costs for most communities. If they are reached, there results a tendency to restrict funds for other equally important public health purposes. It is now generally felt that the stimulus by various well-meaning individuals and voluntary organizations for construction of numerous tuberculosis hospitals has placed too great emphasis on the value of hospitalization *per se* as a preventive measure. Many authorities believe that equally satisfactory results might have been obtained by less expensive methods.

Small tuberculosis hospitals (*e.g.*, less than 75 or 100 beds) are usually uneconomical administrative units.

The therapy of pulmonary tuberculosis has changed radically in recent years. Rest—*absolute rest*—of the lung is the essential feature of treatment and is frequently secured by surgical means. A few clinicians have attempted to carry out simple collapse therapy on patients who remain in their homes. Up to the present, the consensus is that these patients should be treated in the hospital. These modern methods of treatment cannot be furnished in the old type of tuberculosis sanatorium, which had no facilities for surgical treatment and often had no x-ray. The new therapeutic methods require a much better type of tuberculosis hospital construction, but it now seems probable that a smaller number of beds will be needed because of the more rapid turnover of patients. A shorter period will be required for hospital care, so that the total expense for hospitalization should not be prohibitive.

One of the chief advantages of hospitalization is that it teaches the patient to care for himself when he returns home. It also prevents the dispersion of tubercle bacilli by the open case, and separates the active case from his immediate family contacts. This is very important when the patient has a positive sputum.

**Summer Camps.** These institutions are frequently organized by local tuberculosis associations for the prevention of tuberculosis. They are intended to improve the nutrition of children, develop better food habits, and provide storage of vitamins and of fat for the long winter months. They are usually conducted by voluntary organizations, occasionally as an official health department project. Some organizations limit attendance to cases of known or suspicious hilum tuberculosis. These programs undoubtedly have some effect in preventing the development of pulmonary tuberculosis, in that a few of the children may be removed from exposure to an active case for a short period of time. They are not expensive to operate. Their chief value to the children is the improvement in nutrition that is effected in any well organized summer camp.

**Home Care.** Sanatorium care is of little value unless there is an intelligent, well supervised plan for home care after the patient is discharged from the hospital. The most difficult period of adjustment is the rehabilitation of the patient who is able to do a few hours' work a day, but cannot yet assume the responsibilities of a full time job. A health department can save money to the community and prevent relapses with re-hospitalization by developing a simple rehabilitation "workshop" for convalescents.

**Clinic Service.** An average city with approximately 100,000 population should plan for 600 to 800 visits to a tuberculosis clinic a year. This would require a weekly clinic with about 15 patients, or a fortnightly clinic with 30 patients, on the average. The chief of the clinic should be an expert on chest diagnosis. A specialist may be employed by the health department on a part-time basis. The nurses whose services are required for the home visiting in tuberculosis (if the specialized nursing plan is followed) may aid in the clinic. X-ray facilities are most essential. The work may be incorporated in the outpatient clinic service of the general hospital. In this case the hospital may receive a subsidy from the health department. In rural, sparsely populated communities, the state may furnish itinerant clinic service. These clinics furnish expert diagnostic and consultation service, as well as x-ray facilities. They are of little value unless the local rural health department is well organized, and can furnish permanent competent follow-up nursing service. In so far as possible the tuberculosis clinic service should be built around the sanatorium service and closely integrated with it.

**Nursing Service.** The home nursing service is the most important part of the tuberculosis program. It makes no material difference whether the generalized or specialized type of nursing organization is followed. A standard community of 100,000 will require the equivalent of three or four full-time public health nurses to carry out the activities of a tuberculosis program. The nurse keeps in touch with each reported case in her jurisdiction. The sanatorium reports all pending discharges to the health department, so that the patients who are returned to the community can be followed carefully in making home adjustments. Patients on the nurses' active file are visited as often as the individual situation indicates. All patients are visited on the average of once a month. The instructional nursing visit is not only of great value to the patient, but to the family as well. Through the home nursing service, all contacts are watched carefully. A Mantoux test on children in the family is advisable, together with an x-ray of those children showing a positive tuberculin test.

**Case Finding Programs.** As tuberculosis incidence has declined, it has become possible to institute intensive and specific technics of tuberculosis control. These are "sharp-shooting" rather than "shotgun" methods, and correspond to the search for typhoid carriers in the control of typhoid fever.

In a case finding program a special group in the community is selected, and by intensive search, through tuberculin testing and x-ray of all Mantoux positives, or perhaps by x-ray alone, all the active cases of tuberculosis that can be found in the group are picked out.

School programs were developed earliest. All the children whose parents gave consent were given a standard tuberculin test (Mantoux). If the test was positive, then the child was given an x-ray of the chest. The children were then classified as adult type of tuberculosis, hilum tuberculosis, suspicious, or negative. This work was done in the grade schools. This type of survey has been given up as unprofitable because so few cases of tuberculosis were found. It is an excellent educational measure and does find a few cases of active tuberculosis.

The work was then extended to the high school age groups. Even in this highly selected field so few cases of tuberculosis have been found by the screening technic as to throw doubt on the method as a valuable routine administrative procedure. It is now general practice to do one test for tuberculosis during a child's school life. The best period is in the third or fourth high school year, the sixteenth or seventeenth year of age.

The best case finding programs are those which concentrate on those particular groups in the community where most of the tuberculosis is likely to occur. In other words, one looks for tuberculosis where it is probable that the disease will be found.

The highest tuberculosis death rates are, of course, in the lower economic levels of the community. In the larger cities, the Negro section of the city should receive first consideration. In New York City, for example, the tuberculosis death rate of Harlem is three times that of the adjacent Washington Heights district.

An effective case finding program requires an intimate knowledge of the economic, social, and racial make-up of the health officer's jurisdiction. The health officer should know his whole district in great detail, and should confine his efforts in tuberculosis case finding to those groups in the population that will obtain the greatest benefit from the program.

Many of the large industrial organizations conduct a continuous tuberculosis case finding program among their employees. Colleges, and particularly medical schools and hospitals, have extensive and very effective systems for early detection of tuberculosis among their students, interns, and nurses.

**Case Finding Rules.** A few simple rules will be of advantage to the health department in formulating a case finding program: [3]

1. The exposed infant. A baby from birth to 3 years that has been exposed to open tuberculosis must be watched carefully. A periodic tuberculin test should be done, with roentgenogram of the chest if the tuberculin test becomes positive. The length of interval between the tuberculin tests depends upon whether or not the exposure is continuous. If this is the case, then not less than three months should elapse between each tuberculin test.

2. The child of 3 to 10 years. If the child from 3 to 10 years of age has a negative tuberculin test, and if the exposure to tuberculosis has been discontinued, there is no practical reason for continued supervision, and no necessity for retesting with tuberculin during this seven-year period.

3. From 10 to 25 years of age, with a negative tuberculin test. If the exposure to tuberculosis has been discontinued and the tuberculin test is negative, no routine supervision is necessary for this age group.

4. From 10 to 25 years of age, with a positive tuberculin test. If there is a known exposure to tuberculosis at the present time or within a year, then the contact case should be followed routinely: roentgenogram of the chest should be made at least annually, until the twenty-fifth year of life.

If a "parenchymal" lesion is discovered during this period, the contact should be very closely followed. Special attention should be given to the adolescent Negro child, particularly Negro girls.

Medical students, young physicians and nurses, as well as other young people who have continuous and unavoidable exposure to tuberculosis, should have an annual tuberculin test. If this test is positive, they should have an annual chest roentgenogram. If the tuberculin test becomes positive while under observation, they should be given special supervision, with chest X-ray every six months.

5. From 25 to 30 years of age. If the exposure has been broken, and roentgenology of the chest is negative, no further routine supervision is required.

6. After 30 years of age. If roentgenogram of the chest is negative at this age, and the exposure to tuberculosis is not continuous, no further need for supervision of the contact case exists.

It is quite possible that this fairly concise program for supervision by age groups of contacts of cases of tuberculosis may be changed in the near future, because of the rapidly changing epidemiologic features of the disease.

[3] The material on case finding rules is reprinted from the author's *Preventive Medicine and Public Health*, pages 281–283, published by The Macmillan Company in 1946.

**Mass Surveys.** The mass survey for tuberculosis control is an examination of large numbers of apparently healthy persons who have had no known exposure to tuberculosis.

Certain simple principles are involved:

1. The survey is conducted or sponsored by the official health service of the community. The state may aid by supplying a mobile unit, with equipment and capable technicians. Aid may be given by the voluntary tuberculosis association. In some instances where a large industrial group is surveyed, the employers or the labor unions give aid in the conduct and in meeting the cost of the service, but the responsibility for the survey rests with the local health department.

2. Care should be taken in selecting the groups to be surveyed. One should concentrate his efforts on the age and social groups where the disease is most likely to occur. For example, mass surveys of grade school children have been found to be a waste of effort.

3. The value of the clinic is dependent upon (*a*) suitable equipment for taking rapid and inexpensive x-rays of the chest of large numbers of people, (*b*) a trained and competent personnel, and (*c*) availability of facilities to classify promptly and accurately the significance of the lesions found by the x-ray technicians.

4. The health department must assume responsibility for providing proper care of all cases of significant tuberculosis that are found during the survey.

In one large city an extensive mass survey for tuberculosis was carried out, and many unsuspected cases of active tuberculosis were found. But the city had made no provision for the sanatorium care of these patients, nor was it possible to provide for suitable nursing service and home care. Thus the value of the mass survey was greatly diminished.

The mass survey has a definite place in the technic for detection of early tuberculosis. It is also an excellent method in community education. But unless it is properly handled, and widely advertised, it may prove an expensive and relatively ineffective procedure.[4] Special groups that give most information are suggested by Edwards[5] in the order of relative importance:

Group 1. Those living under substandard conditions, unemployed and on the city relief rolls.

Group 2. Negro populations living under congested city conditions.

Group 3. Industrial workers subjected to toxic dusts, particularly silica dusts.

Group 4. Those groups that are subjected to continuous exposure to infection, as young physicians, nurses, and medical students.

[4] See Edwards, H. R.: "The Place of the Mass Survey in the Tuberculosis Control Program." *N. Y. State Jour. Med.* Feb. 1, 1945, p. 269.

[5] Edwards, H. R.: *Yale J. Biol. and Med.* 1940, Vol. 15, p. 424.

Group 5. Patients that are admitted to a general hospital.
Group 6. Young adults seen for the first time in general practice.
Group 7. Inmates of mental hospitals.
Group 8. Pre-employment examination of industrial workers.
Group 9. Applicants for civil service positions, particularly school-teachers and others who come in contact with children.

Routine chest roentgenograms will give precise and valuable information, for these technics will detect many cases of unsuspected tuberculosis, often in the minimal stage of the disease, that otherwise might go unrecognized.

When an individual has participated in a mass survey, and has been found negative, he should be so informed. Those persons who by the screening test indicate that they have a suspicious lesion, should be followed carefully, either by their own private physician or in the public clinic.

The interpretation of the findings is a task requiring long experience. In one half of the lesions discovered, the decision as to whether or not the lesion is active cannot be determined without periodic supervision.

The health officer will find it advantageous to establish certain fairly definite standards for supervision of contacts and diagnosed cases of tuberculosis. The Bureau of Tuberculosis of the New York City Department of Health has instituted certain standards which are suggested as a guide to those who are particularly interested.

**Pasteurization of Milk.** Pasteurization of milk has proved a most effective method of prevention of bovine tuberculosis. Thus, pasteurization of the entire milk supply is a goal of the tuberculosis prevention program. Tuberculin testing of cattle is a function of the department of agriculture rather than of the health department. The importance of the procedure from the public health standpoint is obvious and the program should be fully supported.

## EDUCATIONAL PROGRAM

The educational program in tuberculosis prevention that has been so extensively developed in recent years has been of untold value. The credit belongs in great part to voluntary health organizations, particularly the National Tuberculosis Association. There is scarcely a young adult in the United States who has not received the information that persistent cough, afternoon fever, loss of weight and night sweats are symptoms of tuberculosis. The contagious nature of the disease and the value of the rest cure are fully appreciated, as well as the simple facts that the disease is spread by careless disposal of sputum, and may be cured by proper treatment. This educational work has been concentrated in the schools and has reached into every village and hamlet of the country. It would not have been so successful were it not for the American compulsory public school attendance policy. It has been a great achievement, and is probably the largest single factor in reducing the death rate of tuberculosis in the United States.

**Voluntary Organizations.** The effectiveness of voluntary organizations in rendering valuable aid to official health department programs is best illustrated by the activities of the anti-tuberculosis societies in all parts of the United States. The policy of the National Tuberculosis Association has been to work hand in hand with local health officials. The wise health officer will not only gladly accept this assistance, but through advice and counsel, he will assist the local voluntary organization in planning an effective program that will supplement his own official activities.

## REFERENCES

1. Pratt, J. H. *The Development of the Rest Treatment in Pulmonary Tuberculosis.* N. E. J. of Med. 1932, Vol. 206, p. 64.
2. Opie, E. L. *The Pathogenesis and Transmission of Tuberculosis.* Amer. J. Med. Sciences. 1930, Vol. 179, p. 104.
3. Pope, A. S. *The Discovery and Prevention of Tuberculosis in a Community.* J.A.M.A. 1931, Vol. 97, p. 846.
4. Opie, E. L. and Isaacs, E. J. *Tuberculosis in Jamaica.* Amer. J. Hyg. 1930, Vol. 12, p. 1.
5. *Home Treatment Standards for Tuberculosis Patients.* Cattaraugus County Board of Health Reports. 1927.
6. Bishop, E. L. and Stewart, H. C. *Tuberculosis Control in Tennessee.* J.A.M.A. 1932, Vol. 99, p. 356.
7. Seideman, R. M. *A Comparative Study of Old Tuberculin and the Purified Protein Derivative.* Amer. J. Hyg. 1939, Vol. 30 (Section B), p. 1.
8. Douglas, B. H. and Harmon, G. E. *Results Obtained in an Extensive Tuberculosis Case Finding Program in a Large City.* Am. J. Pub. Health. 1939, Vol. 26, p. 583.
9. Miller, J. A. *The Modern Approach to the Early Diagnosis of Pulmonary Tuberculosis.* N. Y. State J. Med. 1939, Vol. 39, p. 2208.
10. Edwards, H. R. *Tuberculosis Case-Finding; Studies in Mass Surveys.* Am. Rev. Tuberc. 1940, Vol. 41, supplement no. 6.
11. Edwards, H. R. *Tuberculosis Case Finding and Supervision.* Yale J. Biol. and Med. 1943, Vol. 15, p. 423.
12. Edwards, H. R., Rocks, E. and Biorklund, A. V. *The Economics of Mass Examination for Tuberculosis.* Milbank Mem. Fund Quart. 1941, Vol. 19, p. 402.

Every student should be familiar with the following publications of the National Tuberculosis Association, New York:

1. *Diagnostic Standards and Classification of Tuberculosis.*
2. *Chest X-ray Interpretation,* by J. B. Amberson, Jr.
3. *A Manual of Tuberculosis Case Finding.* 1940.

# CHAPTER IX

## VENEREAL DISEASE CONTROL

THEORETICALLY, the venereal diseases should be handled by the health department in the same manner as other communicable diseases. In actual practice, however, this is impossible. These diseases have many things in common with other communicable diseases, but infection is usually contracted through sexual irregularities. Thus a moral significance is introduced, which complicates an otherwise simple matter. The public considers such infections to be a social disgrace, and the patient makes every effort to keep his misfortune a secret. Preventive and control measures are so intimately related to social and moral issues that the public health administrator is unable to proceed in a logical manner. Thus one state health department had to cut off all venereal disease control appropriations for a time because the budget committee felt, in essence, that sufferers of venereal disease were simply paying the penalty of their own misdeeds. It is true that venereal diseases are usually acquired through sexual ignorance or social maladjustment, and are often closely related to commercialized vice and prostitution, but these facts do not relieve the health department of the responsibility of preventing their spread by the most vigorous and effective means.

The epidemiological factors of the venereal diseases which relate to their control are unusually simple and clear-cut. They have much in common, but will be discussed separately.

### SYPHILIS

**Mode of Spread.** The causative agent is the *Treponema pallidum*. The disease is spread by intimate personal contact, usually sexual contact, occasionally by articles freshly soiled with the discharges of the patient.

**Prevalence.** One can only make an estimate of the prevalence of syphilis in any community. Well-meaning health educators have, by frightening implication, frequently indicated—though it has never been so stated authoritatively—that one person in 10 has syphilis. This is, of course, a gross exaggeration. In certain prison populations the positive Wassermann rate may be 25 per cent. But a Wassermann survey of the students of a whole state university will not show one positive reaction in a thousand students.

A syphilitic survey [1] of Birmingham, Alabama, has given us an excellent community-wide picture of syphilis prevalence in a typical American industrial city. This city has a higher proportion of Negroes than many American cities, but the data have been separated on a race, age, and sex basis.

Serologic tests for syphilis were carried out, in a mass survey in 1945, on 264,823 persons, and an infection rate of 12.3 per cent was found.

An analysis by sex and race gave the following information:

|  | Persons Examined | Infection Rate |
|---|---|---|
| White males | 64,487 | 2.5% |
| White females | 96,593 | 2.0% |
| Negro males | 41,969 | 27.0% |
| Negro females | 61,624 | 28.9% |
|  | 264,673 |  |

The survey omitted, for the most part, persons under 14 and over 50 years of age. All other ages were well represented, except males from 20 to 30 years. Many of these young men were absent in military service, but sufficient numbers in these age groups were obtained to give adequate comparative data.

Fig. 14 gives the percentage distribution of total syphilis infection by age, sex, and race.

The authors have divided the discovered cases of syphilis into

Group 1. primary and secondary
Group 2. early latent syphilis
Group 3. total infections which include groups 1 and 2 and all other cases of chronic syphilis infections, most of which are presumably non-infectious.

From an administrative point of view, these are very important distinctions, since persons from Group 1 are the chief sources of community infection. Group 2 is almost of equal public health importance.

There were only 61 cases of primary and secondary syphilis discovered in 161,080 white persons examined: a ratio of 38 per 100,000. In the Negroes, there were 645 cases of primary and secondary syphilis in a total of 103,593: a ratio of 623 per 100,000 population that were tested.

The data on primary and secondary syphilis in whites are too small to analyze on an age and sex basis.

In Table 2 is presented the distribution in Negroes by age and sex of primary and secondary syphilis.

A similar table has been constructed for whites, which includes Groups 1 and 2, *i.e.*, primary, secondary, and early latent syphilis.

These data, together with a great deal of further valuable informa-

[1] Smith, W. H. Y. and Denison, G. A.: "Blood Testing and Treatment Program in Jefferson County, Alabama." *Jour. Vener. Dis. Inform.* 1946, Vol. 27, p. 94.

tion that was derived from this study, are most illuminating. They supplement most effectively the results that were secured from an analysis

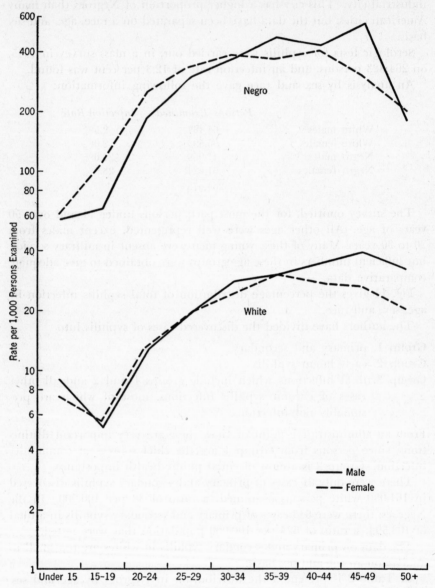

FIG. 14. *Rate of Infection of Syphilis in Jefferson County, Alabama, 1946.* By Age, Sex, and Color. Data from Alabama State Department of Health and Jefferson County Department of Health.

of the nation-wide serologic examinations for syphilis in young men who were drafted in the armed forces for World War II.[2]

[2] Smillie, W. G.: "Syphilis in the United States Primarily a Negro Problem." *J.A.M.A.* 1943, Vol. 122, p. 365.

## TABLE 2

### Primary and Secondary Syphilis in Negroes

| Age | Males | | | Females | | |
|---|---|---|---|---|---|---|
| | No. Cases | Persons Examined | Rate per 1,000 | No. Cases | Persons Examined | Rate per 1,000 |
| Under 15 | 0 | 1,324 | 0 | 10 | 1,430 | 7.0 |
| 15 – 19 | 36 | 6,874 | 5.2 | 135 | 9,355 | 14.4 |
| 20 – 24 | 57 | 3,148 | 18.1 | 157 | 9,123 | 17.2 |
| 25 – 29 | 38 | 3,954 | 9.6 | 87 | 8,786 | 9.9 |
| 30 – 34 | 26 | 5,304 | 4.9 | 26 | 8,760 | 2.9 |
| 35 – 39 | 24 | 5,988 | 4.0 | 14 | 8,894 | 1.5 |
| 40 – 44 | 13 | 6,589 | 1.9 | 6 | 7,034 | 0.8 |
| 45 + | 9 | 8,352 | 1.1 | 7 | 7,501 | 0.9 |
| Totals | 203 | 41,533 | | 442 | 60,883 | |

Total cases, 645; total persons examined (including those of unknown age, not shown above) 103,593; ratio, 623 per 100,000.

Data from Alabama State Dept. of Health

## TABLE 3

### PRIMARY, SECONDARY, AND EARLY LATENT SYPHILIS IN WHITES

| Age | Males | | | Females | | |
|---|---|---|---|---|---|---|
| | No. Cases | Persons Examined | Rate per 1,000 | No. Cases | Persons Examined | Rate per 1,000 |
| Under 15 | 7 | 2,301 | 3.0 | 8 | 2,297 | 3.5 |
| 15 – 19 | 37 | 10,258 | 3.6 | 58 | 14,283 | 4.0 |
| 20 – 24 | 36 | 3,720 | 9.7 | 144 | 15,539 | 9.3 |
| 25 – 29 | 40 | 5,533 | 7.2 | 85 | 14,240 | 5.9 |
| 30 – 34 | 38 | 9,151 | 4.1 | 56 | 13,569 | 4.1 |
| 35 – 39 | 19 | 9,967 | 1.9 | 23 | 12,993 | 1.8 |
| 40 – 44 | 25 | 10,364 | 2.4 | 12 | 10,955 | 1.1 |
| 45 + | 17 | 12,624 | 1.3 | 17 | 11,767 | 1.4 |
| Totals | 219 | 63,918 | | 403 | 95,643 | |

Only 61 cases of primary and secondary syphilis in 161,080 white persons examined; a ratio of 38 per 100,000

Data from Alabama State Dept. of Health

From these analyses we are able to draw new and important epidemiological conclusions concerning syphilis in the United States.

The most striking conclusion is that syphilis in the United States is overwhelmingly a disease of the Negro. It is more than 10 times as prevalent in the Negroes of both sexes and all age groups as in the corresponding group of whites. Furthermore, the cases of presumably infectious syphilis, i.e., Group 1, in the Negro race outnumber the cases of infectious syphilis in white persons by 15 to 1.

The peak of incidence of syphilis occurs at a very early age, 20–24 years. Nearly 20 per cent of all primary syphilis occurs before the victim's eighteenth birthday. The disease appears one to two years earlier in girls than in boys, but women in the 30–40 age group have less primary syphilis than men. Practically all—90 per cent—of primary and secondary syphilis in Negro and white men as well as women, occurred before the persons had reached their thirty-fifth birthday. Thus serious consideration need not be given to control of the spread of syphilis by individuals who are 40 years of age or older.

All these various epidemiological factors have an important bearing on the planning of a syphilis control program.

**Index of Syphilis Prevalence.** Let us imagine that an administrative area has 100,000 population, with 10 per cent Negroes and a normal age distribution. If we apply the Birmingham data (which included persons from 15 to 50 years of age) and 87 per cent of all syphilis (estimated), then the prevalence of syphilis would be approximately as follows:

*Make-up of Population*

Group 1. From birth to 14 years ......................... 30,000
Group 2. From 15 to 34 years of age ................... 35,000
Group 3. From 35 to 49 years of age ................... 20,000
Group 4. 50 years of age and over ...................... 15,000

Total population ...................................... 100,000

*Total Syphilis Prevalence*

$$\text{Whites} \quad \frac{100}{87} \times \frac{2.25}{100} \times 49,500 = 1280 \text{ persons}$$

$$\text{Negroes} \quad \frac{100}{87} \times \frac{28}{100} \times 5,500 = 1770 \text{ persons}$$

Total   3050 persons with syphilis

From the point of view of the public health administrator in control of syphilis, only groups 2 and 3 require consideration, with a special interest in group 2. Thus the actual numbers of total syphilis infection in the community which require consideration may be calculated as follows:

*Primary and Secondary Syphilis*

$$\text{Whites} \qquad \frac{38 \times 49,500}{100,000} \qquad = 19 \text{ persons}$$

$$\text{Negroes} \qquad \frac{623 \times 5,500}{100,000} \qquad = 34 \text{ persons}$$

$$\text{Total} \qquad\qquad 53 \text{ persons}$$

A similar analysis can be made which includes early latent syphilis:

*Primary, Secondary and Early Latent Syphilis*

$$\text{Whites} \qquad \frac{386 \times 49,500}{100,000} \qquad = 191 \text{ persons}$$

$$\text{Negroes} \qquad \frac{6,519 \times 5,500}{100,000} \qquad = 358 \text{ persons}$$

$$\text{Total} \qquad\qquad 549 \text{ persons}$$

This detailed analysis brings out the astonishing fact that in the whole community of 100,000 people, there are only 19 whites and 34 Negroes with infectious syphilis, with a total of 549 persons who have primary, secondary and early latent syphilis. The syphilis control program of the health department should obviously center its attack on these few (53) very dangerous sources of infection, and should also make full provision for treatment of the 549 cases of early latent syphilis. The remaining (2501) cases of chronic disease are, for the most part, non-infectious cases of syphilis. They are the special responsibility of the clinical facilities, rather than the public health facilities of the community—namely, the private physician, the private and public hospitals, and clinics. The health department would not refuse to treat these cases of course, but it should be clearly understood that in doing so, the health department is not performing a specific public health function.

In communities where the Negro population reaches 25 per cent to 30 per cent, the syphilis control program becomes manifold. In any area with 50 per cent or more of Negroes in the population, the control of syphilis becomes by far the outstanding feature of the whole communicable disease control administration.

**Immunity.** Contrary to popular opinion, one attack of syphilis does not give permanent immunity. Second infections do occur, particularly if the first infection has been treated vigorously during the early stages of the disease.

**Infectivity.** Syphilis is highly infective during the early stages of the disease. A case of latent syphilis has little infectivity, but relapses are common, and the open lesions of late stages of the disease may be infective. Authorities believe that the disease can be cured; certainly most cases can be rendered non-infective rapidly, if the patient is under expert care and guidance.

**Diagnosis.** The diagnosis of syphilis is relatively simple. The dark field illumination technic is a valuable diagnostic aid in the early stages, and the Wassermann or some of the related blood tests almost always give a positive result within three or four weeks after onset. The Wassermann test is not only a very reliable diagnostic test, but is of great practical importance in determining the stage of the disease and the probable degree of infectivity.

**Trend of Syphilis.** There is some evidence that syphilis is declining in the United States. Deaths from sequelae, such as general paresis, have declined in recent years, and congenital syphilis has almost disappeared. These results have been due to earlier diagnosis and better treatment. Better diagnosis may confuse the issue, and give evidence of actual increase in numbers of infected persons, when, in fact, the disease is on the decline. Up to 1941 there were many indications that control measures were effective. Among these were: decline of the rate of positive blood Wassermann tests in prenatal clinic services, decline in premarital syphilis indices, decline in the death rate of infants under one year from syphilis, and many other data which suggested that syphilis was less prevalent than it had been in the past.

The World War changed this trend. A true epidemic of venereal disease occurred as a concomitant of the disturbed social conditions brought about by the war. Syphilis increased not only in the military personnel, but also throughout civilian life. This has been true of all wars throughout history, so that health administrators were not surprised nor unprepared for this emergency. The development of better technics in specific therapy for syphilis, and also the other venereal diseases, was an outgrowth of medical research that was stimulated by the war, and new technics in prevention and control of venereal disease were developed, so that in the long run the outlook is hopeful.

General measures for administrative control of syphilis will be discussed at the end of this chapter.

## GONORRHEA

The causative agent is *Neisseria gonorrhea*. The disease is much less serious in its effects on the individual and the community than syphilis, but is much more difficult to control. Many of the epidemiological features of gonorrhea are similar to those of syphilis. It is spread in the same manner. From the practical point of view almost all cases are acquired by sex contact (except ophthalmia neonatorum and vulvo-vaginitis of childhood).

**Prevalence.** The true prevalence of gonorrhea in the United States is not known. Many infected persons never consult a physician; many physicians do not report their cases to the health department. It may be said with certainty that the attack rate is at least three or four times as high as the attack rate for syphilis. The disease is more common in men than in women; more prevalent in Negroes than whites; more common in the urban centers than in the rural population, with a special predilection for the lower economic groups of society. The age group showing highest incidence of infection is 20 to 30 years, affecting somewhat younger age groups in females than males. Vonderlehr estimates that there are over 1,000,000 fresh cases of gonococcal infection each year in the United States, with an urban attack rate twice that of the rural areas. He sees no evidence of any downward trend.

**Immunity.** One attack produces little or no immunity to subsequent attacks. The duration of the disease is usually short, but may be prolonged. The patient remains infective so long as the gonococci persist in the discharges.

**Diagnosis.** Diagnosis of gonorrhea is a relatively simple matter. The clinical picture is characteristic and is verified by standard bacteriological methods. It is difficult to determine, by any method, at just what point the patient finally becomes non-infectious.

Treatment by sulfanilamide has created a paradoxical situation in relation to gonorrhea. The drug rapidly relieves the patient of symptoms, and its results are so immediate and striking as to lead to extensive self-treatment. But the patient may remain infectious, though symptoms disappear promptly. Cultural technics have been developed to so satisfactory a degree that they can and should be widely adopted in determining when a patient is no longer infectious to others.

During the early years of sulfonamide therapy, great hopes were entertained of elimination of this infection, since 90 per cent of all strains of gonococci were affected by the drugs. Soon sulfonamide resistant strains appeared, so that by 1945, over 50 per cent of all gonococcus infections were resistant to sulfonamide therapy. Penicillin is an excellent supplement to sulfonamide therapy, but here too, it seems clear that drug resistant strains will emerge.

Gonococcal vaginitis of little girls, once a very troublesome administrative problem, has been adequately solved by the discovery that the condition clears up promptly following the administration of estrogens.

## LYMPHOGRANULOMA VENEREUM

This disease is due to a filtrable virus. It is not a new infection, but only recently has it been recognized as a distinct clinical entity. The development of the Frei test [3] has made us aware of the high prevalence and relative importance of this disease. Epidemiologically it follows closely the pattern of syphilis and gonorrhea. It is acquired by direct sexual contact, and all those community groups that show a high prevalence of these diseases will also have a high prevalence of lymphogranu-

[3] Shaffer, M. L., *et al.: Am. J. Syph., Gonor. and Ven. Dis.* 1941, Vol. 25, p. 669.

loma venereum. Surveys of prostitutes give up to a 45 per cent infection rate.

The incubation period of the disease is from 14 to 21 days. It produces a chronic suppurative local lesion, and its victim may remain infectious for a long period of time.

The most important complication is an extension of the lesion to the ano-rectal region, leading to cylindrical stricture of the rectum.

The disease is frequently confused with syphilis, and also frequently accompanies this disease. It is a good general rule to do a Frei test on each newly discovered case of syphilis.

Many authorities have had excellent therapeutic results with the sulfonamides. General measures for control of the disease are the same as for the other venereal diseases.

## CHANCROID

This troublesome, but relatively easily controlled, venereal disease is due to *Hemophilus ducreyi*. The disease is acquired by direct sexual contact, and has a short incubation period, 3–10 days. It comprises less than 5 per cent of all venereal disease infections. The diagnosis is easily made by direct microscopic examination of smears from the lesion. It must not be forgotten that syphilis may accompany chancroid, so that dark field examination of the local lesion should also be taken.

The disease responds rapidly to sulfonamide therapy. Other general measures for the control of chancroid are the same as for other venereal diseases.

**Granuloma inguinale** is a venereal disease that is seldom encountered in the United States. It is due to a Donovan body, which produces a chronic ulcerative indolent lesion, after a long incubation period. Treatment is usually ineffective.

## ADMINISTRATIVE METHODS OF CONTROL

For purposes of simplicity and because all the venereal diseases can be handled in much the same manner, the general administrative control measures for these diseases may be considered together.

**Reporting.** The reporting of the venereal diseases becomes better each year, though it is much more complete in syphilis. Because of moral implications and the fear that their secret misfortune may become public knowledge, patients give false names, and physicians neglect to send reports to the health department. In some states, reports are not made to the local health officials at all, but directly to the state health department. It is generally conceded that reports should be made directly to the local health officer by number or symbol. The report should be mailed in a sealed envelope; not on a postcard. The name should not be reported by the physician, unless the patient lapses treatment. If the patient persistently refuses to continue proper treatment until he is no longer a menace to society, then the physician should report the patient's name to the health department and the health officer should assume responsibility for protection of the public.

**Diagnostic Service.** A laboratory for serological and bacteriological diagnosis of the venereal diseases is an essential part of the venereal disease control program. Small local laboratories should not attempt to make the serological diagnosis of syphilis. This service should not be organized unless at least two thousand blood specimens are to be tested annually. In a community of 100,000 people approximately 5,000 to 10,000 Wassermann tests may be requested each year. The most satisfactory procedure in any but the very large cities is to send the bloods that are to be tested to a large central state laboratory. The laboratory service should be free—irrespective of the economic status of the patient. Direct dark field examination is an important diagnostic laboratory aid. Facilities for making dark field examination should be a part of the equipment of every syphilis clinic. A few state laboratories have adopted the technic that has been developed in New York State whereby properly collected serum from suspected lesions may be mailed to the central laboratory for dark field examination.

**Clinic Service.** The prevention of venereal disease is a joint responsibility of the individual and his family physician, and the community as represented by the health department, together with allied social agencies. The primary purpose of the health department is to prevent the spread of infection; secondly, to prevent the ravages of the disease, once it is acquired.

**Prevention of Spread of Infection.** From the Birmingham data, it is clear that the great proportion of cases of syphilis in a community are not a menace to others. Only a small proportion are sources of infection. Obviously the health department's efforts should be concentrated upon control of the infection in this group.

The major objective is to render infectious cases non-infectious as rapidly as possible. The most difficult and important part of the program is to find the sources of infection, and also to follow the immediate contacts of newly discovered cases. Thus the director of a venereal disease clinic must be not only a good diagnostician and thoroughly familiar with the therapy of venereal diseases, but must also be a good epidemiologist and carry out his work from this point of view.

Adequate, prompt treatment is a most effective method in the prevention of the spread of venereal disease. Because of the great expense of the prolonged treatment which is often required, and because most of the patients are in the lower economic groups, many infected persons are unable to obtain adequate treatment. In large centers of population, health departments have stimulated, subsidized or actually conducted free venereal disease clinics. In a city of 100,000 people, one or two clinics a week for men and one for women are sufficient. These facilities will care for 800 to 1,000 patients annually, each patient averaging 10 to 15 visits to the clinic. The cost of the clinic must be borne, in great part at least, by the local health department. A clinic of this type would have the following personnel:

1 or 2 physicians (part-time).

1 male nurse.

2 nurses (part-time) for the clinic service.

1 full-time social service worker—preferably a nurse with social service training.

The annual cost of this clinic is approximately $7,000 or about $0.50 per visit. The patients may be asked to pay for a part of the cost.

The most important individual in the clinic personnel is the nurse who has charge of the social work. She should admit the cases to the clinic, and become familiar with their special problems. Patients who lapse treatment may be sent first a letter of reminder. This is followed by a personal visit, which is usually effective. Sources of infection are searched for and brought to the clinic. Family contacts of patients are given serological tests and put under treatment, if necessary. All this work represents, in fact, a true epidemiological investigation. The extraordinary results that have been secured by a tactful, sympathetic, competent nurse in the venereal disease clinic represent a real achievement in preventive medicine.

**The Follow-Up Work.** This should be directed by the physician in charge of the clinic, but is actually carried out by a well qualified public health nurse, or by a medical social worker who is skilled in solving family and social problems. The important part of her work is to find the source of each newly acquired infection, to trace the direct sexual contacts of the case itself during the infectious period, and also to trace sexual contacts of the original source of infection. This may prove to be an exacting and very difficult task, requiring great tact and ingenuity, but it is a task well worth the effort. It is not as overwhelming an effort as first appears, since the actual numbers of infectious cases in any community at any given time is quite small.

Clinic services should be free to all, irrespective of their ability to pay for this service. Patients with ample funds may be referred to private practitioners for continuation of therapy after they are rendered non-infectious, but clinic care is the chief available method for determining sources of infection in the community.

Pre-marital examinations for the detection of syphilis and other venereal diseases are now required by most states. This has been an excellent educational measure, and has detected many unsuspected cases of early syphilis. This examination should not be cursory, but should include not only a blood test for syphilis, but also careful direct inspection of the genital organs.

**Pre-natal Examinations.** Many states require physicians to make a serologic test for syphilis on all expectant mothers. This sensible rule has resulted in the discovery of many hidden syphilitic infections. If the mother is properly treated, her baby will not develop congenital syphilis.

**The Social Aspects of Venereal Disease Control.** The health department cannot ignore the fact that the venereal diseases are true social diseases, in that their incidence is directly related to unfavorable social conditions. The diseases invariably have a higher prevalence in the lower economic groups of the community—the poor, the underprivileged, those living in crowded slum conditions with little opportunity for wholesome recreation and normal family life. Ignorance, poverty, social upheaval, war, and any other factors that tend to break down a normal wholesome family and community life are all factors in a higher incidence of venereal diseases.

The control of these factors should not rest solely upon the health department. Sex education is a responsibility of the family itself, the school, the church, and voluntary social and welfare agencies in the community, as well as the health department.

**Small Communities.** Except under exceptional circumstances, it is not feasible to establish a separate venereal disease clinic service in a population of 25,000 to 30,000 people because of public curiosity and the chances that abound for disclosing the secrets of infected individuals. This difficulty is met by incorporating the service into the general hospital outpatient clinic. The work may be supported by a small subsidy to the clinic from the health department.

**Epidemiological Investigations.** Munson, late district health officer of New York State, demonstrated that syphilis and, to some degree, gonorrhea, may be controlled effectively by careful epidemiological investigation of sources of infection. This is true because the actual sources of infection in any community are few and the period of infectivity may be cut short by prompt detection and adequate treatment. Syphilis and gonorrhea are not uniformly distributed through the community at all times, but occur in a series of sporadic and localized epidemics. Thus it is well worth while for the epidemiologist to determine the sources of infection and check the spread of the disease at its source, as in any other communicable disease. As has been stated in the foregoing, some of the best epidemiological results have been obtained through employment of a nurse with social service training, who is attached to the venereal disease clinic.

An example of this type of investigation may be taken from the records of the New York City Health Department.[4] A diagram of an interesting epidemiological investigation of a localized outbreak of syphilis in the Harlem District of New York City is illustrated by Fig. 15. A survey of the results of this study showed that, beginning from the initial

[4] Weinstein, Joseph: *Jour. Social Hygiene.* 1938, Vol. 24, p. 21.

case, and working from this point, the names of fifty-two possibly exposed persons were obtained, forty-five located and examined, and nineteen cases of syphilis found. Seven of the cases occurred in males, twelve in females, ranging in age from six months to forty-two years. Thirteen of the cases were acquired by way of normal sexual intercourse, one through homosexual practice, one by way of kissing, and four cases were congenital in origin. Five of the infections were discovered with primary lesions on the penis, two with lip chancres, three with secondaries, four were early asymptomatic, and five were late cases. Twelve were new and seven were known to the Health Department. Sources of infection were established in eleven or 58 per cent of the nineteen cases. Twenty-two household contacts were examined, all of whom were negative for syphilitic infection. Six delinquents among old cases were persuaded to return for further treatment; the seventh case could not be located. The entire group, with one exception, was brought under medical treatment and supervision.

Turner and his associates were able to discover forty-six contact cases from each original 100 cases. All were previously unrecognized and 30 per cent of the newly discovered cases were in the infectious stage. These authorities estimate that it costs $10 to bring each unrecognized case under medical care, and about $18 to discover and treat each infectious case.

The State of Georgia, in conjunction with the United States Public Health Service, has developed a most effective plan of case finding and treatment of syphilis in a rural area with a large Negro population. A mobile clinic travels from settlement to settlement on a regular weekly schedule. Blood tests for syphilis are given; approximately 30 per cent of young adults 15 to 30 years of age are found to be positive. Therapeutic results are somewhat more expensive but are more satisfactory than in the stationary clinic, because more people are reached. The convenience of the service makes lapses in treatment less frequent. Standard epidemiological technics would probably not be successful in this population group. The Georgia experiment illustrates the important point that the program must be planned to fit each population situation.

Rosenthal notes that the special epidemiological problems in a large city are:

1. Transients who lapse treatment and cannot be found.
2. Clandestine prostitutes who give false addresses.

Of 577 persons, mostly young women, whose names were given to the investigators as sources of infection in one year, 37 per cent could not be located because of frequent removal or false address.

Practical results of follow-up were surprisingly good. Of 728 named sources of infection, 54 per cent were found and examined. Sixty-one per cent of over 2,000 lapsed treatment cases were found and returned to the clinics. Ninety per cent of household contacts were found, with a 17 per cent infection rate.

**General Educational Methods.** The health department should conduct a continuous information service for the general public in relation to the prevention of venereal disease. This may be done through suitable posters, pamphlets, and lectures.

The most important groups to be reached are young men and women of high school age, because the attack rate in both gonorrhea and

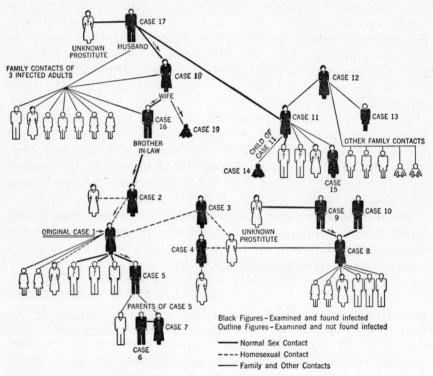

FIG. 15. *Investigation of a Localized Outbreak of Syphilis in New York City.* Source: Weinstein, Joseph: *Journal of Social Hygiene.* 1938, Vol. 24, p. 21.

syphilis is highest in the younger age groups. The press has now overcome its aversion to the use of the words "gonorrhea" and "syphilis" and has become a most efficient instrument of proper education in the prevention of the venereal diseases. Some state health departments have stressed the dissemination of information concerning personal prophylaxis in prevention of venereal disease. Unfortunately, personal prophylaxis is not an effective method in preventing either gonorrhea or syphilis under civilian conditions, despite the favorable results secured under a military regime.

Routine Wassermann surveys of large groups of the population are not an effective control or preventive measure. A pre-employment Wasser-mann reaction for persons who have direct and personal contact with people, as for example food handlers, nurses, domestic employees, bar-bers, employees of beauty parlors, is an often-recommended procedure, but is not an effective public health measure. A positive serologic test for syphilis should not exclude the individual from employment as a food handler, domestic servant, etc. If the individual is non-infectious and under appropriate medical care, he may continue his employment with complete safety to the community.

**Law Enforcement.** The abolition of houses of prostitution under police regulations has been of real value in preventing venereal disease. Medi-cal supervision of prostitution has not been effective. Isolation of in-fected patients by arbitrary law enforcement has proved a futile gesture in an attempt to control venereal infection. It may be successful in the individual case, but the sources of infection are driven to cover, and all subsequent or similar infections will be very carefully hidden. It is possible to make treatment compulsory in a given case, but this method should be used only as a last resort. Rather every effort should be made to safeguard the secrets of the patient and win his confidence and co-operation. Compulsory means should be taken only when the recalci-trant individual flagrantly betrays confidence and willfully exposes the community to infection.

Special aid to state-wide venereal disease control programs may be obtained by State Boards of Health from the Federal Government through the United States Public Health Service, under authorization of the Venereal Disease Control Act of 1938.

The State health officers have worked out a comprehensive plan, in conjunction with the United States Public Health Service, for the con-trol of venereal disease in the United States, and there is every reason to believe that this plan will bring about results that are commensurate with the effort and funds expended.

**Sex Education.** The education of the public, and particularly the children, in matters relating to sex and sex hygiene is a function of the parent, teacher, religious leader or voluntary social hygiene organization rather than the official health department. The health department should furnish suitable information in printed or other form, and aid in every possible way in presenting proper scientific material to the parents and teachers for purposes of instruction.

### REFERENCES

1. Munson, W. L. *Epidemiology of Syphilis and Gonorrhea.* Amer. J. Pub. Health. 1933, Vol. 23, p. 797.
2. Turner, G. B., Gelperin, A. and Enright, J. P. *Results of Contact Investiga-tion in Syphilis in an Urban Community.* Amer. J. Pub. Health. 1939, Vol. 29, p. 768.

3. Burney, L. E. *Control of Syphilis in a Southern Rural Area.* Amer. J. Pub. Health. 1939, Vol. 29, p. 1006.
4. Rosenthal, T. and Weinstein, J. *Epidemiology of Syphilis in New York City.* Amer. J. Pub. Health. 1939, Vol. 29, p. 1034.
5. Vonderlehr, R. A. and Usilton, L. J. *Present Status of the Epidemiology of Gonorrhea.* Amer. J. Syph. 1938, Vol. 22, p. 537.
6. Parran, Thomas. *Shadow on the Land: Syphilis.* 1937.
7. Clarke, C. W. *Newer Research Findings for Dealing with Syphilis and Gonorrhea.* Amer. J. Pub. Health. 1939, Vol. 29, p. 761.

Public health education bulletins and pamphlets in relation to the prevention and control of syphilis and gonorrhea may be secured from the American Social Hygiene Association, New York City, the Metropolitan Life Insurance Company, the United States Public Health Service, the Massachusetts Social Hygiene Society and various other sources.

"Social Hygiene" issued by Social Hygiene Committee of N. Y. Tuberculosis and Health Association, 386 Fourth Avenue, New York City. Particularly, *The Syphilis Clinic—Organization and Management.* 1944.

"Journal of Venereal Disease Information" issued by United States Public Health Service.

# CHAPTER X

## ACUTE RESPIRATORY INFECTIONS

### "COLDS"

THE various acute respiratory infections which are called "colds" are the most common of all the infectious diseases in the United States. They are a major causative factor in loss of time from illness in industry. They cause enormous absenteeism in public school attendance. It is quite evident that there has been little decline in their incidence despite many recommended preventive measures.

Whenever an epidemic of colds appears in a community, the health administrator is in a dilemma. The great popular demand requires that he take some action in an attempt to prevent the spread of the infection. He is compelled by this pressure to recommend some program of action. The intelligent health officer realizes fully, however, that his program will be of little or no avail in prevention of disease, though he may be able to alleviate suffering.

Patient investigation is being pursued which gives some indication that we shall be able to determine some of the hidden secrets of the epidemiology of the acute respiratory diseases. We are at about the same stage with this group of diseases now as we were with diphtheria and allied diseases fifty years ago. Certain sound advice can be given, however, and certain pitfalls avoided, if the health officer understands the condition fully and is aware of his limitations.

The weight of evidence indicates that colds are initiated by a filtrable virus. The disease is highly communicable, infection is by direct contact, and carriers are very rare or non-existent. Colds are self-limited, but are frequently followed by secondary complications, such as sinusitis, bronchitis, otitis media, etc., which are much more troublesome than the original infection. The duration of immunity following a cold is short, sometimes only 6 weeks; more commonly 3 to 4 months. The incubation period of a cold is about 36 hours. The patient may transmit the infection to others before symptoms appear, and for about three days thereafter.

Colds may occur at any time of year, but are less common during the summer months. The epidemic peaks are in the fall—October or November—and in the spring, usually about the end of February. The first epidemic peak is not followed by a marked increase in pneumonia and other serious secondary infections. The spring peak is invariably fol-

119

lowed by an increase in pneumonia, with a lag of about one week.

The sequelae and complications of colds are produced, in great part at least, not by the virus, but by the invasion of secondary organisms which are commonly found in the nasopharynx. The pneumococcus is by far the most common offender. Environmental factors undoubtedly play a part in this secondary invasion. The low relative humidity of super-heated homes in winter seems to have an influence upon complications of colds. Chilling of the body surface may also influence the incidence, degree, and duration of these secondary infections.

**Control Methods.** Many of the statements that have been made by public health educators concerning the prevention of colds have little basis in fact. There is no statistical evidence that methods for training the heat regulatory mechanism, such as taking cold baths, or sleeping on outdoor porches, are of any value in prevention of colds. Ultra-violet light radiation or special dietaries have no proved value. The avoidance of sources of infection, which is so often recommended, is almost impossible in modern busy industrial life. Infants and invalids are especially subject to the ill effects of colds. They can and should be protected from contact with persons who are in the communicable period of a cold. Others cannot avoid this contact, no matter how careful they may be.

Any factors which prevent intimate personal contact in community life would, theoretically at least, aid in prevention of transmission of colds. As examples, one may note:

   *a.* Regulations forbidding overcrowding of theaters, public buildings, vehicles of transportation, schools, etc.
   *b.* The proper spacing of desks in offices and working benches in factories.
   *c.* The sterilization of dishes and all utensils in public eating places, etc.

Continuous education in the proper use of the handkerchief by individuals who are sneezing or coughing may prevent the spread of infection. Individuals should be urged to isolate themselves at home and in bed during the early stages of a cold, both for their own protection and for the protection of the public. Children in the early stages of an acute cold should not go to school, but remain at home for at least two days. School children will, of course, take advantage of this rule and the school attendance officers will object to it seriously, but in the long run, it is a good policy. A large hospital has kept a record of time lost by nurses and physicians from colds. The nurses were taken off duty at the first sign of a cold and put to bed. The interns kept at work as long as they could stand. At the end of the year, the time lost per intern from colds and their sequelae was greater than the time lost by nurses.

During the course of a cold the individual should take every precaution to avoid chilling of the body surface, exposure or exhaustion. Serious complications, particularly pneumonia, may occur in the course of a cold, if the individual suffers from exposure or chilling.

**Vaccines.** Clinical evidence seems to indicate that "cold" vaccines are of little effect in prevention of colds. Experimental evidence had suggested that the vaccines might prevent invasion by secondary organisms, and thus prevent the sequelae and complications of colds, but clinical trials have, on the whole, been disappointing.

Diehl and his colleagues [1] vaccinated 272 University of Minnesota students and held 276 as controls. They were observed an entire winter. No student knew whether or not he was a control. The difference in incidence of colds in the two groups was not significant.

It may be possible to reduce the incidence and severity of colds by air sterilization technics. (See Chapter XXII.) The airsols, and also ultraviolet light, will undoubtedly destroy the cold virus that is floating in the air, but most colds are probably acquired by direct droplet infection contact. Furthermore, it will not be feasible to sterilize the air of an individual's whole environment at all times.

**Treatment.** The sulfonamides [2] and penicillin do not prevent colds and should not be given indiscriminately during a cold in the hope of preventing a secondary pyogenic infection. This type of specific therapy should be held in reserve for treatment of the secondary infection, if it should occur.

**Public Health Education.** There are no administrative procedures that a health officer can employ to prevent or alleviate colds. His chief function is the development of an educational program which will teach the individuals in his community all we know about the etiology and epidemiology of colds, as well as the few proved methods which aid the individual in the avoidance of infection.

## LOBAR PNEUMONIA

Lobar pneumonia is one of the commonest of all the infectious diseases, and is one of the leading causes of death in the United States. We have no accurate index of the exact prevalence of the disease in the United States, as it has not been well reported.

Britten [3] has analyzed the incidence of pneumonia as recorded in the National Health Survey of 1934–36, and has brought out some important epidemiological information. The annual frequency of all types of pneumonia in this study of over 700,000 people—chiefly city dwellers—was 5.4 per 1,000 white persons. No great difference was encountered in different geographic areas, but the rate was slightly higher in rural communities.

[1] Diehl, H. S., Baker, A. B. and Conway, D. W.: *J.A.M.A.* 111:1168, 1938.
[2] Cecil, R. L., Plummer, N. and Smillie, W. G.: *J.A.M.A.* 1944, Vol. 124, p. 8.
[3] Britten, R. H.: "The Incidence of Pneumonia As Recorded in the National Health Survey." *Pub. Health Rep.* 1942, Vol. 57, p. 1479.

Highest frequency was in early childhood and old age. There was no marked increase in incidence in Negroes, but a close association between bad housing, overcrowding, and unfavorable social conditions was encountered. This report includes all types of pneumonia, and does not attempt to differentiate the lobar pneumonia from other types.

Ungerleider [4] and his associates have studied the incidence of pneumonia in 100,000 industrial workers throughout the United States, including various types of industry. They found an annual incidence of 3.0 per thousand employees, and present some evidence that the unfavorable social conditions, such as overcrowding, that were brought about by war conditions, had increased pneumonia incidence throughout the United States. Their most striking finding was the remarkable drop in the case fatality rate in five years—20.8 per cent in 1935 to 3.9 per cent in 1941—and they calculate that "the advent of sulfonamide therapy has proved a boon to industry, saving the lives of some 25,000 workers annually. A further annual saving of over a million working days has resulted from shortening of the period of illness."

All studies have shown that lobar pneumonia is more prevalent in men than in women.

There can be no question that the case fatality rate from pneumonia has declined rapidly. It was declining before the introduction of sulfonamides and penicillin therapy, but this decline has been greatly accentuated in recent years. (See Fig. 16.)

Certain industrial cities, notably Pittsburgh, have much higher death rates from lobar pneumonia than have other cities of similar size.

Deaths from pneumonia in 1910 in New York State were 160 per hundred thousand population; whereas 30 years later the death rate per hundred thousand was less than half this rate. This decline does not necessarily mean a decline in incidence, for the effective work in relation to pneumonia has been in the prevention of *deaths* rather than the prevention of infection.

The disease has a distinct seasonal prevalence, reaching its peak in the United States late in February or early in March, with the lowest incidence in August. The rate may be greatly increased during epidemics of influenza.

The total pneumonia death rate throughout the United States at the present time is less than 40 per hundred thousand population. We are not sure what proportion of these deaths is due to lobar and what proportion to bronchopneumonia, as the distinction between these two diseases is not always clear cut.

**Etiological Agent.** The pneumococcus is the etiological agent in 95 per cent of the cases of lobar pneumonia. This organism has been divided

[4] Ungerleider, H. E., Steinhaus, H. W. and Gubner, R. S.: "Public Health Aspects of Pneumonia—A Comparison with Pre-sulfonamide Years." *Am. Jour. Pub. Health.* 1943, Vol. 33, p. 1093.

according to specific characteristics into more than 50 divisions, or types; but few of the higher types are important factors in the causation of pneumonia. The types of pneumococci that cause lobar pneumonia are encountered in the following order of prevalence: Types 1, 2, 3, 8, 5, 7, 4, and 14. This order may vary in different communities and from year to year. Type 1 is, in all studies, the most common in adults; types 4, 7, and 14 are frequently encountered in children. Type 3 lobar pneumonia

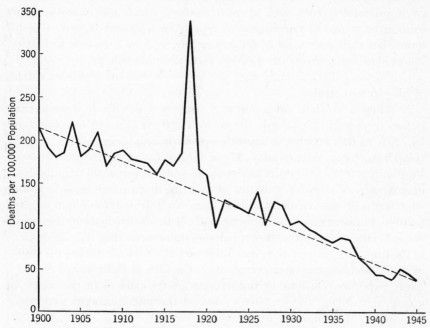

Fig. 16. *Pneumonia Death Rate, State of New York, 1900–1945.* Combined Rate for Lobar and Bronchopneumonia. Data from New York State Department of Health.

is a very fatal disease of elderly people, but is not a very serious infection in the young adult.

Case fatality rates in the pneumonias due to these different types vary tremendously. In former years, 40 per cent to 60 per cent of all Type 3 infections were fatal, whereas Type 2 had about a 40 per cent case fatality rate and Type 1, 25 per cent. In general, it may be said that formerly the case fatality rate of all types of lobar pneumonia was approximately 25 per cent. Newer methods of treatment have completely changed these figures.

**Epidemiological Factors That Affect the Control of the Disease.** Whenever a person develops lobar pneumonia, we must ask ourselves: where did this particular infection come from? We know that at least 60 per cent of the population are carriers of some types of pneumococci at any one time, but in most instances the organisms found in the normal throat belong to the higher types and are relatively avirulent. Suddenly a type-specific, highly virulent organism appears out of nowhere and produces a serious illness. The patient is seldom infected from direct contact with an actual case of pneumonia. We must assume that he was infected by a carrier.

Are there insidious, dangerous permanent pneumococcus carriers, "Pneumonia Marys" comparable to the notorious "Typhoid Mary"? May a carrier of a virulent strain transfer the infection to others, implanting the organism without producing disease? Are there any measurable environmental factors, such as overcrowding, which influence the ready transfer of a specific pneumococcus type from a patient or carrier to his immediate contacts? Some of these questions we have been able to answer; others remain unanswered. Certain facts are established:

1. The case of pneumonia does not, as a rule, become a chronic carrier of his virulent strain.

2. When a virulent pneumococcus invades a family, it spreads from person to person. Frequently the entire family is affected: one may have an otitis media, another a sinusitis—perhaps only one member will develop true lobar pneumonia. These family invasions frequently occur concomitantly with a family outbreak of colds. Some of these individuals may remain carriers for a matter of months, and undoubtedly it is they who transmit the virulent strains from an infected to a non-infected family. Transfer seems to be more ready if the individuals in the family are suffering from colds. A virulent pneumococcus that may be present in the upper respiratory tract may increase tremendously during the course of a cold and become most prevalent on the fifth or sixth day of the cold. Thus, exposure, chilling, or indiscretion by the patient in the course of a cold and during the invasive period of the pneumococcus may result in subsequent pulmonary involvement.

3. Different individuals, even members of the same family, possess varying degrees of resistance to the pneumococcus. This resistance seems to be specific for given types, rather than general for all types.

**Control of Pneumonia.** Formerly, when the health department took an active part in the pneumonia control program, serum therapy required determination of the type of offending pneumococcus, and extensive laboratory facilities were needed for rapid typing of pneumococci. Many health departments made provision for type specific sera, and also provided expert consultation service in diagnosis and therapeutic administration of serum.

These procedures have all been abandoned. The discovery of the sulfonamides, and later penicillin, has completely changed and simplified the technics of pneumonia therapy.

**General Measures for Control of the Spread of Pneumonia.** The measures recommended by Finland [5] are so succinct that they may be

[5] Finland, Maxwell: "Recent Advances in the Epidemiology of Pneumococcal Infections." *Medicine,* 1942, Vol. 21, p. 307.

given in their entirety. They are based on measures recommended by O. T. Avery [6] and his associates at the Rockefeller Institute in 1917.

"*Education* of the medical profession and of the public concerning the danger of the spread of pneumonia by contact with cases, direct or indirect, is essential.

"General *compulsory reporting* of cases is recommended in order to ascertain the incidence and focal distribution of cases.

"Since certain types are particularly important, the widespread application of *pneumococcus typing* by hospital and health department laboratories is highly desirable. This would supply additional important epidemiologic data.

"Each case should be regarded as a possible focus of spread, and measures found useful in other communicable diseases should be applied. The patient should be isolated from other persons as far as possible.

"Since pneumococci spread mostly by way of the secretions of the mouth and respiratory tract, care should be taken in collecting sputum and burning or disinfecting containers. All utensils, handkerchiefs, bed clothing, etc., which are likely to become contaminated through contact with the mouth should be sterilized before they are used again.

"Frequent cleansing of the sickroom, carried out in such a way as to minimize the amount and spread of dust, is important. The sickroom should be cleaned thoroughly after it is vacated by the pneumonia patient.

"While the control of convalescent and healthy contact carriers of disease-producing types of pneumococci through isolation would be desirable, it is not practicable. Carriers, however, may be instructed to avoid promiscuous spitting.

"Under conditions which are most suitable for the spread of pneumococci, namely, in dormitories, barracks, hospitals, asylums, labor compounds, prisons, etc., these preventive measures may be especially important and should be applied as soon as the first cases are recognized. Search for carriers among the contacts of the cases should be undertaken immediately. Isolation of the carriers, or at least precautions instituted to prevent further spread by them, should be carried out."

**Carriers.** It was hoped that small and continuous doses of sulfonamides would be a satisfactory method for clearing up the carrier state. Experiments with this technic have been disappointing.

**Community-Wide Immunization.** It is quite possible to increase resistance against invasion of specific virulent pneumococcus strains by injection of appropriate antigens. One or two injections are sufficient; no serious reaction occurs, and the immunity lasts for at least a year. It is not a suitable routine public health procedure, as the case incidence of the disease in the general population is low. It may prove effective in certain groups that are apt to contract pneumonia—as, for example, army

[6] Avery, O. T., Chickering, H. T., Cole, R. and Dochez, A. R.: Rockefeller Institute for Med. Research, Monograph No. 7, 1917.

recruits who may be called for winter service. Hodges and MacLeod's [7] studies of epidemic pneumococcal pneumonia in army camps demonstrated the value of pneumococcus vaccination in a special and particularly vulnerable population.

It must be confessed that with our present knowledge of the disease, much more effective results are obtained in the prevention of deaths from the infection than in the prevention of actual incidence.

## BRONCHOPNEUMONIA

No direct method of attack has been devised which has any proved utility in the prevention of bronchopneumonia. It must be remembered, of course, that more than 50 per cent of all bronchopneumonia is due to the various types of pneumococci. These are often of the relatively avirulent higher types.

The disease is nearly always a secondary and complicating factor in some debilitating illness. Terminal bronchopneumonia is encountered in a large proportion of those who die a lingering death. Obviously any measures that are taken to sustain a patient's strength during a debilitating illness will lower the incidence of bronchopneumonia. Penicillin or sulfonamides, if given with skill and good clinical judgment, will often prevent bronchopneumonia in a person who is suffering from a critical illness, or who has had an operation, or serious accident.

A good local health service which gives special consideration to postponement of attacks of measles and whooping cough from the period of infancy to later childhood will undoubtedly obtain some reduction in the incidence of bronchopneumonia. Good health education programs, intelligent and adequate public health nursing service, and especially a carefully conceived infant hygiene service, should have an appreciable effect in lowering the incidence and also decreasing the number of deaths from bronchopneumonia.

The best chance for reduction of morbidity and mortality from bronchopneumonia is to attack those primary causes which, in the end, may produce, or at least may result in, this secondary—often terminal—infection.

## PRIMARY ATYPICAL PNEUMONIA

This is not a new disease, but has been recognized only recently and separated as a clinical entity from other pneumonias. Formerly it was called grippe, bronchitis, influenza, or a severe cold. The extensive utilization of the x-ray has demonstrated that it is a separate disease, with a clear-cut epidemiology.

[7] Hodges, R. G. and MacLeod, C. M.: "Epidemic Pneumococcal Pneumonia. I. Description of the Epidemic; V. Final Consideration of the Factors Underlying the Epidemic." *Am. Jour. Hyg.* 1946, Vol. 44, p. 183, 237.

Experimental studies [8] of human transmission of the disease give strong evidence that the disease is due to a filtrable virus. The incubation period is long—2 to 3 weeks. Transmission is the same as in colds and influenza. The onset is insidious: often the respiratory symptoms are absent at first; clinical symptoms are fever, malaise, fatigue and deep muscle pain, with a dry cough. The diagnosis is usually confirmed by the x-ray. Mild infections often go unrecognized.

The disease occurs in epidemic form, at any time of year. It is common in young adults. Numerous outbreaks have been encountered in university students, and in the army camps during the training period in the United States in 1941. In 1945 the annual attack rate in army camps was 2.6 per cent. The death rate is very low, and incidence in the general population during an outbreak is also low.

Measures for control of this infection have not been developed. The usual general measures that are employed in prevention of the spread of colds and influenza should be used for this disease. Penicillin and sulfonamides are ineffective in the treatment of this infection.

## INFLUENZA

"Influenza is an acute infectious respiratory disease of epidemic nature which is of variable extent and severity. It is characterized by rapid dissemination, high morbidity, sudden onset with fever, chills, leukopenia, and inconstant bronchitis or pneumonitis" (Francis). The mortality of the disease is low as a rule, and recovery is fairly prompt. In most instances, the temperature returns to normal within three or four days. Convalescence is prolonged and weakness may persist for weeks or months.

**Etiology.** Human influenza is caused by a filtrable virus. Shope first showed that swine influenza, which is similar in its clinical characteristics to human influenza, is due to a filtrable virus. He also demonstrated that symbiosis with the swine influenza bacillus was essential to the epidemiology of the disease. The virus alone caused a relatively mild disease in pigs, and the influenza bacillus alone was not injurious, but when the two were combined a typical epidemic occurred. The discovery that ferrets and mice are susceptible to the influenza virus has greatly facilitated the study of the disease. Smith, Andrewes, and Laidlaw discovered that ferrets are susceptible to the human virus.

Francis and Magill, as well as others, have demonstrated that mice and ferrets develop active immunity after infection. This immunity may be complete or partial. Studies in young children show a low degree of immunity to the influenza virus, but this immunity tends to increase with age. Nearly 50 per cent of a group of individuals chosen from various cities were determined by Francis and Magill to have a high immunity against the virus, and 30 per cent more gave partial protection. These

[8] Dingle, J. H.: "The Present Status of the Etiology of Primary Atypical Pneumonia." *Bull. N. Y. Acad. Med.* 1945, Vol. 21, p. 235.

data explain readily the epidemiological characteristics of the disease. These authorities have also shown that human influenza virus can be introduced subcutaneously into human beings without causing any evidence of infection. The subjects develop antibodies against the virus which persist for at least five months, and the vaccination produced as high an immunity as resulted from naturally acquired infection.

One great difficulty in producing immunization with the influenza virus vaccine is that the different strains vary antigenically. Magill and Francis have shown that there is a rough grouping of strains, and that similar strains tend to be found in single epidemics; but it does seem clear that the human influenza virus contains a mosaic of antigens, and all strains may not contain antigenic components of other strains.

The incubation period of influenza is from one to three days, and the period of communicability of the patient is short—seldom more than three or four days. The disease is probably spread by direct contact only, but is very highly communicable.

The most commonly encountered strains of influenza virus in the United States have been named virus A and B. It is probable that other strains occur. There is some evidence [9] that epidemics due to strains A and B occur in cycles, virus A having a periodicity of 3 years and virus B, 4 to 6 years. Virus A epidemics always result in a greater increase in the community death rate than virus B.

These viruses are grown readily on chick embryo, and a vaccine may be prepared from this material which gives a high degree of specific immunity from infection. This immunity is of short duration. If given in the late fall, it lasts during the period of greatest prevalence of respiratory infection, but probably does not carry over with complete effectiveness for a full year.

Influenza always occurs in epidemic form. It may be restricted to a relatively small area, or may sweep rapidly across the whole country. Great pandemics occur at intervals. The last was the devastating pandemic of 1918. We have no knowledge of the actual cause of this pandemic, but have every reason to believe that it will be followed by another equally extensive pandemic at some future time. From 1918 to 1944 some eighteen major or minor epidemics of influenza occurred in the United States. [10] Thus scarcely a year passes that the disease is not reported in epidemic form from some part of the nation. Often 25 to 50 per cent of the population of an invaded community are affected during an epidemic. There is great variation in severity of the disease. It may range from the mild symptoms of a temporary cold to very severe pneu-

[9] "The Periodicity of Influenza." The Commission on Acute Respiratory Diseases, Fort Bragg, North Carolina. *Am. Jour. Hyg.* 1946, Vol. 43, p. 29.

[10] Collins, S. D.: "Age and Sex Incidence of Influenza in the Epidemic of 1943–1944 with Comparative Data for Preceding Outbreaks." *Pub. Health Rep.*, 1944, Vol. 59, p. 1483.

monia and death. The case fatality rate, even in severe outbreaks, is less than 3 per cent, but the incidence of the disease in a community epidemic is so high that the death rate is always elevated appreciably.

**Control Measures.** We have given a good deal of consideration to the epidemiological features of influenza because they offer some hope that measures may be developed for the control of this most baffling disease. Personal prophylaxis is almost impossible for the active individual during epidemic periods of influenza. The same measures that have been suggested for the control of colds may be followed, and it may be possible to avoid the sequelae and complications of influenza by simple measures that may be taken by the individual patient during the early stages of the disease.

**Community Program.** The protective measures that have been suggested during epidemics of influenza in the past have not been of any great value in the prevention of the spread of the disease. Isolation of certain community units has been successful occasionally, particularly in instances where natural barriers to communication exist. Masks are of no value. Closing of schools, churches, and other public places has no measurable effect in the control of an epidemic when it is raging, or in diverting an epidemic when it is expected.

The extensive studies [11] of the value of influenza vaccine by the Surgeon General's Commission on Influenza, headed by Dr. Thomas Francis, proved that it was practicable to immunize an entire community against influenza. The vaccine that was used in this large human experiment consisted of a mixed virus A and B suspension from chick embryo cultures, killed by formalin. One cubic centimeter was given intracutaneously to 6,263 young soldiers, with a similar number of controls. A single injection only was administered. The reactions were negligible. Immunity was built up rapidly, reaching its peak in about two weeks. An epidemic of virus A pneumonia appeared shortly after the vaccine was given. The attack rate in the controls was 7.1 per cent, and in the vaccinated 2.2 per cent. The disease, when it occurred in the vaccinated, was milder than in the controls.

These studies, together with much subsequent work, indicate strongly that it may be possible to control the ravages of influenza, to some degree at least, by extensive specific immunization procedures.

Furthermore, the death rate from influenza can be greatly reduced through the well-planned utilization of sulfonamides and penicillin. These drugs have no effect upon the virus, but death in influenza is almost always due to secondary invaders which do respond to this type

[11] Commission on Influenza. Board for the Investigation and Control of Influenza and Other Epidemic Diseases in the Army, Preventive Medicine Service, Office of the Surgeon General, United States Army: "A Clinical Evaluation of Vaccination against Influenza." *J.A.M.A.* 1944, Vol. 124, p. 982.

Francis, Thomas, Jr.: "The Development of the 1943 Vaccination Study of the Commission on Influenza." *Am. Jour. Hyg.* 1945, Vol. 42, p. 1.

of therapy. It does not seem advisable to administer sulfonamides or penicillin as a prophylactic to each person who develops influenza. Rather these drugs should be held in reserve, to be utilized as therapeutic instead of prophylactic agents.

We can be sure of one thing—that pandemic influenza will return. It may appear within a few years or may postpone its ravages for many years; but come it will. There is reason to believe, from research that has already been carried out, that when it does occur, the virus of the pandemic will be quite homogeneous. Under this condition, it should be possible—in theory, at least—to prepare a suitable vaccine and to utilize it extensively in immunization of the population ahead of the march of the pandemic.

This, of course, may be simple wishful thinking, but if the advances in the study of the disease are made as rapidly in the next few years as they have been in the past, there is every hope that some control of the next pandemic may be instituted. In case of an epidemic of influenza the health officer must assume leadership in planning for the coming disaster. From information which he receives from Federal and State health officers, he can determine not only the probable date the epidemic will arrive in his community, but also the probable number of cases that will occur, the probable duration and intensity of the epidemic and, within certain limits, the probable number of deaths in his community. Suitable preparation should be made to meet the emergency and a skeleton organization formed well in advance of the outbreak to cope with the situation when it arrives. This matter is discussed in detail in the chapter on "Disaster Relief."

## REFERENCES

### "COLDS"

1. Paul, J. H. and Freese, H. L. *An Epidemiological and Bacteriological Study of the Common Cold in an Isolated Arctic Community.* Amer. J. Hyg. 1933, Vol. 17, p. 122.
2. Van Volkenburg, V. A. and Frost, W. H. *Acute Minor Respiratory Disease Prevailing in a Group of Families Residing in Baltimore, Md., 1928–30.* Amer. J. Hyg. 1933, Vol. 17, p. 122.
3. Dochez, A. R., Mills, K. and Kneeland, Y. *Study of the Virus of the Common Cold and Its Cultivation in Tissue Medium.* Proc. Soc. Exp. Biol. and Med. 1931, Vol. 28, p. 513.
4. Long, P. H., Doull, J. A. *et al. The Etiology of Acute Upper Respiratory Infection.* J. Exper. Med. 1931, Vol. 53, p. 447.
5. Milam, D. F. and Smillie, W. G. *A Bacteriological Study of "Colds" on an Isolated Tropical Island.* J. Exper. Med. 1931, Vol. 53, p. 733.
6. Cecil, R. L., Plummer, N. and Smillie, W. G. *Sulfadiazine in the Treatment of the Common Cold.* J.A.M.A. 1944, Vol. 124, p. 8.

INFLUENZA

1. Smith, W., Andrewes, C. H. and Laidlaw, P. P. *Influenza: Experiments on Immunization of Ferrets and Mice.* Brit. J. Exper. Med. Feb. 1934, Vol. 59, p. 201.

2. Francis, T., Jr. and Magill, T. P. *Immunological Studies with Virus of Influenza.* J. Exper. Med. Oct. 1935, Vol. 62, p. 505.

3. Francis, T., Jr. and Magill, T. P. *The Antibody Response of Human Subjects Vaccinated with the Virus of Human Influenza.* J. Exper. Med. Feb. 1937, Vol. 65, p. 251.

4. Stokes, Joseph J., Chenoweth, Alice D., Waltz, Arthur D., Gladen, Ralph G. and Shaw, Dorothy. *Results of Immunization by Means of Active Virus of Human Influenza.* J. Clin. Invest. March 1937, Vol. 16, p. 237.

5. Magill, T. P. and Francis, T., Jr. *Antigenic Differences in Strains of Epidemic Virus: Cross-neutralization tests in mice.* Brit. J. Exper. Path. 1938, Vol. 19, p. 273.

6. Rickard, E. R., Thigpen, M. and Crowley, J. H. *The Isolation of Influenza A Virus by the Intra-allantoic Inoculation of Chick Embryos with Untreated Throat-washings.* Jour. of Immunology. 1944, Vol. 49, p. 263.

7. Commission on Influenza, Bd. for the Investigation and Control of Influenza and Other Epidemic Diseases in the Army, Prev. Med. Service, Office of the Surgeon Gen., U. S. Army: *A Clinical Evaluation of Vaccination Against Influenza.* J.A.M.A. 1944, Vol. 124, p. 982.

8. Hirst, G. K., Rickard, E. R. and Friedewald, W. F. *Studies in Human Immunization Against Influenza.* Jour. Exp. Med. 1944, Vol. 80, p. 265.

9. Salk, J. E., Pearson, H. E., Brown, P. N. and Francis, T. *Protective Effect of Vaccination Against Induced Influenza B.* Proc. of Soc. for Exp. Biology and Medicine. 1944, Vol. 55, p. 106.

10. Hirst, G. K. *Direct Isolation of Influenza Virus in Chick Embryos.* Proc. of Soc. for Exp. Biol. and Med. 1945, Vol. 58, p. 155.

11. Francis, Thomas, Jr. *The Development of the 1943 Vaccination Study of the Commission on Influenza.* Am. Jour. Hyg. 1945, Vol. 42, p. 1.

12. Commission on Acute Respiratory Diseases, Fort Bragg, North Carolina. *The Periodicity of Influenza.* Am. Jour. Hyg. 1946, Vol. 43, p. 29.


PNEUMONIA

1. Orenstein, A. J. *Vaccine Prophylaxis in Pneumonia.* J. Med. Assn. S. Africa. 1931, Vol. 5, p. 339.

2. Cruikshank, R. *Pneumococcal Infections.* Milroy Lectures. Lancet. 1933, March 18, 25, and April 1, pp. 563, 621 and 680.

3. Smillie, W. G. *The Epidemiology of Lobar Pneumonia.* J. Amer. Med. Assn. 1933, Vol. 101, p. 1281.

4. Smillie, W. G. and Leeder, F. S. *The Epidemiology of Lobar Pneumonia.* Amer. J. Pub. Health. 1934, Vol. 24, p. 129.

5. Felton, L. D. *The Concentration of Anti-pneumococcus Serum.* J. Amer. Med. Assn. 1930, Vol. 94, p. 1893.

6. Smillie, W. G., Warnock, G. H. and White, H. J. *A Study of a Type I Pneumococcus Epidemic at the State Hospital at Worcester, Mass.* Amer. J. of Pub. Health. 1938, Vol. 28, p. 293.

7. Heffron, R. *Pneumonia: with Special Reference to Pneumococcus Lobar Pneumonia.* 1939. The Commonwealth Fund.

8. *An Institutional Outbreak of Pneumonitis.* I. *Epidemiological and Clinical Studies by J. W. Hornbrook and K. R. Nelson.* II. *Isolation and Identification of Causative Agent by R. E. Dyer, N. H. Topping and I. A. Bengtson.* Reprint No. 2203 from Pub. Health Reports, 1940, Vol. 55, p. 1936.

9. Finland, Maxwell. *Recent Advances in the Epidemiology of Pneumococcal Infections.* Medicine. 1942, Vol. 21, p. 307.

10. Commission on Acute Respiratory Diseases, Fort Bragg, North Carolina. *Epidemiology of Atypical Pneumonia and Acute Respiratory Disease at Fort Bragg, North Carolina.* Am. Jour. Pub. Health. 1944, Vol. 34, p. 335.

11. Plummer, Norman, and Ensworth, H. K. *Primary Atypical Pneumonia in General Hospitals and in Private Practice.* Bull. N. Y. Acad. Med. 1944, Vol. 20, p. 292.

12. Moore, N. S., Wightman, H. B. and Showacre, E. C. *Primary Atypical Pneumonia.* I. *A Statistical Report of 196 Cases.* N. Y. State Jour. Med. 1944 (Apr. 15), p. 869.

13. Dingle, J. H. *The Present Status of the Etiology of Primary Atypical Pneumonia.* Bull. N. Y. Acad. Med. 1945, Vol. 21, p. 235.

# CHAPTER XI

## ADMINISTRATIVE CONTROL OF SMALLPOX

No administrative problem in relation to communicable disease can cause more exasperation to the health officer than the control of smallpox. It should be a very simple matter to prevent the disease from entering his jurisdiction, yet it is often extremely difficult. The methods of control of smallpox are understood better than those of any other disease. The disease has a definite incubation period, the diagnosis is not difficult, and there are no carriers. Epidemiological work is simple, since every case has been in contact with a recent case of the disease. Isolation and quarantine are effective measures of control. Most important of all, prophylactic measures for combating the disease are practically perfect in their results. The very fact that the disease has been controlled in the past has produced a sense of security in communities that are now highly susceptible to an epidemic of smallpox. Furthermore, in recent years, the prevailing type of smallpox in the United States has been very mild, with a case fatality rate of only 0.1 to 0.2 per cent, in contrast to the severe type of the disease that prevailed in the earlier years of the national development. Many people will state frankly that they prefer to contract this mild type of smallpox rather than be vaccinated. Thus, compulsory vaccination, which has proved time and again to be a simple, but perfectly effective, procedure in preventing smallpox in any community is gradually losing ground. Its enforcement meets with constant opposition from the general public for a variety of reasons; most important of which is that a regulation enforcing compulsory vaccination is an infringement on personal liberty.

## EPIDEMIOLOGICAL FEATURES OF SMALLPOX WHICH RELATE TO ADMINISTRATIVE CONTROL

**Etiology.** The disease is due to a filtrable virus which is present in the lesions of the skin as well as in the secretions from the nose and throat.

**Transmission.** Smallpox is one of the most readily communicable of all diseases. It may be transmitted in the early stages of the disease, before a skin eruption appears. Smallpox is spread by contact with a case. Air-borne transmission probably occurs, and the disease may also be transmitted indirectly through materials contaminated by the patient, or may be carried by flies. The virus lives but a short time outside the human host, so that the secretions or objects contaminated by the patient remain infective for a short time only.

**Incubation.** The incubation period of smallpox is usually 14 days; rarely is it so short as 7 days; occasionally as long as 21 days.

**Immunity.** Natural immunity to smallpox does not exist. One attack practically always produces life immunity, though a few instances of second attacks have been reported. Immunity following vaccination is practically complete for at least one year. The immunity gradually declines year by year, though some degree of immunity persists throughout life. In general, an individual who is successfully vaccinated during the first year of life, and revaccinated on entering school, has a permanent protection against the disease. During an epidemic it is always a wise precaution to revaccinate all persons who have not been recently vaccinated. Those who are immune will have practically no reaction from the vaccination and the non-immune will be protected. Immunity of any individual may be determined by the "reaction of immunity," which is a characteristic reaction occurring within 36 to 48 hours at the site of revaccination.

**Prevalence.** Smallpox is rapidly disappearing from the United States, and to the clinician it has become a disease of great historical interest, but of little practical importance. He may never see a case in a lifetime of practice.

But the health officer must keep the disease constantly in mind, and retain a permanent barrier in the community against invasion.

The disease fell below 1,000 total cases in the United States for the first time in 1942. Many states now pass an entire year with no cases of smallpox reported. Some few states with lax control laws, and particularly those states bordering upon Mexico, are subject to invasion of the disease from time to time.

The secret of success in the maintenance of a low smallpox incidence lies in continued vigilance by the health department authorities in a continuous program of adequate vaccination.

Well vaccinated communities are immune to epidemics of the disease, but areas in which vaccination is not widely practiced for one reason or another will have outbreaks of smallpox. The disease is most prevalent in the late winter months, with its lowest incidence in summer. In recent years the type of disease in the United States has been very mild. Many patients are not seen by physicians and are not ill enough to be confined to their beds. They are, of course, often undiagnosed. The case fatality in these outbreaks may be less than one per thousand. From time to time serious localized outbreaks occur which resemble in every particular the former type of smallpox, with severe, often fulminating symptoms and a case fatality rate of 15 to 30 per cent.

## ADMINISTRATIVE METHODS IN CONTROL OF SMALLPOX

**Reporting.** All cases in which there is any question of a possible diagnosis of smallpox should be reported immediately to the local health department. The effective control of an epidemic lies in early recognition, immediate reporting, and early and accurate diagnosis.

When a case of smallpox has been diagnosed, the information should be given to the community at once, by newspapers or otherwise. One of the greatest mistakes made by authorities is the attempt frequently made to cover up the presence of smallpox in a community because of its effect on business, or for other reasons.

**Diagnosis.** The local health department should furnish diagnostic facilities through a physician skilled in the differential diagnosis of smallpox and chickenpox, as well as other diseases which may be confused with smallpox (as syphilis).

Certain characteristics of smallpox must be borne in mind.

| A. *Distribution of Rash* | *Smallpox prefers:* | *Chickenpox prefers:* |
|---|---|---|
| Location of rash | The face and extremities | The trunk |
| Distribution of rash | Outer surfaces preferred to inner. Rare in groin, arm pits, abdomen, sides of chest | General distribution, less profuse on extremities |
| *In very scanty eruption:* | | |
| | *Smallpox* | *Chickenpox* |
| Count spots on both arms | Many | Few |
| Count spots on trunk | Few | Many |
| B. *Appearance of Rash* | *Smallpox* | *Chickenpox* |
| | Spots similar in age, size and shape | Spots vary in age, size and shape |
| Appears first | Face and forehead | Trunk |
| Growth of spot | Slow. Requires days | Rapid. Requires hours |
| Spread | Wave from face to feet | New spots appear in among the old |
| C. *History of Case* | Sharp illness, then improvement, then rash | Rash appears at onset of illness |

The differential diagnosis in many instances is difficult and must be made with caution. One must remember that the severity of clinical symptoms is no index; smallpox may be very mild; chickenpox, particularly in an adult, may be severe. The individual lesion in smallpox may have a characteristic shot-like appearance, and aid in differential diagnosis, but this cannot be relied upon as a clear-cut differential point.

**Isolation.** The patient should be isolated from susceptibles completely until all lesions are free from the primary crusts. Three weeks is usually sufficient. Isolation in a contagious hospital is the best procedure. The room must be screened from flies, and careful concurrent disinfection of all materials soiled by the patient should be insisted upon. This includes disinfection of bedding, utensils, clothing or any article that may have come in contact with the patient. Gowns completely covering the clothing of attendants or visiting physicians should be used. Placarding is a good procedure. In some health departments, the traditional yellow flag of quarantine is reserved for smallpox.

**Quarantine.** The family and all immediate personal contacts should be quarantined and vaccinated at once. They may be released after the vaccination reaction has begun to subside. If vaccination is refused, the quarantine of contacts must be continued until 17 days after last exposure. If the patient remains in the home, this represents a quarantine of nearly six weeks. All contacts should be vaccinated whether they have had previous successful vaccination or not.

Some health departments permit release from quarantine of contacts who have had a successful vaccination within five years, and who submit to revaccination, if they leave the household at once. This procedure may be followed, if these contacts are kept under observation for a period of two weeks.

Vaccination should be urged on all persons who may have had even a remote contact with the patient during the early stages of the disease. Once smallpox has become established in the community—that is, if a second crop of cases follows an initial case—the only procedure is to urge everyone to be vaccinated at once. Revaccination should be urged for those persons whose last successful vaccination was more than a year before.

Since vaccinia has such a short incubation period and the reaction is full-blown in eight days, a successful vaccination given as late as four days after the initial exposure to a case of smallpox will prevent the development of the latter disease.

**Vaccination.** The health department should furnish a potent vaccine free of charge to every physician requesting it. During an epidemic, the department should organize a clinic for free vaccination of all indigent persons.

An ideal program for the complete protection of the community is compulsory vaccination of all children before the first birthday, with revaccination required before the child enters school. A very effective method for community protection is a regulation requiring vaccination of all children entering school. In those states where this simple law is in effect, smallpox has vanished.

**Vaccination Technic.** Vaccine is obtained by inoculating calves with cowpox virus. The lymph must be fresh and must be kept below freezing until the hour it is used. It should be shipped in dry ice and preserved below freezing. The skin of the arm at about the insertion of the deltoid muscle is thoroughly cleansed with *acetone* and allowed to dry a few seconds. Alcohol should not be used, as it may injure the virus. A drop of lymph is placed on the dry skin and a single scratch about 1 cm. long is made through the lymph with a sterile needle. The puncture method may be used, of thirty light punctures with the needle held parallel with the skin. The point is not driven into the skin, but with each pressure the elasticity of the needle will pull a tiny part of the epidermis over the point of the needle. The arm is exposed to the air for five minutes and no dressing is used. The vaccination should be inspected on the sixth day. Bacteria-free virus has been developed by the Goodpasture and also by the Rivers technic. This virus is introduced intracutaneously. Donnally reports that the Rivers virus did not produce strong and lasting immunity. Ellis and Boynton compared Goodpasture, Rivers, and calf lymph virus in 9,000 students at the University of Minnesota. They report that the calf virus give a higher percentage of primary takes, with little difference in the size of the scar in the intracutaneous and multiple puncture technic. Local reactions were slightly less severe with the Goodpasture virus. Theoretically, there are many reasons why bacteria-free intracutaneous vaccination should be preferable, but in practice calf lymph virus is very satisfactory.

Sepsis following vaccination occurs very rarely. It is usually due to contamination of the vaccination wound in the pustular stage. Postvaccinal encephalitis has caused grave concern in some of the European countries, but is very rare in the United States. Symptoms develop 10–13 days after vaccination and the disease has a case fatality of about 25 per cent.

Distinguishing characteristics of this disease, in contrast to lethargic encephalitis, are that meningeal symptoms predominate in postvaccinal encephalitis, and when recovery occurs, it is complete. The condition is rare in infants, occurs most frequently in children of school age and prevails in the spring months. Symptoms are probably not due to vaccinia, but to a latent infection which is activated by vaccination.

**Epidemiological Investigation.** The occurrence of an initial case of smallpox in a community calls for an immediate epidemiological investigation. The activities of the patient during the previous 14 days must be carefully checked:

1. The source of the original infection should be determined.
2. Casual contacts of the patient during the period of contagion should be determined if possible.
3. Contacts should be vaccinated. If vaccinated within 4 days of contact, they will be protected. If the period has been longer than four days,

the two conditions, vaccinia and smallpox, may run their respective courses simultaneously.

4. Suspected contacts should be kept under observation two weeks and daily temperatures should be taken. Since every case of smallpox is due to a direct contact within two weeks with another actual case of the disease, it is often possible to retrace the course of the infection, discover unrecognized cases, and check the further spread of the disease.

5. If the suspected source of infection is in some other state, that state health department should be given the details of the epidemiological investigation.

**Education.** Educational measures in relation to prevention of smallpox should be continuous, rather than concentrated at the time of an outbreak. In recent years these educational efforts have fallen on deaf ears because of the sense of security that prevails so generally, due to the absence of major catastrophes. Educational methods must be restrained and dignified, for there is a very general feeling that the health officer has exaggerated the importance of compulsory vaccination and most people are willing to take a chance of infection. Many persons believe that the disease is mild in any case, and they may postpone vaccination until the event of an outbreak. The obvious fallacy of this argument is that virulent smallpox is a constant menace that may suddenly appear at any time and in any community.

## REFERENCES

1. Chapin, C. V. and Smith, J. *Permanency of the Mild Type of Smallpox.* J. Prev. Med. 1932, Vol. 6, p. 273.
2. Armstrong, C. *Post Vaccinal Encephalitis with Special Reference to Prevention.* U.S.P.H. Reports. 1932, Vol. 47, p. 1553.
3. Thompson, R. *The Etiology of Post Vaccinal Encephalomyelitis.* Arch. Pathology. 1931, Vol. 12, p. 601.
4. Rivers, T. M. and Ward, S. M. *Further Observations on Cultivation of Vaccine Virus for Jennerian Prophylaxis in Man.* J. Exper. Med. 1933, Vol. 58, p. 635.
5. Goodpasture, E. W., Woodruff, A. M. and Buddingh, G. J. *Vaccinal Infection of Chorio-Allantoic Membrane of Chick Embryo.* Am. J. Path. 1932, Vol. 8, p. 271.
6. Donnally, H. H. *Smallpox Vaccination of Infants.* J. Amer. Med. Assn. 1939, Vol. 113, p. 1796.
7. Ellis, R. and Boynton, R. *Comparison of Vaccines and Techniques.* U. S. Public Health Reports. 1939, Vol. 54, p. 1012.
8. *Vital Statistics of the United States, 1944.* Part II. Washington, D. C., U. S. Gov't Printing Office. 1946, p. 482.

## CHAPTER XII

## MALARIA

We shall limit this chapter to a discussion of the administrative control of malaria within the United States, and shall exclude consideration of malaria control in the insular possessions. In general, the disease is the same in all parts of the world and the mode of transmission is the same: namely, through the bite of the anopheles mosquito. But methods of control in different parts of the world vary greatly, depending on economic and social factors and also upon the particular species of anopheles that is responsible for the infection in each area. The different species of anopheles have different seasonal prevalence, different breeding and biting habits, as well as other variable characteristics, so that those control measures which may be carried out in one area may be unsuccessful in another.

Malaria was formerly a very important communicable disease throughout practically the whole of the United States. It was distributed from New England to Florida and westward as far as civilization extended. The infection in the Ohio Valley was particularly heavy, as it was in the valleys of all the main tributaries of the Mississippi River. In Massachusetts there were great epidemics in 1647–1650 and 1680. The disease occurred in epidemic form chiefly in the northern tier of states, but was heavily endemic in the south. The wide distribution of the disease was due to many factors, most of them incident to a pioneer civilization. Some of these important causal factors were:

1. The location of the settlements along the water courses.
2. The slave trade, which continually introduced new carriers of the parasite.
3. The haphazard clearing of the land.
4. The damming of the water courses for small grist and power mills,— thus producing ideal breeding places for anopheles mosquitoes.
5. The flimsy structure of the habitations.
6. The small number of cattle and livestock.
7. A low standard of nutrition.
8. Inadequate treatment of cases of malaria.

With the advance of civilization and the retreat of the frontier, malaria retreated rapidly, so that by 1945 it had almost completely disappeared from the northern states and was seldom seen in the larger cities and towns in the south.

The great decline of malaria occurred after the Civil War and was due to many factors, among which were:

1. Fixation of the population. The people developed permanent homes, cleared the land properly, drained the lowlands, and moved from log cabins to more substantial houses.

2. Development of transportation. Railways were extended, waterways were abandoned and the older, small wayside inns were replaced by hotels in the larger centers.

3. The spread of agriculture from the bottom lands to the uplands.

4. The abandonment of the water-driven grist mills, and consequent disappearance of the millponds, subsequent to the development of large power mills in the great cities.

5. The increase in the number of cattle on farms.

6. The great decline in rice culture.

7. The invention of screens.

8. The discovery of the mode of transmission of the disease.

This last remarkable achievement, made by Ross in India in 1897, made possible an intelligent and directed effort toward control of the disease.

The malaria zone has now been narrowed to such a degree that the disease is endemic only in the Atlantic seaboard south of Washington, the Mississippi valley south of Springfield, Illinois, and westward in Texas to the point where the annual rainfall is less than 30 inches. A few isolated endemic spots are found in irrigated areas in New Mexico, California and the Valley of the Rio Grande. Even in these areas, malaria has been completely controlled in zones with a dense population, and has become a strictly rural disease.

As recently as 1920 it was authoritatively estimated that over a million cases of malaria occurred in the United States each year. It is impossible to make an accurate estimate, as the physicians do not report the disease well. Many patients are not seen by a physician at all, but are given treatment at home. At present, there are probably not more than 200,000 cases in the United States in an average year.

Both aestivo-autumnal and tertian forms of malaria occur in the United States. The former is limited to the subtropical sections of the country and is much less prevalent than the tertian type. Quartan malaria does occur, but it is rare.

## EPIDEMIOLOGICAL FEATURES OF MALARIA WHICH AFFECT CONTROL MEASURES

Certain clinical features of malaria must be understood if control measures are to be carried out successfully. Diagnosis of malaria is not always a simple matter, for the parasite is not easily found in the blood smears. The two common types of malaria in the United States are quite distinctive in their symptomatology.

**Tertian Malaria.** This disease is differentiated by its characteristic temperature curve and a striking clinical picture. The paroxysms of fever occur at regular intervals with normal periods intervening. The disease is chronic in type, with partial recovery followed by relapses. Two years of normal life may intervene followed by a true relapse. Eventually, recovery occurs spontaneously. Splenomegalia is the rule, especially in untreated cases; anemia is a characteristic symptom. The disease usually begins with an irregular increasing temperature, which follows an incubation period of 10 to 14 days. The first febrile period lasts 3 to 5 days and is followed by daily fever with chills. This second period of the disease lasts perhaps a week. The intermittent fever, tertian in type, then manifests itself and is of variable duration, usually continuing for weeks, if the patient is not treated. The case fatality rate is from 3 to 5 per cent. The adult forms of the malaria parasite, with which the mosquitoes are infected, appear in the blood early in the disease and may persist long after clinical symptoms have abated.

**Aestivo-autumnal Fever.** This disease is much more malignant than tertian malaria. The incubation period is about the same as in tertian malaria, and is followed by a period of about a week's duration of daily high temperature with rigors. Freedom from fever then occurs for a few days followed by a second attack more severe than the first. Four or five of these periods may occur at 10- or 12-day intervals. During the attack the patient has a fluctuating temperature which usually does not return to normal. The case fatality rate in untreated cases is very high, 25 per cent or more, but the disease is less chronic than tertian malaria.

Relapses from both types of malaria may occur following a variety of conditions, including insufficient food, gastro-intestinal disturbances, fatigue, injury, change of climate or sudden exposure to dampness or cold.

Absolute natural immunity to malaria is rare, though some degree of racial resistance to the effects of the parasite exists, most markedly among the Negro race. Different strains of parasites occur, within a given species. Immunity to one strain does not always represent immunity against subsequent infection. Boyd and his associates have shown that immunity to *P. falciparum* will occur following injection of a given strain, but reinoculation with a different strain of the same parasite may result in an even more severe attack than the first. In the case of *P. vivax* infection, heterologous immunity does occur.

Frequent exposure to the disease produces some immunity. The resistance to malaria of old residents in a highly endemic area is well known. Children in hyper-endemic areas have a continuous reinfection with marked enlargement of the spleen up to 12 or 14 years of age. The blood of the older children may be full of parasites continuously, but splenomegalia in these children may disappear in adolescence. Parasites may be found in the blood of all adults in a hyper-endemic area, without the occurrence of splenomegalia, fever, or a marked degree of anemia.

The common species of anopheles mosquito in the eastern United States are: *A. quadrimaculatus, A. crucians,* and *A. punctipennis.* In the western states, particularly California, *A. maculipennis* and *A. pseudopunctipennis* are found. Formerly, it was assumed that all species of anopheles mosquitoes transmitted malaria. Darling's work in the Canal Zone proved that some species cannot be implicated as vectors of the disease. It remained for Carter of the United States Public Health Service to demonstrate that the important vector of malaria in the United States is *Anopheles quadrimaculatus.* In the laboratory the other species may be infected, but in nature they are not of great importance. (*A. maculipennis* is the vector on the Pacific Coast.)

In planning malaria control measures in the United States, therefore, the administrator can more or less ignore other anopheles mosquitoes and concentrate on the control of *A. quadrimaculatus.* This is known as "species control."

*A. quadrimaculatus* is easily distinguished from other anopheles mosquitoes by certain wing markings. The bionomics of the mosquito have been studied extensively. The geographic distribution is known, as well as the seasonal prevalence. The life cycle, breeding habits, biting habits, and the range of flight have all been determined. It prefers clear fish ponds or impounded rivers.

*A. quadrimaculatus* possesses many characteristics that are common to other anopheles mosquitoes. Certain individual characteristics of this mosquito are important from the point of view of control of malaria. They are:

1. It is most prevalent in late summer and disappears with the first cold weather.

2. The larvae are found chiefly in impounded areas of fresh water. They are not found in running streams—even sluggish streams—nor in stagnant pools, borrow pits, etc.

3. The characteristic resting place of this mosquito is in the immediate environs of habitation or actually within the home. Its flight range is about one mile.

The larvae of *A. quadrimaculatus* are very similar to other anopheles larvae found in the United States, but have certain minor anatomical variations, which make it possible to distinguish them under the microscope (Russell).

## ADMINISTRATIVE METHODS OF CONTROL OF MALARIA

It is not possible to describe in this text in suitable detail the various technical procedures that must be followed in a malaria control program. General principles only will be developed.

A local health organization should not undertake a program of malaria control, without first securing expert advice. The state health departments of those states which have a malaria problem should be equipped to furnish this expert consultation service to local health departments and should furnish, also, facilities for making diagnostic examinations of thick and thin blood films that are collected in the field. It is not necessary to establish a separate state division of malaria control. The three divisions most concerned are epidemiology, laboratories, and sanitary engineering. Each in turn will be called upon for advice.

**Preliminary Survey.** The first step in a malaria control program is a preliminary survey of the area in question to determine the extent and degree of the malaria problem. Three indices are commonly used.

*History index.* Death certificates of the area are not a good index, as case fatality is low. Physicians' reports are of some value, but the physicians do not see more than half of the cases. House to house visits, to obtain a probable history of malaria of the inhabitants, are of real value as an index of malaria in any community, if the data are evaluated with discretion.

*Spleen index.* Children under 12 years of age only are selected. The degree of splenomegalia as determined by palpation is noted. This is a very valuable index in the United States, particularly if taken in the late fall or early winter. In an area of high endemicity the spleen index may be misleading and of little value. Clark, in Haiti, found a much higher blood than spleen index.

It must be remembered that the spleen index is not a definite indication of presence or absence of malaria in the individual, but is an index of the prevalence of malaria *in the community*.

*Parasitic index.* The prevalence of parasites in the blood of individuals in a community is not a very valuable index of malaria prevalence in areas of low endemicity—as in most of the United States. The results depend, to a great extent, on the time of year the index is taken, and the methods used. Both thick and thin film samples should be taken and they should be examined by expert technicians.

The splendid *Manual for the Microscopical Diagnosis of Malaria in Man,* published by the U. S. Public Health Service, is highly recommended for its clarity in description of technics, and for the beautiful colored illustrations.[1]

**A spot map** of the area should be prepared showing the location of the residence of each case of malaria. A card is prepared for each case, giving name, age, sex, color, location of residence, duration of the disease, the history of previous malaria, and history of other cases of malaria in the family.

This preliminary survey will make it possible to determine the probable

[1] Wilcox, Aimee: *Manual for the Microscopical Diagnosis of Malaria in Man,* National Institute of Health Bulletin No. 180, U. S. Government Printing Office, Washington, D. C. 1943.

endemic foci of malaria in the area. Each endemic focus should be treated as a unit, in instituting control measures.

**Endemic Foci.** When the extent of the endemic focus has been determined, a detail map of the area is provided.

1. An accurate spot map of each new case of malaria is posted as it occurs.

2. Mosquito catching stations are established at strategic points in the area and visited at regular intervals during the *A. quadrimaculatus* season. This procedure has two purposes:

   *a.* To determine the density of *A. quadrimaculatus* in the area, and to enable the health officer to estimate the effects of mosquito control measures that will be carried out in the future.
   *b.* To give indications of probable sources of mosquito breeding.

3. Larvae dipping stations are established in numerous areas where *A. quadrimaculatus* breeding is suspected, and are visited at regular intervals. Careful records are kept of mosquito and larvae catches.

The data obtained by the above means enable the health department to determine:

   *a.* The actual amount of malaria in the area.
   *b.* The breeding places which are responsible for the vectors of the malaria.

The local health department should then consult with the state health department's division of sanitary engineering and epidemiology to determine the methods of elimination that are most feasible for that particular area. In general, it may be said that anopheles control is always possible, but frequently is not practicable or economically feasible.

The decision as to best methods for developing a control program depends on many factors:

1. The degree of endemicity of malaria.

2. The density of *A. quadrimaculatus* breeding.

3. Determination of natural fluctuations in malaria.

4. The density of population in the endemic area and the per capita wealth.

5. The land values of the area and particularly the land value of the area that may be salvaged by drainage.

6. The cost of initial measures and particularly the cost of maintenance.

In large centers of population complete anopheles eradication is feasible at small per capita cost; whereas, in sparsely settled rural communities or temporary construction camps, it is often not practicable at all.

In some areas, a single permanent control measure will eradicate the disease. Usually a combination of various methods is required.

**Control of Anopheles.** The control measures that may be employed against anopheles are varied and must be adapted to suit the needs of any given situation. Hackett's classification of these various factors is an excellent summary:

"*Natural.*—Restriction of anopheline breeding or contact with man by natural environmental conditions.

"*Artificial.*—Restriction of anopheline breeding or contact with man through conscious human intervention:

|  | Against Aquatic Stages | Against Adults |
|---|---|---|
| "I. *Mechanical:* | e.g., Ditching and drainage | e.g., Screening |
| [2] "II. *Toxic:* | e.g., Paris-greening | e.g., Insecticide sprays |
| "III. *Naturalistic:* |  |  |
| (a) Chemical | 1. Pollution of water | 1. Creating repellent barriers of odorous plants |
|  | 2. Changing salt content of water | 2. Administering drugs like sulphur which cause odorous perspiration |
| (b) Physical | 1. Natural fills, warping, silting | 1. Destruction of shelters, clearing |
|  | 2. Sluicing | 2. Creation of plant barriers to flight |
|  | 3. Flooding | 3. Rendering bedrooms or dwellings unattractive as resting-places |
|  | 4. Fluctuating water-levels |  |
|  | 5. Intermittent drying |  |
|  | 6. Agitating |  |
|  | 7. Stagnating (ponding) or setting water in motion |  |
|  | 8. Muddying |  |
|  | 9. Shading or clearing |  |
|  | 10. Drying by planting |  |
| (c) Biological | 1. Natural enemies (predatory enemies) | 1. Introduction of natural enemies |
|  | 2. Changing flora and fauna | 2. Deviation by animals |
|  | 3. Off-season attack | 3. Winter killing." |

**Prophylactic Quinine.** Quinine sulphate in therapeutic doses is a very valuable agent in checking the ravages of malaria. It will not reduce endemicity, or check the march of an epidemic of malaria, but it will save lives and prevent much suffering. *Prophylactic quinine* is given in 10 grain doses daily during the period the individual is exposed to the disease. It is a useful protective measure for individuals who must spend a limited time in highly malarious areas. It is not a true prophylactic, but actually is a therapeutic agent, and is given in therapeutic doses.

[2] World War II studies showed that D.D.T. was an effective toxic spray, both for mosquito larvae and adults. For a discussion of the technics of insect repellents and insecticides, see Chapter XXII.

**Treatment.** Several drugs are employed in the treatment of malaria. All are important from the public health point of view, since they not only prevent suffering and death, but also reduce the sources of parasites, from which anopheles become infected.

**Quinine.** The recommended therapy is 1.3 grams of quinine sulphate daily for 5 to 7 days. All relapses are treated in the same manner. This drug was used almost exclusively for treatment of malaria for a great many years. It became unavailable during the war in the South Pacific in 1942, and as a result, substitutes were utilized. Atabrine proved even more effective than quinine.

**Plasmochin.** Plasmochin is a gametocide. This drug may be toxic, and must be administered with care. Plasmochin has particular value as a gametocide for *Plasmodium falciparum* in malignant tertian malaria.

**Atabrine.** Atabrine has been used widely in the tropics for some years for the treatment of malaria. The drug is a synthetic quinoline derivative which is administered daily in 0.3 gm. doses for five days.

The advantages claimed of atabrine are that the drug is almost immediate in its effect on clinical symptoms, relapses are rare, and the patients rapidly become non-infective to their fellows. The drug is relatively non-toxic. It sometimes leaves a deposition of a yellowish dye in the skin following treatment. This gives the patient a very peculiar and somewhat alarming appearance, but is a matter of no serious consequence.

Atabrine may be taken as a prophylactic during a period of unavoidable exposure to malarial infection and for four weeks thereafter. The dose is 0.1 gm. daily.

During World War II, Dr. Francis R. Dieuaide, working under the Surgeon General's Office, made remarkable progress in the development of chemotherapy of malaria. These new drugs proved to be much more effective, and less toxic, than atabrine or quinine.

Paludrine has been developed by English scientists. It has the great advantage of being both curative and preventive. These studies have thrown the whole field of malaria therapy wide open to rapid advancement and great improvement.

## EDUCATIONAL MEASURES

Malaria control programs will not be successful unless the people are fully informed as to the mode of transmission and methods of prevention of the disease. A large proportion of the population does not believe as yet that malaria is transmitted by mosquitoes. Large control projects may be undertaken under special conditions, such as in labor or army camps, without popular support; but, as a general rule, any malaria control program must be preceded by an educational program, and all subsequent steps which are taken must be fully explained to the persons who may be concerned.

The control of malaria during World War II, particularly in the very adverse conditions that were encountered in the South Pacific area, is one of the miracles of modern public health practice. In the very early stages of the war, malaria was devastating, but as the campaign advanced, the disease completely lost its power. It was necessary to use every available known malaria control measure, and to devise new measures to meet unexpected conditions.

Perhaps the outstanding innovation was the introduction of highly potent insecticides and insect repellents.

These campaigns proved that when necessary, malaria can be controlled, even under the most difficult natural barriers and apparently insurmountable obstacles.

The utilization of insecticides and insect repellents is discussed in another chapter. (See page 254.)

## REFERENCES

1. Boyd, Mark F. *Introduction to Malariology.* Harvard University Press. 1930.
2. Darling, S. T. *Relative Importance in Transmitting Malaria of A. Quadrimaculatus, Punctipennis and Crucians, and Advisability of Differentiating between These Species in Applying Control Measures.* South. Med. J. 1925, Vol. 18, p. 452.
3. Darling, S. T. *Splenic Enlargement as a Measure of Malaria.* Annals of Clinical Medicine. 1926, Vol. 4, p. 695.
4. Smillie, W. G. *Studies of an Epidemic of Malaria at the Gantt, Alabama, Impounded Area.* Amer. J. of Hyg. 1927, Vol. 7, p. 40.
5. Public Health Bulletin No. 158. Transactions of Fifth Conference of Malaria Field Workers. Several valuable papers upon administrative control of malaria.
6. Symposia of the National Malaria Committee, reprinted from the Southern Medical Journal. See particularly: 1937, Vol. 30.
7. *Use of Fish for Mosquito Control.* 1924. Publications of International Health Board of the Rockefeller Foundation.
8. *Regulations Governing the Impounding of Waters.* 1927. Publications of the Alabama State Board of Health.
9. Malaria Commission of the Health Section of the League of Nations. Publications of the Health Section of the League of Nations, Geneva. See Fourth General Report. 1937, No. 6.
10. Boyd, M. F., Stratman-Thomas, W. K. and Kitchen, S. F. *On Acquired Immunity to Plasmodium Falciparum.* Amer. J. Trop. Med. 1936, Vol. 16, p. 139. (See also numerous articles by Boyd and associates on the immunology of malaria.)
11. Hackett, L. W., Russell, P. F., Scharff, J. W. and White, R. S. *The Present Use of Naturalistic Measures in the Control of Malaria.* Quarterly Bulletin of the Health Organization of the League of Nations. December, 1938, Vol. VII, No. 6, p. 1016.
12. Hackett, L. W. *Malaria in Europe.* 1937. Oxford University Press.
13. Sawyer, W. A. *A Proposed Program to Prevent the Spread of Malaria in*

*the United States from Infected Individuals Returned from Abroad.* Jour. Nat. Malaria Soc. 1944, Vol. III, p. 61.

14. Boyd, M. F. *Present Day Problems of Malaria Infections.* J.A.M.A. 1944, Vol. 124, p. 1179.

15. Herms, W. B. and Gray, H. F. *Mosquito Control: Practical Methods for Abatement of Disease Vectors and Pests.* Second Edition. New York: The Commonwealth Fund, 1944.

16. Nelson, A. A., Draize, J. H., Woodard, G., Fitzhugh, O. G., Smith, R. B. and Calvery, H. O. *Histopathological Changes Following Administration of D.D.T. to Several Species of Animals.* Pub. Health Rep. 1944, Vol. 59, p. 1009.

17. Bishopp, F. C. *The Medical and Public Health Importance of the Insecticide D.D.T.* Biggs Memorial Lecture, N. Y. Academy of Medicine, April 5, 1945.

18. Simmons, S. W. and Staff. *Tests of the Effectiveness of D.D.T. in Anopheline Control.* Pub. Health Rep. 1945, Vol. 60, p. 917.

# CHAPTER XIII

## RABIES

RABIES in human beings is a very rare disease, but the administrative measures for prevention of rabies in dogs are an important and disproportionately troublesome feature of any health officer's work. Theoretically, it should be a very simple matter to prevent rabies; practically, control of the disease is very difficult. The horror in which the disease is held by the general public is, paradoxically, the chief reason why it is so hard to control. When the disease appears in any community, the excitement is great, and a wave of popular sentiment demands the formulation of regulations in regard to dog quarantine, or muzzling, that are unenforceable. Then interest dies, and the health officer is left to face sentimental dog lovers who resist every effort that is made to restrict the freedom of their pets.

Rabies is endemic in dogs in most parts of the United States. It remains quiescent for a period, then breaks out in epidemic proportions. Not every rabid dog bites a human being, and not every person bitten by a rabid dog would develop rabies,—in fact, not more than 10 per cent—even if the Pasteur treatment were not available. But the symptoms of the disease in human beings are so horrifying and the outcome so inevitable that any health officer is confronted by a serious situation whenever the disease appears in dogs within his jurisdiction.

**Inciting Agent.** Rabies is primarily a disease of dogs, and only incidentally a disease of human beings. The course of the disease, incubation period, symptomatology, and outcome are similar in man and animals. The disease is due to a filtrable virus, which must be introduced into the body through some break in the integument, usually the skin, and which travels to the central nervous system along the nerve trunks.

**Incubation Period.** The incubation period may be prolonged. The average period in man is 40 days; in dogs somewhat less. Bites on the face and neck may result in symptoms within three weeks, and the longest authentic incubation period is less than one year. Rarely is it longer than three months in dogs or man.

**Symptoms.** The disease in dogs is characterized by three stages:
*First stage.* Irritability.

The dog becomes restless and irritable. His eyes are active, following every movement in the room. He is sensitive to sudden noise and may

149

bark for no apparent reason. This period may last for 15 to 24 hours.
*Second stage.* Fury.

The dog refuses food. He has some difficulty in swallowing. He usually has a dry, ropy salivation. He may not recognize his master and is not clearly conscious of his surroundings. He has a peculiar, unnatural howl, rather than his natural bark. He runs aimlessly about the countryside, snapping at every moving thing; such as the moving shadow of the leaves, or the lawn sprinkler in the yard. He does not snarl or growl as he fights with other dogs, but bites or snaps and runs away. He will go out of his way to snap at a group of playing children, or at animals in the pasture. This stage may last for three or four days and the dog may wander many miles from home.

*Third stage.* Paralysis.

Paralysis develops slowly. The dog cannot swallow and becomes very thirsty and greatly emaciated. He is no longer a serious menace, as his legs become completely paralyzed and he cannot run about. The pupils become widely dilated, coma develops and the animal dies.

Sometimes the furious stage does not develop, but the animal passes directly from stage one to stage three. This type of disease is called "dumb rabies." Both types of rabies may appear in the same epidemic. House pets are more likely to develop "dumb rabies"; the stray dog is more likely to become furious and is the greatest menace.

**Diagnosis.** The diagnosis of rabies in dogs is easily made by means of the characteristic symptoms, together with examination of fresh brain tissue. Proper staining brings out the "Negri bodies" in the brain tissue, which are diagnostic of the disease. The examination of the brain tissue should be done by a trained technician who is familiar with rabies diagnosis.

The virus of rabies occurs in the salivary secretions of the dog throughout the active stage of the disease, but does not appear in the saliva more than three or four days before definite clinical symptoms develop.

**Treatment.** Pasteur treatment is a very successful method of preventing the development of rabies in humans that are bitten by rabid dogs. The treatment must be begun as soon as possible. The usual method now adopted is called the Semple method—a carbolized fixed virus—which is given in 14 divided doses, one treatment being given daily. The carbolized virus is injected subcutaneously into the anterior abdominal wall. Some swelling and pain will occur about the point of injection. Immunity develops about 21 days after treatment is initiated. Thus, individuals bitten about the face and neck may not be saved by the standard method. Some authorities recommend shortening the 24-hour interval between doses in particularly urgent cases.

Under usual circumstances, one can assure the patient with practical certainty that the Pasteur treatment will be protective.

A League of Nations summary in 1928 of 5,000 cases treated by the

Semple method showed only five deaths and only one real failure of the treatment. Rarely, encephalitis follows rabies vaccine administration, as it sometimes follows other virus therapy. The League of Nations report (1927) found only one case of paralysis per 3,538 persons treated with the vaccine.

**Administrative Measures in Control of Rabies.** Control of rabies depends upon a reasonable restriction and control of dogs in all communities. The disease occurs in wild animals, such as foxes, coyotes on the western plains, and skunks; but the real endemic reservoir is the domestic dog. Most effective measures are:

*Registration of all dogs.* This procedure is simple in municipalities, but difficult to enforce in rural areas.

*Regulations* requiring that all dog bites of any nature be reported to the local board of health. An investigation is made in each case to determine if the dog has evidenced any symptoms of rabies. The dog should be restrained and kept under observation for two weeks. If alive at the end of that time, any consideration of danger to humans exposed may be dismissed even though the animal may later die of rabies. If the animal dies on or before the fourteenth day, its head should be packed in ice and submitted for microscopic examination.

The animal should not be killed unless absolutely necessary for its capture or for protection of humans. If killed, a negative laboratory diagnosis means nothing for the animal may have been rabid but Negri bodies insufficiently developed in the brain for discovery by microscopic examination. *Confine, do not kill the suspected animal.* The longer it lives the less likelihood of rabies.

a. If the dog should show any suggestive symptoms, he should not be killed, but kept under observation and restraint. If the dog is mad, characteristic diagnostic symptoms will develop inevitably. The dog should then be killed and the head removed and shipped entire to the diagnostic laboratory. The brain should not be removed from the head. It must be packed in sawdust and ice to prevent decomposition, or better, in "dry ice," which is readily available in most communities.

b. The health officer must check carefully the history of the activities of the dog during its rabid stages to learn, if possible, if it has bitten any other persons or other dogs. He should also trace, if possible, the original source of infection.

c. All dogs known to have been bitten by the rabid dog should either be destroyed, or should be kept under rigorous quarantine for at least 90 days. A valuable dog may be given the standard Semple treatment, and the disease will be prevented in exactly the same manner as in human beings. If this treatment is begun within 36 hours after the bite, the results are very satisfactory.

**General Measures.** Accurate information should be given to the community in which there is a rabies scare, in the form of news items in the local papers. This method is useful as a general educational measure, and serves also as a means of quieting the general alarm. In any community that has been visited by a rabid dog, no one can tell what other dogs have been bitten, so that the only logical measure is to restrain all dogs for a period of three months. It is almost impossible to enforce this regulation in rural areas.

Active immunization of dogs by the use of prophylactic vaccine has been applied extensively. A single injection immunizes the animal in about 21 days, and the immunity lasts for one or two years.

Some health departments, for example Nassau County, New York, have offered free clinics for rabies vaccination of dogs, when the disease existed in the community. In some instances health departments have lifted the restrictions on confined dogs, in the presence of an epidemic. The rules are:

All dogs must be restrained as follows:

*a.* Thirty days after the dog's immunization.
*b.* Any dog that has not been vaccinated within one year.
*c.* Any dog that has been bitten by, or been in contact with, a rabid animal (4 months' restriction).
*d.* Any dog that has bitten a person (2 weeks' restriction after the bite).

Each dog that is at large must have a tag indicating the date that vaccination was given.

The State of New Jersey has a state dog tax which provides funds that are used solely for control of damage caused by dogs and for control of epidemics in dogs. Rabies is given primary consideration. We suggest that the health administrator who has a special interest in these matters consult the New Jersey laws on rabies control.

**Treatment of the Patient.** Great discretion must be used in treating any dog bite wound. If there is any reason to suspect that the dog which bit the individual was mad, the wound must be cauterized. The ordinary disinfectants are of no value. The wound should be treated with fuming nitric acid or actual cautery. These measures are of little value if applied more than 6 hours after the bite.

Wounds cauterized in this manner are seldom followed by rabies. This treatment is particularly important in wounds of the face or neck, where the Pasteur treatment may fail. Great objection will be encountered to cauterization of face wounds, because of the resulting scars, but the bite itself is sure to produce a scar, which will not be accentuated by the cautery.

If the head of the dog has been secured, it is usually not necessary to begin Pasteur treatment until a laboratory report has been received.

This represents a delay of one or two days at most. If the report is negative and the dog has had no clinical symptoms of rabies, no Pasteur treatment need be given. If positive, treatment should be begun at once. The patient need not go to a central station, as was formerly the universal practice, but may be treated at home by his family physician. If the patient is indigent, the Pasteur treatment should be furnished by the local health department. In some states, the local health officer actually administers the treatment to indigent persons; in other places, the health department pays the local private physician for this service. In some states, the Pasteur treatment is furnished free to all physicians who may apply for it, if there is ample evidence that the dog which bit the patient had rabies.

In many instances it is impossible to trace the dog which bit an individual. A child may come in from the playground with an obvious dog bite, yet be unable to give a coherent story of the accident. Here a well balanced judgment must be employed. Were the children annoying the dog? Had it some provocation, or was the dog really rabid? In other instances an individual may have been in intimate contact with a rabid dog, but may not have been bitten. Sometimes the initial symptoms suggest that the dog has a bone in his throat and attempts are made to remove it. Did the individual have any open lesions on his hand that might permit entry of the virus? In making a decision in regard to the administration of Pasteur treatment, a good general rule to follow is: —in case of doubt, it is best to recommend Pasteur treatment.

This rule must be followed with discretion. Dowling and his associates in Birmingham, Alabama, who have probably had as much practical experience with rabies as any one in the United States, believe that rabies vaccine is given too indiscriminately. They recommend that the virus *be not advised* in the following instances:

1. Contamination of old cuts, sores, abrasions, scratches, or hangnails with saliva of known rabid animals.
2. "Pinches" in which skin is definitely broken but the clothing neither torn nor penetrated.
3. Handling, eating after, sleeping with, kissing or other intimate exposure to rabid animals.
4. Drinking milk of rabid cows, eating meat of rabid animals.
5. Bites of any animal living fourteen days from the time of biting.
6. Bites from fleas from rabid animals.
7. Any exposure to a case of human rabies other than an actual bite, or direct contamination of fresh open wounds.
8. Any exposure to a nonrabid animal just bitten by a rabid animal except when infected saliva is directly transmitted to a fresh open wound.

These authors use the criteria that rabies vaccine need not be given unless:

1. The person suffers from an actual bite or scratch from a suspected animal, or

2. There has been known contamination of a fresh, open wound with saliva of the suspected animal.

## REFERENCES

1. Semple, D. *The Preparation of a Safe and Efficient Anti-rabies Vaccine*. 1911. Scientific Memoirs. Gov. of India. No. 44.
2. *Results of Treatment by the Semple Method*. Studies of the Health Section of the League of Nations. 1928. Supplement to Ann. de l'Inst. Pasteur.
3. Rosenau, M. J. *Rabies. The Treatment of Wounds and the Prevention of the Disease*. N. E. J. Med. 1928, Vol. 198, p. 787.
4. Denison, G. A. and Dowling, J. D. *Rabies in Birmingham, Alabama*. J. Amer. Med. Assn. 1939, Vol. 113, p. 391.
5. Johnson, H. N. *The Significance of the Negri Body in the Diagnosis and Epidemiology of Rabies*. Ill. Med. Jour. 1942, Vol. 81, No. 5.
6. Johnson, H. N. *Rabies*. Jour. Med. Assoc. of St. of Ala. 1944 (Nov.).

# CHAPTER XIV

## POLIOMYELITIS

THE attempts that have been made by health officers to control poliomyelitis have met with little success. No prophylactic measures have been developed, specific therapy has not been entirely satisfactory, and quarantine is of little avail. The disease resembles cerebrospinal meningitis in that many unrecognized temporary carriers of the infective agent occur in the community in epidemic periods, and no practicable method has been developed for detecting these carriers.

Poliomyelitis occurs throughout the United States. It is more prevalent in the northern states, decreasing progressively as one reaches the subtropical portions of the country. The disease is most prevalent in the late summer and fall. It recurs each year, disappearing almost entirely in the winter, appearing again in the summer. Several years may pass with a low endemicity, followed inevitably by an epidemic year in which the disease reaches severe proportions.

### EPIDEMIOLOGICAL FEATURES OF POLIOMYELITIS
### WHICH AFFECT CONTROL MEASURES

Anterior poliomyelitis is due to a filtrable virus. The initial symptoms of the disease are those of a mild general infection with gastro-intestinal disturbances. Headache may occur, with nausea and vomiting, a mild fever and perhaps diarrhea. The duration of this phase of the disease is about three days. No further symptoms may develop and the disease may pass undiagnosed or unnoticed. The virus may localize in the nervous system and produce the characteristic symptomatology of the disease. The second phase is characterized by headache, drowsiness and a coarse tremor, with stiffness of the neck, followed by weakness and paralysis. Any group of muscles may be affected, depending upon the localization of the lesion in the spinal tract. The degree of paralysis depends upon the extent and severity of the process in the cord.

Diagnosis is made by the characteristic symptoms and verified by spinal puncture. The spinal fluid is under moderately increased pressure, shows an increase in globulin and cells, with a normal sugar content. Diagnosis may be made from the spinal fluid puncture before definite paralysis has developed. In inter-epidemic periods, the diagnosis of poliomyelitis is seldom made before the appearance of nervous symptoms, but in epidemic periods a definite diagnosis is often made in the pre-paralytic phase of the disease, since physicians are on the alert for any suspicious symptoms, and make a spinal puncture on these cases.

The incubation period of the disease is from 7 to 14 days. The virus is transmitted by direct contact with a case, or much more commonly, by contact with a healthy carrier. A few milk-borne epidemics of the disease have been recorded which seem to be authentic.

The virus is found in the discharges from the nasopharynx and intestines of the actual case. Paul and also Kramer have demonstrated the virus in the sewage outlet of institutions in which cases of poliomyelitis were under treatment. They believe that the intestinal discharges may be an important source of community infection. The prevalence of this virus in any community during normal periods is not known, but during epidemics it is certain that a large number of people harbor the virus for an indefinite length of time. As in meningitis, only a small number of those individuals who are invaded by the virus actually develop the symptoms of the disease. Thus the temporary carrier of the virus is a far more important factor in the spread of poliomyelitis than the actual case. Unfortunately, there is no practicable routine public health laboratory method of determining the presence of the virus in the nasopharynx or intestines of the normal individual.

Pearson [1] and his colleagues, under the direction of Dr. Thomas Francis, made an extensive study of the distribution of poliomyelitis virus in a community (Fort Worth, Texas) in 1943 during an epidemic period.

Stool specimens from 524 persons were tested for poliomyelitis virus by monkey inoculation. The following table summarizes the results:

|  | No. | Virus of Polio. | Households Invaded % | Contacts |
|---|---|---|---|---|
| Households containing family contacts with poliomyelitis | 8 | 6 | 75% | 27 |
| Households containing non-family con-tacts, e.g., school contacts, etc. | 45 | 8 | 18% | 80 |
| Households containing no known direct contact with poliomyelitis | 127 | 2 | 1.6% | 374 |

These data indicate clearly that the virus is distributed in the community during an epidemic in direct relation to immediate contact.

As Pearson and Rendtorff [2] note in their study of the distribution of poliomyelitis virus in a small town, "personal association was the principal factor involved in the spread of infection within the community."

[1] Pearson, H. E., Brown, G. C., Rendtorff, R. C., Ridenous, G. M. and Francis, Thomas, Jr.: "Studies of the Distribution of Poliomyelitis Virus. III. In an Urban Area During an Epidemic." *Am. Jour. Hyg.* 1945, Vol. 41, No. 2.

[2] Pearson, H. E. and Rendtorff, R. C.: "Studies of the Distribution of Poliomyelitis Virus. II. In a Small Town." *Am. Jour. Hyg.* 1945, Vol. 41, No. 2.

A great deal of epidemiological speculation has centered in the possibility of an animal vector of poliomyelitis. Insects have been considered many times as possible transmitters of this infection. Furthermore, the fact that the virus is in the intestinal tract and has frequently been isolated from community sewers, has led to the speculation that polluted drinking water might be an important source of infection with poliomyelitis.

Certainly water is a possible source of epidemics of poliomyelitis, but all the available evidence indicates that the epidemics of poliomyelitis that have occurred in the United States have not been transmitted through water as a vehicle of infection.[3]

The disease spreads radially by direct contact from person to person, from family to family, and community to community. "The disease is on the wane in the central focus while it is still ascending in the outer concentric zones." [4]

There is great variation in susceptibility to infection. Aycock[5] believes that this is due to "constitutional type," and points out that family aggregation of poliomyelitis may be due to greatest family susceptibility.

An excellent study[6] of the epidemiological features of an outbreak of poliomyelitis in a rural upper New York State area by a district health officer is especially recommended for study by the health officer in a rural area who is faced with an epidemic of this disease.

Poliomyelitis is essentially a disease of young children. There is some evidence that in recent years the age distribution has shifted to the older age groups. Adults may develop the disease. Infants are usually immune. There is little immunity to the disease in children from one to five years. After this age, immunity gradually develops to such a point that most adults in the community are completely immune to the disease.

Mortality rates vary greatly in different epidemics. Probably many children develop only the preliminary symptoms of the disease, and these cases are not recognized as poliomyelitis. The case fatality rate of recognized cases in an epidemic may be as low as 3 per cent or as high as 20 per cent, or sometimes even higher.

## ADMINISTRATIVE METHODS IN CONTROL OF POLIOMYELITIS

It must be recognized that those methods that have been used in the control of poliomyelitis have been unsatisfactory. The reasons for this

[3] See Maxcy, K. F.: *Am. Jour. Pub. Health.* 1943, Vol. 33, p. 41.

[4] Perkins, J. E.: "The Epidemiology of Poliomyelitis." *N. Y. State Jour. Med.* 1945, p. 159.

[5] Aycock, W. L.: "Constitutional Types and Susceptibility to Paralysis in Poliomyelitis." *Am. Jour. Med. Sciences.* 1941, Vol. 202, p. 456. *Ibid.:* "Familial Aggregation in Poliomyelitis." *Am. Jour. Med. Sciences.* 1942, Vol. 203, p. 452.

[6] Conway, J. A. and Bigwood, D. E.: "Observations Made During a Poliomyelitis Epidemic in 1944 in the Hornell State Health District, New York." *N. Y. State Jour. Med.* 1946, Vol. 46, p. 275.

are clear from the discussion of the epidemiology of the disease. The following measures have some value.

**Reporting.** All cases should be reported immediately to the health department. This should include the reporting of suspected cases as well as the frank cases. The patient should be removed to a hospital, if possible.

**Diagnostic Facilities.** The local health department should furnish diagnostic facilities through an experienced physician who is trained in the differential diagnosis of poliomyelitis, meningitis, etc. The procedure which is followed is exactly the same as in meningitis control. The diagnostician makes his visit on request of the family physician and accompanied by him. The diagnostician should have available at all times suitable materials for making a spinal puncture, and should take to the bedside the portable laboratory equipment, in order that a presumptive diagnosis may be made on the first visit. This diagnostic service should be without cost to the patient. Treatment of the case is the responsibility of the family physician and not the health officer, but the health department should do everything possible to facilitate diagnosis and treatment.

**Treatment.** Convalescent serum has been used extensively in treatment of poliomyelitis, but has largely been given up. Its value is questioned by most authorities, who feel that there is not sufficient evidence to prove that the serum is of actual benefit in treatment of poliomyelitis, even if given early in the disease.

**Isolation.** All cases should be isolated during the febrile period of the disease. Concurrent disinfection of all discharges and the usual bedside prophylactic procedures in relation to disinfection of bed clothing, food remnants, etc., should be followed. Special attention should be given to the intestinal discharges. They should be treated with chlorinated lime or other suitable disinfectant before disposal in the sewer.

**Quarantine.** Formerly it was customary to quarantine all children in the household, when poliomyelitis had occurred, for a period of three weeks, together with all adults who handle food or who come in frequent contact with children, such as school teachers. Placarding also was a common procedure, but has no obvious advantages. During epidemics, quarantine measures are more or less of a gesture, since we have no evidence that the quarantine of contacts of a case has been of any particular value in checking the march of the outbreak. It is obvious that, with the number of normal, unknown carriers in an infected community exceeding the number of suspected carriers by the ratio of at least 10 to 1, quarantine of known contacts will be wholly ineffective as an attempt to check the epidemic.

It is possible, as in epidemics of meningitis, to use quarantine effectively under certain circumstances. For example, the disease may be kept within bounds when a whole community may be quarantined, as an orphanage, or some children's institution.

Partial isolation of normal young children from contact with the general population is a valuable procedure during an epidemic. This can be carried out only by intelligent, understanding co-operation of parents and is not a direct function of the health department.

**Orthopedic After-care.** Some health departments have assumed responsibility for organization of the orthopedic after-care of poliomyelitis. The local public health nurse does the case finding work, and organizes the clinic.

The children are seen at regular intervals by the orthopedic surgeon in the clinic. The public health nurse may aid the parents in carrying out the physician's orders, by giving the suitable muscle exercises to the child, and by procuring appliances for the prevention of deformities.

The care of crippled children has a particular appeal to any community and the local health officer and nurses will have no difficulty in obtaining financial aid from voluntary organizations, such as men's clubs, women's organizations, etc., to pay for necessary orthopedic appliances or hospital expenses of orthopedic operations for the indigent child who has been crippled by poliomyelitis. The Social Security Act of 1935 has greatly assisted states and local communities in promoting the proper care of children that are crippled by poliomyelitis.

**Rehabilitation.** A continuous and effective rehabilitation program for those persons who have been crippled by poliomyelitis is an important community responsibility.

Some communities, notably Rochester, New York, have developed "Industrial Workshops," where the crippled are trained and given an opportunity to develop their talents, even though they may be seriously handicapped.

**Education.** Educational methods are of little value in control of poliomyelitis. During an epidemic the community is thoroughly alarmed and should be kept informed in regard to the current state of affairs, and reassured as much as possible. Publicity may be used for the purpose of giving information as to best methods of avoiding infection of the children. In so far as possible, young children should be kept from contact with the general population. There is nothing to be gained by closing schools, theaters, churches, etc., though it may seem best to close crowded summer playgrounds and swimming pools, where large numbers of children come in close personal contact. During an epidemic the wise mother will avoid travel and keep her brood of small children in as quiet and isolated a place as possible, realizing that the epidemic will have disappeared by early fall.

**Vaccination.** Community immunization by vaccination has been tried, but the methods have been unsuccessful. Even if a method should give perfect protection and have no inherent danger, nevertheless the procedure probably would not be incorporated in public health practice, as it would be necessary to vaccinate at least 10,000 children to prevent one case of paralysis from poliomyelitis.

Poliomyelitis may follow an operation for removal of tonsils. Thus it is recommended that children who require a tonsillectomy should not be operated upon in August or September. June is probably the month of choice.

## REFERENCES

1. Kramer, S. D. *Active Immunization against Poliomyelitis.* Jour. Immunology 1936, 31:191.
2. Kramer, S. D., Gilliam, A. G. and Molner, J. G. *Recovery of Virus of Polio-myelitis from Stools of Healthy Contacts in Institutional Outbreak.* U. S. Public Health Service Reports. 1939, Vol. 54, p. 1941.
3. Paul, J. R., Trask, J. D. and Culotta, C. S. *Poliomyelitis Virus in Sewage.* Science. 1939, Vol. 90, p. 258.
4. Aycock, W. L. *Constitutional Types and Susceptibility to Paralysis in Polio-myelitis.* Am. Jour. Med. Sci. 1941, Vol. 202, p. 456.
5. Aycock, W. L. *Familial Aggregation in Poliomyelitis.* Am. Jour. Med. Sci. 1942, Vol. 203, p. 452.
6. Nelson, N. B. and Aycock, W. L. *A Study of the Reporting of Paralytic Poliomyelitis in Massachusetts, 1928–1941.* Am. Jour. Hyg. 1944, Vol. 40, p. 163.
7. Perkins, J. E. *The Epidemiology of Poliomyelitis.* N. Y. State Jour. Med. 1945 (Jan. 15), p. 159.
8. Pearson, H. E. and Rendtorff, R. C. *Studies of the Distribution of Poliomye-litis Virus.* II. *In a Small Town.* Am. Jour. Hyg. 1945, Vol. 41, No. 2.
9. Pearson, H. E., Brown, G. C., Rendtorff, R. C., Ridenous, G. H. and Francis, Thomas, Jr. *Studies of the Distribution of Poliomyelitis Virus.* III. *In an Urban Area During an Epidemic.* Am. Jour. Hyg. 1945, Vol. 41, No. 2.
10. Conway, J. A. and Bigwood, D. E. *Observations Made During a Poliomyelitis Epidemic in 1944 in the Hornell State Health District, New York.* N. Y. State Jour. Med. 1946, Vol. 46, p. 275.

# CHAPTER XV

## MENINGOCOCCUS MENINGITIS

EPIDEMIC cerebrospinal meningitis is of relatively little importance to the health officer, under normal conditions. He may be concerned with isolated cases which may occur from time to time in children, but seldom are there more than one or two secondary cases following the first one.

In any community, however, an epidemic of meningococcus meningitis will appear sooner or later. The epidemic may be mild and of short duration, or may be severe and linger for several years. The disease is extremely difficult to control because of the high degree of prevalence of the specific organism during epidemic periods and its low degree of invasiveness. In other words, a very large proportion of the population will harbor the organisms in the nasopharynx for a short period during the epidemic, whereas only a relatively small proportion of those who are infected will develop the disease. This is a characteristic of a few diseases, which always puts the health officer on the horns of a dilemma. The health officer can seldom quarantine the whole infected community; if he isolates the sick individuals and quarantines only their contacts, his efforts are futile.

## EPIDEMIOLOGICAL FEATURES OF THE DISEASE WHICH RELATE TO ADMINISTRATIVE CONTROL

Meningococcus meningitis is due to *Neisseria intracellularis*. This organism belongs to the general group of gram negative diplococci. The organism may be divided into a variety of types, according to certain specific characteristics of agglutination (as with pneumococcus). There are four main groups. Usually, one group preponderates in any single epidemic; though two or more types may be prevalent in the same major outbreak. These organisms invade the body through the nasopharynx. In the early stages of the disease, the meningococci may be found in the blood stream. This septicemia may continue for weeks without localization. In a typical case, an early localization occurs in the cerebrospinal system.

The disease is characterized by sudden onset of fever, which is preceded in some instances by nasopharyngitis. Headache is severe, as well as nausea and vomiting, which is sometimes projectile in type. The most

161

striking symptom is the rigidity of the neck, together with other signs of meningeal irritation. Often there appears an irregular petechial rash on the body, these areas sometimes fusing into a profuse eruption. This type of rash is common in the fulminating cases which are seen in a severe epidemic.

A definite diagnosis is made by intra-spinal or intra-cisternal puncture. The cerebrospinal fluid contains large numbers of polymorphonuclear leucocytes and the typical meningococci are found both inside and outside the white cells, and may be cultivated on suitable media (5 per cent blood agar plates).

The disease occurs most commonly in young children, but may occur in adults, particularly during epidemics. Cerebrospinal meningitis is much more common in winter than in summer. During an epidemic the incidence may decline in the late spring and the disease may disappear completely in August, only to reappear in October or November, perhaps with increased prevalence and virulence.

The case fatality rate varies greatly in different epidemics. Sporadic cases have a relatively low fatality rate. In the past, some epidemics have had fatality rates of 25 per cent; in others over 60 per cent of the patients died, despite careful observation and treatment.

During normal periods meningococci may be found in the nasopharynges of a limited number of the population; during an epidemic a large proportion of the population will harbor the organism at one time or another. In most people the carrier state persists for one or two weeks and produces no symptoms. The more crowded the living conditions, the higher will be the percentage of temporary carriers. The incubation period of the disease is short, 2 to 8 days, but certain individuals may carry the organisms in their throats for two or more weeks and then develop the disease following exposure or fatigue, or for other reasons.

The silent temporary carriers keep the disease going in any community. The actual case of meningitis is not a great source of danger to others, as his contacts are limited, and the organisms usually disappear from his throat before the clinical symptoms of meningitis have ameliorated.

Susceptibility to the disease seems to depend upon the virulence of the strain of organism, the dosage, and the general physical condition of the individual. Natural immunity to implantation of the organism in the nasopharynx is low, but resistance to invasion of the cerebrospinal system is high, even in epidemics. Thus in crowded barracks, during an epidemic among the soldiers, over one half of the nasopharyngeal cultures taken at random may show typical meningococci, but less than 10 per cent of the men develop the actual disease. The organism dies very rapidly, if removed from its natural habitat—the human nasopharynx—so that the secretions from a patient (or carrier) are a menace for a short period of time only.

Specific prophylaxis has not been attempted on a large scale, though, theoretically, it would be feasible. In a Brazilian barracks, where meningitis was prevalent, an autogenous vaccine was prepared and given to all the soldiers. The epidemic ceased abruptly, but when these same soldiers were moved to a new territory, meningitis broke out in the civilian population, indicating that carriers persisted in the troop despite absence of disease.

**Treatment.** The treatment of cerebrospinal meningitis has been revolutionized through the development of the sulfonamides, penicillin, and other types of specific therapy. The results have been so spectacular that they are almost unbelievable. Only the older clinicians who have had to face the heart breaking ineffectiveness of therapy in an epidemic of meningitis can fully appreciate the miracle of sulfonamide therapy in the treatment of a serious case of cerebrospinal meningitis. Furthermore, these drugs may be used effectively in control of the carriers of the infection.

**Prophylaxis.** During World War II sulfonamide prophylaxis was used extensively in preventing meningitis in young recruits during the training period.[1]

Six hundred thousand men stationed at eight training centers were given 0.5 gm. to 1 gm. of sulfadiazine daily during a training of 7 weeks. Five cases of meningococcal meningitis developed in the group—three occurring within 24 hours after prophylaxis was begun. In the control group there were 146 cases of meningitis.

Penicillin is also a very effective drug in the treatment of meningococcal meningitis, and may be utilized as supplementary therapy.

## ADMINISTRATIVE CONTROL OF THE DISEASE

**Reporting.** All suspected cases should be reported immediately to the local health department.

**Isolation.** The patient should be isolated, preferably in a hospital (for therapeutic reasons). Sulfonamide therapy is very valuable in treating the case, but the drug must be given rapidly, and in effective doses. Penicillin may be utilized if immediate results are not secured by sulfonamides. Isolation is usually continued for two weeks.

**Diagnostic Facilities.** The local health department should furnish diagnostic facilities through a physician skilled in the differential diagnosis of various types of meningitis, poliomyelitis, etc. He should be connected officially with the Division of Communicable Diseases and be on continuous call, so that his services are available to any practicing physician at any time. This diagnostic consulting service should be free to all. The diagnostician of the health department should not take charge of the patient, but should make his visit on the request of the family physician and accompanied by him.

[1] Cheever, F. S.: "The Control of Meningococcal Meningitis by Mass Chemoprophylaxis with Sulfadiazine." *Am. Jour. Med. Sci.* 1945, Vol. 209, p. 74.

The consulting diagnostician should have ready the necessary equipment for spinal puncture, and also a portable laboratory equipment, so that provisional diagnosis may be made at the bedside. The health department should also supply diagnostic laboratory facilities for direct examination of spinal fluid, and for bacteriological cultivation of the organisms that may be found in the spinal fluid.

**Treatment.** Sulfanilamide, and if necessary penicillin, also should be made freely available by the health department to all physicians, for treatment of those patients who are unable to purchase the drugs.

Concurrent disinfection of all discharges of the patient should be carried out, with a final cleansing of the room after the patient has recovered. Placarding of the case is a common procedure, but has little theoretical justification.

**Quarantine.** Quarantine of meningitis is the rock on which most health officers stumble. Many health departments require quarantine of all contacts of a case until two negative nasopharyngeal cultures are obtained, or, if cultures are not made, for a period of two weeks.

It is undoubtedly true that the healthy carrier is the important source of distribution of the disease, but during an epidemic, a large proportion of the population will become carriers, sooner or later. The quarantine of *known* positive carriers is of little avail in checking the march of an epidemic, for only one healthy carrier may be under quarantine while ten are walking the streets. Thus a bacteriological check as a method of control of carriers has not proved practicable, because of the very enormousness of the undertaking.

In institutions, barracks or construction camps, where meningitis prevails, it may be feasible to quarantine the whole camp for an arbitrary period, but we have very little evidence that quarantine *per se* has ever been effective in checking the progress of an epidemic of cerebrospinal meningitis.

Control of the temporary carrier by sulfonamide prophylaxis is a much more satisfactory technique. Two grams daily for 5 days will be sufficient in most instances to render any carrier free. In family contacts and in soldiers' barracks, it is a good policy to consider all close contacts as potential carriers, and to give each the necessary prophylaxis.

Overcrowding is probably the most important factor in the spread of the disease in jails, prisons, barracks, sleeping quarters on board ships, institutions, etc. The simple procedure of increasing the distance between beds in a barracks may be effective in checking an epidemic.

General regulations in regard to housing are important factors in preventing the spread of meningitis; particularly those regulations that relate to overcrowding of sleeping quarters in tenements, in orphanages, children's homes, etc.

Specific educational methods concerning the prevention of cerebrospinal meningitis are of little avail. Instruction in measures of general hygiene and personal cleanliness are important, particularly in relation to avoidance of close personal contact and avoidance of droplet infection.

During an epidemic certain precautions may be taken. Exposure to severe cold, exhaustion, an alcoholic debauch, or other debilitating factors often precipitate an attack of meningitis. These are apparently autogenous, and it may be assumed that the patient under normal conditions would have resisted the invasion. Thus, anyone who may have been exposed to the infection should avoid exposure to wet and cold weather, or to fatigue.

## REFERENCES

1. Ismail, A. *The Use of Antimeningococcus Vaccine in the Prophylaxis of Cerebrospinal Meningitis.* Bul. Offic. Internat. d'Hyg. Pub. 1933, 25: 1725.
2. Norton, J. T. and Baisby, I. E. *Meningococcus Meningitis in Detroit in 1928–1929.* Paper IV. *Carriers.* J. Prev. Med., 1931, 5:357. (See also three previous papers by these authors and associates, on the same epidemic.)
3. Riding, D. and Corkill, N. L. *Prophylactic Vaccine in Epidemic Meningococcal Meningitis.* Amer. J. Hyg., 1932, 2:258.
4. Schwentker, F. F., Gelman, S. and Long, P. H. *Treatment of Meningococcal Meningitis with Sulfanilamide. Preliminary Report.* J. Amer. Med. Assn., 1937, 108:1407.
5. McKhann, C. F. *Meningococcus Meningitis in Infants.* New Eng. J. Med., 1930, 202:520.
6. Phair, J. J., Schoenbach, E. B. and Root, C. M. *Meningococcal Carrier Studies.* Am. Jour. Pub. Health. 1944, Vol. 34, No. 2.
7. Miller, C. P., Breadenkopf, W. G., Peck, D. and Robbins, M. W. *A Survey of Chronic Meningococcus Carriers in a Semi-permanent Population.* Jour. Inf. Dis. 1944, Vol. 74, p. 212.
8. Cheever, F. S. *The Control of Meningococcal Meningitis by Mass Chemoprophylaxis with Sulfadiazine.* Am. J. Med. Sci. 1945, Vol. 209, p. 74.
9. Boor, A. K. and Miller, C. P. *The Effect of Penicillin on the Lethal Action of Meningococcal Endotoxin in Experimental Animals.* Science. 1945, Vol. 102, p. 427.
10. Strong, P. S. and Blumberg, J. M. *Treatment of 56 Meningococcus Carriers with Chemotherapy.* Military Surgeon. 1943, Vol. 92, p. 59.

# CHAPTER XVI

## INTESTINAL PARASITES

### HOOKWORM DISEASE

THE control of intestinal parasites is an important duty of the health officer in certain portions of the United States, and offers particular administrative difficulties. In some areas, the intestinal parasites, particularly hookworms, cause greater mental and physical retardation in children than all other factors combined. Hookworm disease and, to a lesser degree, ascariasis are the most important members of this group of diseases. In the United States both are essentially diseases of children, though adults may, of course, be affected. The epidemiology of hookworm disease is somewhat different from that of ascariasis, and therefore the methods of control are not identical. Certain general hygienic principles may be developed which aid in the control of the whole group of intestinal parasites. These methods aid also in the control of various other infections which are due in great part to inadequate systems of disposal of human feces; as, for example, typhoid fever, bacillary and amebic dysentery, etc.

### EPIDEMIOLOGICAL FEATURES OF HOOKWORM DISEASE WHICH RELATE TO ITS CONTROL

Hookworm disease in the United States is due to *Necator americanus* (except in a small area in California). The adult parasite lives in the upper part of the small intestine where it is attached to the mucosa. Each parasite sucks blood from the host, so that the essential clinical picture is one of anemia. The degree of clinical symptomatology depends in general upon the number of parasites harbored. Age, nutrition, intercurrent infection and other factors may be variables which influence this general rule. Ova are discharged in the feces and hatch only on exposure to the air. The larvae live in the soil, and pass through several moults until the infective stage is reached. Under favorable conditions this free living stage may last three months. Invasion of the host occurs in practically every instance through the bare skin, usually of the foot. The larvae penetrate to the lymph circulation, thence through the general circulation to the lungs. They pass through the alveoli to the bronchial tree and are carried up to the posterior nasopharynx and swallowed. Once in the small intestine, the adults fasten themselves to the mucosa and are removed with difficulty. They may live for five years or longer. The parasites as a rule are "slowly acquired and slowly lost," so that children under four years seldom develop clinical disease. There are exceptions to this rule, for instances of massive infection following a single exposure have been reported.[1] Negroes have a marked degree of immunity to infection.

The weak link in the life cycle is the free living stage. The larvae are readily killed by drying, and by cold. They do not migrate through the soil laterally, but follow the ground water, moving in a perpendicular direction. Thus the zone of pollution of the soil from any single source is relatively limited. The disease is limited to the southeastern portion of the United States, since the larvae require a long, warm, moist season. Tight textured soils are unfavorable to larval life, so that the disease is of chief importance in areas with a sandy soil. Hookworm disease is now uncommon in cities and towns or even small villages because of the development of suitable systems of disposal of feces. Even in heavily infected areas, adults usually have a light degree of infection because of the protection of shoes. Thus, hookworm disease, as a serious menace, exists in those areas in the United States that have an annual rainfall of at least 30 inches, a temperature which does not fall below 50° F. for at least three months, and which have a sandy soil, and possess a rural population that is without an adequate system of disposal of human feces.

The diagnosis is readily made by a microscopic examination of the feces for characteristic ova. The degree of infection can be estimated by one of the various modifications of the Stoll ova count method. In general, light infections produce no measurable injury. Fifty worms or even more (*Necator americanus*) may produce no symptoms, even in small children. Thus it is a good general rule to consider any individual with an infection of 25 worms or less as a carrier only. One need not attempt complete eradication of the parasites from all persons, but simply reduce the average intensity of infection to the point where they produce no appreciable harm. Good nutrition, and particularly a diet rich in foods containing iron, will alleviate greatly the symptoms of hookworm infection, even without removal of the parasites. Rhoads and Castle in Puerto Rico, showed that the anemia of hookworm disease is very effectively treated by the simple administration of suitable doses of iron.

Cort and his associates, in experiments with dogs, have proved that the animals develop a relative immunity to superinfection with hookworms. If the dogs are given a deficient diet, this immunity is lost, but it may be regained if the animals are given an abundant diet. It is probable that the same rules hold true in human infections with hookworms.

The worms may be removed from the intestinal tract by treatment with

[1] Ashford, Payne, *et al.: Jour. Am. Med. Assn.* Sept. 9, 1933, 101: p. 843.

a suitable vermifuge. The ideal vermifuge is one which will remove all parasites from the intestinal tract in a single administration and without inconvenience to the host. This ideal has not been attained, for all vermifuges that have been developed so far have some degree of toxicity. Tetrachlorethylene has given excellent results in removing hookworms. Hexylresorcinol or one of its derivatives is an excellent drug in the treatment of both ascaris and hookworm infections. It is less toxic than other vermifuges and is very easy to administer.

### Administrative Control of Hookworm Disease

From the epidemiological discussion it is evident that true hookworm disease is limited essentially to rural white children of school age in certain areas of the southern part of the United States, particularly in those areas that have a preponderance of sandy soils.

The health officer's first step in attempting control is to determine the extent and intensity of the infection in his jurisdiction. Hookworm surveys of the rural school children by routine feces examination as part of the general school health program will soon reveal the importance of the disease. These stool specimens may be sent to the central state laboratory to determine not only incidence, but intensity of infection.

All children harboring an estimated number of 25 worms or more should be given treatment. Heavily infected children—500 worms or more—may require two treatments. The parents may be advised to take such a child to their family physician, or the consent of the local medical society may be secured and a treatment clinic may be organized at each school in co-operation with the medical society. Parents should not be given the vermifuge to administer to the children at home since all effective vermifuges have some degree of toxicity, and should be administered under the watchful eye of a physician.

Relief following treatment is almost immediate, but the results are temporary. If the child remains under former environmental conditions he will become reinfected to the previous degree within a few years. Recovery will be hastened, if iron is supplied therapeutically in the diet.

An essential step in the control of the disease is an active educational program which will emphasize the simple epidemiological features of the disease.

The most satisfactory method of permanent control of the disease is the installation and use of sanitary privies. Since the families most affected are over-conservative and often very poor, the type of privy which is suggested must be as simple and inexpensive as is consistent with reasonable permanence.

This matter has been given a great deal of consideration by competent sanitary engineers and a standard pit privy has been developed, with concrete floor, and iron or concrete riser, which is both cheap and permanent. The greatest difficulty encountered in the whole program is in securing the installation and use of this pit privy by all members of the family and all families in the community. Patient, persistent and continuous effort is required. The least detail in regard to construction of the privy must be furnished each family, and, in some areas, actual subsidies have been given to the rural people in the form of materials, or through assistance by the sanitary inspector of the health department in the actual construction of the privy.

The slow and often discouraging results that are secured by the sanitation program may seem disproportionate to the effort that has been exerted by the health department, and there is a tendency for the health officer to become disheartened. He is often tempted to introduce a compulsory regulation requiring universal installation of suitable pit toilets. Experience has shown that such a regulation is ineffective, since it is impossible to compel the people to use these toilets after they have been constructed. It must be remembered that one is attempting to remold and modify the customs and habits of generations. This may be possible if the individual is uprooted from his old environment and has gone to make his home under entirely new conditions, as in a city. So long as the family remains under ancestral conditions, the change of habits and customs will be slow.

Leathers and Keller have demonstrated conclusively that the active hookworm control measures that have been carried out through the endemic area in the United States during the past 25 years have been very effective. But the disease is not yet under control, and in the infected areas constant vigilance will be required for many years to come.

## ASCARIASIS

### Epidemiological Features of the Infestation

Ascariasis is due to *Ascaris lumbricoides*. This large worm lives in the human intestine. Enormous numbers of ova are deposited in the feces by each female worm, so that persons harboring only a few worms may distribute the disease over a wide area. The ova are very resistant to sunlight, drying, and cold, and may persist in the soil for a long time. The ova become embryonated after about two weeks—under summer conditions—and infection occurs through swallowing ova in this infective stage. The larvae hatch in the intestine, penetrate the intestinal tract, reach the general circulation and are carried to the lungs. Here they penetrate to the alveoli, as do the hookworm larvae and are carried up the bronchial tree. In passing through the lungs, the larvae may produce symptoms of respiratory infection. They are carried up the trachea, are swallowed and finally reach maturity in the intestine after a period of some two months' migration.

The degree of infection varies from a single worm to very many. Four or five hundred worms have been removed from a single child. In the

United States young children are usually more heavily infected than adults or children of school age.

The disease does not have the same geographic distribution as hookworm disease. The endemic centers are chiefly the Appalachian chain of mountains in the southeastern United States, from West Virginia and the southwestern part of Virginia down through the mountainous regions of eastern and central Tennessee, Kentucky and western North Carolina, northern Georgia and Alabama.

The disease is spread because of inadequate systems of feces disposal, and particularly through poor household sanitation and improper habits of personal hygiene on the part of young children. It is the custom of the small children in many rural areas to deposit their feces on the soil in the immediate environs of the house. Eventually, the ova from the infected feces are carried far and wide and have even been found in the dust of the household floor. Children playing about in the yard get the embryonated ova in their mouths. The ova are swallowed and thus the worms gain entrance to the body.

The adult worms may be removed from the intestine by treatment with oil of chenopodium or better by hexylresorcinol. A single treatment is often effective in removing all the worms. Oil of chenopodium may be very toxic for small children and when used in treatment of ascariasis should always be mixed with castor oil. Success in treatment of intestinal parasites is dependent upon meticulous attention to details. The instructions given in Volume II of *Nelson's Loose-Leaf Medicine* are useful for reference.

### ADMINISTRATIVE CONTROL OF ASCARIASIS

Ascariasis is directly associated with improper methods of disposal of human feces. It may be controlled through:

1. Installation and use of sanitary toilets by the whole population.

2. Education of children and parents, and particularly mothers, as to the epidemiological features of the disease. If a mother understands just how her small children become infected with ascaris, the struggle for control of the disease is already half won.

School children in the areas of infection should have a routine feces examination as a part of the school hygiene program; but the heaviest infections occur in preschool age, so that this is a relatively ineffective control method. Parents in the endemic areas should be encouraged to secure feces examinations of their young children. This laboratory service should be offered free through the local health department. The positive cases should be referred to their family physician, or, if the local medical profession agrees, the health department may hold clinics and actually administer treatment.

Since the ova are widely distributed and survive for a long period, mass treatments of ascariasis by the clinics are of limited value, since reinfection will occur, if the children return to their former environmental conditions. The two major elements of the control program are education of the parents as to the mode of infection, and installation of proper systems of feces disposal. The pit privy which has been widely recommended as a method of hookworm disease control is also the simplest and best feces disposal system for the average rural home in the areas where ascaris infestation prevails.

**Oxyuriasis.** Pin-worm infection has a nuisance factor which is completely out of proportion to its relative innocuousness. It never killed its victim, although the author knows of an instance in which one of its adult victims actually contemplated suicide because of the intolerable itching that was produced by the parasites. It is the despair of the distraught parent, and has wrecked the professional reputation of many a pediatrician. It is a disease which refuses to stay cured.

The work of Hall and his associates at the National Institute of Health awakened new interest in the epidemiology of this troublesome disease. They developed a simple and very effective cellophane anal swab, which has greatly simplified and facilitated the diagnosis of oxyuriasis. Using this technic, they demonstrated that the infection is much more widespread than had ever been realized.

*Control.* Control of *Enterobius vermicularis,* like that of scabies, is primarily a matter of family hygiene. Every member of the family that suffers from the infection should be treated at the same time. Bed clothing and the underclothing of all the patients should be boiled. Woolen clothing that has been in contact with the skin should be pressed with a hot iron. Each patient should keep his nails short and should scrub his hands after each trip to the bathroom and before each meal.

Hall and his associates also developed a very effective therapy. Hexylresorcinol pills, 0.1 gm. for each year of age, are given by mouth, followed by a hexylresorcinol enema (1/1000) and application of this drug in a jelly to the buttocks; this is an excellent treatment.

Gentian violet has also been employed most successfully in the removal of the parasites. The therapy consists of a 1 grain tablet of gentian violet crystals, given before meals three times a day for 6 or 7 days.

## REFERENCES

Discussions of trichinae infection, and also of the beef tapeworm, are included in the section of food inspection. (See page 247.)

1. Smillie, W. G. *Nelson's Loose Leaf Medicine.* Vol. II, Vol. VII.
2. Cort, W. W., Stoll, N. R. *et al. Investigations on the Control of Hookworm Disease.* 34 separate papers. See General Summary No. XXXIV. Amer. J. Hyg. 1925, Vol. 5, pp. 49–89.
3. Stoll, N. R. Same Series. No. XV. Amer. J. Hyg. 1923, Vol. 3, p. 59. No. XVIII. Amer. J. Hyg. 1923, Vol. 3, p. 156.

4. Smillie, W. G. and Augustine, D. L. *The Relation of Type of Soils of Alabama to Distribution of Hookworm Disease.* Amer. J. Hyg. 1926, Vol. 6, p. 36.

5. Lamson, P. D., Brown, H. W. *et al. Field Treatment of Ascariasis, Ancylostomiasis and Trichiniasis with Hexylresorcinol.* Amer. J. Hyg. 1931, Vol. 13, p. 803.

6. Cort, W. W. *Recent Investigations on the Epidemiology of Human Ascariasis.* J. Parasit. 1931, Vol. 17, p. 121.

7. Lamson, P. D., Caldwell, E. L. *et al. Hexylresorcinol in the Treatment of Human Ascariasis.* Amer. J. Hyg. 1931, Vol. 13, p. 568.

8. Rhoads, C. P. and Castle, W. B. Journal of Clinical Investigation. 1932, Vol. 11, p. 809.

9. Leathers, W. S. and Keller, A. E. *Investigations Concerning Hookworm Disease in Southern States, with Suggestions for Continued Control.* South. Med. Jour. 1936, Vol. 29, p. 172.

10. Foster, A. O. and Cort, W. W. *Further Studies on Effect of Generally Deficient Diet upon Resistance of Dogs to Hookworm Infection.* Am. J. Hyg. 1935, Vol. 21, p. 302.

11. Hall, M. C. *Studies on Oxyuriasis: Types of Anal Scrapers, with a Description of an Improved Type of Swab.* Am. J. Trop. Med. 1937, Vol. 17, p. 445.

# CHAPTER XVII

## A MISCELLANEOUS GROUP OF DISEASES OF PUBLIC HEALTH IMPORTANCE

### UNDULANT FEVER (BRUCELLOSIS)

UNDULANT fever has undoubtedly been fairly prevalent in the United States for many years, but only recently have health departments begun to recognize its frequency and importance. There is some evidence that the disease is increasing, although it seems more probable that the increase is apparent and is due to better diagnosis and thus more frequent recognition.

**Etiology.** Undulant fever is due to *Brucella melitensis*. There are three common strains, the caprine, bovine and porcine. The caprine strain is highly virulent to humans, but fortunately it prevails in only a few restricted areas in the United States. The bovine strain has a relatively low virulence for human beings. The porcine strain occupies an intermediate place, less virulent than the caprine strain, more virulent than the bovine strain.

**Prevalence.** Undulant fever in man has a wide distribution throughout the United States. It has been reported from every state in the Union, but is much more prevalent in those states that have a large cattle and hog industry. Hardy has studied over 800 cases from Iowa. *B. abortus* and *B. suis* varieties of the organisms are about equally responsible for morbidity. The disease is most common among rural male adults.

**Mode of Infection.** In urban regions the disease is transmitted chiefly through raw milk from cattle that are infected with the abortus variety of Brucella. Hardy believes that most of the persons who develop the disease in Iowa are infected from direct contact with infected hogs or cattle.

**Incubation Period.** The average incubation period of the disease is two weeks, but may vary from five days to four weeks.

**Diagnosis.** Undulant fever is important to the health officer, not only because it is a preventable disease itself, but also because it is frequently confused with typhoid fever, malaria, tuberculosis, influenza and other febrile conditions. The disease is characterized by an evening rise in temperature, accompanied by weakness and associated with chills and night sweats. The febrile period may be as short as three weeks or may

173

last for many months. The case fatality rate is low, but the patient may lose weight and strength and become a chronic invalid. The disease is characterized by a leukopenia and the spleen may be palpable. There may be a long period of quiescence followed by a relapse with return of all the typical symptoms.

Definite diagnosis is made by suitable blood agglutination tests. The specific agglutinins are usually present in the blood by the tenth day of the disease and by the end of the third or fourth week the agglutination titer is sufficiently high so as to leave no doubt as to the cause of illness.

Many persons in the community have some immunity to the infection, as evidenced by agglutinins in the blood. In communities where pasteurization of milk is not a common practice, a large proportion of the population will develop agglutinins.

Blood cultures are not a satisfactory diagnostic procedure.

**Control.** The disease is almost never transmitted from person to person. Thus isolation and quarantine measures are not required. Laboratory infections in those scientists who have studied these organisms show a high incidence, with many severe infections. Proper pasteurization of milk is the most effective measure in prevention of undulant fever that is available at present. State departments of animal industry have taken active measures in many states to rid infected herds of *Brucella* infection. In some districts the infection rate in cattle is very high and elimination of the infection is a slow process. A few dairies that produce certified milk have succeeded in completely eliminating abortus infection from their herds; but the basic preventive measure is milk pasteurization.

**Vaccines.** Huddleson has prepared a vaccine which he believes is of real value in cutting short the attack of the disease. Prophylactic vaccination in the United States is not a feasible procedure because of the relatively low attack rate.

Along the French Mediterranean Coast, where the caprine form of the bacillus prevails, with a case fatality rate of 7 per cent, the authorities have recommended vaccination for all those who are specially exposed—particularly goat and sheep herders. Huddleson has written a comprehensive review of the whole subject of undulant fever. Students are referred to this authoritative source for detailed information concerning this important group of diseases.

## BUBONIC PLAGUE

Bubonic plague is historically one of the great destroyers of mankind. It has invaded the United States many times in the past, causing sharp epidemics in the vicinity of seaports, but until recently it did not become endemic in this country. The disease is primarily an infection of rodents, and is transmitted from animal to animal by the bite of a flea. Man is infected more or less incidentally, and epidemics in man only follow extensive epizootics in rats.

The infection has been introduced into Pacific Coast ports many times before and since the San Francisco epidemic of 1900, and strenuous efforts have been made to prevent the infection from spreading to the interior. These efforts have not been successful. The infection has been spread, by ground squirrels chiefly, and is now found in at least ten species of these rodents. The infection is now known to exist in endemic form in at least nine of the far western states, exclusive of California. It has been found on the eastern slope of the Great Continental Divide and is beginning to spread to the great plains east of the Rockies.

Cases of human infection are rare. The disease is spread without detection over a wide area in the wild rodents that have little contact with man. Prairie dogs, chipmunks, marmots, and many other rodents aid as agents of dispersion. Domestic rats as yet have not been infected in recent years except in the cities on the Pacific Coast.

**Control.** Control of plague resolves itself into a continuous fight against the transmitter of the infection—the rodent. Eradication of ground squirrels is an endless task, expensive, and, because of the nature of the terrain, relatively ineffective.

Thus, there is now widely established in the United States an endemic plague focus that will remain as a potential menace for years to come. It is possible that the rats of some large interior city may become infected. If this occurs, an epidemic of plague in human beings may follow. Sporadic cases of human infection will occur annually in the remote mountainous regions of the country.

The great dread of bubonic plague that has prevailed through the centuries has now been dispelled, in great part, through the discovery that sulfadiazine is an effective therapeutic agent in this disease. Penicillin has little effect on the organism, but streptomycin readily controls the plague bacillus, even in high dilutions of the drug.

The reader who has a special interest in the control of sylvatic plague in the United States is referred to a splendid discussion of the subject by K. F. Meyer, "The Prevention of Plague in the Light of Newer Knowledge," reported at the New York Academy of Sciences, Section on Biology, in March 1946.

## TULAREMIA ("RABBIT FEVER")

Tularemia is due to *B. tularense*. This organism is pathogenic to a great many wild animals, including some game birds, but practically all human infections are acquired from contact with infected rabbits. The disease was first discovered in Tulare County, California, and was thought to have a somewhat limited distribution, but is now widely spread throughout the United States. Better diagnostic methods may have played some part in this increase, but other factors have certainly contributed to it. Sportsmen have introduced western rabbits throughout the eastern seaboard, thus implanting the infection in virgin territory, so that all parts of the country are now infected. In the fall of 1938 the State of Illinois alone reported 501 cases of tularemia during the rabbit hunting season, with a case fatality rate of 7 per cent. The disease occurs in rabbits in widespread epizootics at intervals of several years. It is spread from animal to animal (and sometimes to man) by insect bites. Ticks are the most common transmitting agent in animal infections.

The disease in the rabbit is characterized by numerous whitish-gray spots in the liver and other organs. The animal may appear sick or sluggish, but often shows no noticeable signs of illness. Man is infected, as a rule, through a scratch or other break in the skin, while handling infected wild rabbits. The incubation period of the disease is about three days, followed by chills, backache, prostration and high fever of two to three weeks' duration. Often there is a persistent glandular enlargement of the lymphatic area draining the primary lesion. Diagnosis is made by positive agglutination tests.

**Control.** Control measures are largely educational. Every hunter should know that he should use heavy rubber gloves whenever he "dresses" wild game. Foshay [1] has recommended the use of a vaccine in those persons particularly exposed, as for example, meat handlers, handlers of wild rabbits and other game. The vaccine is given in three doses at weekly intervals, and protects for about one year. The internal organs of game should be examined for the characteristic lesions, and in any suspicious case the carcass should be buried. The thoroughly cooked meat is, of course, harmless as food, so that the only damage that occurs is in the handling of the carcass.

In 1939 Baltimore had such a bad experience with tularemia—31 reported cases and 8 deaths—that the health department prohibited entirely the importation and sale of wild rabbits and hares.

Streptomycin has been discovered [2] to have a dramatic effect in the treatment of tularemia. It is given intramuscularly in 1 to 2 gram doses every 4 hours until the disease is under control.

## EQUINE ENCEPHALITIS

An epidemic of encephalitis that occurred in young children in Massachusetts in the summer of 1938 focused attention on the danger of equine encephalitis to man. Equine encephalitis is primarily a disease not of horses but of fowls and birds. It is transmitted to horses by the bite of an *Aedes* mosquito. The mosquito bites the infected animal during the active stages of the disease, passes through an incubation period of four or five days, and then remains infectious for life.

The disease is due to a virus, and there appears to be an eastern and a western strain. A disastrous epizootic occurred in American horses in

[1] Foshay, L.: *Arch. Int. Med.* 1937, Vol. 60, p. 22.

[2] Howe, Calderon, Coriell, L. L., Bookwalter, H. L. and Ellingson, H. V.: "Streptomycin Treatment in Tularemia. *J.A.M.A.* 1946, Vol. 132, p. 195.

1938, which caused great loss to western farmers. A very successful vaccine for prevention of the disease in horses has been developed under the direction of Tenbroeck and his associates at the Rockefeller Institute.

Infection of human beings with equine encephalitis was first noted in 1938 in Minnesota. The outbreak, of some 40 cases, in children in Massachusetts, reported by Wesselhoeft and his co-workers, had a high case fatality rate. The disease is transmitted from animals to man by the bite of a mosquito, and infection occurs, therefore, in the environs of an animal epizootic of the disease. Birds and wild fowl are believed to be the reservoir of infection with this virus.

**Control Measures.** Community-wide immunization of horses will presumably serve as a protection against human infection. The health officer should do everything in his power by educational means and otherwise to aid the agricultural department in securing complete vaccination of all horses in any infected area. Human vaccination has not been used widely because of the low attack rate. All measures that are taken to control mosquitoes should presumably aid in prevention of this infection. There are no available methods for prevention or control of post-influenzal encephalitis, nor encephalitis following measles or smallpox vaccination.

## EPIDEMIC ENCEPHALITIS

Encephalitis sometimes follows such common virus diseases as measles and vaccinia. A world-wide epidemic followed the pandemic of influenza in 1918–20, and seemed at that time to be related in its epidemiology to influenza.

In 1933 an extensive epidemic of epidemic encephalitis occurred in St. Louis, with over a thousand cases. It was primarily a disease of adults. This disease occurred in the summer and was due to a virus. The disease resembled Japanese *B encephalitis,* but the viruses of the two diseases, though similar, are immunologically distinct.

## ROCKY MOUNTAIN SPOTTED FEVER

The staff of the United States Public Health Service deserves great credit for its tenacious attack on Rocky Mountain spotted fever. The epidemiology of the disease has been worked out very carefully, the etiology determined, and a specific prophylaxis developed. These studies were confined in great part, in the past, to the Bitter Root Valley, Montana, for the disease had a very limited distribution.

Then, for unknown reasons, the disease spread to various parts of the United States, as far as the eastern seaboard, and has now been reported in almost every state in the Union.

In the eastern states the disease is spread by the bite of the dog tick, *Dermacentor variabilis,* and therefore, potentially, the disease may now be considered as present wherever this tick is found. In heavily infected

Montana areas one tick in 300 is infected with the virus of the disease.

The incubation period of the disease in man is from 4 to 14 days. The onset is sudden, with a chill followed by a rapid rise in temperature, and severe headache. A rash appears three or four days after the onset, first on the arms and legs and then spreading to other parts of the body. The case fatality rate is high—10 per cent to 25 per cent.

**Control.** A very effective method of personal prophylaxis, in tick-infested areas, is to institute a search for ticks every night immediately on return from the forest or field. The danger of infection is greatest if the tick has fed for 6 to 8 hours. If it is removed quickly—within two to four hours—there is little probability of infection. One should look carefully under the arms, in the groin, at the hair line at the back of the neck, and behind the ears. The ticks should be removed with forceps and should not be crushed in the fingers. After the ticks have been removed, the area bitten and also the hands should be washed with alcohol.

A very effective vaccine has been developed as a preventive in Rocky Mountain spotted fever. It should be given once a year, preferably in early May. It has no value unless given at least ten days before the bite of the infected tick.

Widespread vaccination is not advisable. The use of the vaccine should be limited to known heavily infected areas and should be given to those who are most exposed to the bites.

In heavily infected areas, various measures that have been employed to reduce the tick population have met with considerable success.

The Pacific campaign of World War II demonstrated that it is quite feasible to protect a man against ticks by the use of insect repellents. Dimethylphthalate and benzyl benzoate are both very effective. A forester or other person who has a constant exposure to tick bites may protect himself very effectively by impregnation of his trousers with benzyl benzoate. Persons subject to casual exposure may simply spray the repellent about their ankles and legs to the knees. (See Chapter XXII on insect repellents.)

## ENDEMIC TYPHUS FEVER

*Epidemic* typhus fever, which has devastated Europe and invaded the United States many times during the past century, is not a serious menace to this country at the moment. It is related to extreme poverty, over-crowding, war, and human desolation. The vector is the human body louse.

The remarkable success that was obtained in the control of typhus in the Mediterranean area by the United States of America Typhus Commission during World War II was one of the brilliant epidemiological achievements of the war. The utilization of DDT and other insecticides was responsible for this result. It has revolutionized administrative methods in the control of typhus, and undoubtedly saved a great many lives, particularly in the civilian population that was devastated by the war.

*Endemic* typhus fever maintains itself in the rat as a reservoir and is transmitted to man by the rat flea. The disease either did not exist or was not recognized until its epidemiology was worked out by Maxcy, Dyer, and other epidemiologists of the United States Public Health Service.

More than 2000 cases [3] are known to occur annually. The disease is found chiefly in the southern tier of states and occurs in both rural and urban areas. The case fatality rate is low: 5 per cent to 10 per cent.

After an incubation period of twelve to fourteen days, the disease begins with severe headache, chills, and high fever. Mental and nervous symptoms may be marked. Prostration is severe.

The rash, which appears about the third day of the fever, is small, pinkish, discrete, and appears first on the abdomen and chest, later spreading to the arms, legs, and back with little involvement of the head. A crisis occurs about the fourteenth day.

The disease is frequently confused with Rocky Mountain spotted fever, cerebrospinal meningitis, and sometimes with typhoid fever. In its early stages the disease is often called influenza. The characteristic rash is a valuable aid in differential diagnosis. A positive Weil-Felix blood test is of value in diagnosis, but it does not appear until late in the second week of the disease.

**Control.** Successful vaccine has been prepared for endemic typhus, but the present low endemicity of the disease does not warrant community-wide immunization procedures, even in the most heavily infected areas of Georgia, Alabama, and Texas.

Intensification of rat control through destroying rat-breeding places and decreasing available rat food supply is the method that offers great promise of success in the control of human infection with this disease.

Control of rat fleas and other insects by DDT sprays has also been recommended as a useful measure in control of endemic typhus.

**Rickettsialpox.** An extensive outbreak [4] of a new disease resembling

[3] 1938 reports of endemic typhus fever were as follows:

|  | Cases | Deaths |
|---|---|---|
| South Atlantic States .......... | 1,278 | 77 |
| West South Central States ...... | 525 | 35 |
| East South Central States ........ | 390 | 24 |
| Pacific States .................. | 21 | 0 |
| Middle Atlantic States .......... | 13 | 0 |
| East North Central States ...... | 4 | 1 |
| New England States ............ | 2 | 0 |
|  | 2,233 | 137 |

[4] Huebner, R. J., Stamps, P. and Armstrong, C.: "Rickettsialpox: A Newly Recognized Rickettsial Disease." *Pub. Health Reports.* 1946, Vol. 61, p. 1605.

typhus fever was discovered in New York in 1946. It is an infection of mice which is transmitted to man by a rodent mite.

## PSITTACOSIS AND ORNITHOSIS

Psittacosis is primarily a disease of birds of the parrot family, but has been transmitted to canaries and other pet birds. It is a virus disease which is transmitted by contact with sick birds and with healthy carriers. Transfer of the disease to man is quite frequent wherever there is contact of man with birds of the parrot family. Several serious outbreaks have occurred. The disease in man has been confused with pneumonia, with typhoid fever, and with influenza. The case fatality rate is high—20 per cent to 40 per cent.

Restriction of importation from the tropics of birds of the parrot family has not controlled the disease, because the infection became endemic in the parrakeet (love bird) industry in Southern California.

**Control Measures.** The control measures that have been enforced with considerable success are:

1. Destruction of all birds from infected aviaries, and thorough disinfection of contaminated premises.
2. Licensing of aviaries and issuance of shipping permits. Each healthy bird has an identifying leg band, indicating its source and date of shipment.
3. Quarantine of all birds of the parrot family that come to the United States from foreign ports.

Despite these rigorous regulations, an outbreak of human psittacosis occurred in a large eastern city. It was discovered that the "love birds" carrying the epidemic had been shipped from California under a forged permit and with illegal leg bands. Following this episode, several states prohibited entirely the importation or sale of birds of the parrot family within their jurisdiction. This is the policy now recommended by most health officers.

Ornithosis is due to a psittacosis-like virus. It is an infection of pigeons, chickens, ducks, turkeys, and other domestic and wild fowl. The disease is transmitted readily from the sick birds to man, but is seldom transmitted from man to man. An atypical pneumonia is produced which is sometimes very difficult to differentiate from other types of atypical pneumonia. The virus is found in the respiratory secretions of sick animals and man. In some instances, an apparently healthy bird carrier has transmitted the disease to man. A diagnosis of the disease may be made by animal inoculation of the infected secretions.

Epidemics of ornithosis have been reported in man, but more commonly the disease occurs endemically, and if followed carefully, may be traced to contact with infected birds.

The interested reader is referred to an extensive literature on this and related diseases at the end of this chapter.

## TETANUS

*Cl. tetani* is an anaerobic spore-bearing organism which is found normally in the intestinal tract of horses. It finds favorable opportunity for development in human beings in injured and macerated tissues, producing a strong toxin which is absorbed along the nerve trunks. It was at one time a greatly dreaded disease, fairly prevalent, and highly fatal. Its disappearance is due in large part to modern industrial motorized development, but also to better understanding of the nature of the disease, better surgical technic in débridement of wounds, and almost universal use of potent tetanus antitoxin following deep, destructive wounds.

The antitoxin is given as soon as possible after the wound has occurred. Only a small dose is required as a passive immunizing agent, but a second dose may be required when the passive immunity wears off after two or three weeks. Many health departments furnish prophylactic tetanus antitoxin to all indigent patients who have been injured and may be in need of protection against tetanus toxin.

**Alum Precipitated Tetanus Toxoid.** Utilization of alum precipitated tetanus toxoid is a logical development, following similar work with diphtheria toxoid. The results are highly satisfactory.

Active immunization against tetanus was universal in American soldiers during World War II. The results were striking. Practically no cases of tetanus occurred in the wounded soldiers, despite the heavy exposure in the European battlefields. Standard military immunization practice during World War II was:

1. Initial immunization. 0.5 cc. of alum precipitated toxoid; two injections given intramuscularly not less than 4 or more than 8 weeks apart.

2. Routine "booster" immunizations. One year after initial immunization, each individual is given 0.5 cc. of alum precipitated toxoid, and thereafter every 4 years.

3. Emergency "booster" immunization. Individuals who are wounded or receive a severe burn in battle, or who receive punctured or lacerated non-battle wounds, are given an emergency immunization of 0.5 cc. of alum precipitated toxoid.

Tetanus antitoxin is reserved for clinical treatment of tetanus, and as a passive immunization of those who have not, for any reason, received active immunization with tetanus toxoid.

This technic produced a very high degree of immunity against tetanus infection.

Rogers has recommended its use in private practice for:

1. Asthmatic persons, particularly those who are sensitive to horse serum and who live in the country.

2. Persons who are in constant contact with horses and frequently exposed to possible infection.

Tetanus vaccination is not an essential health department procedure because the chance of infection of the average person at the present time is not great.

Many pediatricians incorporate tetanus immunization in their routine program of childhood immunization. It is a simple protective measure, and is quite justified as a procedure in preventive medicine.

## INFECTIOUS HEPATITIS (CATARRHAL JAUNDICE)

World War II called our attention to the public health importance of infectious hepatitis.

**Epidemiology.** This disease may occur in epidemic form, or may occur sporadically. It is due to a filtrable virus which is present in the fecal discharges of the patient. The incubation period is long—21 days. Havens [5] transmitted the disease to human volunteers. Those fed with feces developed the disease in 20 days, whereas intracutaneous injection of the virus resulted in an incubation period of 64 days, on the average.

The disease is most common in children and young adults, but may occur at any age. The case fatality rate is low, but the disease may be severe and its effects prolonged.

Many individuals undoubtedly have the disease in unrecognized form, and it seems most probable, from its epidemiology, that carriers occur. Stokes and Neefe [6] described an extensive epidemic that occurred in children in a summer camp, and which was probably due to infection of the camp water supply. They also produced evidence that administration of gamma globulin to the exposed children prevented the disease in many of the exposed individuals.

The disease may be transmitted to a recipient of a blood transfusion from a donor who seems perfectly well.

Murphy [7] has described an epidemic due to polluted raw milk. (See page 204.)

**Control.** Measures which are taken to promote adequate disposal of human feces and other secretions certainly will aid in prevention of the spread of infectious hepatitis. Reporting of the disease may be considered as a worth-while procedure by the health officer, particularly if facilities and personnel are available to investigate possible sources of infection. Isolation of the patient during the first week of his illness is a reasonable precaution. However, few cases have been traced to contact with an acute case of this illness. Proper disposal of the discharges of the patient is important.

[5] Havens, W. P., Jr., Ward, Robert, Drill, V. A. and Paul, J. R.: "Experimental Production of Hepatitis by Feeding Icterogenic Materials." *Proc. Soc. Exp. Med. and Biol.* 1944, Vol. 57, p. 206.

[6] Stokes, Joseph, Jr. and Neefe, J. R.: "The Prevention and Attenuation of Infectious Hepatitis by Gamma Globulin." *J.A.M.A.* 1945, Vol. 127, p. 144.

[7] Murphy, W. J., Petrie, L. M. and Work, S. D.: "Outbreak of Infectious Hepatitis, Apparently Milk-borne." *Am. J. Pub. Health.* 1946, Vol. 36, p. 169.

# REFERENCES

## UNDULANT FEVER

1. Huddleson, I. F. *Undulant Fever*. 1934. Publication of the Commonwealth Fund, New York City.
2. Hardy, A. V., Jordan, C. F. *et al. Undulant Fever, with Special Reference to a Study in Iowa*. National Institute of Health Bulletin. 1930. Dec., p. 158.
3. Evans, A. C. *Further Studies on Bacterium Abortus and Related Bacteria*. J. Inf. Dis. 1918, Vol. 22, p. 580.
4. Readers are also referred to the *Symposium on Undulant Fever* by various authors. J. Amer. Pub. Health Assn. 1931, Vol. 21, p. 491.
5. DuBois, C. and Sollier, N. *Inefficiency of Legislation against Brucellosis*. Bulletin of Academy of Medicine of Paris. 1939, Vol. 121, p. 256.

## BUBONIC PLAGUE

Eskey, C. R. and Haas, V. H. *Plague in the Western Part of the United States*. Public Health Reports. 1939, Vol. 54, p. 1467.

## EPIDEMIC ENCEPHALITIS

1. Matheson Commission, Third Report. *Epidemic Encephalitis: Etiology, Epidemiology Treatment*. Columbia University Press. 1939.
2. Eklund, C. N. and Blumstein, A. *Relation of Human Encephalitis to Encephalomyelitis in Horses*. J. Amer. Med. Assn. 1938, Vol. 111, p. 1734.
3. Wesselhoeft, C., Smith, E. C. and Branch, C. F. *Human Encephalitis: 8 Fatal Cases, with 4 Due to Virus of Equine Encephalomyelitis*. J. Amer. Med. Assn. 1938, Vol. 111, p. 1735.

## PSITTACOSIS AND ORNITHOSIS

1. Enders, J. F. *Psittacosis in Virus and Rickettsial Diseases*. Cambridge. Harvard University Press. 1940.
2. Meyer, K. F. *The Ecology of Psittacosis and Ornithosis*. Medicine. 1942, Vol. 21, p. 175.
3. Eddie, B. and Francis, Thomas, Jr. *Occurrence of Psittacosis-like Infection in Domestic and Game Birds of Michigan*. Proc. Soc. Exp. Biol. and Med. 1942, Vol. 50, p. 291.
4. Levinson, D. C., Gibbs, J. and Beardwood, J. T. *Ornithosis as a Cause of Atypical Pneumonia*. J.A.M.A. 1944, Vol. 126, p. 1079.

## TETANUS

Rogers, R. P. *The Use of Tetanus Toxoid in Private Practice*. Bulletin of N. Y. Academy of Medicine. 1939, Vol. 15, p. 553.

# PART III

# BASIC ACTIVITIES OF A HEALTH ORGANIZATION

# CHAPTER XVIII

## VITAL STATISTICS

"The force of mortality pressing upon a people may in some degree be weighed and measured by accurate enumeration of the number and ages of the living and the location, circumstances and causes of death, and intelligent abstract of these facts."[1]

Vital statistics is the science which considers the application of statistical methods to certain vital facts. The science is a part of a very much broader subject; namely, the science of demography.

"Broadly speaking, demography is a statistical study of human life. It deals with vital facts, such as birth, growth, marriage, sickness and death, and incidentally with political, social, religious, educational, sanitary and medical matters" (Whipple).

The health officer is interested in all phases of demography, but certain divisions of the subject are his special responsibility. For example, the field of demography includes a study of eugenics and genealogy. The health officer may have more than an academic interest in these subjects, but they do not concern his work directly. On the other hand, the measurements of human growth and development are a subdivision of the science of demography which has a direct application to the field of child hygiene, and is thus of direct interest to public health. Pathometrics is a study of pathological conditions of mankind. This subdivision of demography is of primary interest to the pathologist and clinician, but also of direct interest to the alert health officer. His special responsibilities in the field of demography are (a) registration and (b) biometrics.

The science of biometrics deals with the application of mathematical methods to vital data. These two phases of demography—registration of vital data and their analysis—comprise the field of *vital statistics*. Because of their direct relationship to the health and welfare of the people it has gradually become recognized that they are a direct governmental function and, as such, have been incorporated in official health department practice.

The recognition by the various governments in the United States, local, state and federal, of the importance of vital statistics as a governmental function is a comparatively recent event. Such elemental governmental functions as simple registration of births and deaths have not been re-

[1] Lemuel Shattuck. *Census of the City of Boston.* 1845.

187

quired of local communities in many of our states until very recent years. Even when registration is required by law, the laws have not been enforced. Thus, a great portion of the vital statistics data of the nation from its early history up through the end of the last century are in a chaotic state. Even at the present time births and deaths are not reported satisfactorily and completely in a few of the states.

Statistics are facts expressed in figures. For example, a birth report recorded officially is not a vital statistic, but a vital fact. These facts may be expressed by figures, classified, tabulated and arranged in various ways for study and comparison. These tabulations and classifications may be visualized by the use of graphs. The various mathematical processes that are used in analysis of the vital facts make it possible to formulate generalizations and to draw logical conclusions or inferences from the basic data.

The primary responsibility of the health department is the collection and analysis of vital facts that have a direct bearing upon the public health. Certain essential steps must be taken to secure a satisfactory result:

1. Census. A complete enumeration of the population.
2. Registration. Accurate recording of vital facts.
3. Statistical analysis of vital facts.
4. Logical interpretation of the analysis with conclusions.

**Census.** The health department must have a fairly complete enumeration of the people within its jurisdiction. This is as necessary for the small city or county health department as for the state. The information should include the distribution of the population by geographic areas, as well as the age and sex distribution. Other important information includes: racial distribution of the population, occupation, and, to some degree at least, the distribution of wealth. All these data, together with other valuable information, are obtained at ten-year intervals by the federal census. Through the use of suitable statistical methods a very fair estimate of the above data may be obtained for any area during any given intercensal period.

**Registration.** We have already noted that registration of vital facts is a governmental function, which is a recent conception in the United States. Formerly, this activity was regarded as a semi-religious or a social function. A few of the states have compiled fairly accurate records of births and deaths for over a hundred years. These death records give some indication at least of the causes of death. Each state followed its own method of registration and there was no uniformity of plan, or standard system of classification. It is obviously impossible to secure accurate registration and analysis of vital data on a nation-wide basis without a uniform nation-wide plan of registration.

The national registration area for deaths was initiated in 1880. The Federal Bureau of the Census required for admission of any state to the

national registration area:
1. Satisfactory state laws and a suitable system for registration.
2. At least 90 per cent completeness of reporting.

Various checks are used by the Federal Census Bureau to determine whether a given state has fulfilled all requirements. The national registration area began with the states of Massachusetts and New Jersey, the District of Columbia and nineteen cities. Gradually the various states were admitted by the Federal Census Bureau so that every state is now included in the National Registration Area for Deaths. The National Birth Registration Area was established in 1915. Criteria for admission were similar to those required for admission to the death registration area. All states have met the federal requirements, though a few states have difficulty in maintaining the national registration standards. This formation of national registration areas marks one of the major progressive steps in public health administration in the United States. It was brought about through formulation of a model registrational law which was first presented to the official Association of State Health Officers and approved by it. This model law has gradually been adopted by the various states.

Registration of all births and deaths within the state is a function of the state health department. The state health officer, or some other person on his staff, who is responsible to, and is designated by him, is the official state registrar of vital statistics.

The basis for effective registration is the formation of an organization whereby each birth and each death that occurs within the state shall be recorded immediately on an individual certificate. Standard uniform certificate forms may be used, as well as standard methods of collection of the certificates and standard methods of interpretation of the data. These certificates are filed as a permanent record, and become a part of the state archives.

**Conventional Bases Used in Expressing Vital Statistics Rates.** There are certain simple ratios in expressing vital statistics that have been adopted by international agreement and accepted in international usage, as follows:

*Crude Death Rate* (general death rate) : The number of deaths per 1,000 population.

*Birth Rate:* The number of live births per 1,000 population.

*Stillbirth Rate:* The number of stillbirths per 100 live births.

*Infant Mortality Rate:* The number of deaths under one year of age per 1,000 live births.

*Neonatal Mortality Rate:* The number of deaths in infants under one month of age per 1,000 live births.

*Standardized Death Rate:* The number of deaths that would have occurred per 1,000 in some selected standard population (such as the population of England and Wales in 1901) if its age-specific-death rates were the same as that of a given community.

*Maternal Mortality Rate:* The number of deaths from puerperal causes per 1,000 live births.

*Death Rate from a Specific Disease:* The number of deaths from that specific cause, per 100,000 population.

*Death Rate at a Specific Age:* The number of deaths at that particular age, per 100,000, 10,000 or 1,000 population.

*Morbidity Rate:* The number of cases of a particular disease, per 100,000 population.

*Case Fatality Rate:* The number of deaths from a specific disease, per 100 cases of that disease.

The conventional unit of time observed in expressing rates is one year.

## ORGANIZATION OF REGISTRATION FOR VITAL STATISTICS

The state is divided into registration districts, with an official local registrar for each district. The unit varies in different states. It may include a whole city or town, but is usually a voting district. The local registrar must be more or less familiar with local events, and thus may check unreported births and deaths in the community. The local registrar should be selected by the state health officer or his representative—the state registrar of vital statistics—and should be subject to removal from office by the state health department in case his duties are not performed properly. Wherever there is a well-organized local health service, such as a city health department or full-time county health department, the local health officer should be appointed by the state registrar as deputy registrar of vital statistics for his whole jurisdiction. In this case the local registrars report directly to the local health officer, and become, in reality, part-time members of his staff. In those areas where there is no organized health service with competent personnel, the local registrars report directly to the state. Local registrars are usually paid a fee for each certificate. The rate varies from 25 cents to 50 cents. The local governmental unit, county, township or incorporated city, pays the local registrars annually. The expenditures for vital statistics activities of the state are incorporated in the budget of the state health department.

Deaths are reported to the local registrar by the person who has charge of the interment of the body. A standard certificate, properly filled out, must be filed with the local registrar before a burial permit may be granted. Burial permits are usually issued by the local registrar. Deaths are reported immediately; that is, a reasonable period of 36 to 48 hours is given for filing the report. The medical data of the certificate are filled out by the physician who attended the person in his last illness. The standard International Classification of Causes of Death is utilized for determination not only of the primary cause of death, but also the contributory causes. In most states, some special provision is made for those instances in which the deceased was unattended by a physician during his last illness. The authorized person who shall certify as to cause of death, under these circumstances, may be a member of the staff of the department of health. In some states the coroner system is used, and in others an official medical examiner is employed to investigate all cases of accidental or sudden death, or death from unknown causes.

Births are reported to the local registrar by the person who was responsible for the delivery of the child: physician, midwife or lying-in hospital, as the case may be. The usual period allotted for filing the birth certificate is ten days. These certificates are of great significance, since the child has no real legal proof of existence in the eyes of the state without a proper birth certificate. The state archives of birth certificates are constantly consulted to prove citizenship, to prove exact age, to obtain permission to enter school, or to seek employment under the child labor laws of the state, or to determine whether the individual has reached marriageable age, for determinations of old age benefits, social security benefits, and for many other purposes. The person may wish to prove his right to vote, to hold public office, to inherit property, or to obtain a pension. The state may use the birth certificate to prove liability for military service.

The national Social Security Act proved to be a great stimulus to accurate birth certification. Many people had never considered a birth certificate to be of any importance until old age assistance, unemployment insurance, and other ramifications of the Social Security Act demonstrated to them that it was necessary to have this official proof of their existence. Everyone in the United States is now willing to agree that each child born is entitled to proper certification of its birth. If the person who is responsible for filing the certificate does not do so, he should be penalized. The model law carries a penalty clause for failure to report births and deaths.

Each stillbirth may be reported as both a death and a birth. Many states use a separate type of certificate for stillbirths. In case of plural births, a certificate should be filed for each child. If a child is unnamed at the end of ten days, the certificate should be filed and a supplementary slip sent with the name at some later date, but not later than one year after birth. The local registrars collect the certificates, check them for error, and make a copy of the essential data of identification. These are recorded by serial number. The original certificates are forwarded at monthly intervals to the state registrar. If the city or county health officer has been selected as deputy state registrar, the local registrar sends the monthly collection of certificates to him. The local health department makes a complete copy of the certificate for its own files, and checks the certificate for errors, paying particular attention to errors in the proper classification of the diagnosis of the cause of death. The original certificates are always sent to the state bureau of vital statistics.

Summaries of state vital statistics data are forwarded by each state to the National Bureau of the Census for nation-wide analysis and interpretation.

The commonest errors of physicians in filing death certificates are, according to one experienced registrar of vital statistics,

1. Physician fails to state date of attendance on patient.
   a. If the patient has been attended by the doctor less than 24 hours prior to death, the certificate must be filed by the medical examiner. (New York State.)
   b. If the physician has attended the patient for some time (months or years) but has not seen him alive ten days prior to death, the case should be referred to the medical examiner. (New York State.)
2. Physician fails to give the time of death.
3. Physician fails to write legibly. *This is most important.*
4. Physician fails to fill in the date of onset at the right of the certificate.
5. Physician fails to state principal cause of death in proper place, sometimes giving the final symptoms under cause of death and the actual cause of death under "Contributory causes."
6. Physician uses improper terms for cause of death, such as:

| | |
|---|---|
| Heart disease | Natural causes |
| Heart failure | Senility |
| Pneumonia | Peritonitis |
| Cancer | Pulmonary hemorrhage |
| Convulsions | |

7. Physician fails to refer to the proper authorities deaths due to traumatism. In many states, any death caused by trauma or accidental injury, regardless of the time when the accident occurred, must be reported by the medical examiner. *E.g.:* A patient injured in an automobile accident is in bed for six months due to a fractured pelvis; he contracts a hypostatic pneumonia and dies. The medical examiner must file the certificate, not the attending physician.
8. The family physician should not certify to deaths:

| | |
|---|---|
| Following abortion | Drowning |
| Due to occupation | Electric shock |
| Suicide | Poisoning |
| Homicide | Sudden deaths and persons found dead |

9. Physician fails to fill in properly the question regarding occupation.
10. Physician fails to write his name so that it can be read. Even though the rest of the certificate is legible, some men develop characteristic illegible signatures.

The state bureau of vital statistics checks the certificates for error. The chief difficulties that arise relate to proper classification of the cause of death. It is frequently necessary to correspond with the physician who signed the certificate in order to obtain a true picture of the condition.

The certificates are bound and filed in fireproof vaults and are kept as part of the state archives.

**Morbidity Reporting.** The reporting to the health department of certain diseases dangerous to the public health is required by law in all the states. These morbidity reports bear a direct relationship to mortality reports, but since the machinery for reporting morbidity is quite different from that of reporting mortality, it seems advisable to discuss morbidity reporting under the subject of communicable disease control.

**Registration of Marriage and Divorce.** Registration of marriage and divorce is not a public health function. For purposes of convenience the state registrar of vital statistics in some states is given the responsibility of proper state registration and analysis of the data relating to marriage and divorce.

## ANALYSIS OF DATA BY STATISTICAL METHODS

It is not the province of this text to discuss the details of statistical methodology. Suffice it to say that no health officer is equipped to carry out his work effectively unless he is familiar with the simple fundamental principles of statistical methods. If he uses proper methods, he will be able to avoid many pitfalls; he will not compare things that are not comparable, nor generalize from inadequate data. There are now many excellent texts that cover this field adequately. A list of books that the author has found to be most helpful in this field is given at the end of this chapter.

The proper interpretation of recorded data is the most important feature of the work of the department of vital statistics. It is possible, of course, to draw certain logical inferences, if suitable statistical methods are used, even when the initial recording of data is not perfectly exact. One never gets perfect records. One of the essential functions of the health department, however, is to secure as accurate recording as possible, since, in the end, no conclusions or inferences are stronger than the initial data on which they rest. Statistical methods make possible certain logical conclusions or inferences in regard to trends. They enable the health officer to analyze the effectiveness of the activities of his own department, to compare results secured in the area under his jurisdiction with the results obtained in similar areas elsewhere, and to plan his program so as to meet the special needs of his particular community.

**Compilation and Tabulation of Data.** Standardized criteria should be used in compilation of data. Deaths are classified according to the International List of Causes of Death. Certain standard tabulations are made which are commonly included as a part of statistical practice by all health departments. Special tabulations may be made that relate to subjects in which the health department is particularly interested.

Tabulation of data is a tedious process at best. Most state health departments have tabulating machines, punching machines and other necessary equipment for rapid and accurate tabulations. Some of the larger cities also have the necessary facilities for mechanical tabulation. The Hollerith system is used by most health departments for mechanical tabulation. The sorter will separate 350 properly punched cards per minute.

Whenever the tabulation is purely mechanical, requiring the cross index-
ing of a mass of data which are contained in the original record, the
method is invaluable. Mechanical tabulation has the serious defect that
it is rigid and inflexible. The classification permits no qualitative analysis. It is impossible at times to divide the data into clear-cut categories.
In many instances there may be a shading of one classification into
another. In this case mechanical tabulation may not be suitable.

The smaller health organizations may make their own tabulations,
but a better plan is to request the state health department, which already
has the required data on punch cards, to make any desired compilation
for the local health department. Some cities have their own punching
machines but no tabulating machines. In such cases, when the local

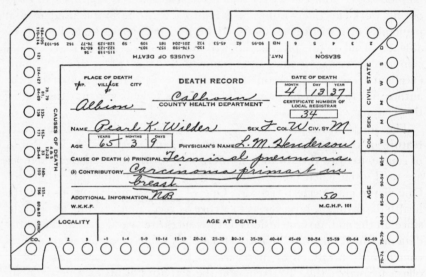

FIG. 17. The Gregg simplified punch card. This card is particularly useful where
the number of units to be analyzed does not exceed 5,000.

health department wishes to make a study of a special subject, the department prepares the punch cards for sorting, and then sends these
cards to the state department of vital statistics for tabulation. In general,
it may be said that it is not feasible to use the punch card system and
mechanical tabulation unless at least 5,000 units are to be analyzed.

A simple system for the analysis of public health data, which was
devised by Dr. Alan Gregg when he was conducting hookworm studies
in Brazil, has been widely adopted when the data to be analyzed do not
exceed 5,000 units, and the individual items are not too numerous. The
standard 5″ × 8″ card has holes punched in the margin and one corner
is cut. (See Fig. 17.) Each item is given an assigned place on the card.
The notches are punched by an ordinary conductor's ticket punch. In
sorting the cards, they are aligned and a rod is run through the desired

hole. The cards are shaken, and all cards in which that hole is punched drop out. For example, in the card given in the illustration, we would find in a very few minutes' manipulation that the person was a native-born married white woman, between 65 and 69 years of age, who died of cancer or other malignant tumor. These cards are particularly useful in analyzing epidemiological data.

Standard statistical tables are prepared by each local department and published in the annual report, where they are filed as a permanent record. It is customary in most of these tables to compare the annual rates with the local or state norm for a five-year period.

More or less standard statistical tables that are suitable for the annual report of any health department, large or small, include:

1. A summary table of total deaths, births (and marriages) analyzed by sex, color and race, with the estimated population and the rate for each group.

2. A table of deaths, exclusive of stillbirths, classified by cause and analyzed by age and sex groups.

3. A summary table of deaths classified by chief cause, and by nativity and sex.

4. A table of deaths, classified by chief cause and by season (or by months).

5. A table of births classified by sex and race.

6. A table of deaths (exclusive of stillbirths) under one year of age, classified by age (in weeks) and by cause.

7. A table of deaths under one year of age, classified by season and by nativity of mother. This may be accompanied by a record of neonatal as well as infant mortality.

8. A table of morbidity, giving actual numbers and also the rate of reportable communicable diseases, classified by season. It is also advisable to include in this table the mortality from these diseases.

States and also the larger cities may tabulate the various data given in the tables suggested above by geographic areas; that is, by counties, wards, etc. Many other tables of important data may be formulated. The health department may be conducting special activities that require emphasis, or the area may have certain problems that warrant special consideration. Essential data should be presented in the annual reports from year to year in a similar form in order that suitable comparisons may be made.

## COMMUNITY PLANNING FOR HEALTH

A health officer must know his district intimately in order to be in a position to plan his work effectively. The community is not a homogeneous mass, but is made up of people—living in larger or smaller families, under a great variety of conditions, with a great variety of resources at their disposal. They may belong to different racial stocks, each with its own peculiar prejudices and customs.

## KIPS BAY - YORKVILLE HEALTH DISTRICT

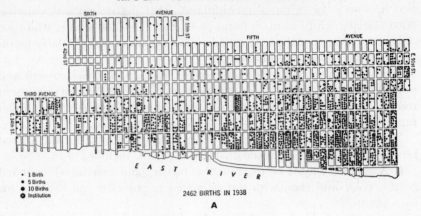

- 1 Birth
- 5 Births
- 10 Births
- ⊗ Institution

2462 BIRTHS IN 1938

**A**

## LOWEST RENTALS......1934

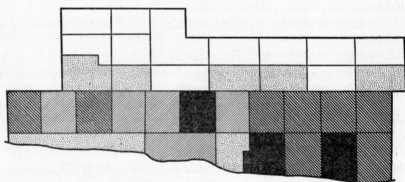

PER CENT OF RENTALS LESS THAN
$7.00 PER MONTH PER ROOM

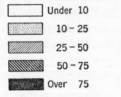

Under 10

10 - 25

25 - 50

50 - 75

Over 75

Source:
N.Y.C. Housing Authority
Real Property Inventory

**B**

FIG. 18. *Community Planning. a.* Map of Kips Bay-Yorkville Health District, with spots showing addresses of families into which babies were born in 1938. *b.* Map of same health district giving economic status of district, by census tracts. Correlation of the data will aid the health officer in planning local health department activities in child hygiene.

The health department should have readily at hand detailed information in regard to all these matters that relate to the social structure of the community. For example, a spot map of the area should be maintained in order to show residence of new-born babies. Another map may indicate concentration of school-age children in the district. Some data on the economic status of the district, zone by zone, should be determined. Frequently the census tract is used as the unit, and the criterion employed is the median family rental. Further spot maps may show the location of grade schools, high schools, hospitals and clinics, playgrounds and recreational facilities, kindergartens, welfare agencies, etc.

If we superimpose one map on the other, it becomes clear that a well-baby station is badly needed in one area, and that there is an over-abundance of clinic facilities in another zone. A study of the data will show just where a health center should be located in order to be most effective and most useful. If trends are followed, it will be possible to predict that in a few years a new school will be needed in a certain area; or that a hospital clinic that has been very active in the past may, within ten years, outlive its usefulness.

All these intimate community details that can be secured only by painstaking effort are valuable aids in promoting an effective community-wide program of adequate health services.

## GRAPHIC METHODS

The graph is a very useful device for the visualization of a compilation of facts. Most people have great difficulty in visualizing figures. To them tables convey very little meaning. A graphic representation of these same tables has a telling effect, even upon the most casual observer.

It is not the province of this text to describe in detail the technic of graphic representation. One principle of graphic methods should be emphasized, namely, the graph must be correct in form and detail, and must tell the true story. Mistakes are frequently made when graphs are used, through improper presentation of the data. Furthermore, it should be noted that different types of diagrams are required to represent different things. One type of graph may be suitable for representation of the trend of events; another type is used to represent things which vary continuously; quite a different type of graph is required to show distribution of things. Many devices are employed, each of which has its own special place, and is particularly suited for representation of certain classification of figures. The bar diagram, the pie diagram, histograms, cyclical time trend, the spot map, the shaded map and other devices all have their logical place in graphic representation of statistical data. The three-dimensional graph has been found to be of special value in enabling the casual observer to visualize in an unforgettable manner the whole course

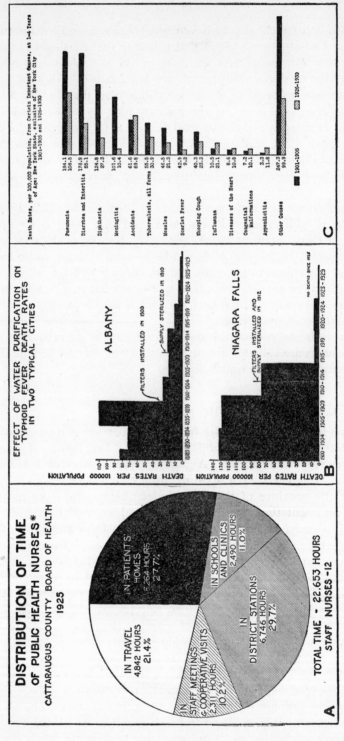

Fig. 19. *Graphic Methods.* Illustrations of different types of graph. *a.* Pie diagram. *b.* Histogram. *c.* Bar diagram. *d.* Time trend line graph. *e.* Spot map. *f.* Shaded map.

198

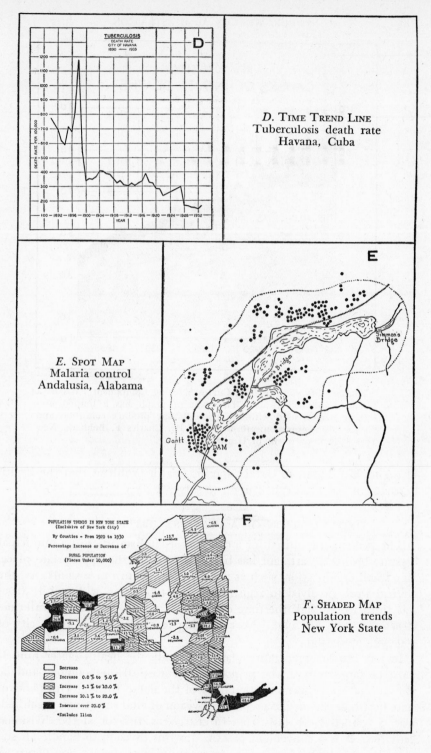

*D.* TIME TREND LINE
Tuberculosis death rate
Havana, Cuba

*E.* SPOT MAP
Malaria control
Andalusia, Alabama

*F.* SHADED MAP
Population trends
New York State

199

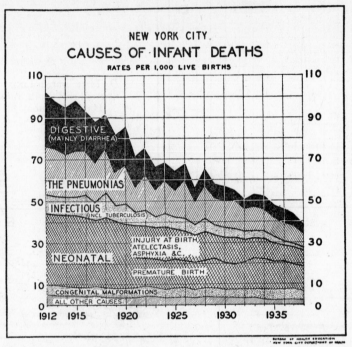

FIG. 20. *Graphic Methods,* Curves Showing Component Parts of a Whole—Combined Graph. This type of graph has a limited usefulness. Unless used with discretion it may produce confusion and give a false impression. (Courtesy of Dr. Charles F. Bolduan, New York City Department of Health.)

of events in relation to certain specific health problems that the health department has been called upon to solve.

## ORGANIZATION OF A VITAL STATISTICS SERVICE

The personnel required for a division of vital statistics in a municipal or state health department has been discussed in the appropriate place. In a small organization, such as a county health unit or a small city, the clerical work involved in registration and tabulation will require from one third to one half the time of the office clerk. One or two full-time clerks can carry the detail work relating to vital statistics for a city of 100,000 population.

In any health organization, large or small, the health officer himself must be familiar with the principles of statistical methodology and be able to make a proper interpretation of the data. In large cities and in state health departments, a separate division of vital statistics is organized, with a trained vital statistician in charge, as director of the divisional activities. It is a convenient practice for this division to handle all statistical computation in relation to communicable disease prevalence, as well as the mortality data. In some instances the director of the division of communicable disease also has supervision of the division of vital statistics. In this case both mortality and morbidity reports are received in the same division, though they are not derived from the same source.

## REFERENCES

1. Whipple, G. C. *Vital Statistics.* John Wiley and Sons. New York.
2. Pearl, Raymond. *Introduction to Medical Biometry and Statistics.* W. B. Saunders and Co.
3. *Manual of the International List of Causes of Death.* Based on the Second Decennial Revision by the International Commission, Paris. Bureau of the Census, Washington, D. C. 1938.
4. Arkin, H. and Colton, R. R. *Graphs: How to Make and Use Them.* Harper and Brothers, New York. 1936.
5. Hill, A. B. *Principles of Medical Statistics.* The Lancet, London. 1937.
6. Davenport, C. B. and Ekas, M. P. *Statistical Methods in Biology, Medicine and Psychology.* John Wiley and Sons, New York. 1936.
7. Mainland, Donald. *The Treatment of Clinical and Laboratory Data.* Oliver and Boyd, Edinburgh. 1938.
8. Brinton, Willard. *Graphic Presentation.* Brinton Associates, 1939.
9. Bureau of the Census, U. S. Public Health Service: Physicians' Handbook on Birth and Death Registration, Washington, D. C., Government Printing Office. 1943
10. Hall, M. F. *Public Health Statistics.* New York, Paul B. Hoeber, Inc. 1942.
11. *Vital Statistics of the United States.* Bureau of the Census, U. S. Public Health Service, Washington, D. C. An annual publication.

# CHAPTER XIX

## EPIDEMIOLOGY

EPIDEMIOLOGICAL investigation is an important function of any health department, large or small. Many health administrators have considered that epidemiological activities were primarily research in nature, of no immediate or practical importance, and had no place in routine health department organization. They have assumed that it was their primary obligation to apply the knowledge that was already well established, but have felt they were not justified in expending public funds for investigative purposes. This has been a serious mistake. The health officer is under obligation, not only to apply the knowledge that is already available, but to unearth fresh information, if for no other reason than the important one that such a policy will render his own activities more effective.

What is epidemiology? What is the scope of the epidemiologist's field? What part does the epidemiologist play in a well-knit, orderly plan of health administration? Stallybrass considers epidemiology as "the science of infective diseases, their prime causes, propagation and prevention. It deals more especially with their epidemic manifestations." This was the original meaning of the term, as clearly indicated by its etymology. As understood at present, however, the field of epidemiology is much more extensive. The word is now loose from its etymological mooring, so that any definition must be considered as more or less subjective. Each person considers himself privileged to define it according to his own ideas and interests. W. H. Welch has defined epidemiology as "the natural history of disease" and Dudley indicates practically the same thing in the statement, "The epidemiologist is a medical ecologist." The American Epidemiological Society has defined epidemiology as "the science which concerns itself with the natural history of disease as it is expressed in groups of persons related by some common factors of age, sex, race, location or occupation, as distinct from the development of disease in individuals." W. H. Frost [1] preferred a definition adapted from Hirsch, as follows: "The science which will give, firstly, a picture of the occurrence, the distribution, and the types of the diseases of mankind in distinct epochs of time and at various points of the earth's surface; and secondly, will render an account of the relations of these diseases to inherent characteristics of the

[1] Personal communication.

individual and to the external conditions surrounding him and determining his manner of life."

Under these definitions, it is obvious that there may be an epidemiology of cancer or heart disease, as well as of diphtheria or plague. The former etymological meaning of the term no longer prevails, and an exact meaning will eventually be determined through fixed usage.

## QUALIFICATIONS FOR AN EPIDEMIOLOGIST

1. One of the most important qualifications for the epidemiologist is that he should be familiar with statistical technics. Unless he is cognizant of the pitfalls that occur when dealing with masses of data, he is sure to arrive at false conclusions, no matter how sound his original premises may be.

This principle was well illustrated in the case of an epidemic of typhoid fever that occurred in one of our large cities. The outbreak was not explosive. The cases were scattered throughout the city and occurred over a considerable period of time. The health department investigation showed that most of the patients had consumed the milk that was sold by a large distributor. This milk was received in bulk from a great number of producers, was pasteurized and distributed in pint and quart bottles. The pasteurizing plant was inspected carefully and was found to be functioning properly. The stools of all the employees of the pasteurization plant itself, together with specimens from the employees of the bottling room and distribution department, were examined, with negative results. It was decided that the milk supply was not at fault, so that other possible sources of infection were investigated, including the municipal water supply, as well as the source of supply of fresh fruits, fresh vegetables, shell fish and many other possible factors. All efforts were without avail. Meanwhile, cases of typhoid fever continued to occur; one here, and one there. The State Epidemiologist was finally called upon for aid. Almost solely on the basis of a statistical analysis of the data and by purely deductive reasoning he concluded:

*a.* That the source of infection must be the milk supply that had been suspected in the first place.

*b.* That the pasteurization process was perfect and that infection with the typhoid bacillus did not occur until after the milk had left the pasteurizer, but before it was placed in the hands of the individual milk men who delivered the milk to consumers.

*c.* That the source of the infection must be in the process of bottling the milk and the person responsible must be an employee who had been working in this particular position for some time.

Having arrived at these conclusions from a statistical analysis of the information at hand it was a simple matter to solve the problem as to just where and how the milk became infected.

The milk was bottled by machinery. A few minutes' observation showed that the machine which capped the bottles did not function perfectly. One operator stood by and when the machine failed, he capped the milk bottles by hand. Repeated examinations of this operator's stools proved that *he was a typhoid carrier*. In the preliminary routine examinations of all the pasteurization plant employees the feces of this operator had been examined once for typhoid bacilli, but the results were negative.

Another example of the value of the statistical approach in solving an epidemiological problem is the study by Murphy [2] of an epidemic of infectious hepatitis in Forsyth, Georgia.

The data were as follows:

2,390 persons exposed, with 10 cases.

950 persons under 20 years of age exposed, with 9 cases.

These data suggested that the community probably had an acquired immunity which was related to age.

Water was suspected as a source of infection, but the disease was limited to white persons, whereas the town had a large Negro population, and water was universally distributed. The possibility of a common food source was considered.

Dairy A supplied 114 persons, with 9 cases.

Other dairies supplied 2,276 persons, with 1 case.

Dairy A supplied 26 households, with 9 cases.

Other dairies supplied 586 households, with 1 case.

Dairy A supplied 38 persons under 20 years of age, with 8 cases.

Other dairies supplied ± 912 persons under 20 years of age, with 1 case.

An investigation of Dairy A revealed very unsanitary conditions, with ample possibility of gross contamination of the milk. Furthermore, the milk was not pasteurized. There had been one case of infectious hepatitis at the dairy farm about April 15, and a second case about May 20. The epidemic of 10 cases occurred from May 21 to June 28. In view of the fact that the incubation period of infectious hepatitis is more than one month, the authors were justified in concluding that the first case of infectious hepatitis at the dairy was a probable source of infection of the other 10 children in the village, and that Dairy A milk was the probable vehicle of infection. Also, it seems probable that the case at the dairy farm on May 20 was infected from the same source, at the same time as the 10 village cases. The most important conclusion is that the source of the infection was, in reasonable probability, contaminated unpasteurized, unsanitary milk.

2. The epidemiologist should be well grounded in the diagnosis of communicable disease. Much of his work will be carried out in the field. He should be able to collect his own data from its original sources with a satisfactory degree of accuracy.

There is no better illustration of brilliant epidemiological work which was a direct corollary of diagnostic acumen than the studies of typhus fever in the southern part of the United States by Maxcy. The disease had undoubtedly been occurring for years in many different parts of the

[2] Murphy, W. J., Petrie, L. M. and Work, S. D.: "Outbreak of Infectious Hepatitis, Apparently Milk-borne." *Am. J. Pub. Health*. 1946, Vol. 36, p. 169.

country, but had been diagnosed incorrectly. Maxcy first established the diagnosis and then worked out the mode of spread of the disease in the rural portion of the southern states.

Tularemia also is a disease which has occurred in many parts of the United States, probably for a long time. Its clinical picture is so characteristic that the physician need only think of the possibility of tularemia to be able to make a tentative diagnosis; yet the diagnosis of this disease is often missed by the public health personnel as well as by practicing physicians. Once the diagnosis has been made, the epidemiological work in relation to the particular outbreak becomes a relatively simple matter.

3. A well-trained epidemiologist should be familiar with the history of medicine, particularly that portion of it that relates to epidemics of disease. The observations that have been made on the epidemiological features of disease, long before the causal agents were discovered, are of interest and importance to the epidemiologist in his study of disease as it occurs in the community at the present time, or as it may occur in the future.

Austin Flint is widely remembered because of a certain heart sound that has been given his name. Few know that he made some very keen and analytical epidemiological observations in relation to the importance of water as a vehicle of transmission of typhoid fever. In the first volume of reports of meetings of the American Public Health Association in 1873, Dr. Flint described an epidemic of typhoid fever that occurred in the hamlet of North Boston, New York, in 1843. He had been asked to investigate the outbreak because a Mr. Stearns was accused of poisoning the community well.

His investigation revealed that a young man had travelled on the stage from Massachusetts, became sick en route and was compelled to stop at the tavern in North Boston on September 21 because of his illness. He died October 19. Between October 14 and 19, twenty-eight of the forty-three persons living in the hamlet contracted typhoid fever and ten died. The family of Mr. Stearns escaped completely. There was a community well adjoining the tavern and belonging to it, but used by all the adjacent cottages except that of the Stearns family. Mr. Stearns had quarreled with the inn keeper shortly before and had been required to give up the use of the tavern well and dig a well of his own. When every family except that of Mr. Stearns became ill, Mr. Stearns quite logically was accused of poisoning the tavern well. Dr. Flint, by autopsy, showed that the disease was not due to poison but was typhoid fever. He assumed the disease was spread by an effluvium, perhaps introduced into the community by the Massachusetts stranger.

Nearly thirty years later, Dr. Flint learned of the studies of William Budd in England on the spread of typhoid fever through contamination of drinking water with discharges from typhoid fever patients. He went back to his old notes on the North Boston epidemic, wrote to the old family physician who was still practicing in the area and built up a complete and comprehensive picture of the outbreak.[3] In brief, he showed that typhoid fever had been introduced into

[3] Flint, Austin: *Relations of Water to the Propagation of Fever.* Reports of the meetings of the American Public Health Association. 1873, Vol. I, p. 164.

a virgin field by a stranger who had come from a town where the disease prevailed at the time. The dejecta of the sick man had been disposed of in such a manner that the community well might easily have been contaminated. Those families that used the tavern well water were all infected with the disease. All twenty-eight of the patients became ill within a ten-day period. The Stearns family and two other families of the village that lived a little distance away and had their own water supply developed no cases of illness. Dr. Flint drew the conclusion that the well had been contaminated from the dejecta of the Massachusetts traveller and the patients had all been infected by drinking the water from the tavern well. If these early observations on the North Boston epidemic by Dr. Flint had been given the attention they deserved; if the simple, but clearcut and logical analysis of the mode of spread of typhoid fever that Dr. Flint developed and the conclusions and recommendations that he presented had been understood and accepted, it now seems quite possible that many subsequent water-borne epidemics of typhoid fever that devastated the United States during the following fifty years might have been avoided.

4. The epidemiologist should have a good knowledge of bacteriology and immunology and a thorough understanding of physiology, particularly in relation to the varied external environmental factors that may influence the health of individuals.

The epidemiologist must remember that an individual is not an objective unit, unrelated to his surroundings. Each and every person is highly dependent upon his environment, and is influenced profoundly by a thousand varied factors that may determine his well-being, or may even bring about his destruction.

It is difficult to conceive of the fact that the texture of the top soil of an area might have a profound and direct influence upon the health of large masses of people. But epidemiologists have shown conclusively that such is the case. The correlation between severe hookworm disease and the sandy coastal plain of Alabama is an excellent example of this principle. The "Black Belt," a heavy textured clay soil, extends across the state in a broad band. The line of demarcation between the two types of soil, sandy loam and heavy clay, is abrupt. The mode of life, the sanitary habits, the type of population, the climatic factors, such as temperature and rainfall as well as many other factors that may influence the population, are practically identical in the two soil areas; yet the people that live on the sandy soils are heavily infected with hookworms and the people living in the Black Belt have little or no infection.

The fundamental environmental factor which has determined whether or not whole masses of people have suffered from severe infection has been the texture of the top soil of the area. The "Black Belt" soil is unfavorable for the development of the hookworm larvae; whereas the light sandy soils offer highly favorable conditions for larval development. Thus those people living in the Norfolk and Greenville sandy loam section were heavily infected with *Necator americanus*.

5. The epidemiologist must develop a point of view which will inter-relate disease processes as they affect *the community as a unit* rather than the individual. Thus he must have a real knowledge of the principles of preventive medicine.

Godfrey's diphtheria studies have brought out very clearly the distinction between *individual immunity* and *community immunity* to diphtheria. The individual may receive a very satisfactory protection by immunization with toxoid. In order to secure individual protection each baby over six months of age should be immunized. But Godfrey's data indicate that community protection may be produced satisfactorily even though many children are not immune to diphtheria. If the health officer can secure immunization of approximately 35 per cent to 50 per cent of the preschool age children of a given community, he may feel fairly sure that even if diphtheria invades his city, it will not spread to epidemic proportions.

Epidemiology is a splendid training ground for the prospective health administrator. Every health commissioner should be well grounded in the principles of epidemiology, if he is to make a success of his work. Each and every bit of detail work that is well done contributes to our knowledge concerning the mode of spread of disease, and thus aids in development of more effective methods of prevention. It is highly desirable, therefore, not only that each health department should organize a good epidemiological service, but also that every medical health officer should be familiar with the principles of good epidemiological work.

## THE EPIDEMIOLOGICAL APPROACH

The epidemiological *point of view* is essential to good health department practice. In fact, most of the health leaders recommend to young men who are interested in making public health a career that they enter public health through the epidemiological approach. Here the opportunities for productive work are most fruitful, and the knowledge gained will be of great value in subsequent years of activity in health administration.

Epidemiology as a science is a relatively new conception, though epidemiological observations have been made from earliest times, long before clinical medicine developed as a science. Brilliant examples of early field epidemiology are Budd's studies of typhoid fever, Snow's studies of the epidemiology of cholera, and the work of Semmelweiss and Oliver Wendell Holmes in relation to epidemics of puerperal sepsis. These men arrived at conclusions that were of immense importance in control of these diseases, even though the actual bacterial causes were not discovered for many years.

Each newly reported case of communicable disease is an unsolved epidemiological problem, related in some manner to the health of other individuals in the community. The solution of these problems is an integral part of health department practice. Dr. Munson, formerly District Health Officer of New York, used to call this work "sole-leather" epidemiology.

A simple illustration of the importance of tracing sources of infection is clearly brought out in the following report of a small outbreak of syphilis in a rural area.

A farmer, living in an isolated section of the county, brought his three year old son to the office of the county health department. The child had a rash and his throat was sore; but otherwise he was not very ill. The diagnosis was secondary syphilis and the primary lesion was on the tonsil. On careful inquiry it was discovered that the family nurse followed the once common custom of feeding the child predigested food. She chewed tough pieces of meat, for example, and then put them in the child's mouth. The nurse was brought to the office and she also was found to be innocently infected with syphilis. The source of infection in the family was the father. He had infected the mother and she, in turn, had been the source of infection of the nurse. A week later a fourteen year old son was brought to the health officer with a primary lesion of syphilis on the wrist, the infection occurring from use of the family roller towel. Further investigation showed that the father had been infected by a promiscuous negress who had cooked for the family. The whereabouts of this source of infection was discovered, and after some difficulty the names of possible contacts with her were obtained. The investigation now ramified in two directions, among white families and negro families. When the investigation ceased because of lack of further leads, some sixteen persons that had been infected from the common source had been discovered and placed under treatment. Some of the cases that were discovered in the investigation had already consulted their physicians and were under treatment, but most of them were receiving no treatment at all.

This rather characteristic community outbreak of syphilis illustrates the fact that a case of acute communicable disease is often related to some unsuspected source of infection in the community and that investigation will often discover unrecognized or unreported cases and will reveal quite surprising modes of spread of infection. In many instances a simple investigation which unearths hidden sources of infection will serve as an important means toward prevention of further spread of a given disease.

This fact has been appreciated for years by the leaders in public health. Some of the best epidemiological work that has been done in the United States has been accomplished by Chapin as municipal health officer of Providence, and Chesley as state health commissioner of Minnesota, by means of careful analysis and interpretation of methodical, more or less routine, communicable disease control activities of a busy health department.

Good epidemiological work need not be limited to the large municipal and state health departments. In fact, there are many advantages which favor the rural health worker, because his situation is less complex, human contacts less frequent and contributing factors more easily determined. This fact was clearly understood by Ezra Hunt, one of the founders of the American Public Health Association in 1872. In his paper on "The Need of Sanitary Organizations in Villages and Rural Districts," [4] he says,

"A great number of cases to observe is in some respects valuable, but confusion and difficulty of study sometimes arises from too great aggregation of disease under the extra artificial conditions of cities, hospitals, etc., and very much is to be learned from a few typical cases occurring under circumstances less complicated.

"There is often not so much to be learned by observing a very great number of cases as by an exhaustive searching into a few cases, all the facts of which are more within the grasp."

The advantage gained through study of an epidemic which occurs under simple conditions and in a relatively sparsely settled area may be illustrated by an outbreak of malaria that occurred on the Yellow River in Covington County, Alabama. There had been no malaria in the area for several years. Suddenly the disease appeared in almost every family living within a roughly circular zone, the diameter of which was about two miles. The farmers thought that the disease had been produced by the carelessness of a Mr. Wood who had cut timber in the east branch of the river bottom and allowed the "slash" to rot in the river. A simple sketch map on which all the homes of the area were plotted, and all the cases spotted, showed that Mr. Wood could not be the responsible person. The source of anopheles breeding must be in the center of the circle; whereas he lived on the outer edge of the infected zone. Larval catches in both branches of the river proved that only *A. crucians* was breeding there, whereas the important vector of malaria in Alabama is *A. quadrimaculatus,* a pond breeder. The obvious place to search for the *A. quadrimaculatus* breeding focus was the center of the circle, and it was soon found. It was a small artificial pond, only a few rods in diameter, hidden away under a hill and built by an old man as a private fishing pond. It had been built for three years without causing any trouble. The year of the epidemic, the owner of the pond had brought a new negro tenant family from a malarious area many miles away. Thus the exact conditions for an epidemic of malaria were produced. The proper anopheles vector was already present in abundance. The parasite was introduced from afar and placed in a house beside the little pond. From this source the anopheles mosquitoes became infected. The normal flight range of this vector is about one mile, so that very soon every home within a radius of one mile from the pond was infected with malaria. Once the source of infection was determined, it was a simple matter to stop the epidemic by opening the dam and draining the artificial pond.

## TYPES OF EPIDEMIOLOGICAL WORK

Epidemiological work may be divided for practical purposes into four main categories:
1. Experimental epidemiology.
2. Investigation of a specific epidemic in the field.

[4] *Reports of Meetings of the American Public Health Association.* 1872, Vol. I, p. 493.

3. Continuous efforts by the local public health personnel to determine sources of infection in the community and the modes of spread of disease.

4. Epidemiological analysis and interpretation of data that have been accumulated by the health department over a period of time concerning specific conditions.

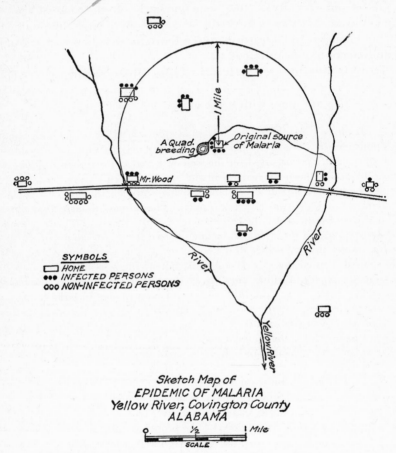

SYMBOLS
▭ HOME
••• INFECTED PERSONS
ooo NON-INFECTED PERSONS

Sketch Map of
EPIDEMIC OF MALARIA
Yellow River, Covington County
ALABAMA

FIG. 21. *An Epidemic of Malaria on Yellow River, Covington County, Alabama.* Illustrates an epidemiological field study.

**Experimental Epidemiology.** An effort toward the study of epidemiology on an experimental basis and from the laboratory point of view is a relatively recent conception. The brilliant pioneer work of Topley and Greenwood, of Webster, and their associates should be familiar to everyone interested in the subject. This approach is very difficult and time consuming, and does not fall within the province of the health officer.

**Field Epidemiology.** The epidemiologist of the official health service is called upon, often at a moment's notice, to investigate an outbreak of disease that has occurred within his jurisdiction.

He will find the community in confusion, distraught by many conflicting rumors and opinions. He must approach his problem with an open mind, quite uninfluenced by the observations of others or by his own preconceived ideas.

The first and most important step is to make an accurate diagnosis of the disease. A sufficient number of cases must be seen to determine this fact. While so doing he will be able to determine a second factor of this particular outbreak, namely, the virulence and invasiveness of this particular infection. Once the preliminary steps have been accomplished, he must review in his own mind the general epidemiological features of the disease in question.

a. The normal epidemic curve of this disease.

b. The effect of secondary factors upon susceptibility to this condition, such as age, sex, race, overcrowding, fatigue, nutrition in the broad sense, climatic and seasonal factors, etc.

c. The most common and probable sources of infection in this disease.

d. The common methods of transmission of the disease.

e. The extreme limits of the incubation period of the disease and the degree of communicability.

f. The most effective methods of control.

The second step in the investigation is to determine the extent of the invasion of the community, the degree to which the disease has already spread. In the investigation of this point he will make house to house visits, and will determine at the same time the various human activities that may have occurred in the community, and the aggregation and dispersion of people which might account for distribution of the infection.

The epidemiologist will then analyze the detailed data he has collected. He should have sufficient information to make it possible to determine, or at least to suspect, the original source or sources of the infection and the method of transmission of the disease in this instance. Further investigation may disclose hidden reservoirs of infection, human or otherwise.

Once the source of the infection has been discovered, and the mode of spread has been determined, all that remains to be done is to establish the well recognized specific prophylactic measures that are in commonly accepted usage. He will attack the reservoirs of infection, and by specific immunization, isolation, quarantine or by other means, prevent further spread of the disease.

A well organized and satisfactorily completed study in field epidemiology is one of the most satisfying results of the health officer's work. Effectual efforts are concrete, the results immediate and highly appreciated, and success is obvious. Failure is usually due to lack of sufficient intelligently gathered information, or lack of knowledge of the epidemiology of the given disease. The whole problem resembles very much a child's jigsaw puzzle. One finds at first a heterogeneous mass of apparently unrelated details, scattered and confused. By patient work, with skillful hands, these may be fitted together piece by piece, so that a complete familiar picture evolves.

**Continuous efforts by the local public health personnel to determine sources of infection in the community and modes of spread of disease.** The field investigation of an epidemic of disease is often an exciting experience and when the source of infection has been determined and the whole chain of events linked together, the results are most gratifying.

If we analyze these epidemiological studies of startling outbreaks of disease, we are struck by the fact that in most instances the damage has already been done before the epidemiologist has even been asked to make the investigation. In many instances the investigation has served to clear up a mystery, but has not saved any lives, nor prevented perhaps a single case of infection. These investigations are a fine example of the old adage about the stable door that has been locked after the horse has been stolen.

The chief value of this type of epidemiological investigation is not that it has aided in stopping the particular outbreak, but that it points out the source of infection and gives a vivid lesson to the stricken community, and to other communities as well, as to how the epidemic might have been prevented if proper conditions had prevailed in the first place, and also how similar epidemics may be avoided in the future.

A much less spectacular, but more fruitful, type of epidemiological work is the continuous effort by the full-time personnel of any health department in a day-by-day determination of sources of infection in the community. The work of the public health nurse serves as a very useful adjunct to this type of epidemiological service. The constant searching for contacts of cases of tuberculosis and syphilis, the discovery of mild and unrecognized cases of diphtheria and scarlet fever, the careful investigation of every case of typhoid fever, all a part of everyday health department practice, will yield far more effective results in prevention of disease than the brilliant investigation of a striking outbreak of septic sore throat or bacillary dysentery. Every member of the health department must always have before him the fact that each new case of communicable disease in the community is an unsolved epidemiological problem, related, in all probability, to some other case in the community and also a potential source of new cases.

This type of epidemiological work cannot be carried on satisfactorily with part-time public health personnel or a partially organized health service. The best work of this type has been done in the rural communities with a well organized full-time health department service and with well trained and alert personnel.

It is quite probable that for years to come emergency studies of striking outbreaks of disease will be an important part of state and local health department practice, and that much new knowledge will be gained from these studies. We must recognize, however, that the far less spectacular day-to-day investigation of the source of infection and the mode of spread of individual cases of communicable disease will, in the long run, yield more important information and much more productive results.

An illustration of the technic whereby a health department may carry on this type of work as an integral part of its health service may be seen in the practices that were developed by the Providence City Health Department.

*Illustration* [5] *of Routine Collection of Epidemiological Data as Practiced in Providence.* Reports of contagious diseases are made to the health department by the private physician through the mail by means of laboratory specimen, personal visit, or, chiefly, by the telephone. Each report contains the patient's name, residence, age, disease, the doctor's name, and the date of the report.

A History Record Form is partially filled out by the clerk from the report slip. She puts in the patient's address, name, age and date of attack, when known, and on the reverse side fills in the doctor's name and the patient's address, and checks with directories on the address. She puts a check mark on the report slip to indicate that the record form has been made out. She also underlines the date of attack to mean that the report slip has been checked.

The History Record Form is taken by the doctor or nurse to the home.

All epidemiological data are secured by the nurse or doctor on the first visit to the case; including names of all members of the family, with ages, occupation or school, previous attacks, milkman, question of exposure, etc. All this information is filled in *at the home.*

The record form is then returned to the office where the clerk enters the cases on the proper school and milk cards. She also excludes the children from school as indicated by the medical inspector.

The clerk uses the following marks as checks:

Red E to indicate exclusion from school.

Red S to indicate record on school card.

Red check at milkman to indicate that notice has been sent to him and has been recorded on his record card. When another case develops in the same family, the clerk enters the case on the school and the milkman's card, and checks through the original red mark with a red line. She also underlines the date of attack on the record form when she makes out the report slip for the secondary case.

The clerk also checks all diphtheria cases and exposures with the immunization records.

Cases are *charted* and entered in the *diary* from the history record form. When a case is entered on the *chronological chart,* a check mark is put through the date of attack. When the case is entered in the diary, a check is put on the upper left hand corner of the record form. *Spot maps* are made from this diary, which is then checked.

All laboratory records are entered in red ink on the record form, negative cultures are indicated by a circle about the date, positive cultures by a plus sign

[5] Personal communication from Dr. Charles V. Chapin.

after the date. All history record forms that show positive cultures are marked on the face with a large red cross, those showing only negative cultures are marked with a large red circle. This helps in tabulation. To assist in tabulating, all records where a person has received serum for measles or scarlet fever, are so stamped with a rubber stamp. Other stamps are used to indicate home living, home death, early hospital, and late hospital cases. When the cases on the history record form have been tabulated according to age and month, the slip is stamped on the reverse side with a rubber stamp. Another rubber stamp is used after they have been tabulated for susceptibles. These stamps and check and tabulation marks do not interfere with the legibility of the records.

Record forms are filed alphabetically according to streets. After tabulation they are filed in cardboard boxes by years.

A more or less routine, simple method, such as the Providence plan of recording communicable disease, is essential to a good epidemiological service. Using these records as a starting point, the epidemiologist can go into the field, secure the necessary additional data, learn of unrecognized cases of the disease, determine the sources of the infection, and thus be in a position to check further spread of the disease in the community.

**Analysis of "Silent Data" in the Health Department Files.** If we return to our original definition of epidemiology given on a previous page, we discover that our discussion of the subject up to the present bears little relationship to our true conception of epidemiology. "Epidemiology gives the picture of the occurrence, the distribution and the types of disease of mankind in distinct epochs of time and at various points on the earth's surface." Thus the most essential factor in advancement of this science is *time*—a long, slow, patient, meticulous accumulation of records of disease as they occur in the community; not by one person or one health department, but by a great many different epidemiologists, working over a long period of time and at many different places, under varying environmental conditions.

Much of the epidemiological data relating to diseases as they have occurred in the United States during the past century are of little value because the records are so incomplete and diagnoses so inexact. Diphtheria, for example, up to 1850, at least, was classified under four different headings. Only in recent years have we begun to accumulate information that can be subjected to critical analysis and interpretation. Thus epidemiology as a science is yet in its infancy. Dr. Chapin was one of the first in the United States to realize the value and import of careful routine collection of epidemiological data as an integral part of health department practice. Many of Dr. Chapin's important contributions to the field of epidemiology have been made from the analysis of data of this type, data that were secured through a careful accumulation of individual records over a period of more than forty years.

The tabulation of the data is a simple matter. In many situations the interpretation of the findings may require all the skill, intelligence and knowledge that the epidemiologist can muster.

## ORGANIZATION

Every division of communicable disease of every health department, large or small, must supply epidemiological service.

**State Health Departments.** Epidemiology is not organized as a separate division of state health service, but is incorporated in the division of communicable disease control. The epidemiologist is more or less of a "free lance," ready to go anywhere at any time to aid local health departments in solving local emergency situations. The service is advisory and consultatory, similar to the function of a state sanitary engineer. In more populous states, two or more full-time epidemiologists may be required. In the smaller states, the director of the division of communicable disease may serve as epidemiologist, and will occupy most of his time with this special activity.

**Municipalities.** Large municipalities, 200,000 population and over, find it advantageous to employ one or more epidemiologists who devote their full time to this field. They are assigned to the division of communicable disease and work under the director of this division. In smaller cities the director of the division of communicable disease carries out this activity.

**County Health Units.** In small health departments, as, for example, county health units, the health officer will take direct charge of all epidemiological activities. He will, of course, receive advice and counsel from the state epidemiologist, and call on him for direct aid when any emergency arises.

**Federal Health Service.** The United States Public Health Service has a large staff of expert epidemiologists. These men are available to State Health Departments upon request, and have been of invaluable aid in solving some of the more difficult epidemiological problems that have arisen from time to time in the United States.

## REFERENCES

1. Stallybrass, C. O. *The Principles of Epidemiology*. 1931. Published by Geo. Routledge and Son Ltd., London. Contains comprehensive and valuable bibliography.
2. Hirsch, A. *Handbook of Historical and Geographical Pathology*. 1885. (Out of Print.)
3. Hamer, Wm. *Epidemiology Old and New*. 1929. The Macmillan Company, New York City.
4. Greenwood, Major. *Epidemiology Historical and Experimental*. 1930. The Johns Hopkins Press, Baltimore.
5. Greenwood, M. and Topley, W. W. C. *Further Studies in Epidemiology*. J. of Hyg. 1925, Vol. 24, p. 45. See also numerous other papers on experi-

mental epidemiology by the authors and their co-workers, especially the following:

6. Greenwood, M., Topley, W. W. C. and Wilson, J. *Contributions to the Experimental Study of Epidemiology. The Effect of Vaccination on Herd Mortality.* J. Hyg. 1931, Vol. 31, p. 259.

7. Delta Omega Series. Publications of Epidemiological Classics.

8. Vaughan, V. C. *Epidemiology and the Public Health.* 1922, 2 Vols. C. V. Mosby Co., St. Louis, Mo.

9. Webster, L. T. *Epidemiology of Fowl Cholera.* J. Exper. Med. 1930, Vol. 51, p. 219. See also numerous other articles by this author and his co-workers upon experimental epidemiology.

10. Brownlee, T. *Investigation into Periodicality of Infectious Disease.* Public Health. 1914, Vol. 28, p. 125. See also numerous papers by this author upon Periodicity of Disease.

11. *Epidemiology.* The Commonwealth. 1933, Vol. 20, No. 3. Publication of Massachusetts State Health Department.

12. Scott, H. H. *Some Notable Epidemics.* 1934. Edw. Arnold Co., London.

13. Budd, William. *Typhoid Fever.* 1860. Republished 1931, Delta Omega Series. American Public Health Association, New York City.

14. Panum, P. L. *Measles.* 1846. Republished 1940, Delta Omega Series. American Public Health Association, New York City.

15. Winslow, C.–E. A. *Conquest of Epidemic Disease.* Princeton University Press. 1943.

16. Frost, W. H. *Collected Papers of.* Edited by K. F. Maxcy. The Commonwealth Fund, New York, N. Y. 1941.

17. Smith, Geddes. *Plague on Us.* Commonwealth Fund, New York, N. Y. 1941.

18. Simmons, J. S. and co-authors. *Global Epidemiology.* J. B. Lippincott Co., Philadelphia. 1944.

# CHAPTER XX

## THE PUBLIC HEALTH LABORATORY

An official public health organization cannot function effectively without its own public health laboratory. The laboratory is an important adjunct to every division of public health activity, and is one of the most valuable means of winning support for the whole health department.

The department of public health is dependent upon practicing physicians in determining when, where and to what extent communicable disease prevails in the community. The physician is dependent upon the laboratory for diagnostic aid. Thus, free laboratory service to physicians is, to some degree, at least, a compensation for their services in the reporting of cases of contagious disease that occur in their practice. Confidence of physicians in the public health laboratory wins their confidence and support of other activities of the general public health program.

### FUNCTIONS OF THE LABORATORY

There are two major types of public health laboratory: first, the municipal or local type of laboratory, which usually is small, and which has limited functions, and serves the immediate needs of the community; second, the larger state laboratory, involving a large jurisdiction and with more extensive functions. There are certain primary activities which are common to state and local laboratories, and which are correlated with the work of other divisions of the health department.

**Communicable Disease.** The laboratory is of paramount importance in aiding in the diagnosis of communicable disease. Its purpose is threefold:

*a.* To detect communicable disease in the individual, to serve as a control of therapy that is administered—as in sulfanilamide treatment—and to give indications for release from isolation.

*b.* To obtain information concerning prevalence of communicable disease in the community, and to aid in search for carriers of infection.

*c.* To furnish means of control.

217

The laboratory does not carry its service directly to the public, but works through the practicing physicians. The diagnostic material is obtained from them, and the laboratory reports back to them directly or through the department of communicable disease.

The epidemiologist is dependent upon the laboratory in checking his field investigations of sources of infection, determination of prevalence of infection, and as an index of the effectiveness of control measures. Thus, the relationship between the division of communicable disease and the laboratory must be very close.

**Division of Sanitary Engineering.** The Division of Sanitary Engineering is dependent upon the laboratory for certain services, particularly in relation to the control of water supplies and sewage disposal plants and allied services related to environmental sanitation. A systematic standard bacteriological and chemical check of public supplies of water and sewage is indispensable in any health organization. Swimming pools require constant bacteriological study, and roadside pumps and springs to which the public has access must be examined by laboratory methods at proper intervals. In addition, the laboratory carries out many other tests for this division.

**Foods and Drugs.** Those who have control of the public health aspects of food control and particularly milk sanitation must rely upon the laboratory to check their field work. Often the laboratory will give the clue that makes it possible to determine the solution of some difficulty, or to corroborate evidence that has been largely circumstantial.

Bacteriological and chemical tests of foods of all kinds, of drugs, beverages, and other substances may be required from time to time, as necessity demands. One of the great benefits that the public derives from the public health laboratory, and that receives little appreciation, is the practically complete abolition of fraudulent adulteration of foodstuffs in recent years throughout the United States. Simple laboratory tests have been developed that furnish incontestable proof of adulteration and give the offenders no loophole of escape.

**Industrial Hygiene.** The laboratory may be a valuable aid in industrial hygiene, through detection of industrial poisoning, through tests of environmental working conditions to determine toxic and harmful working situations, and in many other ways.

**Maternal and Child Hygiene.** The laboratory is utilized in various ways by this division of the health department. The pre-natal clinics may request urine examinations of pregnant women; the laboratories may be requested to furnish arsenicals, silver nitrate ampoules, diphtheria toxoid, measles convalescent serum, whooping cough vaccine, and the like for the protection of the health of mothers and babies.

**Standards of Laboratory Procedure.** One important function of the public health laboratory, particularly the large state laboratory, is that it sets standards of procedure for other laboratories within the jurisdiction of the health department. The quality of the work of the official laboratory must be above reproach; for the local administrative officer must accept its findings in preference to any other. The official laboratory must use its best efforts to raise the standards of work in private, commercial and hospital laboratories within its zone of influence. Small, unsupervised clinical laboratories with inexperienced personnel are all too common; and the result of their poor work may prejudice the physicians against laboratory results in general and injure those reputable laboratories that do accurate work.

Some state health departments have made attempts to standardize and regulate diagnostic laboratory procedures throughout the state. Certain minimum standards of equipment and personnel are required and certain standard procedures are outlined in order that each laboratory may meet the official requirements, and win approval of the state health department. The laboratories must also report on test specimens at intervals. These laboratories which meet the requirements are given a certificate, which must be renewed annually. Laboratories that are handicapped by lack of funds may receive a small state subsidy. This plan serves two purposes: it raises the standards of laboratory procedure, and produces a decentralized state laboratory service of high standards.

**Pathologic Service.** The nature of public health work is changing continuously. It must be modified to meet changing social conditions. As communicable disease has declined, other diseases have increased. Notable in this increase is cancer.

Many states have introduced a tissue diagnostic service for cancer. In some instances the state organizes and subsidizes diagnostic cancer clinics. The biopsies from this clinic service are examined in the central laboratory. In other states, the state laboratory offers a cancer diagnostic service to all physicians of the state who desire to send in properly taken biopsy material.

The development of the technic called the Papanicolaou diagnostic service, particularly for early diagnosis of cancer of the uterus, may open a new field of diagnostic laboratory service.

Certain public health laboratories have also aided physicians in the treatment of diabetics. Quantitative tests for sugar in the urine and blood of diabetic patients is provided, in order that the patients may be handled more adequately.

This type of diagnostic and therapeutic laboratory work seems to many public health administrators as an encroachment on the clinical laboratory field. This matter is discussed further under *Organization of Laboratory Service.*

**Investigation.** All public health laboratories should maintain the investigative spirit. The public health laboratory is frequently swamped by the volume of routine work. If the diagnostic service wins the approval of physicians, the volume of work grows faster than the appropriation. This diagnostic service is an essential function and a primary duty, and must be done well. But strict limitation of the work to routine activities is one of the chief weaknesses of the average official laboratory. A competent director is in a difficult position. He realizes the importance of basic research, and is overwhelmed by the wealth of material and the abundance of problems that continually present themselves for study; yet his routine diagnostic work cannot be neglected. A compromise at least may be made. It may not be possible for the laboratory to undertake complex studies, but every public health laboratory should at least carry out investigations in the development of new tests for the modification of technic, and improvement in practical methods. Public health laboratory directors may well be proud of the contributions of public health laboratories to scientific knowledge, both theoretical and applied. They have proved of great value in the past and will continue to be of increasing importance and fruitfulness in years to come.

**Manufacture of Biologicals.** The manufacture and free distribution of vaccines and sera are one of the developments of the activities of the public health laboratory. The small laboratory cannot manufacture biological products economically. Large volume production is necessary and thus, if it is undertaken, it usually becomes a state laboratory function. The state does not need to make a profit to pay for advertising, charge for overhead, or to replace unused material, as do the commercial laboratories, so that it can often manufacture biological products in large quantities at a lower cost than the most favorable commercial prices. The important principle that has been established is that the community has the responsibility to supply suitable biological products for the prevention of illness in those instances where the individual cannot obtain these benefits for himself or his family through his own resources. It is the responsibility of the health department to provide these biological products as economically as possible.

The criterion as to whether the products should be manufactured by the state or purchased from private companies is briefly stated: If, in the long run, a good quality product can be made by the state laboratory at a lower cost than the contract purchase price of a private laboratory, then the state should make the product. If not, the product should be purchased.

## ACTIVITIES OF THE PUBLIC HEALTH LABORATORY

The activities of the two main types of diagnostic laboratory differ in certain details.

**Municipal or Local Laboratories.** Certain activities may be carried on very effectively by a small laboratory; other procedures can only be followed satisfactorily if done on a large scale. When the important factor in the laboratory diagnosis is speed, the local service should be much more effective than the large central laboratory. For example, diphtheria diagnosis, meningococcus identification or pneumococcus typing may be done best by the local laboratory. Bacteriological examination of milk, also, should be made as soon as possible after the sample is taken. In general, the work of the small laboratory should include:

1. Direct examinations requiring simple equipment.
    a. Diphtheria.[1] Diagnostic cultures and release cultures.
    b. Examination of sputum for diagnosis of tuberculosis.
    c. Smears for diagnosis of gonococci.
    d. Blood films for diagnosis of malaria.
    e. Spinal fluid examination, both direct and cultural, for diagnosis of meningitis.
    f. Stool examination for ova of intestinal parasites.
    g. Examination of animal brain in diagnosis of rabies.
    h. Direct examination for diagnosis of syphilis, if a dark field equipment is available.
    i. Pneumococcus typing. In order to be of any value to the physician or the patient, pneumococcus typing must be done quickly and in the early stages of the disease. The small laboratory can give this service very effectively.

The development of simple technics for the bacteriological diagnosis of typhoid fever and bacillary dysentery has also brought these tests within the scope of the local laboratory. Some authorities believe that "cough plate" diagnosis of whooping cough should be included in the schedule of the small public health laboratory.

Culture of the tubercle bacillus has now become a simple and very important laboratory procedure, and culture of the gonococcus for determination of the cure of the patient is a simple and very satisfactory local laboratory test. Other diagnostic methods are constantly being introduced which may be incorporated in local laboratory services.

The simple administrative principle is to utilize the local laboratories in tests that give immediate and direct results, and that do not require elaborate equipment or highly specialized skills.

In addition, the small laboratory may make standard bacteriological tests of:

a. Water samples.
b. Milk samples.

as well as total fat determinations and other simple standard chemical examinations of milk and milk products.

---

[1] Some authorities believe that diphtheria diagnosis is no longer the province of the local laboratory. The diagnosis is difficult and requires constant practice. Diphtheria is becoming so infrequent that the test has become an "unusual laboratory procedure," and the technician of the small laboratory lacks sufficient experience to be confident of results.

The small laboratory should *not* attempt:

*a.* Wassermann examinations or serodiagnosis of syphilis unless one hundred or more specimens are received weekly.

*b.* Chemical examination of water and sewage.

*c.* Preparation of any biological products.

It is questionable, also, if the small laboratory should attempt the more unusual diagnostic procedures that are required at irregular intervals. Included in this group are diagnostic methods for undulant fever, for tularemia, for typhus fever and other similar tests.

2. Distribution center.

The local laboratory should be a depot for distribution of vaccines and sera that have been prepared or purchased by the central laboratory, and should also have charge of the distribution of laboratory containers, so that they are placed in readily accessible places throughout the area for the use of the local health officials and practicing physicians.

**Central Laboratory.** The large central laboratory carries out the same activities as the small local laboratories and, in addition, has special activities that are feasible only when done on a large scale, or which actually require highly specialized skill. Diagnostic services of communicable disease are:

*Diphtheria.* Rapid results are essential. The service is of little value if the laboratory is more than six hours by quickest delivery route from the most remote area to be served. The plain, sterile cotton swab is the most satisfactory method of obtaining the specimen. The direct examination, the eight hour culture and the eighteen hour culture examination are made. Positive results should be reported by telegram.

Release cultures should follow the same procedure except that the direct examination is omitted and reports may be sent by mail. Virulence tests for diphtheria carrier release is also an occasional procedure.

All the usual direct, microscopic laboratory tests are made by the large laboratory, including gonococcus smears, malaria blood films, examination of animal brain for rabies, feces examination for intestinal parasites, sputum examination for tuberculosis, etc.

Cultural examination of blood, feces and urine for diagnosis of typhoid fever, as well as Widal tests, and cultural examination of spinal fluids in diagnosis of meningitis are within the scope of the activities of the large laboratory.

One of the chief activities of any large laboratory is the serodiagnosis of syphilis. A good technician can make 500 to 1,000 tests a week without difficulty.

Chemical and bacteriological examination of public water supplies and of sewage effluents are routine procedures of the large laboratory. Most public health laboratories also make chemical and bacteriological analyses of foods.

*Vaccines and Sera.* Preparation of vaccines and sera play an increasing part in the activities of some of the larger state public health laboratories. Among the products that have been produced with profit are:

1. Typhoid vaccine.
2. Diphtheria toxoid and toxin for the Schick test.
3. Silver nitrate ampules.
4. Smallpox vaccine.
5. Rabies treatments.
6. Collection and preparation of convalescent sera.
7. Collection of normal whole blood, with processing of serum globulin.

Less frequent activities are: preparation of diphtheria antitoxin, tetanus antitoxin and pneumococcus anti-serum. It should be re-emphasized that the health department may find it cheaper in the long run to purchase rather than manufacture biological products.

**Private Clinical Laboratories.** The functions of the private clinical laboratories are quite distinct from those of the public health laboratory and there need be no misunderstanding or disagreement between them. The clinical laboratory carries out clinical tests to determine individual disability, or the clinical progress of a disease in the individual. The public health laboratory limits its activities to diagnosis of those conditions that are of importance in protection of public health. Thus, examination of municipal water supplies or of water supplies to which the public has access is the function of the health department; but it is not feasible for the official laboratory to furnish free laboratory tests of all private wells of the jurisdiction. It is generally conceded also that routine urine examination, differential blood counts or total leucocyte counts and other clinical diagnostic tests are not the function of the public health laboratory.

The chief exception to these general rules has been the free diagnostic cancer service that has been given by some of the municipal and state laboratories.

**Extension of Public Health Laboratory Activities.** There is an unmistakable tendency to extend public health laboratory technics to include other fields. Cultivation of gonococci to determine duration of infectiousness has been adopted in some laboratories. Cultivation of the tubercle bacillus is recommended rather than standard animal inoculation tests. Tissue diagnosis in suspected cancer is an accepted public health laboratory test in many communities, and physicians are constantly asking for public health laboratory facilities for determination of blood levels of sulfanilamide and its derivatives, determination of blood nitrogen, of blood sugar, and other clinical tests.

There seems to be more demand for development of laboratory diagnostic service on a community-wide and community-supported basis than for almost any other medical service. In general, it is fair to say that these requests have come from the medical profession rather than from the public. Some physicians believe that this represents an opening wedge for "state medicine." If this is true, the fact remains that the physicians themselves have made the request.

## ORGANIZATION

The organization of the public health laboratory depends upon density of population and facilities for transportation. The laboratory is a direct link between the health department and the public, and can make or mar the reputation of the whole organization. It is one of the most expensive units of the health department, because of the high cost of equipment, and because of the higher salaries that must be paid for well-trained, experienced technical assistants.

A poor laboratory is worse than no laboratory at all. It is not feasible, therefore, to establish a laboratory with one technician only, working without supervision. Some states have encouraged the inclusion of a trained bacteriologist in the personnel of a county health unit. This is feasible only in the larger, more prosperous counties. The smallest effective laboratory unit consists of one director, one technician and one helper. This unit can carry a volume of 10,000 to 15,000 specimens a year. As the work grows, the personnel may be increased by the addition of a technician and a clerk. This unit will serve the needs of from 50,000 to 100,000 persons and requires a budget of approximately $8,000.

If only 10,000 specimens are done by this laboratory annually, the per specimen cost is 80 cents, which is excessive.

One plan that has worked effectively in some small health jurisdictions is the organization of a joint public health and clinical laboratory service. The local hospital, for example, and the health department join forces, arrange a joint budget and establish a laboratory in space furnished by the hospital. The objections to this plan from an administrative point of view are obvious. If the hospital is a community hospital in the true sense of the word, with a bed capacity of 100 or more, and serving a population of 50,000 or more, then it may be quite possible to develop a community-supported laboratory service that will meet all the needs of the people, including the clinical laboratory tests that may be required, and also the various public health laboratory procedures.

If a community health and hospital service is organized as a single administrative unit, then the administration of the public health laboratory service is very simple. All the clinical and public health laboratory activities are organized in a single well co-ordinated service which carries out both the clinical and public health laboratory requirements of the community, with no fine distinction as to which service is or is not a public health responsibility.

**The Small Laboratory.** Some small jurisdictions have provided an excellent simple laboratory service with one technician only. The laboratory is in the community hospital, and the laboratory technician does the clinical diagnostic tests, the simple public health laboratory work, and may also serve as x-ray technician. This type of laboratory service is quite inexpensive, but can only function effectively if it is closely linked with a central laboratory which is under a capable director. This central director must give close supervision of the activities and standardization of technics in the local branch laboratories.

**Cost.** The proportional cost of the state laboratory should not be greater than 15 to 20 per cent of the total budget of the state health department. The local laboratory will absorb less than 10 per cent of the total health department funds.

A state laboratory serving a million people, more or less, is best organized as a separate bureau of the health department, with a full-time director. It is advantageous if the director has a medical degree in addition to his technical laboratory training. Four chief divisions of activity are usually organized, each with a competent technical assistant in charge. An organization may be planned as follows:

DIRECTOR

| *Administration* | *Bacteriological* | *Serological* | *Chemical* |
|---|---|---|---|
| Receiving specimens. Mailing containers. Recording and tabulating data. Reporting results to physicians and local health officers. 2 or 3 clerks. | Diagnosis of communicable disease. 5 technicians. 3 or 4 helpers. | 2 or 3 technicians. 1 helper. | 2 chemists. 3 helpers. |

The budget for this organization is approximately $40,000 to $60,000. This laboratory would examine about 100,000 specimens a year at 50 cents per specimen. This represents 1 specimen examined for every 10 persons, and about 50 specimens examined for each physician practicing in the state.

The per specimen cost in a well organized laboratory should not be greater than 35 to 40 cents. It is impossible to make a fair comparison of various laboratories on the basis of per specimen cost. The important factors are accurate technic and availability of the service. It is a bad policy to cut the per specimen cost of the service at the expense of quality.

**Decentralized Laboratory Service.** One central state laboratory cannot give adequate service in states with a large area. In New England and some other smaller states, such as Delaware and New Jersey, where the population is dense, communication rapid and distances are not great, one central laboratory will suffice. In states with a widely scattered population the difficulty has been met by establishment of branch laboratories under control or supervision of the central laboratory. Such a system is in operation in nine or ten states, as well as some of the provinces in Canada, the Philippine Islands and Hawaii. The plan seems to be universally adaptable. It has the advantage of uniformity of methods, unification of administration under single responsibility, better service at a lower per specimen cost, and maintenance of high standards of service.

In some states a co-operative arrangement for branch laboratory service has been made with some of the state institutions, such as state university laboratories or state hospitals. Where this occurs, there is a tendency for the branch laboratory to lose its identity with the public health department.

The system of decentralization of laboratory service developed in Alabama by Havens is singularly free from the defects and criticisms which are common to most state health laboratories. The branch laboratories are located in railroad centers or strategic junctions where they can serve the territory most effectively. Each laboratory is a part of the local health department and is thus identified with local health activities. The local health department furnishes space, as well as electricity and gas for laboratory requirements, and in some instances contributes toward the budget of the laboratory. The branch laboratory is equipped to make the same diagnostic tests as the central laboratory. The branch laboratories are under close supervision of, and are responsible to, the central laboratory. Technic and methods are uniform. Supervision is maintained in three ways: by personal inspections, by test specimens at frequent intervals, and by monthly reports. This policy has resulted in a highly effective service, which is within ready reach of the entire population of the state. This plan gives a close contact with the medical profession, a uniformity of laboratory standards, a high degree of efficiency, and a co-ordination with other local and state health department activities. If community medical centers are developed in various parts of the United States, not on a proprietary basis, but rather as sound, community-supported institutions, then the logical corollary development is the establishment of local laboratories in each of these community medical centers.

Under such a plan, much of the work of the central state department laboratory can and should be transferred to the local laboratories. Under this de-centralizing laboratory system, the central laboratory division of the state would serve as a supervising and standardizing agency; only those few special activities would be carried out in the central laboratory that could not be done effectively in the local community laboratory.

**Interpretation of Results.** One important administrative principle must be emphasized in relation to public health laboratory practice. The laboratory *must not interpret* the results of the laboratory to the physician or to the various divisions of the health organization to whom reports are made. A blood specimen is reported as a positive Wassermann, not as a positive diagnosis of syphilis; a throat culture is reported as negative for diphtheria bacilli, and should not be interpreted as absolute proof that the child is suffering from some other disease than diphtheria. The water analysis is reported according to the bacteriological and chemical findings to the Department of Sanitary Engineering. The sanitary engineer then puts together all other data that he has accumulated and makes the proper interpretation.

The laboratory is a very important aid in making a diagnosis, whether it be of a clinical case of disease, or study of a source of an epidemic; but the laboratory should not make the diagnosis nor interpret the results. It is the function of the laboratory to carry out the technical procedures as accurately as possible and report these results. The clinician or epidemiologist must interpret them and make the final diagnosis.

**Educational Requirements for Public Health Laboratory Workers.** Men and women with a great variety of training and experience are employed in the public health laboratory. In 1945, about 1,500 workers in the professional grades were employed in the official public health laboratories of the United States. There is every reason to believe that this number will increase.

The minimum training for appointment to the professional staff of a public health laboratory is a bachelor's degree, with major training in one of the scientific fields that is embraced in laboratory work. The higher laboratory positions require long experience or post-graduate study leading to a doctorate. The directorship of a laboratory service is a responsible position, with many administrative duties, and requires a doctor's degree with special public health training in administration, epidemiology, and vital statistics. There are many advantages to a medical degree for persons who direct large state or municipal laboratories.

The educational qualifications of public health laboratory workers have been carefully and clearly defined by the Committee on Professional Education of the American Public Health Association. They are given in detail in the Appendix.

## REFERENCES

1. Havens, Leon. *The Developments and Results of a State-wide Laboratory Service.* South. Med. J. 1925, Vol. 18, p. 521.
2. *Public Health in New York State.* Publication of the New York State Health Department, Albany, New York. 1933.
3. Wadsworth, A. B. *Standard Methods of the Division of Laboratories and Research.* (3rd edition.) 1946. New York State Health Department. Published by Williams and Wilkins Co. Baltimore, Md. Contains comprehensive bibliography.
4. Kolmer, J. A. and Boerner, Fred. *Approved Laboratory Technic.* (4th edition), D. Appleton-Century Co. New York. 1945.
See also current publications of the American Public Health Association relating to standard laboratory methods, as, for example:
    Standard Methods for Examination of Water and Sewage. 9th edition. 1946.
    Standard Methods for the Examination of Dairy Products. 1947 (9th edition).
    Diagnostic Procedures and Reagents: Technics for the Laboratory Diagnosis and Control of the Communicable Diseases. 2nd edition. 1945.

# CHAPTER XXI

## PUBLIC HEALTH NURSING

PUBLIC health nursing is an organized service (not for profit) rendered by graduate nurses to the individual, family and community.[1] This service includes the interpretation and application of medical, sanitary and social procedures for the correction of defects, prevention of disease and the promotion of health, and may include skilled care of the sick in their homes.

No individual plays a greater part in the development of the public health program than the nurse. Any health organization that does not incorporate the work of the public health nurse as an integral part of its program is sure to be ineffective. Her services are utilized by all divisions of activity including communicable disease, maternal and infant welfare, preschool and school hygiene, industrial hygiene and health education. Even the division of vital statistics, the laboratory and division of sanitation rely upon her for part of their information and for the effectiveness of their work.

The nurse enters most intimately into the lives of the people, wins their confidence and interprets the purposes of the health department to everyone in the community. Thus her services are indispensable.

In any well organized modern local health department, one half the personnel and nearly one half the total expenditures are devoted to the public health nursing service. The initiation and growth of public health nursing has occurred in recent years. Many administrative difficulties have been encountered and, in many instances, the work has been developed with untrained and incompetent personnel. As public health nursing has increased in quantity and quality, certain general principles in regard to public health nursing personnel have been developed:

1. Only those nurses that have graduated from a recognized school of nursing, and have been registered according to state requirements, should be utilized in a public health nursing program.

2. Public health nurses should have special public health training in addition to their general hospital course.

3. Provision should be made for maintenance of a high standard of technical performance of duty. This can best be insured by a plan of continuous supervision of technic by a qualified supervisor.

[1] Definition of the National Organization for Public Health Nursing.

4. A continuous program of education should be maintained for the nurse who is at work in the field.

## QUALIFICATIONS FOR PUBLIC HEALTH NURSES

Minimum qualifications for public health nurses have been established by the National Organization for Public Health Nursing. These standards have been accepted in full by the Committee on Professional Education of the American Public Health Association. They are given in detail in the Appendix.

## THE FUNCTIONS OF A PUBLIC HEALTH NURSE

The duties of the nurse touch every phase of the public health program. There are certain portions of the work that are her special field. The details of technic of public health nursing may be found in the good textbooks on the subject.[2] We shall do more than enumerate some of the public health nurse's activities to demonstrate the scope of her work.

**Communicable Disease Control.** The special function of the nurse in communicable disease control is to assist in the prevention of the spread of disease through instruction in isolation, quarantine and in immunization. She assists in obtaining medical supervision of a case, provides or supervises nursing care in the home, and emphasizes the importance of convalescent care in the prevention of sequelae. In some health departments the nurse carries out the isolation technic in the home. Her work is of direct aid in obtaining complete reporting of communicable disease, and the information secured by her in the home is of great value to the epidemiologist in determining sources of infection.

*Tuberculosis.* The chief burden of tuberculosis prevention falls on the public health nurse. She should keep an active file of all cases of tuberculosis in her jurisdiction, and should visit each of these patients at suitable intervals. She should arrange for medical supervision of the case in the home. It is her duty to teach the patient and the family the necessary technic of partial isolation of the patient in the home. She should arrange for institutional care of patients in her territory and assist in rehabilitation. The nurse should keep in touch with family contacts and secure their medical examination. She may aid in finding early cases of tuberculosis, and may assist also in securing complete reporting of the disease. The nurse helps to organize the tuberculosis clinic, and arranges means of transportation for the patients who have difficulty in attending. In brief, all the tuberculosis cases of her jurisdiction, as well as their families, should be kept under constant, watchful supervision.

*Venereal Disease.* The increasingly important part that the nurse plays in a venereal disease prevention program is being recognized. By tactful, sympathetic understanding, she may aid in securing continuous attend-

[2] The Public Health Nursing Manual, published by the National Organization for Public Health Nursing, is an excellent text.

ance at the clinics of infected individuals in her territory, to the end that each patient will receive adequate care. She may follow up cases that have lapsed; she tries to arrange for the examination of family contacts, and instructs the family in suitable measures for isolation of the infective individual at home. She may determine the sources of infection and get them under proper treatment. Indirectly, the nurse may aid in securing better reporting of both syphilis and gonorrhea.

**Maternity Service.** Maternity service includes prenatal care, postnatal care and care during delivery.

The objective of maternal care is to get in touch with all prospective mothers as early in pregnancy as possible and to arrange for adequate nursing and medical supervision throughout the prenatal and postnatal period. The nurse may arrange for medical examination of the mother, instruct the mother in maternity hygiene and in infant care, give instruction in proper preparation for delivery, and may aid also in arranging for nursing care during and after delivery. Public health nurses frequently carry out the actual bedside nursing service during delivery and make a suitable number of visits to the mother and baby for a fortnight after delivery. Usually, this service is provided by a voluntary rather than by an official health organization.

**Infant Hygiene.** Children under 1 year. The nurse instructs the mother in the hygiene and daily regimen of the baby. She arranges with the parents for medical supervision and instructs the mother in carrying out the doctor's orders in relation to feeding the baby. The line between the province of the family physician and the function of the nurse is a close one, but the tactful public health nurse will have the confidence of the physicians in the community, and will supplement the labor of the physician and relieve him of many of the minute details of instruction in baby care that are so important, but so time-consuming to the busy physician. The nurse must carry out her work without usurping the physician's authority or suggesting procedures that are contrary to his wishes. The nurse should aid in securing smallpox vaccination and diphtheria immunization during the baby's first year, and assist also in securing more complete registration of births.

Continuous bedside nursing of a sick infant is not considered a function of the public health nurse in most communities. In the future, bedside nursing instruction for the sick may well be incorporated in a public health nursing service. It is usually impossible, under present conditions, for the nurse to devote her full time to the care of one sick child, but the nurse may give a demonstration to the mother of proper nursing care and may make provision, if necessary, for continued bedside nursing care by some intelligent person who will follow the instructions of the physician and the nurse.

**Preschool Hygiene.** Ages 1 to 6 years. We have made a serious mistake in dividing the child's age periods too arbitrarily. There is a distinct change in the child's whole life when he enters school,—usually at about 6 years of age; but before this time the health service should be a continuous and not a broken chain. The same type of service that is rendered to infants is continued for the older children by the public health nurse. The older child is seen less often, and the problems are somewhat different. At the end of one year the baby is fairly launched in life; dietary habits have been established, and the period of communicable disease has begun.

The nurse aids in securing medical supervision of the older child, so that any defects that may develop may be corrected as early as possible. She may actually plan suitable arrangements whereby defects may be corrected, through tonsil clinics, etc. The mother is taught the principles of child hygiene and the daily routine of healthy living. The nurse assists also in control of communicable disease by securing proper immunization procedures during the preschool age and by detecting early symptoms of the contagious diseases in the children of her territory.

**School Hygiene.** The nurse is the connecting link between the school medical service and the home. She works with the teacher, the school physician and the parent for the betterment of the health of the child. Actual instruction in hygiene and public health is given by the teacher. The nurse may aid in promotion of sanitation of the school plant, and may furnish suitable material to the teachers for instruction purposes; but unless she is trained in pedagogy she would not be expected, as a rule, actually to teach hygiene to the children. Usually, the nurse aids the school physician in the medical examination of the school children. Her special function is the interpretation of the results of the medical examination to the teacher and parents. She assists also in securing correction of the defects found. She should aid in control of communicable disease in the school by early recognition of symptoms of contagious disease and by securing immunization.

**Mental Hygiene.** Mental hygiene is an integral part of the general program of the public health nurse. It permeates all phases of her work, particularly through the early age groups.

She should be familiar with the principles of psychology and understand normal and abnormal variations in human behavior. She should be on the alert to recognize the early symptoms of definite mental deficiencies in a child. She must be familiar with the resources at her command for the early diagnosis and treatment of children who manifest abnormal behavior, and she should aid in securing proper care for them. She should aid the parents also in adjusting the home life of the child in order to correct habits and tendencies that, if allowed to develop, may result in serious consequences in future life.

**Orthopedic Service.** The public health nurse has a special responsibility in caring for the crippled and handicapped in the community, particularly the crippled children. She should keep a complete card index of all children in her jurisdiction who have orthopedic defects, should secure proper medical care for them and provide means for correction of the defects, in so far as possible. She may actually give the after-care to poliomyelitis victims, and teach the muscle exercises to the patient and the family, thus aiding and instructing them to carry out the physician's orders. She should arrange for rehabilitation of orthopedic cases and secure means of education through vocational guidance.

The Social Security Act has greatly improved the facilities for the care of crippled children throughout the United States. The nurse should utilize these facilities to their fullest extent, and should keep up a continuous search for cripples in her community. The earlier a crippled child receives proper care, the better will be his chances of becoming a useful member of society. The neglected cripple often develops a sense of social injustice and a mental maladjustment that is difficult to overcome. The public health nurse meets a great community need in this field. No other phase of her work has a more popular appeal, or meets with greater sympathy.

## MORBIDITY SERVICE

Morbidity service, or bedside nursing care, is concerned primarily with actual care of sick persons. In the United States this service has been developed in great part as a function of private organizations. Usually, the patients pay for this nursing care, in so far as they are able. In those communities where bedside nursing is not adequately developed by private agencies, there is a tendency for the public health organization to develop a morbidity nursing service. Because of the many demands on official public health nurses, particularly in relation to health supervision, it is usually impossible for the public health nurses to make daily bedside visits to the sick. The purpose of the morbidity service is to give instruction to the family in the proper technic of nursing care of the patient who is ill at home. Whether or not the nursing care of the sick in the home should be a charge on the public treasury is a debatable question. There is no question but that the official health organization should assume responsibility for the control of preventable disease, but it is often very difficult to draw the line in a given case between care of the ill and prevention of future illness and disability. Confronted by this difficulty, the health officer has usually assigned all activities relating to *bedside nursing care* of the *sick* to voluntary private agencies, and has limited the activities of the public health nurse to *prevention* of *illness* and *disability*. This distinction is very confusing to the public, and is a constant source of trouble to the health department. How this administrative difficulty will be solved is a matter for the future to determine. At present, the public health nurse of an official agency cannot give constant bedside care of the sick and carry out her other work as well. If the health department had one nurse for each 2,000 population, it would be possible, but the expense would be much greater than the public has been willing to bear.

## ORGANIZATION OF A PUBLIC HEALTH NURSING SERVICE

The organization of a public health nursing service depends, in some degree, upon the size of the unit. No unit, however small, should develop public health nursing as the only function of the health department. This has been done frequently, and is a serious mistake. On the other hand, no health department is complete without nursing service. Many small health departments have very inadequate nursing service, with only one public health nurse to 30,000 or 40,000 population. But so long as the health officer realizes that his nursing service is inadequate, and outlines a framework for the expansion of his nursing program, he can begin with one nurse and add more as soon as his finances permit. To simplify the discussion as to the organization of an adequate nursing service, a standard community of 100,000 population may be selected. Two chief plans of organization have been developed:

**The Specialized Plan.** The specialized plan requires that each nurse shall develop some special field of work and be assigned to a specific division of the health department; as, for example, the division of communicable disease, tuberculosis control, school hygiene, etc.

From fifteen to twenty public health nurses would ordinarily be employed in a city of 100,000 population, their services divided as follows:

| | |
|---|---|
| 1. Communicable Disease Control | 2 or 3 nurses |
|     *a.* Tuberculosis | 2 or 3 nurses |
|     *b.* Venereal Disease | 1      nurse |
| 2. Maternity, Infancy, Preschool | 5 or 6 nurses |
| 3. School Nurses | 5 to 7 nurses |
| Total | 15 to 20 |

Each nurse would work under the direction of the division chief, as would any other individual of the health department staff. Each person in the division, including the nurse, has a clear-cut function, with a definite province of activity and a responsible head of the service.

This has been a common form of public health nursing organization in the United States in the past and theoretically is most advantageous from an administrative point of view. Practically, it is very unsatisfactory. The community is not divided into cases of tuberculosis and venereal disease, or into groups of school children, but into *families.* The family is the unit of life in the United States. Some member of the family may have tuberculosis, some members of the family go to school. Thus the nurse, to be efficient, must work with the *family* as a unit, and with the whole community within her sphere of influence, rather than with the individual as a specific case.

The specialized plan in actual operation results in great overlapping of activities. Two or three public health nurses may visit the same home on the same day; one to visit an infant, another to secure a correction of a defect in a school child, another to see the father who has incipient tuberculosis. There is no standardization of technic under this plan, and no proper supervision of the nurse's activities, for there is no division of public health nursing and no supervisor. If a supervisor is appointed, she has no authority, for each nurse must work under the director of her special department. Otherwise, the nurse has two directors: the director of her specific activities, who is the chief of her division, and the nursing supervisor, who has technical supervision of her work.

**The Generalized Plan.** The generalized plan requires that a public health nurse be assigned to a definite geographic area in the community with a specified number of families in her jurisdiction.

The usual plan is to assign one nurse to approximately 1,200 families. Thus, for a city of 100,000 people, approximately 16 to 20 nurses would be required, with one supervisor. The great advantages of this plan are its simplicity of administration and cohesion of service. Each nurse carries out all types of public health service in her territory. Thus she becomes familiar with the family problems and the social structure of every part of the community and is known personally by every individual. Her office is in the center of her district and she keeps definite office hours, when the people know they can find her.

The plan is elastic and can be contracted or expanded to meet changing needs. The director of nursing is the connecting link in the service, giving continuous instruction and standardizing the technic and content of the nursing visits. The great difficulty with the plan is, of course, that the work is not organized on a functional basis as is the rest of the health department. For example, the only connecting chain between the nurse who is engaged in communicable disease as part of her activities, and the director of the division of communicable disease, is the nursing director.

To be successful, therefore, the plan requires that the director of the nurses must be a most capable and well-trained person, who has the same status as other divisional directors. She should attend all health department conferences, be familiar with the policies and projects of each divisional director, and must develop the work of the nursing service so that it interlocks with the general program of the department. Under this plan the nurses are directly responsible to the director of nurses and not directly responsible to the divisional directors of specific services. Thus, unless there is the closest co-operation and understanding between the director of nurses and the other divisional directors, the plan will not be successful administratively. Other objections to the plan are obvious. Among other things, many health officers object to a plan which permits one nurse to carry on communicable disease control work and maternity and infancy work at the same time. Some health officers feel that generalized service represents lower quality of service, because the nurse who specializes in one type of work acquires a high proficiency in that technic that is not obtained in general work.

**Small Health Departments.** In small health departments, the *general plan* of public health nursing is the only feasible one. In most county health units, for example, only five or six nurses are employed, often for a population of 35,000 to 40,000 people. Under such conditions, the nurses do the very best they can to cover the whole public health nursing field, but usually they must concentrate on some special activity, such as school hygiene and maternity and infancy work. The capable trained public health nurse will concentrate on health supervision activities, and will select those which are most important to the particular area in which she is situated. The nurse is responsible to the health officer for her program, but her technic and the quality of her service are supervised, as a rule, by a supervisor from the state department of public health nursing. Her functions are the same as those of her sister who works in the large city, but her activities will be less intensive and she must be more resourceful and more capable of initiating and planning her own work.

**Large Health Departments.** The tendency in the health department organization of very large cities has been to develop a certain amount of specialized nursing service, even where the generalized plan has been adopted. Where the health service of the schools is under the direction of the department of education, the specialized plan is adopted almost of necessity. If the school nursing service is not included in the official health department activities, the generalized plan cannot be complete or effective. Many health officers feel that contagious disease control, tuberculosis nursing and particularly maternity and infancy work, require a specialized technic that only long experience can give, and prefer to develop these services on a specialized basis with nurses assigned to these specific activities.

**Combined Plan.** In some of the large cities a virtual combination of the two plans has been devised. A department of public health nursing is organized, with a director who supervises the work of the nurses and standardizes the content of each nursing visit. The nurses are directly responsible to her for their nursing technic. Where large numbers of nurses are required, as in the big cities, the nursing organization consists of a director and a corps of supervisors. Good nursing practice requires one supervisor to every 15 or 20 staff nurses. In addition, the director may have specially trained assistants, such as nutritionists, mental hygienists, and the like, who aid in the continuous in-service teaching program for the staff nurses.

The director of each functional division of service in the health department makes his annual plans, which may require the services of a stated number of nurses. After conferring with the nursing director, the desired number of nurses are assigned to duty in his division, and become responsible to him for the carrying out of certain of the activities of the department. Thus the nurses who are assigned to a department become responsible to the division director for carrying out certain activities, and responsible to the supervisor for their technic. The administrative difficulties of such an arrangement are obvious.

**Industrial Nursing Service.** Industry itself has become a large employer of public health nurses. A remarkable expansion in this field occurred during the tremendous industrial activities of World War II. An increase from 5,512 industrially employed nurses in 1942, to 11,220 in 1944 brought a realization by the nation that the public health nurse has a special contribution to make in this field. Many of these nurses had no proper training for their work. Certain standards of qualifications for industrial nurses have been formulated by the Committee on Professional Education of the American Public Health Association[3] which are of great aid to industry in selecting nurses and planning this health service.

The functions of the industrial nurse and the part she plays in community health protection are discussed in the section on Industrial Hygiene.

**State Health Department Nursing Service.** A few state health departments have very large public health nursing organizations, and carry out a local public health nursing program which is directed from the central office. Except in the very small states, this is not an economical or effective procedure. The chief function of the state health nursing service is to aid local health departments in developing an effective public health nursing service.

The state director of public health nursing must have exceptional qualifications. She must possess qualities which win the confidence and respect of local health officials and particularly the nursing directors of both the official and the voluntary agencies in the state. In fact, she must be generally recognized as the best qualified public health nurse in the state.

Her department need not be large. Depending upon the size of the state, she should have two to six supervising nurses under her direction who have definite geographic assignments. They visit local health departments, confer with health officials in regard to nursing programs, advise local nursing directors concerning the supervision of the technic of the local public health nurses, and aid in the betterment of the local program. Their function is to advise rather than to direct.

The state director of public health nursing should aid in the formulation of a continuous plan of education for the public health nurses in the state. She should aid local health departments also in the selection of their personnel. This latter function is the key to good public health nursing service in the state.

[3] See Appendix.

It is obvious that the most essential factor for success in the state nursing programs is that the state director of public health nursing shall possess qualities of leadership. All the public health nurses in the state, from both the official and the voluntary agencies, should look to her for guidance and advice in all matters pertaining to their work.

## NATIONAL PUBLIC HEALTH NURSING SERVICES

**Federal Services.** There are some eleven or twelve agencies of the Federal Government that employ public health nurses. The two most concerned are the United States Public Health Service and the Children's Bureau. These two organizations employ highly qualified public health nurses, whose major activity is consultant service for state health departments. In addition, some nurses are required for the epidemiologic and other field studies, such as nutrition, investigation, and the like. The Emergency Maternity and Infant Care Program of the Children's Bureau during the war years called for special nursing consultant services throughout the nation.

**The National Organization for Public Health Nursing.** The real leadership in the field of public health nursing in the United States is found in this splendid national organization which was founded in 1912. It has maintained standards of training and qualifications for public health nursing which are revised every five years, and which have been of great value not only in improving the quality of nursing services, but more important, in delineating the functions of a public health nurse and formulating administrative procedures which promote a more intelligent and effective nursing service.

**Red Cross.** The Red Cross maintains a nursing service which has as a major function the provision of public health nursing care to remote areas that are in special need. This has been a pioneer nursing service which has been of great value. Administratively this service has caused considerable misunderstanding, since the service is directed from national headquarters and the nurses have not been assigned to work under the direction of the official health agency of the area in which they are stationed.

## VOLUNTARY NURSING ORGANIZATIONS

Public health nursing is really an outgrowth of the splendid voluntary nursing service that has been developed so successfully by private organizations in many of our larger cities. This work was initiated as a service for the care of the sick in their homes, but the need for preventive work was so obvious that most of the district nursing organizations have gradually assumed public health functions. Much later, public health nursing has been established as an official function of the health department.

The health officer will find it advantageous to utilize the facilities of these established voluntary health organizations, in some instances by adding workers from his department to their staffs, or by otherwise subsidizing their work. Gradually the official health department will assume all responsibility for public health nursing supervision, but the transition will be slow. Most of the voluntary district nursing associations have been glad to relinquish the accepted health supervision phases of their nursing programs as soon as the official agency has been willing to assume them, in order that they might concentrate their efforts on bedside nursing care and do pioneer work in new and untried fields. Best results are secured for the community, if the health officer develops his activities in close co-operation with the voluntary health organizations, serves on their executive boards and aids in directing their policies. He may even delegate certain definite fields of public health nursing, such as prenatal and postnatal care, to the voluntary organizations, so long as they carry out a satisfactory program.

The Tuberculosis Association of any community may be a tower of strength and aid to a local health officer in making his anti-tuberculosis program more effective. The purpose of this organization is essentially educational, but in many communities the society has undertaken the nursing care of the sick, the development of rehabilitation programs for the tuberculous and other handicapped persons in the community, and many other worth while public health activities.

The co-ordination of these activities of voluntary agencies with official health activities is not inconsistent with good administrative methods. The tactful health officer will utilize to the fullest extent the talent and enthusiasm of the people who are interested in the control of tuberculosis, or any other health activity in his community, without sacrificing any of his official prerogatives.

## TRENDS IN PUBLIC HEALTH NURSING [4]

The place of the public health nurse in the social order is just beginning to emerge. An ideal administrative plan for any community would be a single unified community service which would supply all the required medical care. This would include hospital and home nursing, industrial nursing, school nursing, and other services that are now classified as public health nursing.

It has been estimated conservatively that one nurse per 2,000 to 2,500 population would furnish reasonably adequate community nursing service. This would include all the activities now carried out by public health nurses, and also provide for an hourly nursing bedside care service for the sick in their homes.

[4] An address by Miss Alma Haupt to the Committee on Medicine and the Changing Order of the New York Academy of Medicine entitled "Public Health Nursing and the Changing Order" on May 26, 1944, furnished the author with many of the basic ideas expressed in the following paragraphs.

The number of public health nurses in the United States in 1945 was about 20,000. The comprehensive nursing plan would require 65,000 public health nurses, with an increase in budget of over $120,000,000 annually.

**Nursing Personnel.** Not only would a comprehensive nursing service require a great increase in the number of nurses employed, but a different quality of service as well. Mountin [5] has suggested four types of workers for the performance of nursing duties:

1. Administrators, educators, and therapeutic technicians.
2. Staff nurses who "minister to personal needs which are peculiar to sick people."
3. Practical nurses.
4. Housekeeping aids who perform household and simple nursing tasks.

If an organization can be set up which will divide the tasks of nursing, then the highly trained and skilled personnel of groups 1 and 2 can be used to greatest community advantage.

In rural communities with a community hospital which is administered by the director of health services of the community, it becomes quite possible for all nursing services of the area—intra- and extramural—to be organized on a unit basis under the supervision of a single capable administrator. This plan could not be carried out effectively on a fee-for-service basis, but would be organized as part of a community-wide prepayment plan for comprehensive medical care. This type of organization should be admirably suited to local administrative units of 50,000 to 100,000 population, such as municipalities and county health units.

In large cities, it is quite possible to organize a similar type of comprehensive nursing service, but the organization and administrative problems would require great skill and real foresight.

It seems probable that in the near future the private organizations that now conduct public health nursing programs will fuse their activities with those of the official health agencies. Private organizations which give bedside care of the sick on an hourly basis, with fee for service, may well be continued in the larger cities at least, as an active and effective community agency. Under a comprehensive plan for prepaid medical care, these organizations might render nursing care under contract with the central medical care agency of the community.

**National Planning.** Nursing care is a direct service to the people. Obviously it must be organized and administered by the local community. But the development of comprehensive nursing service is only a part of a community plan for comprehensive medical care.

Community planning requires great foresight and skill. This can be rendered best through a strong state advisory service. Furthermore, a

[5] Mountin, J. W.: "Suggestions to Nurses on Postwar Adjustments." *Am. Jour. Nursing.* 1944 (April), Vol. 44, p. 321.

proper division of services to all parts of the nation requires an overall national planning and advisory service. This can be provided best by a federal organization that gives advice and aid to the states, and through them to each of the local communities in formulation of detailed direct service programs.

This matter is discussed in some detail in other sections of this text, but is repeated here, since public health nursing is such an integral and important part of the whole health service of the local community.

The first steps in future planning in public health nursing are:

1. Better geographic distribution of present public health nursing facilities.

2. Better integration of official and voluntary public health nursing agencies.

3. Inclusion of hourly bedside nursing service in prepayment medical care plans.

4. Broader training of public health nurses to meet the needs of the future. This requires provision for special and continuous instruction of public health nurses in the fields of mental hygiene, nutrition, sociology, health administration, and other fields.

5. A continuous program of community education concerning the true functions of a community nursing service, and the development of a community-wide appreciation of the value to the people of this work.

## REFERENCES

1. Gardner, Mary L. *Public Health Nursing.* The Macmillan Company. 1936. 3rd edition.

2. Beard, Mary. *The Nurse in Public Health.* Harper & Brothers. 1929.

3. *Manual of Public Health Nursing.* Prepared by the National Organization for Public Health Nursing. The Macmillan Company, New York City. 1939. 3rd edition.

4. *Board Members' Manual.* Prepared by the National Organization for Public Health Nursing. The Macmillan Company, New York City. 1937.

5. Hodgson, Violet H. *Supervision in Public Health Nursing.* Commonwealth Fund, New York City. 1939.

6. Grant, Amelia. *Nursing: A Community Health Service.* W. B. Saunders Co., Philadelphia. 1942.

7. Freeman, Ruth. *Technics of Supervision in Public Health Nursing.* W. B. Saunders Co., Philadelphia. 1944.

8. Emory, F. H. M. *Public Health Nursing in Canada.* The Macmillan Company. 1945.

9. McGrath, B. J. *Nursing in Commerce and Industry.* Commonwealth Fund, New York City. 1946.

10. Gardner, M. S. *Katherine Kent: A Biography of a Public Health Nurse.* The Macmillan Company, New York. 1946.

The valuable, carefully prepared publications of the National Organization for Public Health Nursing, 1790 Broadway, New York City, should be consulted on all matters relating to details of public health nursing administration.

# CHAPTER XXII

## SANITATION AND SANITARY INSPECTION

THE term "sanitation" as it is commonly used in health department practice is a comprehensive one, for it includes all those matters that relate to hygiene of the environment.

Formerly, sanitary inspection was the most extensive of all the activities of a well-organized local health department, but in recent years the emphasis has shifted to other equally important health functions. In the minds of many people, sanitary inspection is still the chief function of an official health service. As a matter of fact, in more primitive areas or in less advanced organizations, sanitary inspection service still absorbs a large proportion of the budget as well as of personnel.

The great emphasis formerly placed on sanitary inspection service was dependent upon the theory of the miasmatic origin of disease, which postulated a bad effect upon community health as a result of bad odors and decaying animal or vegetable proteins. This thesis presumed that filth and untidiness *per se* produced disease. Thus, many, even most, of the activities of the health department were related to abatement of nuisances and waste removal. We now know that these activities are beneficial to the community from the esthetic point of view, but have little public health importance. A good example of this change in viewpoint is the attitude toward garbage disposal service. Formerly, this activity was considered an essential function of the public health department. Even in recent years a large proportion of the budget of many municipal health departments was used for garbage disposal. We now realize that this activity, whether carried out well or poorly, has no measurable influence upon the prevention of disease in the community. Nevertheless, health officers have had great difficulty in transferring this function to the Department of Public Works, where it really belongs.

Later, gaseous fumigation was developed. This public health activity was dependent upon the theory that most communicable diseases are airborne, and that the infectious agent could be destroyed in the environs of the infected individual by gaseous fumigation. Thus fumigation became an important and expensive function of the local health department. Some cities developed elaborate and very efficient systems of gaseous fumigation and terminal disinfection. This practice has now been abandoned almost completely. It has a limited value and is still used somewhat in destruction of vermin, such as rats on board ships, bedbugs, cockroaches, etc. Though we have known for years that this activity had little or no value as a health measure, nevertheless the practice of gaseous fumigation was not abandoned until about 1930 by the health departments of some of our large municipalities.

Thus, the activities of a division of sanitary inspection are constantly changing. It may be stated as a general rule that, as the general level of civilization of a community is elevated, and the general "sanitary conscience" is improved, less and less emphasis need be placed by the health department upon those environmental factors which relate to the protection of the public health. The various problems gradually are solved, as environmental sanitation passes through the pioneer stage to one of relative stability.

It must not be forgotten, however, that environmental sanitation is a basic activity of any local health department, and must always receive primary consideration. It is a poor policy for any health officer to devote too great a proportion of his personnel and budget in carrying out the refinements of a health program, while the elementary features of the program in his community have not yet been fully developed.

Thus, in a primitive community, where the budget is limited, sanitary inspection may be more important than nursing service. No health program is complete without a nursing service, but often the work must develop a step at a time, and it is advisable to establish the most elementary services first.

A good illustration of this principle was the development of a health service for rural areas of Yugoslavia at the end of the First World War by Stampar. He worked on the basis that in a virgin field it was more essential to develop dairying and to build manure pits than to study the epidemiology of meningitis, and more important to expend the efforts and funds of his department in construction of community wells than to install preschool clinics or branch laboratories. He did not minimize the importance of other activities, but developed environmental sanitation first.

## FUNCTIONS OF A SANITARY OFFICER IN A LOCAL HEALTH DEPARTMENT

We shall make no attempt to give in detail the various technics that are followed in a well-developed health department sanitation program. A number of standard reference books may be consulted which deal with these subjects adequately. We shall simply outline the different functions and indicate the means and personnel that may be required to carry out the necessary essential activities. From our previous discussion, it becomes quite clear that the activities of a sanitary officer in a given local health department may vary greatly in scope in different parts of the country, and are changed or modified from year to year in the same city. These variations depend upon the size of the area and the density of population, and also upon the degree to which essential activities have been developed in the community. Some jurisdictions have special sanitary problems that are peculiar to the area; *e.g.*, anopheles control in malaria prevention. Certain activities are more or less common to all local health departments. Some of these activities are:

**Supervision of the Water Supply**

*Public Supplies.* Many of the larger cities and towns have a separate division of city government which has charge of the water supply, and which is administered by its own special board. In many instances the water supply company is privately owned and does not belong to the municipality at all, but operates under franchise. Other cities have a water commissioner. In any case, the health department should not administer the collection and distribution of water to the people. The chief concern of the health department is that the water supply shall come from an unpolluted source, shall be adequate for the needs of the people, and shall be safe to drink. This requires frequent inspection of the watershed or other source of supply by the health department to determine and prevent possible sources of pollution. This inspection must include storage reservoirs and water purification plants.

Water purification is a highly technical procedure, so that the responsibility for supervision must devolve upon a competent public health engineer. The larger cities may have their own public health engineers. In smaller plants, the division of engineering of the state department of health may give supervisory service. This official may delegate certain routine inspectional activities to the local sanitary inspector.

The local sanitary inspector should take suitable samples of public water supplies at regular frequent intervals for bacteriological and chemical analyses. The chemical examinations are usually made at the state laboratory. Daily bacteriological tests are usually made at the local laboratory. The sanitary inspector should be able to interpret the results of the laboratory findings, and to apply appropriate corrective measures, should they be necessary.

*Private Water Supplies.* The sanitary inspector should understand the principles of construction and suitable methods of protection of private water supplies, and should make recommendations and give advice to home owners in regard to construction of individual wells. Roadside wells and other individual water supplies to which the public has access should be given the same consideration as public water supplies. Many states have developed systems of routine inspection and certification of the roadside wells, because these wells are so freely used by tourists.

*Springs.* The location of springs that are used by the public as a source of drinking water should be known to the sanitary inspector, and he should understand the principles of construction for the protection of springs against contamination. He should have supervision of the sanitary quality of commercial bottled waters, and also the sanitary supervision of the manufacture and marketing of ice.

**Sewage Disposal.** Supervision of a municipal sewage disposal system is a highly technical procedure which should be under the direction of a trained public health engineer. Large municipalities usually have a separate administrative division for this activity with its own public

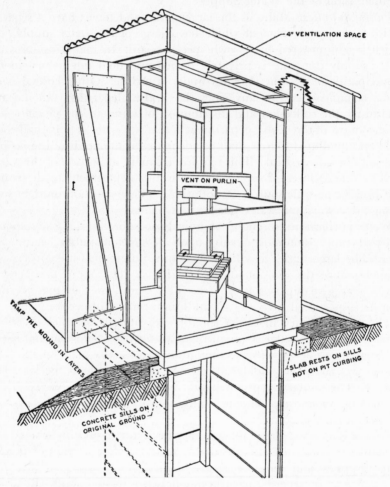

FIG. 22. *U.S.P.H. Service Model Sanitary Privy.* This type of privy is strongly built, is relatively inexpensive and constructed on scientific principles.

health engineer. Smaller municipal plants may receive supervision from the state department of public health engineering. The routine inspection of these plants and collection of samples for laboratory examination may be delegated to the local sanitary officer.

*Sewage Disposal in Individual Homes.* The sanitary officer should have a thorough knowledge of the proper construction and maintenance of the common methods of sewage and waste disposal for private homes. These methods include septic tanks, cesspools, and various types of outdoor privies. He should be familiar with the advantages and disadvantages of each type, the approximate cost of initial construction and of maintenance, and should give advice not only as to the best type for each individual home, but should actively encourage home owners toward betterment of their own sanitary facilities.

He should understand the general bacteriological principles concerned with soil pollution and the nitrogen cycle; he should understand the importance of ground flow, and be ready to give proper advice in regard to the location and construction of suitable types of privies for the rural home. The administrative principles in relation to construction of these privies are simple. The privy must be durable, inexpensive, simple in operation, and its construction must be based on correct scientific principles, and suited to the particular location.

In rural areas, the major portion of the activities of the sanitary officer may be concerned with installation of sanitary toilets and proper construction and protection of wells and other water supplies. These matters, though apparently quite simple, are, in fact, highly technical. Thus, the local health department should utilize fully the expert advisory service of the state department of public health engineering in the determination of any general policies concerning safe water supplies and adequate sewage disposal facilities.

**Plumbing Inspection.** The epidemic of amebic dysentery in Chicago awakened health departments to the fact that cross connections and faulty plumbing continue to be a serious menace to community health. Special danger occurs when large numbers of people have access to the polluted water supply. Thus, industrial plants, public buildings, hotels, stores, and, in fact, all water and sewage connections including those of private homes, require close supervision of installation and maintenance. The epidemic of undulant fever at the Michigan State College in 1939, due to defective plumbing, and the large outbreak of typhoid fever at a state institution for the insane in Illinois during the same year, apparently due to pollution of the institutional water supply from defective plumbing, only served to emphasize the necessity for the establishment of an effective plumbing inspection service by the local health department. The state department of public health engineering should be in a position to supervise this service, and should prepare a state-wide plumbing code to apply to all buildings to which the public has access. Some state engineers believe that their departments should examine plumbing plans for public buildings just as such departments now pass on all plans for community water supplies and sewage disposal plants.

Licensing of plumbers should not be a function of the health department, but should be under the general division of administration, or a special licensing board.

**Milk Sanitation.** The protection of the milk supply of the community is a primary function of the local health department. The local sanitary inspector has authoritative supervision of the methods that are employed for protection of milk and milk products from contamination, and is directly responsible for the cleanliness, purity and safety of the milk supply. Inspections of the dairies, milk collecting stations and pasteurization plants that supply the people within his jurisdiction are made at regular intervals. These inspections are carried out to ensure proper sanitation at each dairy, to determine the suitability of the facilities for rapid cooling of the milk, as well as to make certain that proper methods are being employed in pasteurization and marketing of the milk. As the dairy industry has grown and the population has become more dense, the source of supply has receded farther and farther from the consumer. In many municipalities it is no longer possible for the sanitary inspection service to supervise adequately all the dairies, collecting stations and pasteurization plants that supply milk to the area.

This difficulty has been solved by establishment of state-wide milk sanitation regulations. The sanitary inspection service of dairies is carried out by the state department of health, the state department of agriculture, or by the two departments acting jointly. The Federal Government has assisted greatly in the establishment of uniform state-wide dairy sanitation regulations.

It is now generally conceded that the routine testing of cattle for tuberculosis and undulant fever is not a function of the health department, but of the department of agriculture or animal husbandry. Because of the importance of this work in the protection of health, the local health departments should be thoroughly informed concerning these activities and should aid these programs in every possible way.

When state-wide dairy sanitation regulations are in force and the dairies are all inspected by the state officials, the local health departments need not delegate inspectors to visit dairies at all. Milk and milk products are not admitted to the jurisdiction of the local health department unless they come from approved sources. At most, the local sanitary inspectors will make dairy inspections for special reasons only; as, for example, in the checking of unsatisfactory conditions as determined by the laboratory tests, or in conducting an epidemiologic investigation. The local sanitary officer places a check on all supplies by frequent sampling for bacteriological and chemical tests, thus giving double protection to the consumer. If any dairy is furnishing an unsatisfactory supply, as indicated by the laboratory tests, special inspections should be made, of course. The great safeguard to community health from infection through its milk supply is through pasteurization, so that it is essential that all pasteurization plants should have close supervision.

**Meat and Meat Products.** Formerly, the local sanitary inspector devoted considerable time to ante- and post-mortem inspection of slaughtered products. Since most abattoirs now produce meats for inter-state shipment, the Federal Government has assumed responsibility for a great portion of this activity. Large municipalities often employ their own veterinarians, part or full-time, for meat inspection service. The chief activities of the sanitary officer in meat inspection service relate to proper handling, refrigeration and marketing of meats and meat products, the inspection of storage facilities, the inspection of retail meat establishments and of public markets.

**Parasitic Infections That Are Spread through Meat.** Parasitic infections of meat that are of medical importance in the United States are limited to three infections: trichinosis, beef tapeworm infection, and echinococcus disease.

*Trichinella infection* has been discovered by the United States Public Health Service research workers to be very common in the United States. Bits of human diaphragm muscle, taken at random from over a thousand autopsies, have shown a trichinella infection rate of from 12 per cent to 25 per cent. Most of these persons have had no past history of the disease. In many other instances the infection has been so slight as to pass undiagnosed. In others, serious illness from trichinella has been diagnosed as typhoid fever or other infection.

The disease is primarily an infection of swine, and man becomes infected only incidentally through improperly cooked pork. Grain-fed hogs of the middle west show almost no infection—less than 1 per cent of western hogs are infected. These have very few larvae in the tissues. The heavy infections occur in the garbage-fed hogs on the eastern seaboard of the United States. In some herds 10 per cent or more of the hogs are found to be infected. This infection of garbage-fed hogs results from eating raw, infected pork scraps.

The incubation period of the disease in man varies from three days to a week or more. Onset as a rule is sudden.

The disease is difficult to diagnose at its onset because it has no characteristic symptoms. The headache, fever, prostration, and diarrhea suggest typhoid fever. Eosinophilia may give the first clue to the real cause of the infection. The larvae invade the muscles, causing intense pain and tenderness; and biopsy of muscle tissues at this stage of the disease will give the exact diagnosis. Search for the larvae in the circulating blood is a waste of time.

Accuracy of diagnosis in trichinosis has been greatly aided by the development of the intradermal test with trichinae antigen. This test has been utilized with accuracy in the diagnosis of trichinosis infection in garbage-fed hogs, but this technic has not been widely adopted.

Family epidemics of trichinosis are not uncommon, and frequently a single source of infection will produce all types of the disease: in one case the symptoms will be slight, in another they will be rapidly fatal. As in many other helminth invasions, the dosage of infection is an important factor in prognosis. No specific method of therapy has been developed for trichinella infection.

*Control.* The obvious and most effective method of control of the disease in hogs rests in requiring suitable procedures for cooking garbage before it is fed to hogs. Federal regulations for processing, heating, refrigeration, and other operations in the curing of pork products have been highly effective in destroying the encysted larvae in infected pork. The rapid low-temperature processing of meat is very destructive to trichinae larvae, but this procedure injures the quality of pork. Simple cooking kills the larvae in a few minutes.

*Tenia saginata* infection (beef tapeworm) is becoming more uncommon year by year because of three factors:

1. Improved and more universal meat inspection technics.

2. Improved community sanitation with proper disposal of human feces.

3. Improved refrigeration of beef.

The standard twenty-one-day retention period of beef at usual refrigerator temperature is not sufficient to destroy all the parasites, but 30 days is effective. An alternate and frequently adopted method is preliminary freezing of the meat 15° F. for five or six days.

*Tenia solum,* or pork tapeworm, is very rare in human beings in the United States.

*Echinococcus Infection.* Echinococcus infection has now become rare in the United States. It is, of course, primarily a disease of sheep and of dogs. Man is infected only incidentally. The infection in sheep is readily determined by rigid meat inspection, and some authorities believe that decrease in the infection is due to better meat inspection technic. It seems more probable that the decline in this disease in man and animals is due to our changing methods in animal husbandry.

**Shellfish, Oysters, Clams, Lobsters and Other Sea Food.** Since most of the sea food is prepared for interstate shipment, the federal regulations in regard to sanitation of these products protect the public adequately. The sanitary inspector has the supervision over local storage, handling and preparation of these articles of food and must be fully informed concerning the federal regulations relating to these products. In certain seaboard states, the state health department must devote special attention to the sources and sanitary production of sea foods.

**Food as a Vehicle of Infection**

Adulteration and falsification of food are essentially fraudulent procedures and do not come within the province of the health department, as a rule; though, in some municipalities, the prevention of adulteration of foods is considered a public health function.

The diseases that are due to foods, or are transmitted through food as a vehicle, may be divided into several categories:

**Toxins.** The commonest bacterial toxin in food is staphylococcus enterotoxin. The toxin produces an illness that is characterized by a short incubation period and a high incidence in those exposed. Major symptoms are nausea, vomiting, acute prostration, and diarrhea. Not all staphylococci produce the toxin, but this organism is ubiquitous and finds ready entry to food. The organism is readily killed by heat, but the endotoxin itself is quite heat resistant. Ordinary refrigeration—4° to 6° C.—will hold the growth of the staphylococcus in check; thus improper storage and handling of foods that serve as a culture medium for staphylococci are a common cause of this illness. The chief food offenders are cream-filled pastries, chopped meat sandwiches, and a wide variety of other mixed foods that are prepared by hand and kept at room temperature.

**Botulinus endotoxin.** This toxin is produced by a spore-bearing anaerobe, *Clostridium botulinum*. The organism is encountered in the soil, and is saprophytic. It produces a toxin of very high toxicity, which has a special affinity for the central nervous system.

The incubation period is from several hours to several days. Symptoms are neurological: diplopia, blurring of vision, headache, difficulty in swallowing, prostration, and paralysis of various muscles. Finally respiratory paralysis occurs, and death follows. The case fatality rate is high, even in persons who receive antitoxin.

The chief sources of botulinus poisoning are home-canned foods, particularly non-acid vegetables such as string beans and corn.

The toxin is readily destroyed by heat. Thus home-canned foods should always be brought to a boil before use. All canned food that has a bad odor or shows signs of gas formation should be destroyed. Adequate methods of commercial canning have removed the danger of botulinus poisoning from this source, but home-canning methods do not always destroy the spores.

**Infections.** *Salmonella* infection of food is of common occurrence. It may come from several sources:

(1) Sick animals. Meat, fowl, eggs, or other food may actually contain the organism.

(2) Contamination. The food may be contaminated by excreta from rats or other animals that are carriers of the infection.

(3) Occasionally food handlers may contaminate the food with salmonella, for carriers of this organism do occur.

The symptoms of the disease are similar to those of staphylococcic enterotoxemia, but the incubation period is longer—7 to 72 hours after eating the infected food. The infected food does not as a rule have a "spoiled" odor or taste. Ordinary cooking destroys the organism, but improper preparation of food, and particularly unsatisfactory refrigeration, is a factor in the production of this type of illness.

*Bacillary dysentery* and *typhoid fever* are also frequently transmitted through food, but these matters have already been considered.

**Chemicals.** A wide variety of food poisoning may be produced by chemical substances. The most common causes are: arsenic (usually from insecticides), lead, cadmium (from cooking utensils), fluoride (from insect powders), mercury, cyanides (from silver polish), and others.

Certain foods may be intrinsically poisonous, as for example certain mushrooms, shellfish, particularly certain mussels, fish, as well as favism from fava beans, ergotism from fungus-infected rye, etc.

**Control of Illness Due to Foods.** The rules for food sanitation are quite simple, but are often difficult to enforce. They are dependent for the most part upon elementary bacteriologic principles.

Prevention of food poisoning requires clean food, free from all contamination with human and animal wastes. It must be handled as little as possible, and preferably should be consumed while fresh. Foods that are prepared for hours before serving, and that are allowed to stand at warm (room) temperatures, become excellent culture media for bacteria. This is one reason why food poisoning so often follows large banquets.

Furthermore, cooked products often become contaminated, if allowed to stand, unless kept at refrigerator temperature. They may become sources of infection. Infection may come from soiled hands, unclean utensils, or from contaminated water. Meat, fish, or fowl may be infected antemortem. Food may be contaminated by flies, rodents, and by general unsanitary conditions. Moisture, warmth, and suitable media are bacterial requirements. If the bacteriologic principles of cleanliness and sterilization are followed in food sanitation, then food poisoning will be minimized.

The most important sanitary measures in food handling are heat, *i.e.*, cooking of the food thoroughly to at least 100° C.; steam for the sterilization of utensils; and refrigeration to prevent multiplication of infectious agents.

Supplementary food sanitation measures include the use of chemical agents in cleansing food utensils, drying, ultra-violet light, or simple sunshine.

Food preservatives have been used extensively in the past, and are still important factors in food sanitation. Salting, pickling, drying, corning— all are food preservation methods. For the most part these procedures are being given up for more modern methods of "deep freeze" refrigeration and various types of commercial food sterilization by the "canning" process.

We have barely touched the problems of the food sanitarian in this brief section. All the meticulous details of the food sanitarian's program will be found in a discussion of these subjects in texts that are devoted entirely to these matters.

**Restaurants and Food Handling Establishments.** Supervision of the general cleanliness and sanitation of food handling establishments is a routine activity of the sanitary inspector. This includes suitable methods of preparing food in the restaurant, lunch room and hotel kitchens, methods for the sterilization of dishes and other utensils, etc. Some health departments have attempted to make an annual physical examination of food handlers, including examination for the typhoid carrier state, for open tuberculosis and for venereal disease. This is a very expensive procedure that has many practical difficulties, and, if carried out as a routine measure, does not contribute materially to a reduction in morbidity in the community. A few large city health departments have required each food handler to secure a health certificate annually. The usual plan is to require that a physician must certify that the food handler is free from obvious communicable disease. (Stool examination for the enteric pathogens is sometimes required.) The food handlers present their physicians' statements to the health department and are given a lecture and demonstration (in classes of 20 to 30) concerning the modes of transfer of infection through carelessness, and they are taught the simple technic of the hygiene of food handling.

The chief benefit of this annual certificate plan is the opportunity that it gives for specific health education of the special group.

**Housing.** It seems absurd that a text book on public health should contain only one short section on housing. One authority has stated that housing is the most important single unsolved public health problem in the United States. The direct relationship of housing to public health lies basically in the prevention of overcrowding; and thus, indirectly, the prevention of tuberculosis, cerebrospinal meningitis, the respiratory infections, and the contagious diseases of childhood are involved.

All students of housing recognize that there are certain minimum facilities that are essential for a healthful home environment. These include an adequate water supply of pure quality, proper sanitary sewage disposal, good ventilation, sufficient light, space for normal family life, screening or other protection against mosquitoes and flies, absence of excessive dampness, protection from fire and other hazards, and adequate recreational facilities for both children and adults.

We have a strong belief that optimum housing conditions promote good physical and mental health, and actually prevent certain infectious diseases. But it is very difficult to prove these points.

Britten [1] made an extensive analysis of the relationship of housing to illness, from data that were based on the National Health Survey. The correlation between illness and bad housing was based on a house-to-house canvass of over two and a half million people, and the information that was assembled covered a period of one year. Illness was encountered

[1] Britten, R. H. and Altman, I.: "Illness and Accidents among Persons Living under Different Housing Conditions." *Pub. Health Rep.* 1941, Vol. 56, p. 609.
*See also* Britten, R. H.: "The Relation Between Housing and Health." *Pub. Health Rep.* 1934, Vol. 44, p. 1301; Winslow, C.-E. A.: "Housing as a Public Health Problem." *Am. Jour. Pub. Health.* 1937, Vol. 27, p. 56; Britten, R. H.: "Housing and Health." *Am. Jour Pub. Health.* 1938, Vol. 28, p. 957.

more commonly in crowded homes, *i.e.,* houses with more than 1½ persons per room, than in households with less than one person per room. Pneumonia was strikingly more prevalent in the lower income groups where overcrowding prevailed. Communicable diseases of childhood occurred at an earlier age. Influenza, tuberculosis and rheumatism were more common in persons with substandard housing, and disabling accidents were more prevalent.

But these data do not prove that bad housing was solely responsible for the higher incidence of illness in the lower income groups. People live in substandard housing, for the most part, because they are poor. Poverty is often a concomitant of low intelligence and inferior training for life's work. Often previous accident or illness has crippled the breadwinner, with resultant poverty and consequent substandard housing. In other words, the illness resulted in poor housing, rather than poor housing producing the illness.

McGonigle and Kirby [2] have even suggested that a slum clearance program may actually be deleterious to the health of the very persons that it was intended to benefit. One hundred and fifty-two families in the Stockton-on-Tees slum clearance program were followed over a period of 5 years. A control of 289 families that remained in the old slums was also studied. At the end of 5 years it was determined that there was a higher death rate in the new model housing area than in the control area of old slums. All criteria gave a higher illness index, except infant mortality. The authors conclude that the rents in the new area were out of proportion to total income. Thus the people in the slum clearance had insufficient funds to purchase food, and suffered from malnutrition, though their housing conditions were optimum.

This report is cited to emphasize the point that there are many contributory and complicating factors which may produce illness in the family, such as differences in income, educational and intellectual level, racial customs, family mores, housekeeping efficiency of the mother, and many others.

The important thing to remember is that good health is much more than the absence of a specific disease. Rather it is a state of being in which all physical and mental faculties are blended in a harmony of optimum efficiency and life enjoyment. In the larger sense, therefore, good housing promotes good health.

Thus, even though we cannot prove that bad housing produces disease, the fact remains that housing is a public health responsibility. Every student of public health should familiarize himself with the *Basic Principles of Healthful Housing,*[3] as set forth by the Committee on the

[2] McGonigle, G. C. and Kirby, J.: *Poverty and Public Health.* Victor Gollancz, Ltd., London, 1936.
[3] *Basic Principles of Healthful Housing.* Committee on the Hygiene of Housing. American Public Health Association. 2nd ed., May, 1939.

Hygiene of Housing, published by the American Public Health Association.

The health officer should keep in close touch with the housing authority, and should promote improved housing in his community in every possible way. It must be granted that housing is essentially a public welfare rather than a public health function of government, but the field impinges upon the province of the health department at many points and in many ways, and there should be co-ordination between the health services and the housing authority. The social implication of housing and the technical ramifications of the subject are so complex that the author feels that the matter deserves special and more detailed considerations than can be given in this text.

**Swimming Pools.** The sanitation of swimming pools and public bathing places is a specialized technic. General policies in regard to these matters are usually determined by the state department of health. The local sanitary inspector has supervision of the purification of the water in the pools. This is checked by frequent bacteriological examination. He has supervision also of proper facilities for the prevention of cross infection in the bath house and in the dressing room.

**Barber Shops.** In some municipalities the sanitary inspector has supervision of the sanitation of barber shops. This activity plays little part in disease prevention.

**Abatement of Nuisances.** The great variety of activities that are included under the term "nuisance abatement," and which are a part of the duty of the sanitary inspector, are a heritage from former years. These activities bear little relationship to health protection. Most of them may and should be transferred to other departments of government, particularly the police department, the fire department, and the department of public works.

**Control of Insects and of Insect-Borne Diseases.** The prevention of illnesses that are transmitted by insects is the responsibility of the department of sanitation.

The most important insect vectors of human disease are: (1) mosquitoes, (2) house flies, (3) fleas, (4) body lice, (5) ticks,[4] (6) mites,[4] (7) biting flies.

This text is not the appropriate place to discuss in detail the methods of control of these insects. A general discussion of the principles that are involved may, however, be presented briefly.

**Mosquitoes.** The effective control of diseases that are transmitted by mosquitoes is dependent upon a thorough knowledge of the life history of the insect. Complete control of all mosquitoes is often quite impractical; thus "species" control is employed. Usually measures must be directed first toward destruction of the larvae. Once the larval history

---

[4] Ticks and mites are not, strictly speaking, insects, but for all practical purposes may be placed in this category.

of the mosquito is known, the sanitarian uses his ingenuity and imagination in combating each particular situation. Secondary measures that are employed are: (1) destruction of adult mosquitoes, (2) protection of carriers of infection, and (3) protection of susceptible host from the bite of the offending mosquito.

**House Flies.** These insects, which formerly were important vectors of intestinal infections, have now been brought under control in most communities. The secret of success in house fly control lies in destruction of the habitat of the larvae. Flies breed abundantly in manure piles and in similar organic waste material. About 10 days are required for larval development, so that protection of manure piles from fly egg deposits, and frequent removal of manure, solves this problem easily. Secondary measures are: (1) protection of houses by screening, and (2) destruction of adult flies.

**Fleas.** The most important flea, in transmission of disease, is the rat flea, *Xenopsylla cheopis*. This insect transmits bubonic plague. The most effective method of control is through control of the rodent host. One of the sanitary developments of World War II was more efficient methods for destruction of rats and other rodents. These methods are constantly being improved. The most recent technics for rat destruction may be secured by writing to the Superintendent of Documents, United States Government Printing Office, Washington 25, D. C. Secondary methods in flea control relate to actual destruction of adult fleas and their larvae.

**Body Lice.** *Pediculus vestimenti* is the important transmitter of typhus fever. All types of human infestation with lice, including head lice and pubic lice, are due to lack of personal cleanliness. Under normal conditions of life, the average family can rid themselves easily from lice infestation; but under disturbed social conditions, particularly during war or other disasters, it often becomes impossible to employ the usual methods of personal and household cleanliness.

**Insect Destruction.** The Second World War developed many new methods of attacking disease; among other discoveries of the war was that of D.D.T.

D.D.T. (dichloro-diphenyl-trichloroethane) is a dry powder which is relatively non-toxic to man, and which is a powerful insecticide. When applied to clothing, it is extraordinarily effective against body lice: one application protects the wearer for 4 weeks. It may be used in the hair, to destroy head lice. It is also extraordinarily effective against adult mosquitoes, house flies, bed bugs, ants, and many other insects. If sprayed over a pond, it will destroy mosquito larvae. Whole islands were rendered free of insect life in the South Pacific during the war with the Japanese, by the simple expedient of spraying D.D.T. over the islands with airplanes. The drug, if ingested, may be quite toxic, and troublesome skin rashes have been reported in those who were employed to spray D.D.T. in houses for mosquito control. The action of the drug is cumulative, obviously, and it must be used with caution, but its potentialities in control of insect hosts of disease are enormous.

D.D.T. is highly destructive to house flies, and has been used effectively in destroying rat fleas in the vicinity of human habitation. Thus it has become the duty of every sanitary officer to familiarize himself with modern methods of insect control, and to learn in some detail the technics in distribution of D.D.T.

**Ticks, Mites, and Biting Flies.** Tick eradication is a very difficult undertaking. Man is only an incidental host, and thus only by "accident" does the tick transmit disease to man. The most effective method of preventing disease that may be transmitted by ticks is the employment of insect repellents. These are used by those persons who are directly exposed to tick bites.

World War II developed at least two excellent insect repellents: (a) dimethylphthalate, and (b) benzyl benzoate. Each has its appropriate use.

Insect repellents are most useful in preventing tick bites and also mite bites, if the clothing is impregnated with the repellent. These drugs are relatively non-toxic and may be used directly on the skin with effectiveness, but their repellent value on the skin is lost after a few hours. The drugs will remain in clothing for weeks. They are useful not only in repelling mosquitoes, but also all the common biting flies.

The normal host of the various mites that may transmit disease to man is a small rodent, usually a mouse. Destruction of the host, and particularly destruction of the breeding places and food supply of the rodent host, is one of the effective methods for control of mites. Mites are susceptible to D.D.T., and are repelled effectively by dimethylphthalate.

The reader who is particularly interested in this field is referred to the extensive reports on insect and rodent control that were published by the U. S. Army during and after World War II on this and related subjects.[5]

**Garbage Disposal.** Proper disposal of garbage is not a function of the health department and has been transferred from the health department budget to the department of public works in most cities.

**Industrial Sanitation.** Supervision of the sanitation of working conditions is an important activity of the sanitary officer in any industrial city. This activity includes prevention of industrial poisoning, inspection of safeguards against accident, supervision of suitable working conditions for the personnel, etc. This subject has been discussed in more detail in a separate chapter.

**Vacation Sanitation Problems.** In certain areas, the population is increased tenfold during a short period of the year. This influx puts a great burden on existing sanitary facilities, thus requiring special vigi-

[5] *Methods for Insect and Rodent Control.* Publication of Second Service Command, June 11, 1945. T. M. 5–632, *Insect and Rodent Control.* U. S. Army publication, Oct. 16, 1946.

lance. There is an unfortunate tendency among vacationists to revert to primitive habits of life. Thus special attention must be given to sanitation of tourist camps, summer camps of all types, roadside wells, etc.

Most states have developed a code for the sanitation of camps, which follows closely the standard procedures outlined by the Federal Government for the National Parks. In most states, the local health authorities are responsible for the enforcement of the code. States having a large vacation population or migratory labor camps have found it necessary to place camp sanitation under state health department control, in order to maintain uniformity and effectiveness of procedures.

**Sanitation of the Air.** The Commission on Air-borne Infections of the United States Army Board for the Investigation of Epidemic Diseases was instrumental in pointing out the fact that a great deal of transfer of infection from person to person may occur through the air. It also demonstrated that practical methods may be devised to check this transfer.

It is clear that respiratory diseases cannot be checked by air sanitation in the same comprehensive manner that gastrointestinal infections have been checked by the sanitation of water and food. The reason is that practically the entire water and food supply of a population can be controlled, whereas all transfer of infection through the air cannot be controlled. One reason is that much respiratory infection is transferred by "direct contact." The probability of transfer of an infectious agent from a case or carrier of influenza, for example, bears a direct ratio to the square of the distance from the source of infection to the susceptible host. That is to say, if a person in the infectious stages of acute respiratory disease is within a few feet of a susceptible person, the chances of acquiring the infection by "direct" and immediate transfer is great, and no air sterilization procedures could check this transfer.

Nevertheless a great deal of transfer of infection may occur from the source, over a considerable radius, through the air in closed rooms and buildings, and particularly in places where people congregate in large numbers. Thus measures that may be taken to sterilize the air in hospital out-patient departments, in schools, theaters, public buildings, and in offices and large commercial dwellings, should be of great assistance in preventing the spread of air-borne infection.

Robertson and his co-workers [6] of the Commission on Air-borne Infections demonstrated that in soldiers' barracks such simple procedures as oiling the floors, treatment of blankets, and other methods for the control of dust dispersion, were effective in reducing the prevalence of pathogenic factors in the air.

Robertson and his co-workers [7] also demonstrated that triethylene

[6] Robertson, O. H., Hamburger, M., Loosli, C. G., Puck, T. T., Lemon, H. M. and Wise, H.: "A Study of the Nature and Control of Air-borne Infection in Army Camps." *J.A.M.A.* 1944, Vol. 126, p. 993.

[7] Puck, T. T., Hamburger, M., Robertson, O. H. and Hurst, V.: "The Effect of Triethylene Glycol Vapor on Air-borne Beta Hemolytic Streptococci in Hospital Wards." *Jour. Inf. Diseases.* 1945, Vol. 76, p. 216.

glycol in 1 part to 4 hundred million parts of air would quickly and effectively destroy respiratory pathogens in the air, including such viruses as influenza. Ingenious methods were devised for the continuous distribution of triethylene glycol in the ventilating system of buildings, and automatic controls of the vapor dispersion were invented. These authors also proved that the drug, in this high dilution, had no deleterious effect on animals or man.

Wells [8] developed a different system of air sterilization that has many advocates. He utilizes ultra-violet light, and with Mrs. Wells, has conducted extensive experiments with this method for the control of respiratory infections.

The reader who is interested in this field is referred to the extensive literature on this subject, particularly to the Report of the Commission on Air-borne Infections of the United States Army Board for the Investigation of Epidemic Diseases,[9] and to the Wells' studies.

It is a new field for sanitary engineering, but promises to be a productive one.

**Health Education.** The education of the people in better methods of general sanitation is an important function of the sanitary inspector that too often is forgotten. The activities of the inspection service are usually dependent upon or related to local rules and regulations of the health department that have the force of law and carry certain police powers. Thus, the tendency is to use force rather than persuasion. It is a much better policy for the sanitary inspector to consider each of his actions as an educational measure. He should attempt in each instance to convince the persons concerned that his recommendations are not simply arbitrary rules, but are for the best interest of the persons that are affected by the measure, as well as for the community as a whole.

## PERSONNEL REQUIRED FOR A SANITATION INSPECTION SERVICE

The sanitary inspection activities of a municipality of 100,000 population will comprise a total of approximately six to eight thousand separate inspections of all types annually. Three or four thousand inspections will be necessary for milk sanitation; while food handling and all other inspections will total about three or four thousand. Thus, a municipality of 100,000 population would require approximately the following full-time personnel:

2 Milk Inspectors

1–2 Food Inspectors

1–2 General Sanitary Inspectors

[8] Wells, W. F., Wells, M. W. and Wilder, T. S.: "The Environmental Control of Epidemic Contagion." *Am. Jour. Hyg.* 1942, Vol. 35, p. 97.

[9] *History of the Commission on Air-borne Infections.* Army Epidemiological Board, U. S. Army, 1941–1945. To be published.

This plan does not provide for such activities as garbage or refuse disposal, plumbing inspection, special mosquito control activities, or technical supervision of water supplies or sewage disposal plants. If the statewide system of dairy inspection is introduced, the personnel and activities of local health departments would be curtailed in consequence. The general trend in relation to divisions of sanitation is to employ a smaller number, but higher type, of personnel, to pay higher salaries and to demand a higher quality of performance.

## TRAINING AND TECHNICAL QUALIFICATIONS OF THE PERSONNEL

One of the weakest spots in the health organization in the United States is the low standard for qualification and training of sanitary inspectors. We have insisted upon a high degree of technical skill for the medical health officer and the public health nurse, but required little or no technical training for the sanitary inspector. It is often stated that any reasonably intelligent man in the community may qualify for this work. Too often the positions are filled to pay political debts.

The contrast with the system adopted in Great Britain is striking. There the sanitary inspector not only is required to complete a well-formulated curriculum of technical training, but also must pass a rigid examination before certification.

It is obvious that no sanitary inspector can carry out intelligently all the various activities outlined in the previous pages without suitable technical training. But, with a few exceptions, no comprehensive courses of training are offered anywhere in the United States, where persons who wish to qualify properly for this type of work can do so.

In fact, the very term "sanitary inspector" in the United States has, in the past, carried the connotation of an untrained, political appointee. Governmental authorities have had this point of view so firmly in mind that educational authorities have despaired of raising the standards for sanitary inspection personnel and have suggested a new term, "sanitarian," or "sanitary officer" to represent a qualified individual who has been trained in sanitary science and who is capable of carrying out the various functions and activities that are required in a good sanitation program.

Some health officers have met the difficulty by developing a program of required continuous instruction for those sanitary inspectors who are actually employed in their health departments, thus gradually improving the quality and intelligent application of sanitary inspection service within their jurisdiction.

## STATE BUREAU OF SANITARY ENGINEERING

The state bureau of sanitary engineering should be a separate division of the State Department of Health. Because of the wide scope of its activities a better term would be *State Division of Sanitation*. The major functions of this bureau are:

1. Supervision of all public water supplies and all public sewage disposal plants in the state. All plans for initial construction or for modification of existing plants by municipalities or for any other public supply must be submitted to the State Department of Sanitary Engineering for its approval.

2. The bureau serves in an advisory capacity all local divisions of sanitation of the various local health departments, aiding them in the establishment of policies in relation to sanitation of cities, schools, individual homes, and in all other matters relating to their work.

3. The bureau should furnish a continuous educational service to local sanitary inspectors in order to enable them to meet their own local difficulties and solve their own problems more intelligently.

The local sanitary officers are, of course, under the administrative direction of the local health officer and are responsible to him for all their activities. The state bureau of sanitation should give the technical advice to the sanitary officer, and, in case of emergency, should render direct aid to the local health department.

The director of the State Division of Sanitation should be a trained, competent public health engineer—a man who holds the confidence and respect of all the engineers and health officers of the whole state. He must be highly qualified, for he is a key person in reduction of mortality and morbidity throughout all parts of the state.

It is generally agreed that all those state activities that relate to environmental sanitation should be administered by one central division of the state health department. It is a poor administrative policy to organize a division of sanitary engineering which is concerned chiefly with problems of public water supply and sewage disposal, and a separate division of sanitation which is concerned with milk sanitation, food sanitation and the like.

It is also generally agreed that the State Bureau of Sanitation should not maintain a separate laboratory for this bureau. Some states have developed a laboratory for the bureau of communicable disease, a separate laboratory service for food and milk, with perhaps a third laboratory for water and sewage examinations. A better administrative procedure is the development of a state bureau of laboratories as a separate bureau of the state health department. This bureau should carry out all laboratory procedures for all the various divisions of the state department of public health.

The organization of the Division of Sanitation of a state department of health, the personnel, the budget, the activities and the interrelation of this division with other divisions of the state health service are discussed in a subsequent chapter on state health department administration.

## THE PUBLIC HEALTH ENGINEER

The public health engineer, as Morton has pointed out, has not out-grown the fact that his work originated in two separate fields: sanitary engineering and sanitary inspection. Sanitary engineering is related primarily to the design of water works plants, the construction of sewage disposal plants, or the operation of garbage incinerators. Sanitary inspection, on the other hand, was an activity that was planned to modify environmental factors in order to reduce health hazards. In the past, it has been quite unscientific and wasteful. For the most part these activities have consisted in routine law enforcement in the abatement of nuisances, many of them of little importance in relation to public health.

Public health engineering is comprehensive, in that it includes the essential public health aspects of both sanitary engineering and sanitary inspection. "The prestige and potentialities of public health engineering are based upon the close relation of environment to human health, and upon the further fact that adjustment of the environment involves the application of engineering principles" (Morton).

While the basis of this professional activity is engineering, its major objective is the promotion of human health.

There has been a good deal of confusion in relation to the administration of public health matters relating to environmental control, because of failure to understand the expanding role of engineering in the public health field. The health officer has failed to appreciate and utilize these newer concepts, and many of the engineers who have entered public health have a restricted concept of the place of the public health engineer in the health program.

Public health engineers have clearly presented their concepts of the chief objectives of public health engineering. They are:

1. An effectual educational program concerning environmental sanitation.

2. A comprehensive plan of investigation in the relationship of environmental factors to human health.

3. Unification of the federal, state, and local planning in relation to all problems relating to environmental sanitation.

4. Improvement of engineering technics and administrative procedure to meet the changing needs of the community.

Schools of public health engineering have been developed rapidly in recent years, to prepare qualified personnel to meet the demands of modern public health trends.

The Committee on Professional Education of the American Public Health Association has formulated excellent educational standards which are required to prepare a public health engineer for a career in his chosen field. These standards are given in the Appendix.

## REFERENCES

1. Ehlers, V. M. and Steel, E. W. *Municipal and Rural Sanitation.* McGraw-Hill Book Co., New York. 1943 (third edition).
2. Jacobs, M. D. *The Chemistry and Technology of Food and Food Production* (2 Vols.). Interscience Publishers, New York. 1944.
3. Herrick, A. D. *Food Regulations and Compliance.* Brown Publishing Co., New York. 1944.
4. Schrader, J. H. *Food Control, Its Public Health Aspects.* John Wiley and Sons, Inc., New York. 1939.
5. Dack, G. M. *Food Poisoning.* Univ. of Chicago Press, Chicago, Ill. 1943.
6. *Standard Methods of Water and Sewage Analysis.* American Public Health Association, 1790 Broadway, New York City. 1940 and subsequent editions.
7. *Manual of Recommended Water Sanitation Practice.* United States Public Health Service Reprint 2240. 1943.
8. *Milk Ordinance and Code.* United States Public Health Service Bulletin 220. 1936.
9. *Report of Committee on Sanitation of Swimming Pools.* American Public Health Association, 1790 Broadway, New York City. 1940.
10. *Manual of Recommended Practice for Sanitary Control of the Shellfish Industry.* Public Health Bulletin No. 295, U.S.P.H. Service. U. S. Gov't Printing Office, Washington, D. C.

### HOUSING

1. *An Appraisal Method for Measuring the Quality of Housing.* American Public Health Association, 1790 Broadway, New York City. 1945.
2. *Basic Principles of Healthful Housing.* (2nd edition.) American Public Health Association, 1790 Broadway, New York City. 1939.
3. Britten, Rollo H. *Housing and Health.* Am. Jour. Pub. Health. 1938, Vol. 28, p. 957.
4. Winslow, C.–E. A. *Preventive Medicine in Modern Practice.* (Chapter on the Hygiene of Dwellings.) New York Academy of Medicine, New York. 1942.

# CHAPTER XXIII

## CHILD HYGIENE

ALL general public health measures affect directly the health of the children in the community. A good example of this obvious fact is the influence upon child mortality rates of certain sanitary procedures, such as sewage disposal, and the sanitary control of the milk supply. The regulation of housing is of more importance to children than to any other age group. The control of communicable disease has had great influence in lowering the morbidity and mortality rates in childhood. Reduction of the diarrheal diseases of infancy is a striking achievement, resulting in great part from general public health procedures. These general functions of a health service that may have influence upon child health have been discussed elsewhere. Supplementary to these general health activities that affect all age groups are certain health activities that are aimed specifically toward promotion of the health of the child. Often these special functions have been initiated by voluntary organizations, or by private enterprise, rather than by official health agencies. Gradually, however, health departments have realized the importance of this type of work, and have assumed more and more responsibility for the development of official child hygiene programs.

We are gradually beginning to realize that child hygiene activities are by far the most important single element of the public health program. As has been pointed out in another chapter, those public health measures that are undertaken to improve the health of adults are alleviative and ameliorative in their very nature. Best results in preventive medicine are secured in the early formative years of the individual's life. After the age of 25 the pattern of life has been drawn and little can be done to correct physical defects, improve mental attitudes or promote healthful habits of life. Prejudices have been formed and opinions concerning the value of public health measures have become fixed. The individual at 25 has already had most of the communicable diseases that he is likely to have, including venereal disease, but excluding the upper respiratory infections. He has learned almost all he will ever know about preventive medicine. Thus the administration of public health activities must be concentrated upon that age period in which greatest results can be obtained; namely, during the developmental period of life. Not only are the actual services that are rendered of great effectiveness during childhood, but also the health information that may be imparted is best assimilated at this time.

The subject of child hygiene is of such great importance and the details of the technic which are involved are so intricate that the author of this text has not considered it advisable to attempt more than a meager description of the functions and administrative principles of a child hygiene program. We feel fully justified in this omission, since the subject is so adequately covered in many excellent books, pamphlets, brochures, etc., that are readily available and that deal solely with this special subject. In this text we shall present an outline only of a community program in child hygiene and shall point out the manner in which the organization and administration of such a plan may be integrated with a well balanced official health organization.

**Functions of a Child Health Program.** We are accustomed to separate the functions of child hygiene into various divisions, such as prenatal activities, infant hygiene, preschool hygiene, school hygiene, etc. These divisions do not represent separate compartments of activity. They have arisen because the administrative technics in child hygiene are often quite different for the various age periods. These more or less artificial divisions have resulted in uneven development of functions, with a general tendency to emphasize activities in the school age period and with relative neglect of the age period from two to six years. The divisions are convenient, if it is thoroughly understood that they are artificial, and that an adequate program requires a continuous, comprehensive and individualized supervision of the child.

## MATERNAL HYGIENE

The purpose of maternal hygiene is to protect the mother against the well recognized perils and difficulties of the gestation period, and to assure the unborn infant the best opportunity for normal development.

**Ideal Maternal Hygiene Program.** The ideal maternal hygiene program toward which we should strive has been set forth most succinctly by the Report of the New York State Commission.[1]

It should give medical and nursing instruction, supervision and care from the beginning of pregnancy until the mother can resume her usual activities. The service should be given as a unit, under the direction of the same physician, who should carry it through the antepartum, intrapartum and postpartum phases. It should include the following activities:

1. Complete examination by the physician as soon as the mother becomes pregnant. This examination should include a careful measurement of the pelvis. A Wassermann test should be performed as a routine part of the physical examination. At this time plans are made for the puerperium.

---

[1] *Public Health in New York State.* 1932, p. 285.

2. Regular subsequent visits by the pregnant woman to the physician for examination and advice, as well as regular home visits by the nurse, who should report to the physician in charge. The purpose of these procedures is:

   a. To watch the development of the baby.
   b. To observe the signs and symptoms of the physical and mental condition of the mother.
   c. To give instruction concerning due preparation for the reception and future care of the new baby.

3. Regular visits to the dentist to prevent advance of the dental caries, which so frequently accompanies pregnancy.

4. Provision, if necessary, for proper nutrition of the mother in order that necessary food elements may be supplied to insure proper development of the child.

5. Aseptic delivery by a physician with a nurse in attendance.

6. Nursing and household aid during the postpartum period for the purpose of securing:

   a. Rest in bed for the mother for at least 10 days.
   b. Gradual resumption of the responsibilities of the home by the mother.
   c. Necessary instruction of the mother in proper care of the baby.

7. Postpartum examination of the mother by a physician to determine and correct any bad effects of pregnancy or delivery.

This complete plan of maternity hygiene is now available for a certain proportion of mothers who can afford to pay for this service. The goal of a satisfactory public health organization is to make these various services available to all mothers in the community.

We are still very far from reaching this goal. Nevertheless, a surprising advance has already been made during the short time that has elapsed since the community began to realize its responsibility in this important matter.

A great deal of uncertainty exists at the present time as to the actual degree of community responsibility for the development of a satisfactory maternal hygiene program. What part should the family play? What is the function of the local medical profession? The voluntary nursing association? The community hospital? The local health department? The state? How far has the ideal plan been realized? Who has already assumed responsibility for it? How may the community utilize the existing organizations and facilities to build for the future?

We already have fairly satisfactory answers to some of these questions; others will be answered only as our whole philosophy of community development gradually evolves.

**The Federal Government.** The activities of the Federal Government in the promotion of maternal and child health are assigned to The Children's Bureau. The organization and functions of this bureau have been described elsewhere in the text. (See page 483.)

The Social Security Act of 1935 gave The Children's Bureau sufficient funds to aid each of the states in the establishment of a state bureau of child health and protection, and these state bureaus, in turn, aid local communities in the development of their programs. The Children's Bureau has given no direct services, but does give advice and guidance in the formulation of standards of quality of service and quality of personnel.

World War II brought about an innovation in the activities of The Children's Bureau through the passage of Federal emergency legislation called the Emergency Maternity and Infant Care Program.

**Emergency Maternity and Infant Care Program.** A special plan was devised for maternity care of soldiers' wives in 1943, during World War II, by The Children's Bureau. The general policies of the program were made by the Bureau, and all funds for the service were provided by the Federal Government. Actual administration of the work was centered in each child health division of the individual state health departments. Detailed administration was furnished by each local official governmental agency, usually the local health department.

The E.M.I.C. plan, as it was called, provided for free prenatal service, delivery service, and postnatal care for all wives of members of the armed forces of the lower grades. Certain uniform standards of service were set, and the local health department, in co-operation with the local medical society, was responsible for the quality of the care and for payment to local hospitals and to physicians.

The plan encountered vigorous opposition at first, largely from county and state medical societies. The chief reason was that the plan was an entering wedge for the nationalization of all medical care. In the end, most physicians and hospitals realized the great benefit of the program and supported it fully.

The plan was wisely administered, and met a great national need. Furthermore, many of the young mothers came to understand, for the first time, the advantages of a complete program of prenatal, obstetrical, and postnatal care.

**The State.** The obvious function of the state health department in a maternal hygiene program is to aid local communities in developing sound plans. The state should give leadership, should aid in the development of a local co-ordinated scheme which will secure a uniform and high standard of service, and perhaps give direct aid to certain local communities for a temporary period by subsidy or otherwise to promote a demonstration of some effective type of service.

As noted above, under the original stimulus of the Sheppard-Towner

Act of the Federal Government, and subsequent aid under the Social Security Act, all the state health departments organized divisions of maternal and child health and welfare by means of financial assistance from The Children's Bureau. Thus the nucleus for a state-wide well co-ordinated program exists in most parts of the United States. These divisions have become a potent force in the advance of the hygiene of maternity and infancy.

The child health bureau of the state health department does not carry out local programs, but aids and advises the local communities in this field. In some instances, the state bureau of child health will carry out a demonstration, in local communities, of the value of maternal and child health services, but these demonstrations are so planned that, if they prove effective, they will be assumed by the local community. In areas of special need, actual subsidy for the local program may be a necessary contribution of the state. In some instances, the local demonstration is sponsored directly by The Children's Bureau.

An example of demonstration projects that are developed in states by Federal health agencies, is the maternity care demonstration of The Children's Bureau in Alabama in 1947. The purpose of this demonstration was to show the states, by example, what can be done in giving a comprehensive maternity and child-care service to women and children who, in the past, lacked even elementary care. This demonstration was carried out in an area where per capita income was low, with almost no deliveries of mothers in the hospital, and where much of the maternal care was in the hands of untrained midwives. It was paid for by Social Security funds, and included:

1. The establishment of blood banks at strategic centers to provide for emergency transfusions.

2. Provision of x-rays of the chest for all maternity cases.

3. Funds to care for prematurely born infants in suitable hospitals.

4. Setting up systems of care for crippled children who are victims of rheumatic fever, epilepsy, speech or hearing defects, and other chronic diseases.

5. Granting fellowships in mental health to teachers, in order to provide more mental health services for children.

**Local Health Department.** The exact function of the local health department in the development of a complete maternal hygiene program has not yet been determined.

During the gradual growth of community maternal hygiene programs, certain activities have advanced more rapidly and effectively than others. The whole burden has been divided among many agencies. Prenatal and postnatal service for those who are not well-to-do has been given by practicing physicians, often without charge. Nursing service has been rendered by voluntary agencies for a nominal charge or no charge at all. Formerly, deliveries occurred at home, but more and more, mothers are being delivered in community hospitals. Midwives are disappearing. The plan that has developed to date requires that those who can afford to pay for medical, nursing and hospital care should do so. If they cannot pay, the services are given free as a direct or indirect charge on the community.

The major function assumed directly by the local health department has been an educational one, carried out through the public health nurses.

**Prenatal Nursing Service.** Nursing service to pregnant mothers is fundamentally an educational measure. Under the present plan of organization the trained public health nurse, sometimes from a voluntary agency, sometimes from an official health department, visits the mother at monthly intervals—perhaps more frequently in the latter months of pregnancy—and gives detailed advice and instruction.

In addition to instructional care, the nurse may give actual nursing aid. For example, she may take the blood pressure, get a specimen of urine, observe the general physical condition and carry out other nursing technic. Before giving actual nursing care she should obtain the consent of the physician in charge of the case to carry out specific procedures, and should work under his instructions.

Most of the pregnant mothers will be delivered by private physicians or privately organized maternity hospitals. Part of the educational program of the nurse includes specific instruction to prospective mothers that they should put themselves under the guidance of a physician during the entire gestation period.

Prenatal nursing service has been furnished in great part by voluntary agencies. Since it is primarily educational in nature there is a definite tendency for health departments to assume this responsibility.

**Prenatal clinics** have been organized in many communities for those women who cannot afford the cost of medical supervision during pregnancy. These clinics are usually organized in connection with the outpatient service of the community hospital.

There is some confusion as to the exact responsibility of the official health department for establishment of prenatal clinic service, with obstetricians in attendance. In our opinion, this is not a health department function, for the following reason:

Medical supervision of a mother during the period of gestation should be given by the physician who will have charge of her delivery. Health officials recognize that delivery service and postpartum care are not health department functions. The entire medical supervision of pregnancy, delivery and postpartum care should rest with the physician or the maternity hospital that assumes responsibility for delivery.

Wherever a health department finds it necessary to give prenatal medical supervision for purposes of education, or for other reasons, it must realize that the procedure is a temporary demonstration, and the work must be re-allocated to proper agencies as soon as practicable. There will always be a certain number of prospective mothers in any community who cannot afford to pay for adequate medical supervision during pregnancy. It is obvious that some suitable arrangement should be made for the prenatal care of this group. The health department may find it necessary, in certain instances, to organize prenatal clinics for their benefit. In such instances the patients should be admitted to the clinic only on the recommendation of their physicians. The physician or maternity hospital that will have charge of the delivery of each patient should be advised by the health department concerning the prenatal clinic findings.

If the health officer is also the administrative officer for a community-wide plan for health protection and medical care, including hospitalization facilities, then a co-ordinated program for maternity care should be a simple administrative procedure.

**Future Development of the Maternal Hygiene Program.** If we followed sound administrative principles, the community maternal hygiene program would be administered as a unit. It is a wasteful and ineffective procedure to scatter the responsibilities among various unrelated agencies. The logical plan is to arrange the work so that the physician who is to deliver a mother in childbirth should assume full charge and should have full responsibility for prenatal and postnatal care, including supervision of the nursing service. If the patient cannot afford to pay for this care, then the community hospital should assume the place of the private physician.

It seems probable that prenatal and postnatal nursing service will be furnished in many communities by the nurses of voluntary agencies for a long time to come. Logically, however, this is a community responsibility and in the future this burden will be carried by the nurses of the public health department. But this does not solve the question of unit control.

We will approach much closer to the ideal administrative plan in maternal hygiene when the community hospital in which obstetrical service is given becomes an integral part of the whole community health service. When this plan is consummated, the same physician who delivers the patient in the hospital will see the patient in the prenatal clinic. The hospital nurses will not devote their entire time to the hospital wards, but will simply use the hospital as their base, and will care for the same patients during the entire period of stress, visiting them in their homes during the prenatal period, giving nursing care during and after delivery in the hospital and visiting them again in their homes during the postpartum period.

## INFANT HYGIENE

The results that have been achieved in reduction of the infant mortality rate in the past 25 years in all parts of the country have been astounding. The infant death rate for the registration area for 1900 was

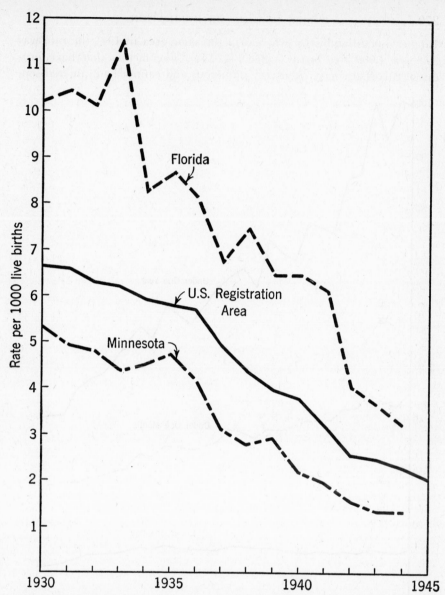

FIG. 23. *Decline in Maternal Mortality in 15 Years, 1930–1945*. States with the Highest and Lowest Rates in 1930 (Florida and Minnesota) Compared with Rates for the United States Registration Area. Source: National Office of Vital Statistics.

## MATERNAL MORTALITY RATES ACCORDING TO RACE

| | U. S. Registration Area | | | Florida | | | Minnesota | | |
|---|---|---|---|---|---|---|---|---|---|
| Year | All Races | White | Non-White | All Races | White | Non-White | All Races | White | Non-White |
| 1940 | 3.8 | 3.2 | 7.7 | 6.5 | 4.9 | 10.2 | 2.2 | 2.2 | 2.9 |
| 1935 | 5.8 | 5.3 | 9.5 | 8.7 | 7.3 | 11.8 | 4.7 | 4.6 | 6.7 |
| 1930 | 6.7 | 6.1 | 11.7 | 10.2 | 8.5 | 14.1 | 5.3 | 5.2 | 15.9 |
| 1925 | 6.5 | 6.0 | 11.6 | 12.1 | 10.2 | 16.3 | 5.3 | 5.2 | 16.4 |
| 1920 | 8.0 | 7.6 | 12.8 | — | — | — | 7.9 | 7.8 | 11.3 |

161 per 1,000 live births, whereas in the same area in 1944 the rate was 39.8 per 1,000 live births. (See Fig. 24.) The factors that have produced this result have been very numerous and cannot be evaluated sep-

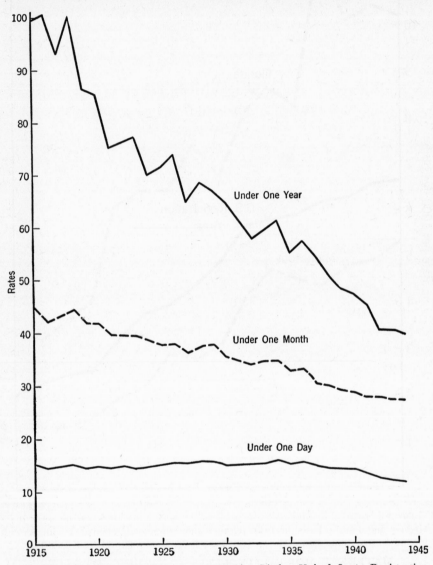

FIG. 24. *Infant Mortality Rates per 1,000 Live Births.* United States Registration Area, 1915–1944. Under One Year, Under One Month, Under One Day. Source: United States Bureau of the Census.

arately. The most important are, probably, (a) improvement in sanitation, particularly water and milk sanitation, (b) improvement in instruction of mothers concerning the care of their babies. The effects of the improvement of milk (and water) sanitation are strikingly shown in the chart which compares infant death rates in New York City for the years 1908–12 and 1928–32, Fig. 25. The peak in infant deaths which formerly came each year in August was due to the diarrheal diseases, which have been almost entirely eliminated. August is now one of the healthiest of months for infants.

The chief gains have been made in prevention of diarrheal diseases and enteritis of infants, prevention of deaths from measles, diphtheria

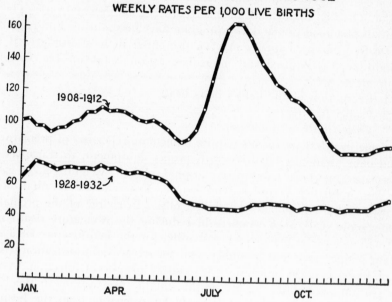

## INFANT MORTALITY IN NEW YORK CITY
### 1908-1912 COMPARED WITH 1928-1932
#### WEEKLY RATES PER 1,000 LIVE BIRTHS

Data from New York City Department of Health

FIG. 25. This chart shows the eradication of an important disease of infants within a period of twenty years.

The peak of infant deaths from July to October in 1908–12 was due to infantile diarrhea. By 1930, infants were healthier in summer than in winter. This has been brought about largely through better sanitation, particularly milk sanitation and pasteurization.

and other communicable diseases, improvement of the technic of infant feeding and promotion of a better standard of general nutrition.

The infant death rate can undoubtedly be reduced much further. It seems probable that this can be accomplished by doing better the things that are now well begun. Great gains may be made by prevention of accidents, more adequate prenatal care, reduction of neonatal deaths in a variety of ways, elimination of diphtheria, and reduction in deaths from measles, whooping cough and pneumonia.

**Neonatal Mortality and Its Prevention.** Over one half the infants in the United States that die during the first year of life succumb during the first 30 days of their existence.

A still greater number are born dead or are reported as stillbirths.

The chief causes of neonatal mortality are:

1. Prematurity.        3. Malformation.
2. Birth injury.       4. Syphilis.

A less important but very distressing cause of neonatal deaths is epidemic diarrhea of the newborn.

**Prevention of Neonatal Deaths.** Prematurity may be prevented to some degree by controlling those factors which produce premature onset of labor. Of chief importance in this regard is good prenatal care. The essentials of a good prenatal care program have been outlined on page 263.

Death from prematurity may be prevented in most instances if the condition is recognized and immediate action is taken. The basic requirements are:

1. Regulation of the baby's body heat.
2. Proper feeding.
3. Protection from infection.

Some health departments require immediate reporting of prematurity, and offer abundant facilities, with proper equipment, to transport the premature newborn baby to the hospital. A baby weighing 2,200 grams or less at birth is considered premature. Provision for hospitalization, with suitable equipment and skilled nurses in charge of the premature baby room, will work wonders in reducing the premature death rate. Provision may be made for breast milk, for the maintenance of a constant temperature and humidity, and for oxygen administration. Isolation under surgical precautions is required to prevent infection. A very important part of the technic is the suitable preparation in the home to receive the baby when it is ready for discharge from the hospital. This is accomplished through a good home nursing service.

*Birth injury,* the second important cause of neonatal death, is preventable in great part. Prevention of death and disability is secured through a good program of prenatal care. Disaster is usually due to disproportion between the size of the pelvis and the baby's head, or to faulty position of the fetus. Knowledge of these facts removes the emergency factor and promotes good obstetrical care.

*Malformation.* For untold generations, people have believed that malformation of a baby at birth was a punishment of the parents for some sin, committed perhaps quite unwittingly. Physicians were almost as fatalistic in the belief that a malformed baby was "nature's mistake," about which nothing could be done.

We are beginning to realize that the study of intra-uterine malformation is a fertile field in preventive medicine.

A good example is *erythroblastosis foetalis.* This disease is due to sensitization of an Rh negative mother with an Rh positive factor which comes from the blood of the fetus in utero. The fetus has inherited the Rh positive factor from the father. The Rh factor is mendelian dominant; thus when the reaction occurs, the father is always Rh positive and the mother Rh negative. About 87 per cent of the population are Rh positive.[2]

Only when an Rh positive man is married to an Rh negative woman is there a possibility of erythroblastosis foetalis. The first child may sensitize the mother, yet be quite normal. Subsequent pregnancies may be disastrous. There are many other factors than heredity that play a part in the incidence of this disease, for it occurs only once in 500 pregnancies. The death of the fetus in utero from this factor is much more common than the disease in the newborn infant, and thus the condition is one which requires careful analysis.

Another example of preventable fetal malformation in utero is the result of research initiated by Australian workers [3] that mothers who have German measles during pregnancy may have malformed children as a direct result of this illness. If this proves to be the case, then a simple exanthematous disease, which has received little consideration in the past, must be guarded against, at all costs, in young pregnant mothers.

*Syphilis* of the newborn is controlled by routine Wassermann tests of all pregnant women and proper treatment of all syphilitic mothers.

In 1945, thirty states had passed legislation relating to requirements for prenatal blood tests for syphilis. In 15 states the blood test is mandatory. In the other 15 states, blood tests are required under special conditions, usually with the consent of the woman.

*Epidemic diarrhea of the newborn* has caused grave concern in many maternity hospitals. The etiology is not determined. There is a severe intestinal toxemia, which is frequently fatal. It occurs equally commonly in breast fed and artificially fed babies. The incubation period is from 2 to 6 days. The importance of this disease is indicated by the fact that in New York City from 1934 to 1946, 151 outbreaks occurred in 65 hospitals. Of 16,000 infants exposed 2,439 were attacked, with 844 deaths. This is a case fatality rate of 35 per cent.[4] Aseptic technic should always be used in handling the babies. When the disease breaks out, the only recourse is to close the nursery and cleanse it completely and thoroughly. The details of a suitable program for prevention of this disease in maternity hospitals will be found in the article by Frant that is cited above.

[2] Wiener, A. S.: "Diagrammatic Representation of Rh Blood Types." *Am. Jour. Clin. Path.* 1946, Vol. 16, p. 233.
   *See also* the editorial in the *J.A.M.A.* 1944, Vol. 125, p. 495, which has an excellent bibliography.
[3] See *German Measles.*
[4] Frant, S., Abramson, H. and Losty, M.: "Problems in Preventing Infections in Newborn Nurseries." *N. Y. State Jour. Med.,* 1946 (Apr. 15), p. 908.

**Postnatal Care** of the baby is the responsibility of the physician, the public health nurse, and the mother herself. The principles of good care are very simple:

1. Maintenance of body temperature.
2. Proper food.
3. Protection from infection.

The carrying out of these principles requires painstaking instruction on the part of the physician and the nurse. One very important rule is that the baby should be shielded from anyone who may be in the early stages of a contagious disease—even a common cold.

Associated factors in the prevention of infant and maternal mortality are the improvement in the quality of general obstetrical practice, and more uniform and stringent regulations governing obstetrical hospital procedure. The licensing of all maternity hospitals should be the responsibility of the State Department of Health, and no license should be given until the hospital has provided standard equipment for the delivery of the mother and proper facilities for handling premature babies.

**Ideal Infant Hygiene Program.** An ideal local program for promotion of infant hygiene should contain at least the following essential elements:

*A.* Continuous, capable medical supervision of the baby. The baby should be seen at monthly intervals during the first three months of life, bi-monthly to the end of the first year and at least semi-annually until school age.

*B.* Public health nursing supervision through home visits at monthly intervals during the first year of life and semi-annually thereafter.

*C.* A well equipped welfare center where mothers can come for advice concerning infant feeding and food habits of children, for mental hygiene —particularly in relation to child training—for dental inspection from the third year of life on, for tests of hearing and vision, and to receive protection against smallpox and diphtheria, etc.

*D.* Adequate facilities in the community for hospitalization—inpatient and outpatient—for the care of sick children and for the correction of physical defects.

Only a few health departments have been able to develop, as yet, the comprehensive type of infant and child hygiene program that has been outlined above and to make these services available to all the children of the community.

It is not enough, however, simply to develop the machinery whereby such a program can be put in operation. A still more important consideration is the quality of the service that is given. A good administrator will not try to develop the whole plan at once, but will take one step at a time and do each activity well, emphasizing the quality of the work done rather than the quantity.

**Development of a Program in Infant Hygiene.** The natural and basic steps in development of an infant hygiene program should be:

1. Instruction of the local public health nurses in the hygiene of maternity and infancy.

2. Supervision and training of midwives.

3. Public instruction of mothers and of prospective mothers in the simple principles of infant hygiene by every possible means, such as letters, radio talks, pamphlets, special classes and personal conferences.

4. Better medical and nursing care through:

   a. Continuous supervision of the work of the local nurses.
   b. Instruction of local physicians in the modern principles and practices of infant hygiene.

Infant hygiene as a function of the health department is essentially an educational measure. Theoretically, at least, it should be possible to make a clear-cut distinction between this function and the medical care of the sick child. The general educational measures in relation to infant hygiene are of great diversity and varying effectiveness. The pamphlets and other educational material of the Children's Bureau are noteworthy. The nursing supervision in the homes is a very effective educational effort, if the nurse has had proper training. The public health nurse usually does not give continuous bedside nursing care to the babies in her jurisdiction, but instructs the mothers concerning proper care of their children. She also aids mothers in carrying out the instructions of their family physician in regard to feeding formulae.

**Well Child Conferences.** Medical supervision of well babies in the community is usually supplied by official or unofficial agencies through well child conferences. Mothers bring their babies to these conferences at approximately monthly intervals during the first year of life of the baby and less frequently thereafter for the purposes of health instruction and medical supervision.

Obviously, this type of medical supervision is not the primary function of the health department, but rather it is the function of the practicing physicians of the community. Enrollment in well baby conferences under official health department sponsorship should be limited to those families in which the parents cannot afford private service. It must be confessed that many practicing physicians are not prepared by training, experience or inclination to assume this activity, and thus many health departments have organized well child conferences on a large scale because of the obvious need, in fact, the insistent demand, for this service by the public.

One major difficulty encountered in well child conferences in which any and all babies in the community may be enrolled, is the inability of the clinic to draw a sharp line of distinction between the health instruction, which may be considered a health department function, and the clinical care of babies that are not perfectly normal, which is clearly not a health department function. The solution of this difficulty would be reached if all practicing physicians offered complete medical supervision of babies as a routine in their private practice. Pediatricians are alive to this need. In fact, the American Academy of Pediatrics has prepared a brochure giving definite and detailed instruction to its members concerning proper technic in the examination and care of well babies. This type of practice is becoming more and more popular among the younger physicians, many of whom now agree to supervise the health of a child during its first year of life for a modest annual fee.

In each community some parents will be too poor to pay for this type of service. This group of children may well be given health supervision by official health department well child conferences, if the baby is referred to the clinic by a practicing physician.

The community services that are required to promote the health of the young child are, in brief:

1. Instruction of the parent in the technics of child care and in the principles of nutrition and methods of protection against illness.
2. Facilities for periodic physical examination for the detection of defects, incipient disease, and the consequences of faulty care and training.
3. Available medical and dental facilities for securing necessary correction and treatment of defects that are found.
4. Immunization against specific infectious diseases, such as diphtheria, smallpox, etc. Ideally, these services may best be given by the practicing physician.

The well child conference plan has been devised for families that are unable to pay for this service.

These conferences are organized to receive all babies from the early weeks of life to school age. The personnel consists of a pediatrician and a public health nurse who participates in the conference and in the home follow-up work. A clerk greatly facilitates the work of the clinic, and a nutritionist and dental hygienist add greatly to the effectiveness of the service. Each enrolled child should be given a physical examination by the physician at least once in three months during the first year of life, and every six months thereafter. Monthly interviews may be held between the physician and parent. At these interviews time should be taken to consider past and present health of the baby, the care, feeding and training of the child, with advice as to changes in the diet or routine such as may be necessary. Effort should be made to arrange for correction of defects whenever they are found. The nurse through her home follow-up visits aids in securing correction of physical defects.

A well child conference functions best if the mothers are trained to come by appointment. In a single afternoon session of three hours, not more than 20 mothers can be seen by one physician. Five of these appointments will be for physical examinations, the remaining 15 for the monthly interview. Except in crowded industrial centers, one physician at each conference is sufficient. If the service grows, the work should be decentralized and the conference brought to the mothers, rather than asking the mothers to come from long distances to the center.

**Advisory Pediatric Committee.** A very useful administrative device in promotion of better well baby conferences is the formation of an advisory pediatric committee. This committee should be appointed by the health officer in co-operation with the local medical society, and should be composed of those physicians in the community who are well versed in pediatrics. These men should advise the health department as to the standards to be set and the procedures to be followed at the well child conferences. They should consider questions such as essentials of diet, proper clothing, the indications for recommendation of special cases to private physicians, the proper technic of general health supervision, etc. They should discuss also the content of a public health nursing visit, the exact function of and the standards of the nursing visit in an infant hygiene service.

**Nursing Service in Infant Hygiene.** The technic of a public health nursing service for infants and the various details of organization of a well child conference cannot be given in this text. They have been amply discussed in the various books on these subjects, to which the student is referred.

**Minor Activities.** Certain minor activities and responsibilities of the health department play an important part in promotion of child health, as, for example:

   *a.* Licensing and inspection of institutions that care for infants.
   *b.* Licensing of midwives.
   *c.* Licensing and inspection of individual homes in which babies are placed by social welfare organizations.
   *d.* Licensing and inspection of lying-in hospitals.

**State Responsibility in an Infant Hygiene Program.** The state health department renders no direct service, except for purposes of demonstration, and for a limited period.

The state should give leadership and guidance of local effort. The state division of child hygiene should elevate local standards of activity, promote more uniform procedures and make a critical analysis of the results that are secured from different types of local effort.

The state should aid in the selection and training of local personnel.

In selected instances the state may, for a temporary period, give a direct subsidy to promising local developments that seem to open the way to more effective methods of work or better type of organization.

## PRESCHOOL HYGIENE

It is customary in public health practice to set apart a special division of activity called "Preschool Work." The age group affected includes all children who have passed the first year of life up through the fifth year of life. While it is true that this particular age group is subjected to special hazards and requires special consideration, nevertheless we must think of the whole child hygiene program as one of continuation. At certain age periods, emphasis is placed on one phase of the work; later, other activities are stressed.

When a child has passed his first birthday, he is fairly well launched in life. The general principles which relate to protection and promotion of the child's health remain the same as when he was an infant, but additional developmental difficulties are soon encountered—difficulties that are inherent in the growth of the child himself and in the broadening of his worldly contacts. Measures along the following lines have been found effective in the promotion of the health of the preschool child:

**Communicable Disease Control.** Children in this age period are particularly susceptible to the communicable diseases. Most of the deaths from scarlet fever, diphtheria, infantile paralysis, whooping cough and measles fall in this age group. Isolation and quarantine are of some avail for this group of children. Immunization procedures, particularly for the prevention of smallpox, diphtheria, as well as the other communicable diseases of early childhood, should be stressed during the preschool age period.

**Nutrition.** Proper nutrition is a subject of major importance in the preschool child. Food habits are formed at this time. The dietary becomes more diverse, and the child's nutritional requirements are exacting. The basis for a sound, healthy, well nourished body is established in the age period of one to five years.

**Mental Hygiene.** The principles of mental hygiene may be applied very effectively in children of preschool age. The public health nurse can be of tremendous aid to mothers in solving the individual problems that arise in relation to promotion of good mental and emotional attitudes.

**Correction of Minor Defects.** Minor physical defects may often be corrected in early childhood. Such efforts will result in immeasurable benefit to the individual in later life. Particularly, attention should be paid to correction of defects of eyesight, hearing, posture, defective tonsils and adenoids, and many other conditions. The care of the teeth of the preschool child requires particular consideration.

The public health nurse is the key person in the community program for promotion of the health of the preschool child. The work is simply a continuation of her infant hygiene activities. The older children are visited less frequently and somewhat different situations are encountered, but the same general principles are involved.

**"Summer Round Up."** "Summer Round Up" is a popular term for a sudden spasm of activity on the part of the health department in which the children about to enter school are "rounded up" and given a physical examination. Recommendations are made to the parents concerning necessary correction of defects in their children, as well as proper immunization procedures that may have been neglected up to this time. The major recommendations relate to dentistry, to foci of infection, and to correction of defects of vision.

This spasmodic activity has undoubted value, particularly if there have been no comprehensive efforts by the health department to care for these children in the community since infancy.

## SCHOOL HYGIENE

School hygiene programs have reached a higher state of development than any other single activity of the local public health service. This is due in great part to the fact that teachers and school authorities are intelligent people, interested in the welfare of the pupils and awake to the importance of the promotion of good health habits, and the advantages of the correction of various physical defects.

The greatest advances have been made in the elementary public schools; the programs for the high schools are less well developed. The purposes of a school health service are:

1. To teach children the rudiments of personal and community hygiene. Good health habits are established in the child. He learns also the various factors that influence a continuous maintenance of good health in after years.

2. To protect the school child from acquiring disease from others.

3. To give assurance that each child is physically fit for the school routine that is imposed upon him.

4. To detect actual disease or physical defects that may impede normal development and progress in school. The last function has little value unless there is a follow-up system to secure correction of defects in those children in which they have been detected by the school medical service.

The school hygiene program should not include corrective work of a definitely medical, dental or surgical nature. Many school hygiene programs include clinic service, such as posture clinics, clinics for preventive dentistry, nutrition clinics, etc. When and if organized, they should emphasize the educational features and preventive aspects of the field, rather than the clinical features.

Baumgartner [5] has summarized a good school health program:

I. An adequate case-finding program.
   A. Periodic medical and dental service by persons who are skilled and trained in the medical and dental problems of children.
      1. The goal of 4 examinations during the child's school life is recommended.

[5] Baumgartner, L., Wegman, M. E., and Wheatley, G.: "Medical, Dental, and Nursing Services for School Children." *Yale J. Biol. & Med.* 1947, vol. 19, no. 4.

> 2. Emphasis should be put on medical examinations for those children that are selected through daily teacher observation, rather than a routine grade selection.
>
> B. Accessory consultation service when indicated by specialists such as ophthalmologists, orthopedists, psychiatrists, etc.
>
> C. Access to diagnostic laboratory service, such as roentgenography, serologic laboratories, etc.
>
> D. Mass testing procedures. Examples are: tests for adequacy of vision and of hearing, and tests for the detection of special conditions such as nutritional status, parasitic (*e.g.*, ringworm) infections, etc.
>
> E. Determination of the immunization status of every child with respect to diphtheria, smallpox, whooping cough, and also tetanus and typhoid fever, when indicated.
>
> II. Follow-up program.
>
> Case finding is largely a waste of time without a good follow-up program. It may be accomplished by:
>
> 1. An interpretation of the case findings and of the recommendations made by the professional staff to parents, children and teachers.
>
> 2. Access to curative services. It is not the function of the school to treat the children. But the school should find ways of making necessary services available to all children.
>
> 3. Access to nursing supervision in the home and in the school. Adequate public health nursing is an indispensable adjunct to a school health service.
>
> 4. Access to psychiatric guidance and to social service.

This plan requires the co-operation of all the community facilities, particularly the whole-hearted and understanding co-operation of the Board of Education with the Department of Health.

The major functions of a school health service are divided ordinarily into four groups:

1. Sanitation.
2. Medical and Nursing Service.
3. Health Education.
4. Physical Education.

**Environmental Sanitation.** The general principles that relate to sanitation of the schools apply to all school plants, from the one room country schoolhouse with a handful of pupils to the largest municipal high school with several thousand students. These principles include such essentials as proper site for the schoolhouse, an ample playground space, a suitable water supply, with a good type of drinking fountain, proper toilet facilities, provision for adequate heating, lighting and ventilation of the schoolrooms, proper adjustable desks and seats, adequate facilities for preparing school lunches, supervised play, security against hazards of fire, and proper precautions for the prevention of accidents.

These various facilities are provided by the school authorities, acting in co-operation with and under the advice of the health department. The health officer or the sanitary inspector of the health department should make regular inspections of these facilities to be sure that everything is in proper working condition.

**Medical and Nursing Service.** A comprehensive school medical and nursing service contains many and varied elements, among which may be included:

a. Communicable disease control in the schools.
b. Health examinations.
c. Follow-up work to secure correction of physical defects.
d. Dental service.
e. Nursing service.
f. Nutritional service.
g. Mental hygiene activities.

**Communicable Disease Control.** Communicable disease control may be divided into several distinct activities.

*Immunization.* Measures that are taken to protect the children against invasion of specific infections, such as Schick testing and subsequent diphtheria toxoid immunization, or cowpox vaccination, are examples of this type of activity. The child should have been vaccinated during his first year of life. A second vaccination on entering school will give him a relatively high degree of immunity for life.

Each child should have been immunized against diphtheria long before his sixth year. Some communities give the Schick test to children on school entrance, and immunize all those who are Schick negative.

*Isolation.* The principle of isolation is secured by a system of *daily inspection.* The teacher of each room should make a daily health inspection. Any of the children that present any of the common signs of infection, such as fever, nausea, pallor, sore throat, skin eruption or any other unusual symptom should be referred to the school nurse. The school nurse, or, in some instances, the school physician should inspect the child and if it seems advisable, should send him home. No diagnosis should be made. The parents should be informed that the child has been sent home because of suspected illness and advised that the family physician should be consulted.

*Readmission to School.* In most schools when a child has had a contagious disease, he is not readmitted to school until he has obtained a health certificate from the school physician. Some schools accept a certificate of health from the family physician. Many schools require also that a child shall not return to school after three days' consecutive absence without a health certificate from the school physician.

These various devices of school exclusion for the purpose of prevention of the spread of contagious diseases have been highly ineffective. School communicable disease control work can be carried out best on the same basis and as an integral part of the regular epidemiological work of the health department. Sporadic activities of the school health service in an attempt to control communicable diseases are of themselves extremely fragmentary and of little or no avail in checking the disease in the school itself or in the community as a whole.

*Special Problems.* The minor skin diseases of children are a special problem in school health work. The most common are scabies, impetigo, ringworm and pediculosis. The nurse should make a careful inspection of all the children for these skin infections when school opens in the fall and again at mid-term. All infected children should be excluded from school until cured. The nurse through advice and practical demonstration can be of real aid to the families of the whole community in getting rid of these very troublesome conditions. It should be noted at this point that no single problem in health work requires greater diplomacy and tact, nor is there any other situation that is so full of potential explosiveness.

**Accidents.** Accidents are the major cause of death in the United States in children of school age—5 to 14 years inclusive.

In 1946 approximately 6,500 school children lost their lives by accidents. A marked decline has occurred in the accident death rate in recent years, but it has not kept pace with the decline in deaths from disease. Thus accidents now account for 40% of all deaths in white school boys and 20% in school girls.

Motor vehicle accidents account for about one third of these deaths in boys, and an even greater fraction of the deaths in girls. The great majority of these accidents occurred while the children were playing in the roadway, or were crossing the street or highway.

Drownings account for nearly one fourth of the accidental deaths of school-age children, while 10% are due to burns, conflagrations or explosions.

These few simple data speak for themselves, and suggest the obvious and simple remedy. A continuous educational program in the schools should train the children in the avoidance of accidents, stressing particularly the methods that must be followed in preventing automobile and highway accidents.

The child who has good training in how to take care of himself in the water in all emergencies, will act automatically when the emergency occurs, and very seldom drowns. The child who appreciates the danger of playing with matches and with firearms is seldom burned in a fire or by an explosion. Prevention of vehicular accidents by education of the children requires a patient and continuous program of training in this field.

This program of child education is a tiresome, repetitious process which is the direct responsibility of the board of education, and particularly the individual schoolroom teachers of the lower grades. If well done, it will bring about excellent results in the prevention of suffering and the reduction of the death rate from unnecessary accidents. The health department should aid and encourage the schools in this program.

**Health Examinations.** Formerly public health authorities recommended that school children be given a medical examination each year. This procedure is required by law in a few states, but is a poor practice, which usually has been carried out in a cursory and ineffectual way. The school medical examination is, at best, a screen which is intended to select those children who require special attention. Some school physicians attain an uncanny ability to pick out the defective child at a glance as he passes by in a single file line. Most authorities now agree that if the examination is conducted at all, it should be done well, and at less frequent intervals.

If the child has had a careful health examination on entrance to school, it will be quite sufficient if this medical examination is repeated twice or three times during his school career. An excellent spacing of these examinations is:

1. Entrance to school—about 6 years of age.
2. Fourth grade—about 10 years of age.
3. Entrance to high school—about 14 years of age.

This is a practical working program and will undoubtedly work injustice to a few children who may develop undetected physical defects during the interval between physical examinations.

The reasons for selecting these ages are: The six-year-old is just entering school. This examination can well be done just before enrollment.

The fourth grade is approximately half way through the average child's school life. He is at the age where he has enough intelligence to correct bad food habits and improve his nutrition of his own volition. Defects in vision and hearing are especially important at his age, and occasionally early rheumatic heart disease is discovered.

Theoretically, the last year of high school would be a better selection than the ninth grade, for thus the young man or woman would go out into the world with all defects corrected and a good start in life. But many boys and girls never complete high school. At 14 they are entering adolescence, with its special environmental problems, including nutrition, and also mental maladjustment.

If the school examination includes a tuberculin test and x-ray of positives, then the best time for this procedure is the last year of high school.

The medical examination should be thorough and unhurried. If possible, one of the parents should be present at the examination to bring out a careful history, and in order that the parent may understand the purpose of the examination and the significance of the recommendations.

**Follow-up Work.** The follow-up service to secure correction of defects that have been found in the medical examination is one of the most important and effective factors of the school health program. This work is the responsibility of the public health nurse. It can be carried out most effectively when the nurse does not limit her activities to school hygiene, but secures correction of defects in school children as part of her general family nursing work. She should be a community nurse, carrying out all phases of the general public health program, with school work as one of her important duties.

**School Nutritional Service, Nursing Service and Mental Hygiene Activities.** These services and activities have been discussed extensively in special chapters, dealing specifically with these subjects. Nutritional service deserves special mention.

A good nutritionist is an indispensable part of a school health program. Nutritional defects and bad food habits are prevalent among school children and are subject to correction in most instances. The activities of the nutritionist, together with those of the public health nurse, the school dentist and the school physician, are all largely educational in nature; but no single technical part of the school health service can be more easily and closely integrated with other school activities than nutritional work.

The nutritionist does not do the actual teaching, but does plan the material and content for the teacher's presentation.

*School lunches.* The school lunch can be made a very important teaching exercise in nutrition. The utilization of the school cafeteria in presenting proper food to children in an attractive way has been seriously neglected. Too often the cafeteria sells an abundance of cheap candy, soft drinks and other unsuitable foods in order to make a profit. The excuses are (*a*) that the cafeteria is used to support some other school activity, and (*b*) that the children will buy soft drinks and candy elsewhere if the cafeteria does not supply them.

The major purposes of the school cafeteria are:

1. To supply the children with wholesome food at cost.

2. To teach by example and precept the essential principles of a well-balanced diet. The cafeteria should be an educational institution, and the school lunch should become an integral part of the teaching machinery in the department of home economics.

**Health Education.** Systematic general education of the school children in regard to health matters is a function of the teacher. The material should be incorporated in the general school curriculum. The health officer and the nurse may be of great aid to the school department in planning the school health program, may furnish material for it, and may teach the principles of hygiene and public health to the teachers. But the teachers themselves must present the subject to the children.

A number of competent authorities have dealt with the various technics of school health education in a series of text books which relate to the various phases of this subject. The author does not feel competent to discuss the theory or the practice of the various methods of health teaching that are recommended in the extensive literature on school health education. An incomplete list of references on this subject is appended at the end of this chapter and also at the end of the chapter on Health Education.

**Physical Education.** Physical training has received a great impetus in recent years in our public school systems. It has been developed by a specially trained, enthusiastic, and competent group of teachers. Their work has been of inestimable value in improvement of physical standards, the development of character, and the inculcation of habits for wholesome enjoyment that may be carried from the school into life.

One fundamental mistake has been made in many schools in the development of physical education. School authorities have assumed that physical education is the keystone of a school health program. This fallacy has at times led to defeat of the whole purpose of health promotion in the schools. Often physical education is the only portion of the school health structure that is given any consideration. In some instances the director of physical education is placed in charge of all the school health work. It should be noted that this misconception has not been limited to the public school administrations, but is evident in its most gross inconsistencies in administration of our large universities. The physical education activities should be an integral part of a well-planned and well-co-ordinated school health service. Otherwise, the results will not only be highly ineffective, but may result in disaster. All too often the boy or girl with a poor heart, with lungs infected with tuberculosis, or with some other serious defect has been urged to take part in strenuous competitive athletics, to the permanent injury of his or her health.

One of the crucial tests of an educated man is that he acts with reason in all things. We have not met this test in the absurd development of competitive athletics as a part of our public school and university health programs.

## ADMINISTRATION OF A SCHOOL HEALTH SERVICE

Many local superintendents of education insist that all phases of the school health program should be under the exclusive administration of the department of education. This is so palpably unsound from the point of view of good administrative practice that it is scarcely necessary to argue the point. No one questions the authority of the department of education in relation to the technic of school health education and physical education; but the medical and nursing aspects of school health work represent an integral part of the whole child health program for the community, and are the province of the health department.

The only excuse for the administration by the department of education of public health medical and nursing service for children of school age has been that health departments have done the work poorly. It is stated that health departments have been, in general, badly organized, with untrained, politically minded personnel, whereas the school department has been free from political pressure and has had the funds to develop the work. In many instances, this has been true. Governmental authorities are only beginning to realize the necessity for well-trained and well-qualified personnel for the health services of the community; whereas the educational department has enjoyed for years the benefits of intelligent, professionally trained direction.

The obvious defects of the present situation should not be permitted to continue. All administrative activities relating to the protection and promotion of the public health should be allocated to a single governmental agency.

There is no real excuse for conflict between the local or state departments of education and of public health in relation to their respective functions. In fact, the activities of one supplement those of the other, and it should be a simple matter to develop a working arrangement which will be mutually satisfactory and advantageous.

We cannot emphasize too strongly, however, that the medical and nursing aspects of school health work should be administered as an integral part of the child hygiene and public health nursing program of the health department. There should be the closest co-operation between the superintendent of the public schools and the health officer, and all plans of the health department for medical and nursing service in the schools should meet the approval of the school authorities and be organized in accordance with the general program of the school department.

For a school population of 20,000 or more children, the employment of a full-time school physician is advisable. In smaller communities, the medical health service in the schools is organized by that physician of the health department who is in charge of the other child hygiene activities of the community. Additional medical and dental service may be purchased by employing local physicians and dentists on a part-time basis.

If the specialized nursing plan is followed, it is generally recommended that one health department nurse should be employed for each 2,000 to 3,000 school children. Under the generalized plan approximately one half of each and every public health nurse's time will be spent in the school work or in related activities.

The cost of the medical and nursing aspects of school health work in different cities in the United States varies greatly. A reasonable allocation for an adequate program is from $0.75 to $1.00 per annum for each child registered in the schools.

### PREVENTION OF HEARING DEFECTS

The best method that has been devised for the early detection of actual or potential defective hearing is the mass audiometer test. These tests can be conducted in the schoolroom, and the whole class of 30–40 children take the test at the same time. The mass audiometer test is simply a method of screening out those children who have *adequate* hearing. The children that have difficulty with the test are then retested, and if an apparent hearing defect is found, the child is referred to an otologist for diagnosis and suitable treatment.

The audiometer test must be made by a person who is skilled in its operation. Large municipalities may employ a full-time person to do this work. In scattered rural areas, the state department of education or the state department of public health organizes the audiometer test program and sends the technician with the equipment into the field. Each child should be tested early in his school life, and at least once again during the grammar school years.

### Tuberculosis Finding

In years past, public schools conducted extensive surveys for the detection of early tuberculosis in school children. With the marked decline in tuberculosis, these programs have been omitted in the schools because the results secured are not commensurate with the effort that is expended. Tuberculosis in children of grammar school age is now encountered very seldom.

A tuberculosis case-finding program in boys and girls of high-school age, particularly the last year in high school, is an excellent educational device. Each youth is given a tuberculin test—the patch test is quite satisfactory for screening purposes—and all children with a positive tuberculin are given an x-ray of the chest. Some health departments offer each high-school graduate an x-ray of the chest, omitting the tuberculin test. Very few cases of tuberculosis will be found by this procedure: perhaps one in five thousand children that are examined. But the effort can be justified on the basis of its value in the education of these young potential citizens concerning the importance of x-ray in the early diagnosis and adequate treatment of the disease.

### Vision Testing

The vision testing program in the schools is similar to the audiometer test, in that it is a preliminary test which screens out those children who have *adequate* eyesight. Any children that have difficulty with the test are referred to an ophthalmologist.

The simplest test is the use of a Snellen Chart. Frequently the test is done by the schoolroom teacher. We are of the opinion that this test should be carried out by a person who is skilled and experienced in the test, and that standard lighting and other conditions must be insisted upon in performing the test.

Annual vision testing is recommended by most school health workers. This is probably unnecessary, as most children with defective eyesight do not have rapidly progressive loss of vision. A carefully done test every third year of a child's school life will probably yield the best results for the most economical expenditure of time and effort.

The reader is particularly referred to: "Suggested School Health Policies"—A Committee Report, which appeared in the *Journal of Health and Physical Education,* May and June 1940, Vol. XI, Nos. 5 and 6.

### DENTAL HEALTH PROGRAM

The promotion of dental health is one of the important functions of the Health Department. It is true that the great proportion of the work that will be conducted in the community for the protection and promotion of dental health will be carried out by the practicing dentists, but the responsibility for the organization of dental health service rests upon the health administrator of the community.

The importance of healthy, sound teeth is unquestioned. We cannot make even an estimate of the injury that results in adult life from the neglect of dental hygiene in childhood. In some instances it is probable that greatly exaggerated statements have been made in relation to the injury that is produced because of bad teeth. We are sure of one thing, however—namely, that dental caries is more prevalent than any other single disease condition. Repeated surveys of school children have been made on the prevalence of dental disease, and they have clearly demonstrated the tremendous extent of dental decay, and the ineffectiveness with which this problem has been met.

The overwhelming magnitude of this problem should not require us to throw up our hands and abandon its solution.

**Etiology.** One important reason why we have not been able to solve the whole problem of dental hygiene is that the etiology of dental caries is unknown. There is convincing evidence that fermentation of carbohydrates in the mouth plays an important part in the chemistry of tooth decay. There is also strong evidence that good nutrition is a definite factor in proper dental hygiene. We are increasingly aware of the fact that if a child has been on a sound nutritional basis during his entire developmental period, from the time of conception and onward through infancy and early childhood, he will tend to have a good dentition. We are also aware that during the periods of increased nutritional requirements of adolescence, and of pregnancy, such demands are put upon the body that dental decay is more rapid than at other times. Nevertheless, we must recognize that children on an excellent nutritional basis have dental caries, and also that the old slogan, "A clean tooth never decays" is colorful but does not tell the truth.

At present our only unquestionably effective method in the prevention of dental caries is to remove the caries of a tooth in its incipiency and replace it with suitable filling material. This is the one method which has proved successful in the prevention of tooth disease and loss.

**Control Program.** In view of our present limitations in dental hygiene, it is obvious that a control program must be based on early recognition of dental caries. Under an ideal plan, the child would visit the dentist before his third birthday, and every six months thereafter throughout life. Corrections should be made when defects occur. In the long run, this program is much less expensive and more effective than the present plan of postponing the visit to the dentist until the tooth begins to ache. It is possible to approach this ideal plan through suitable educational procedures.

Education should be begun with the parents at the birth of the child. The parents should be taught to take their children to the dentist at suitable intervals. Health teaching in the schools is an important factor in the program. This health teaching, to be successful, must be accepted by the school child as an integral part of his learning program, and not as a campaign by the school dentist or the dental hygienist.

Part of the educational program is the examination of the children in the schools. The examination of the teeth should be done by the dentist and not by the school physician as part of the medical examination.

*The dental hygienist.* The dental hygienist's work was initiated as part of the program of school health. Her function was essentially to clean the teeth of the children, and is founded on the fallacy that "a clean tooth never decays." The work of the dental hygienist in the schools can be justified only on the basis of health education. The real and effective place of the dental hygienist is as a valuable and important assistant to the dentist in the dental clinic and in the school. She will relieve him of his simpler tasks, so that he can devote his time to the more important remedial measures.

The whole purpose of the school education plan in dental hygiene is to motivate the child to seek the services of a dentist of his own volition.

**The Health Department's Responsibility in the Dental Hygiene Program.** The procedures which the Health Department should follow in the dental hygiene program are the same as in other disease conditions:

*a.* Case finding.
*b.* Follow-up through the school nurse.
*c.* Early treatment, which shall be given free to the children of those families that are unable to pay for this care.

**Organization.** As has been stated above, the essential preventive measure is early correction of defects. Children in whom dental caries has been discovered, and whose parents can afford dentist's fees, should be sent to the private dentist. The dental clinic of the public health department should be reserved for those children whose families are unable to pay for this care. The clinic should be organized in close relationship with the well child conference service, and mothers who bring their babies to the well child conference should be referred with their babies to the dental clinic for observation before the child's third birthday. Children may also be referred to the clinic by the school health service.

The age limit is usually set at the ninth year. This period is selected, not because children over nine years of age do not require further dental care. On the contrary, the period of adolescence is one of rapid tooth deterioration. The matter is purely one of expediency. The magnitude of the problem is such that it has not been found feasible to organize the clinic service for all the age groups. It is assumed that the adolescent child who has been trained to take pride in his teeth and who recognizes the importance of good dental hygiene will of his own initiative obtain the necessary resources to preserve his teeth.

**State Dental Service.** The State Health Department should give leadership in this field. Under Social Security assistance, by 1947 practically all of the forty-eight states had some type of state dental health organization. The local health departments should use the state dental consultants in the same way as they use the state epidemiologist or the state public health engineer. The function of the State Division of Dental Hygiene is to aid local health departments in the organization of an effective dental health service.

**Community Dental Service.** Larger cities and populous counties may organize a local Division of Dental Hygiene; or in the smaller health departments the dental hygiene program may well be organized as a separate division of the Child Health Service of the local health department. Dental hygienists should be employed on a full-time basis. They act as assistants to the clinic dentists, and may also aid the dentist in the diagnostic examinations in the schools. It is a good routine procedure to conduct an examination of the teeth of the school children at least every other year. (Some health authorities insist on annual dental examination by the Health Department dentist or his assistant dental hygienist.)

All the school children, including those of high-school age, should be included in this examination; and the school nursing service, through suitable follow-up work, should urge the children and their parents to have any defects that are encountered corrected as soon as possible. As has been stated previously, however, it may be necessary to set an age limit for the children who are referred to the health department clinic service.

In the larger cities, a full-time dentist is frequently employed to plan and co-ordinate the dental health program. The essential and basic services of this division are conducted by the clinic dentists, who are employed on a part-time basis. Usually they are paid an annual sum; sometimes they are reimbursed on the basis of actual hours of clinic service.

The chief difficulty that has been encountered in a good dental hygiene program has been inability of the dentists to understand and to handle small children properly. For the most part, dentists have been untrained in the dentistry of children, and many of the older dentists have been unwilling to undertake this type of work. In recent years, however, health departments and dental organizations as well have had remarkable success in providing suitable courses for practicing dentists in the field of children's dentistry.

**A Comprehensive Dental Program.** The Committee on Dental Research of the American College of Dentists has made an attempt to at least evaluate the problems of dental care for children in the United States.[6]

This report estimates that there are 30 million children of school age in the nation. The average child (6–18 years) acquires less than one cavity per year in permanent teeth. (0.8 to 0.9 is the general average, though there is great variation in different parts of the United States.)

The major part of a preventive program at present must consist in the early recognition and prompt relief of caries. Thus it is estimated that one hour of dental service time per year per child, plus one-half hour service for the dental hygienist for teeth cleaning, will be sufficient to meet community needs. It is estimated that approximately 10 per cent of the children will be unable to pay for this service, and thus 10 per cent of the cost would fall on the community. If an average cost of $5 per child for cleaning and filling is allowed, then the annual cost for this service to the health department per annum per 100,000 population is: 25,000 school children divided by 10 = 2,500 children to be cared for by the municipality. At $5 per child, it would cost $12,500 for actual dental services of school children. The Committee believes that if this service is carried on consistently each year throughout the life of the school child (6–18 years) that the total cost of $60 would be much less than the reparative work that would be required throughout adult life, if this program is neglected.

Most discussions relating to dental hygiene are concerned with the conditions as they actually exist in the United States. Prepayment plans for comprehensive medical care have stumbled on this obstacle. How could it be avoided, it is so enormous? The American College of Dentists has estimated that the initial dental care for the average adult in the nation would cost from $50 to $75 per person, with subsequent maintenance care of $12 to $16 per annum. Other estimates for prepayment of service for dental care have been much larger than these figures.

The author is of the opinion that in planning for the future we can give little consideration to the present enormous reserves of neglected oral hygiene. It is water over the dam. Our only hope of success lies in planning for the future and attempting to prevent caries in childhood, so that the next generation will benefit by our efforts. If this point of view is

[6] Treloar, A. E. and Com. on Dental Research, Am. College of Dentists: "Protective Dentristry for Children." *Jour. Am. Dental Assn.* 1944, Vol. 31, p. 322.

*See also* Knutson, J. W.: "An Index of the Prevalence of Dental Caries in School Children." *Pub. Health Rep.* 1944, Vol. 59, p. 253.

accepted, then our efforts in dental hygiene will be concentrated on care of the teeth of children of school and even preschool age.

We have no satisfactory solution of the problem of dental caries. Certain things are clear:

Dental caries varies greatly in different parts of the nation. This indicates that certain environmental factors have a strong influence upon dental caries.

**Fluorine.** Natural fluorine in the water in amounts as small as 1 part per million in the community water supply is accompanied by a low incidence of dental caries in children. It has been suggested that fluorine might be added to community water supplies in these proportions, over a long period of time. Since it has no toxic effect in these proportions, an extensive investigation along these lines is distinctly in order, and in fact is under way in several cities.[7]

Other researches into the cause of dental caries are the most hopeful approach to the solution of this extensive health problem. Meanwhile, efforts must be made to prevent the extension of caries in children by early detection and immediate repair.

*Dental Health Practice of the Future.* Dr. John O. McCall, dean of public health dentistry in the United States and one of the most foresighted thinkers in this field, has presented in summary form his ideas of dental health procedure and dental practice of the future.[8] With his permission, I present them in full:

*Personnel and Methods*
1. Health education, with special emphasis on diet.
    (*a*) Dentist to guide research and provide technical information.
    (*b*) Dental hygienist and classroom teacher in public school and high school, reaching school child and parent.
    (*c*) Health department staff, including public health nurse and allied workers in voluntary agencies, reaching older groups and concentrating attention on maternal cases; also giving attention to infants and preschool children.
2. Protective dentistry.
    (*a*) Dental hygienist, adequately trained, licensed and working under dental supervision to:
        1. Give prophylactic treatment, etc.
        2. Fill teeth of preschool and public school children.
    (*b*) Dentist, fully and adequately trained for:
        1. Diagnostic procedures.
        2. Protective dentistry for high-school group and adults.

[7] Ast, D. B.: "The Caries-Fluorine Hypothesis and a Suggested Study to Test Its Application." *Pub. Health Rep.* 1943, Vol. 58, p. 857.

[8] McCall, J. O.: "Dental Practice and Dental Education in the Future: with Consideration of Social and Health Aspects." *Jour. Amer. Dental Assoc.* 1944, Vol. 31, No. 1.

3. Prophylactic orthodontics and treatment of simpler types of malocclusion.
4. Extractions and minor oral surgery.
5. Crown and bridge work.
3. Denture service.
Dental technician, adequately trained, licensed and working under dental supervision, for denture prosthesis, both full and partial, including taking of impressions.

### MENTAL HYGIENE

Mental hygiene is an essential activity in the child hygiene program of a local health department. This subject has been discussed in another chapter. It is necessary to emphasize at this point, however, that the chief benefits in mental hygiene are achieved in childhood and early youth. The administration of mental hygiene services and the organization of this activity in a local health department thus logically belongs in the division of child hygiene.

### SPECIAL GROUPS OF CHILDREN

**Working Children** require special health supervision. The major matters to be considered are:

a. Restriction of the field or type of work.
b. Prohibition from entering hazardous or repetitive tasks.
c. Control of the hours and conditions of labor.
d. Constant provision for medical health supervision of children at work.

**Crippled and Handicapped Children.** Care of handicapped children is a very special responsibility of any child health service and must be given special consideration.

The administrative problems in relation to childhood tuberculosis and to malnutrition, the importance of summer rest camps, the place of mental hygiene in the child health programs and other related subjects have been dealt with elsewhere in this text. The organization and administration of programs for the care of crippled children were given great impetus by the National Social Security Act of 1935. A discussion of all the various features of this Act is found in Chapter XXXIX.

### ADMINISTRATION OF AN OFFICIAL CHILD HEALTH PROGRAM

Child hygiene is usually organized as a separate division of local health service. Since nurses play so extensive a part in the work, the Division of Public Health Nursing is sometimes combined with the Division of Child Hygiene.

In many municipalities, voluntary agencies have interested themselves actively in promoting child health. The wise health officer will not duplicate these activities, but will correlate his program with those of existing agencies. He may even assign responsibility for certain border line functions to the well organized voluntary agencies, and limit his own program to those activities that are, beyond all question, a definite official responsibility.

In a city of 100,000 people or over, the Division of Child Hygiene should have its own full-time medical director. He may also serve as chief school physician. His work would be almost exclusively administrative and advisory. His division would employ a considerable number of part-time physicians (perhaps five to ten in a city of this size) to carry out the medical aspects of his program, such as medical examinations of the school children, medical supervision of well child conferences, etc. The major portion of the nursing activities of the whole department would be centered in his division. He should work in very close coordination with the superintendent of schools. In some cities the school department gives an actual subsidy to this division for its health work in the schools.

In cities and rural areas with less than 100,000 population a full-time director of child hygiene is seldom feasible. In these smaller populations the health officer himself administers the child hygiene work.

**Public Health Nursing Service.** If the generalized nursing plan is followed, each public health nurse will devote the major portion of her time to child hygiene activities. If the specialized nursing plan is adopted, more than two thirds of the nursing staff will be assigned to prenatal, infant hygiene and school hygiene activities. The organization of this nursing service has been described elsewhere. (See Chapter XXI.)

**Well Child Conference** services should be allocated to meet community needs. No standard of adequate service can be set, since communities vary so in density of population, in economic status, etc.

These well child conferences do not require elaborate clinic equipment or extensive office space. They should be situated as conveniently as possible for the mothers, so that they do not have to bring their children from long distances. Informality is the keynote of success of the service, though the appointment system should be adhered to as closely as possible. The service should include both infant and preschool consultation, so that the mother can make one trip do for both age groups.

These well baby services may be organized by the health department in its own health centers, by voluntary agencies, or in the outpatient department of the community hospital. The health department should require certain standards of equipment and of technic, for, in the end, the responsibility for the accomplishment of this type of work rests upon the official health agency.

**Cost of Child Hygiene Activities.** It is difficult to determine the costs of the entire child hygiene program of any health department. Often one cannot allocate accurately the expenditures for separate health activities that bear some relationship to the promotion of child health. One thing is certain: child health activities are the most expensive part of the whole health program. They are also among the most effective activities and have the greatest popular appeal. A well-knit local health department will allocate from one fourth to one third of its total appropriation to activities that have a direct bearing on child health promotion.

One important recommendation in relation to future developments in child hygiene should be emphasized. As organized at present, the child hygiene program is not well balanced. Too great a proportion of the activities are devoted to the school-age period. Major emphasis should be shifted to the infant and preschool hygiene. The foundations for a healthful and happy life are built before the child reaches its sixth year of life.

The organization of a division of child hygiene within a local health department, and the relationship of the local organization to a state division of child hygiene and to the federal child health service has been given due consideration in other portions of this text.

## REFERENCES

1. Baker, Josephine. *Fighting for Life.* The Macmillan Company, New York. 1939.
2. Holt, L. E. and McIntosh, Rustin. *Diseases of Infancy and Childhood.* D. Appleton-Century Co., New York. (11th edition.) 1940.
3. Gesell, A. and Amatruda, C. S. *Developmentary Diagnosis.* Paul Hoeber, New York. 1941.
4. Spock, Benjamin. *Baby and Child Care.* Pocket Books, Inc., Rockefeller Center, New York City. 1942.
5. Nyswander, Dorothy. *Solving School Health Problems.* Commonwealth Fund, New York City. 1942.
6. Lamkin, N. B. *Health Education in Rural Schools and Communities.* A. S. Barnes and Company, New York. 1946.
7. *Health in the School.* Report of the American Association of School Administration, 20th Year Book. 1942.
8. *Suggested School Health Policies.* J.A.M.A. 1940, Vol. 114, p. 1672.
9. Publications of the Children's Bureau, Washington, D. C., dealing with all phases of child health, are particularly recommended for reference and text.

### DENTAL HYGIENE

1. Carr, M. W. *Dentistry, An Agency of Health Service.* Commonwealth Fund, New York. 1946.
2. Strusser, Harry. *A Comprehensive Dental Health Program.* Jour. Amer. Dental Asso. 1941, Vol. 28, p. 1534.
3. Klein, Henry. *The Dental Status and Dental Needs of Young Adult Males, Rejectable, or Acceptable for Military Service, According to Selective Service Dental Requirements.* Pub. Health Rep. 1941, Vol. 56, p. 1369.
4. *Do You Want Your Baby to Have Good Teeth?* Published by The Murry and Leonie Guggenheim Dental Clinic, 422 East 72d Street, New York City.

5. *Facts about Teeth and Their Care.* Published by National Dental Hygiene Association, Washington, D. C.

6. *The Teacher Improves the Dental Health of the Children.* Published by the Mouth Hygiene Committee, Essex County Dental Society, 91 Lincoln Park, Newark, New Jersey.

*See also Dental Health.* Journal of the National Dental Hygiene Association, 934 Shoreham Building, Washington, D. C.

# CHAPTER XXIV

## PUBLIC HEALTH EDUCATION

No public health program can be completely successful in the United States unless it has the confidence and support of the people who benefit by it. Full support cannot be secured unless the people understand the purposes and objectives of the program. They must not only have confidence in the personnel of the health department, but must understand that its activities represent a direct service to the individual and are of real benefit to the welfare of the community.

Under our social system, it is necessary not only to win the support of the governing body, but to reach into every home, familiarize each family with the functions of the health department, and explain the activities that are being carried out to meet these obligations.

Visitors from foreign lands are amazed at the cumbersomeness of our governmental system, and are appalled at the lack of power of the health officials. In most states, health officers possess little or no compulsory powers whereby they may enforce health decrees. Even if we possessed these theoretical powers, it would not be possible to exercise them. The reason for this is that no governmental policy in this country can be carried out without the full consent of the governed. This is our tradition and the result of our historical development. This consent will not be obtained until the project is generally understood. Thus it is not possible to put into immediate execution the preventive measures that are developed by scientific research. A preliminary step to any advance in preventive medicine or community hygiene is a campaign to acquaint the people with the advantages of the specific methods to be introduced. This presupposes a general and widespread knowledge of the principles of hygiene and community sanitation. This condition does not prevail at the present time. Such an ideal situation would require not only a fairly high general level of intelligence, but also a high level of general education. The system is admirable; in fact, the essence of true democracy, and theoretically should be very effective. People certainly should be willing and anxious to provide for those things which assure them a better individual and community life.

The chief difficulty has been that adults of the present generation did not receive thorough instruction in the principles of hygiene during their elementary school training. Their scientific information is limited and their ideas are often bizarre—founded on superstition, tradition and mis-information. Furthermore, adults are slow to receive new ideas. Their habits and customs have become fixed, prejudices are established, the pattern of their life is formed; old ideas that are well established are changed with difficulty. An excellent example of this fact is the opposition, inertia and obstacles that the health officers of the south have faced in attempting the installation of simple pit privies in rural portions of the southern states for the control of hookworm infection. The people understand the mode of infection of the parasite, they are willing to take treatment, but many of them will not install or use sanitary toilets.

Health education in the United States must, therefore, be divided into two distinct phases:

**1. School Health Education.** This comprises child training in the principles of personal and community hygiene. This training must be given during the formative period of life. The health instruction should not be a thing apart, but should be incorporated in the curriculum of the elementary schools. Special hygiene courses may be introduced in secondary schools and in college training.

**2. Public Health Education** is that part of health education that takes place in the home and the community. This phase of health education is planned primarily for adults. Its purpose is to inform the people of the community concerning current public health problems and to advise them of the policies of the health department in its attempt to solve these problems.

The success of the second half of the health education program is dependent in no small part upon the first. In fact, most public health authorities believe that the most essential feature of health education is proper health training in the schools.

School health education is not the direct responsibility of the health department. This is essentially a pedagogical matter. This material should be presented to the children by the teachers and not by health department personnel. Experience has shown that the teaching should not be given by special public health teachers who may give occasional exercises in hygiene to the pupils. Rather, the materials should be incorporated in the daily classroom work by the regular teachers. To be successful, this plan requires that all school teachers shall be equipped to teach properly the principles of public health. This plan requires, therefore, a systematic training in preventive medicine and community hygiene in teachers' training schools.

The health department may render a real service to the department of education in each community by giving aid in the training of school teachers in public health; through lectures and demonstrations, by furnishing illustrative material to the teachers, by reviewing and criticizing new textbooks and pamphlets, and by formulation of programs for the teachers that may be applicable to the various grades of children that receive instruction. It is not the province of this text to discuss in detail the technic of school health education. The subject has been studied with great care, and a variety of splendid teaching programs has been developed. These various programs of health education have been very successful and have been incorporated in the curricula of all the progressive public schools in the United States. The details of these programs may be found in a large number of textbooks and brochures that are devoted to this subject. A partial list of references is given at the end of this chapter.

We anticipate that the children of the present generation who are being trained in the principles of personal and community hygiene will be receptive to the plans of the health department for community benefit when they become adult members of the community. The influence of this health teaching, though recent in its inception, is already being felt in all parts of the United States.

## OBJECTIVES OF PUBLIC HEALTH EDUCATION

**1. Education About the Health Department and Its Work.** One of the major but often neglected objectives of health education is to inform the citizens of the part played by the health department in the promotion of community welfare. The people should know who the members of the health department are and what they do, and how the department may be of service to them.

**2. Education in the Principles of Personal Hygiene.** This essential resolves itself into a program for health promotion of the individual, in order that the life of each person in the community may be lived more abundantly. This subject covers a very wide range: not simply the narrow field of bodily cleanliness as exemplified by the washing of hands and the brushing of teeth and all those details that have been the concern of personal hygiene for so many years. This field includes such important matters as individual and community nutrition, dental hygiene, mental hygiene, sex hygiene, and so forth.

**3. Education in the Principles of Environmental Sanitation.** Everyone must recognize that one of the basic elements of a health program revolves around those essentials that are required to produce a healthy environment. In many instances, the individual cannot provide these healthy environmental conditions for himself. They are provided for him by the community, but he must know what proper environment is, so that he will be in a position to take proper measures to protect his own health and that of his family in whatever situation he may find himself. He will know also whether or not his community is furnishing him a proper environment in which to live. This field includes a knowledge of the essentials of a safe and adequate water supply, the principles of proper sewage disposal, the requirements for a safe and adequate food supply, a suitable sanitary program for safe milk, the necessity for storage and proper handling and distribution of food. All matters relating to housing and city planning, the prevention of overcrowding, provision for adequate sunlight, public parks and playgrounds, the necessity for proper ventilation of buildings—particularly of schools and public places of congregation—the knowledge of all these things is part of the necessary information of every person in the community. In addition, he should be familiar with the safeguards that protect human life against accident, particularly industrial safeguards.

The control of the intermediate sources of disease transmission is a very important public health matter, and should be part of the knowledge of the people of the land. For example, one may cite the methods that may be employed for the control of the breeding of mosquitoes in the prevention of malaria, the control of house fly breeding, and rat propagation, in the prevention of disease. All these matters relate to community sanitation of the environment and should be taught to the people in a simple and effective way.

**4. The Epidemiology of Some of the Common Diseases.** The people should be informed concerning the basic essentials of the epidemiology of some of the more common diseases. This includes prevalence of the disease, mode of transmission, the incubation period, the case fatality rate, and particularly the methods of prevention and the methods of treatment. These matters must be translated into simple, understandable terms and presented at proper times.

**5. The elements of maternal hygiene and proper child care are** a necessary part of the basic knowledge of every mother or potential mother in the community. These are matters that it is their right to know and our obligation to teach.

**6. The essentials of an industrial hygiene program** should be imparted to every worker in the land. Each individual who is at productive work has the right to expect that his health will be protected and safeguarded. It is essential that he should know the activities and the basic principles upon which this program is founded, and the methods by which they are most properly carried out.

**7. The basic facts relating to the early recognition of degenerative disease** are an important part of our public health information, and are of special interest to a special audience.

**8. Information concerning available agencies** that are responsible for the dissemination of this information to the people is a major but often neglected objective of the health education program. The people should know the various agencies in the community that are in a position to give them the information that they desire. They should understand the place of each organization in the program of health protection of the community. People should know who the members of the health department are, what they do, and how the department may be of service to them. They should know the extent and place of the hospital and clinic facilities. They should know the place of the voluntary agencies in health protection and promotion, and should be in a position to appraise the co-ordination of effort of these various agencies in the whole program for health protection of the community.

## SELECTIVITY IN HEALTH EDUCATION

We have outlined above the simple, basic objectives of public health education in the community. In doing so, it becomes quite clear that it is necessary to be selective in the presentation of this material, since some of it is of major interest to one group and of minor interest to others. It is, of course, a basic principle of education that the individual does not absorb information and incorporate it into his daily living unless it is of direct interest to him and to his family, and is related in some way to his past experience. For example, the early recognition of degenerative disease is a matter that is of primary interest to a special adult audience. A very carefully composed booklet on the prevention of cancer was once prepared *for high-school students.* The publication was written with the greatest care; it met all the necessary technical criteria for a good presentation, and yet in this author's opinion it was inappropriate, and probably quite ineffective, because of the fact that it was addressed to an audience that has little or no interest in the early recognition of degenerative disease.

The essentials of an industrial hygiene program should obviously be imparted to a special group—the adult workers, particularly the younger age groups. This has long been recognized, and the governmental divisions of industrial hygiene, industry itself, as well as labor organizations, are co-operating in the presentation of this subject to the workers in a truly informative and effective manner.

The essentials of maternal hygiene and child care are not matters of general interest. Children certainly are not interested in the slightest degree in this information, and most fathers have a rather vicarious and not very sincere interest in this subject, but the mothers and potential mothers of the community have the deepest interest in all these matters, and it is obvious that the information should be prepared for them and presented to them as directly and effectively as possible.

We have been most successful, perhaps, in our presentation of epidemiology. Often the subject is of topical interest to the entire community. An epidemic strikes a community, may be impending, or perhaps the disease has invaded some other community and has not yet reached our own. Everyone becomes interested and is receptive to information. Influenza may be on the West Coast and seems to be approaching the East with great rapidity; rabid dogs are prevailing in certain counties of one state and may cross the boundary and invade our state at any moment; an epidemic of infantile paralysis in the upper reaches of the Connecticut River gives every evidence of extending to contiguous parts of the country.

People become intensely interested and demand information. They want to know the etiologic agent and the prevalence of the disease in their community; they are anxious to determine how it is transmitted. They learn the incubation period and are especially interested in the case fatality rate. They demand that their health department shall tell them the best methods of prevention and the best mode of treatment. These are the essentials that we wish to teach. This part of the health education program is the function of the health department, although it must be granted that some of the best transmission of epidemiologic information has been done by the voluntary agencies. Prominent in this endeavor are the voluntary associations for the prevention of tuberculosis and venereal disease.

It is clear that here, too, one must be selective in presenting the material to the proper audience. The group to be addressed in the presence of prevailing epidemics of communicable disease is composed essentially of young parents who have little children. There are exceptions to this rule, of course, particularly when pandemics of acute respiratory disease occur, or extensive outbreaks of food poisoning.

Certain epidemiologic information should be presented to very special groups. How useless it is, for example, to broadcast information in regard to venereal disease prevention among individuals over thirty years of age! Venereal disease is a disease of youth, especially children of high-school age and young men and women in the early twenties, and thus health education in these matters should be concentrated where it will do the most good. Tuberculosis we have always considered to be a disease of youth, and health education efforts were centered in this age group. We are now beginning to realize that the source of infection in tuberculosis may now be the older age groups: perhaps it is the unsuspected missed case of chronic tuberculosis that is our major source of infection at the present time. This realization is an excellent example of the fact that it is often necessary to change our emphasis in accordance with the newer scientific knowledge.

Information concerning the available agencies that aid individuals in the community is of chief interest to heads of families, and should be planned to this end, and presented to them as a group.

Environmental sanitation is of much wider interest and is of broader importance than any of the essentials thus far discussed. This information should be part of the knowledge of every person in the community. There is a time, however, when this information is best absorbed, and that is the period when the individual departs from the four walls of his home and is beginning to consider his environment as a place in which to live—the time when he broadens his horizon, and takes an interest in the great world about him. This, of course, is approximately the "teen age," when the child gets away from his home as the center of major interest, and begins to consider his community as his home. This is the time to teach environmental sanitation.

By far the most important objective in the promotion of the health of the individual—and thus indirectly of the community—is instruction in the principles of personal hygiene. This subject matter must be presented in early childhood.

## DEFECTIVE METHODS IN HEALTH EDUCATION

Many methods have been devised to keep the people informed concerning current health problems and health department programs. Some of these methods are ill advised, and in poor taste; others are badly planned. Like the boomerang, they return to the thrower with unexpected violence. One must be very sure of the value of the educational material that is presented. Every policy of health education, every fact to be given out, must be scrutinized. It is very embarrassing to be compelled to retract positive statements or to "unteach" public health practices.

"Swat the fly" campaigns are an example of a public health procedure that was established on an unsound scientific basis, and yet met with enthusiastic popular support. The health officer was on the horns of a dilemma. He must abandon the practice because of its worthlessness; yet, if he did, he would lose the public confidence and esteem which he had won in advocating the measure.

Despite the obvious defects and pitfalls of health propaganda, most experienced health officials in the United States agree that the general dissemination of health information—carefully considered and wisely planned—is one of the most important functions of the health departments; in fact, it is essential to the life and vigor of the department.

**Principles of Health Education in Adult Groups.** Certain broad, general principles should be followed in planning a health education program.

1. The material presented must tell the truth. The scientific data must be accurate, taken from authoritative sources, with supporting evidence at hand within the files of the health department. This principle is the one which is most frequently violated in health department practice.

There are so many examples of bad health education that have influenced the lives of people and affected the advancement of the community to a marked degree, that one should be extremely cautious in the inauguration of any new concept, or any new plan of presentation of public health education material. One of the earliest, and certainly one of the most devastating examples of bad health education was the theory that the decaying of animal and vegetable proteins produced disease. The strongest proponent of this theory was Benjamin Rush, the foremost physician of his time. He lived in Philadelphia and aided in the founding of a great medical school; he was physician to several presidents of the United States—a man who influenced the trend of medicine in this country for a longer period of time and perhaps with greater effect than any physician who ever lived. These theories of Benjamin Rush permeated the whole nation, and are believed by many people right down to the present date. There are still many otherwise well-informed people who are quite sure that bad odors, usually decomposing proteins, are highly inimical to community health and may in all probability produce disease.

Gaseous fumigation was a very popular public health method and was considered highly effective in the control of communicable disease. Formaldehyde gas had a penetrating odor, caused a great deal of inconvenience to the householder, and required a large number of health department employees who had little intelligence, and for this reason could be assigned to the health department by politicians. The gas certainly had been shown, scientifically, to destroy cultures of bacteria, and people accepted it as a splendid means of prevention of the spread of the contagion from its source. But in actual practice, it proved quite ineffective as a control measure in disease prevention.

"A Clean Tooth Never Decays" is a catch phrase that fits in so well with the popular impression of dental hygiene, and seems to be such an effective and easy method of controlling dental caries that it spread over the whole land, and is still taught in many of our health education programs, though well we know its absolute lack of any scientific verity.

Other misconceptions have had their day. We are informed that there will be "No More Tuberculosis by 1960." The radio tells us that the vitamin B complex, or at least one of its components, cures all ills: headache, eye strain, earache, toothache, pleurisy, lumbago, gall stones, sore throat, stomach ache, rheumatism, and others. We have also been told that the draft rejections of World War II are an evidence of serious decadence in our national life; health departments have been derelict; millions of dollars that were spent in health promotion have been wasted; that the nation was worse off in 1941 than it was in 1917, in 1862, or even in 1776.

2. The information must be presented in a dignified manner. Catch phrases and picturesque presentation may attract attention, but do not win the confidence and serious consideration of the audience.

It is not necessary to elaborate on this statement, which is obvious to everyone, although many health educators seem to feel that they must make fools of themselves in order to attract attention. It is true that catch phrases and picturesque presentations attract the eye and catch attention—but what type of attention? It is the attention given to the clowns and to the harlequins. This type of information is not taken seriously; people have no confidence in the information nor in individuals who make themselves ridiculous in order to win momentary acclaim.

3. Presentation must be in sufficiently popular form so that it is readily

understandable. The great tendency is to use long words, involved sentences, and to employ complex scientific terminology that has no meaning to the average lay audience.

4. Material must be selected and presented so that it will have an appeal for the particular group it is desired to reach. No single method of presentation will appeal to all the people.

5. A critical analysis should be made of every bit of health information with the following points in mind: It should be

*a.* Concise.
*b.* Emphatic.
*c.* Interesting.
*d.* Colorful—illustrative.
*e.* Familiar—that is, related to past experience of the audience.

6. The health officer should suit the material to the specific audience that he wishes to reach. For example, the same presentation should not be made to all age groups. Consideration should be given to the social make-up of the audience, to local conditions, local prejudices, and local motivating forces. One must have a knowledge of the psychological peculiarities of the particular group that he may wish to reach, and utilize this knowledge to the fullest extent.

7. Health education must precede legislation in America. We have learned from sad experience that legal restrictions should not be utilized to initiate public health practices. In some of the European nations, one needs to convince only one man that a certain health procedure is sound. An edict is issued, and the desired results are achieved. This is public health education reduced to its simplest elements. But in the United States, a health regulation will be successful only if it is an expression of the popular will. One must admit that this is a very slow and ineffective way in which to accomplish results, but it is the way which we have chosen.

8. The community *leaders* must be fully informed. Derryberry has emphasized the fact that one of the strongest motivations of human as well as animal behavior is "acceptance within the social group to which one belongs." But an outsider does not change the attitudes of a group, unless he can influence the leaders of thought within the group. This principle holds true in all states of human society. The successful health officer of a rural southern area who wishes to improve the health status of the Negroes will cultivate the friendship of the local Negro preacher; the health officer of a large city will win the confidence and support of the labor leaders, as well as the members of the Chamber of Commerce.

9. Health instruction is most effective where the audience has a specific and timely interest in the subject matter.

Not the advice that we believe is required, but the advice that may be requested is the important factor in good adult health education.

The mother who brings her baby to the child health conference, the family that calls the public health nurse in time of a crisis, the person who writes a letter to the health department about a health problem that puzzles him, comprise the best audiences that the educational service of the health department can have.

The health officer may well take a leaf from the book of that past master as a builder of good-will—the politician. *All mail requests for information,* no matter how trivial, should be given close and prompt consideration.

10. Within certain limits, *fear* may be an effective motivation in health education. The well person can see no reason why he should follow public health precepts, when to do so necessitates discomfort, inconvenience, and change in established customs. But the sick person is anxious to regain health, and thus has a strong reason to be concerned with better personal hygiene. Thus, specific health education directed toward those who wish to regain health is an excellent and effective technic.

Some health educators believe it is an unwise policy to stress fear as a motivating force in health education, and point to the damage that may result in developing a widespread horror of cancer, syphilis, tuberculosis, heart disease, etc. They feel unwilling to stoop to the degrading tactics of the patent medicine advertiser and the quack. Others believe that one must use the tools at one's command, as skillfully and judiciously as possible, knowing full well that whenever extensive activity for the welfare of the community is undertaken, some individual injury is sure to occur. Of one fact there can be no question—namely, that fear of illness, pain, and premature death is one of the strongest motivating forces of mankind.

11. Health education is ineffective if the motivation it produces results in dissatisfaction and disappointment. If an individual follows health education advice and gains no benefit therefrom, he and the public as well will consider that the health department is wholly ineffective, and that none of its activities are worth considering. The annual health examination that once was so widely advocated was unsuccessful largely because intelligent men did not feel that the effort and expense that were involved were justified in the results obtained. The person who attends the tuberculosis clinic because of a good health education program, and who receives scant courtesy and little consideration of his personal problems, will not derive any satisfaction from his experience, and will react unfavorably to all subsequent advice from the health department.

## METHODS IN HEALTH EDUCATION

This text is not the appropriate place to present, in any detail, the methods that may be employed in health education. Health education technics are difficult to acquire and necessitate experience, long training, and good judgment. The reader who is interested in the special field of health education technology is referred to the literature that is gradually accumulating in this specialty of public health. He must be warned, however, to use great discrimination, for in the author's opinion much of the work that has been done in this field is unsound. It is based on faulty premises, and developed ineffectively by muddled amateurs.

A great variety of methods is used in transmitting health information. Probably the most effective methods are the day-to-day personal efforts of all the members of the health department, in giving individual health advice and aid.

Mass effort to build up informed public opinion requires the utilization of various mediums that reach large numbers of people. Hiscock has analyzed the more important technics and described their utility. He discusses the value of:

a. Community meetings
b. The newspaper
c. Pamphlets, special articles, and all types of printed matter
d. The radio
e. Exhibits
f. Motion pictures
g. Lectures

Each has its own place, and each reaches an audience that may not be informed in any other way.

Gebhard has emphasized the value of visual aids in health education, and the Cleveland Health Museum in Ohio contains a wealth of information in this particular field. This museum serves as a source of material and of inspiration to health departments throughout the nation.

Intensive drives in certain phases of health education may sometimes be undertaken, to meet emergencies or special needs. The great defect with this type of health education is that it puts undue emphasis on a limited field of work, to the detriment of a well balanced program. Unless the health campaign is timed accurately and used with great restraint, it will in the long run do more harm than good.

**Annual Reports.** The annual report is essentially an account of stewardship. It is most useful as a vehicle for public health education of a selected group. It affords an opportunity to compare the activities and achievements of the health department for the current year with those of previous years, and also to compare results with those of similar organizations elsewhere. The annual report should contain:

1. A description of the organization and functions of the various bureaus, giving the personnel of each division.

2. A summary of the activities of the health department during the year, bringing out the most interesting features of the work and using illustrative material in so far as possible.

3. Suggestions as to means for betterment of the work of the health department by changes in organization or development of new activities.

4. A brief tabular or graphic statistical record of the important vital statistics data for the year. These tables should be uniform from year to year.

5. A concise financial statement.

The annual report is sent to a selected group of influential citizens who are particularly interested in public health work.

**Weekly or Monthly Bulletin.** The weekly or monthly bulletin has more popular interest than the annual report, and is prepared for a larger and more diversified group than the annual report. Articles should be brief and of current interest. It should be illustrative. These bulletins were once a very popular means of transmitting public health information, but their value is questionable. The same audience can be reached by other and more effective means. Some state health departments now utilize the bulletin as a form of news letter to local health departments, thus keeping local health officials informed of current health problems and policies of the state department.

### Health Information through Newspapers

*Newspaper Articles.* News items in local papers are a very effective vehicle for distribution of health information. They should be interesting, brief, vivid, and accurate, and preferably of current importance. They should combine scientific accuracy and human interest. For example, let us imagine that a child in the community has been bitten by a dog. One brief paragraph in the local newspaper may include the following health information. The dog was not killed at once, but held under observation. He developed unmistakable signs of rabies within three days. The dog's head was sent to the State Health Department Laboratory. Diagnosis was made at once and the result reported by telegram. The child is receiving antirabic treatment. The dog may have bitten other children or other dogs, so that parents should be on the alert. A short paragraph giving the above information as a news item has much greater educational value than a long, dry treatise describing rabies and giving methods of prevention and treatment.

*Editorials* concerning public health affairs in the community have real value. They should not be written by the health officer, but by an experienced editorial writer. The health department may furnish the material and urge editorial consideration, but editorial writing is a special talent, which the average health officer does not possess.

*Health Sections or Health Columns.* Many of the larger newspapers publish a column of health information on the same page in each issue. Some of them are very good and have real public health educational value. Many are poor. A few are conducted in the form of a health forum by state or municipal health officers. They have a limited value.

*Special Articles.* Special newspaper articles concerning prevention of certain specific diseases may be written or sponsored by the health department. This type of article is most effective if it is presented when the particular disease is of current interest—especially if an epidemic of the disease is in progress. The reading public will take an active interest in methods of prevention and control of disease under such circumstances, and thus the health department may secure valuable and permanent implantation of public health principles in the consciousness of the community.

**U. S. Chamber of Commerce.** The United States Chamber of Commerce has a Health Advisory Council which is a great source of health education stimulus to local communities. The national organization is in constant communication with each local Chamber of Commerce. The local Chamber is made up of the leading business men of the community, who look to their national organization for leadership and inspiration. The local health officer can utilize this channel of health education most effectively.

**Public Health Pamphlets.** The public health pamphlet, if properly used, is of real educational value. Its subject must be specific and limited. Composition should be attractive and illustrative. Large type should be used, with short, graphic sentences and with no compound words. Distribution of the pamphlets should be very wide, in an attempt to reach and interest every householder. They must be scrutinized for scientific accuracy. Each pamphlet is more effective if distributed when the particular subject is exciting interest at the time. Some of the best examples of effective public health pamphlets have been published by the large life insurance companies and the national voluntary health associations.

**Public Health Exhibits.** Public health exhibits are used where large numbers of persons congregate, as, for example, at State and County Fairs. Their composition is almost exclusively *illustrative*. Colorful posters, interesting models, moving pictures and ingenious mechanical tricks may be employed. The subjects may deal with general public health education, more frequently with a specific subject. Some state health departments maintain portable exhibits that may be shown at various places in the state. One essential feature of the public health exhibit is that there should always be some person in constant attendance to explain the details of the exhibit, to answer questions, and distribute literature.

**Public Health Lectures.** Almost every health department maintains a lecture service. There is no better method of popularizing the work of the department. Lectures must be scientifically accurate, yet be presented in a popular manner and should be planned to suit the particular audience. The subject should be specific, and of current interest. Lantern slides may be used to great advantage. Motion pictures are frequently utilized. Many state health departments have assembled libraries of motion picture films on public health matters which are loaned to various lay organizations in the state. In many cases the motion picture film has supplanted the public health lecture. A good film, like the lecture, must have a specific subject, and be of current interest. Portable moving picture machines are frequently supplied, as well as the films.

**Radio Broadcasting.** The radio is being used more and more for the dissemination of health information. It touches a vast audience that is not reached in any other way. Many people receive a deeper impression from the spoken than from the written word and undoubtedly the method has great value, though it is difficult to estimate just how much real information is transmitted by this means. The technic of radio education is intricate and subtle. It appears so simple that public health educators have made no effort to master it. Experts inform us that public health broadcasts are the dullest and most ineffective of all radio programs. If this very valuable method of health education is to be utilized effectively, it must be placed in experienced hands and directed with finesse and skill. Otherwise "radio health talks" will bring discredit upon sincere and honest effort.

**Personal Letters.** One of the most effective methods of winning the approval of the people and of obtaining the desired results is the use of the personal letter. A series of nine splendid letters for expectant mothers has been compiled by the Federal Department of Maternal Welfare. These letters may be written and mailed to prospective mothers by the local health department at monthly intervals. They are appropriate and valuable. Some health officers use the device of the "birthday letter." The names are taken from the birth certificates. When the child reaches one year of age, the parents are congratulated by personal letter and advised to have the child immunized against smallpox and diphtheria. The variety of devices that may be used is limited only by the imagination of the health officer. The purpose is the same in each; namely, the establishment of the feeling that the health department is personally interested in each individual of the community and is anxious to be of every possible service to him.

## ORGANIZATION OF THE DIVISION OF HEALTH EDUCATION

The activities of a health department relating to health education should be under the close supervision of the health officer. In smaller organizations this work is handled directly by him. Some of the larger organizations have a special division of public health education with a trained director. All publicity material must go through the hands of the health officer for critical analysis.

As we have stated above, an important part of the health department publicity work is not only to inform the people concerning preventive medicine and community hygiene, but also to win public confidence in the health department and support for it by public officials and by the people at large. Proper publicity should not only point out the tangible effects and the advantages of public health work, but also develop the feeling that the health department, as organized and staffed, is thoroughly competent to give the community an adequate health service. This corresponds to the function of a public relations counsel in a business organization.

**The Health Educator.** The health educator is one of the most important members of the staff of the health department. This fact is so well brought out by Glenn Frank in his tribute to the health educator in "Salesmen of Knowledge" that this statement is worth presenting in its complete form:

"The future of America is in the hands of two men—the investigator and the interpreter. We shall never lack for the administrator, the third man needed to complete this trinity of social servants. And we have an ample supply of investigators, but there is a shortage of readable and responsible interpreters, men who can effectively play mediator between specialist and layman. The practical value of every social invention or material discovery depends upon its being adequately interpreted to the masses. Science owes its effective ministry as much to the interpretative mind as to the creative mind. The knowledge of mankind is advanced by the investigator, but the investigator is not always the best interpreter of his discoveries. Rarely, in fact, do the genius for exploration and the genius for exposition meet in the same mind. . . . The interpreter stands between the layman, whose knowledge of all things is indefinite, and the investigator whose knowledge of one thing is authoritative. The investigator advances knowledge. The interpreter advances progress. History affords abundant evidence that civilization has advanced in direct ratio to the efficiency with which the thought of the thinkers has been translated into the language of the workers. Democracy of politics depends upon democracy of thought. 'When the interval between intellectual classes and the practical classes is too great,' says Buckle, 'the former will possess no influence, the latter will reap no benefit.' A dozen fields of thought are today congested with knowledge that the physical and social sciences have unearthed, and the whole tone and temper of American life can be lifted by putting this knowledge into general circulation. But where are the interpreters with the training and the willingness to think their way through this knowledge and translate it into the language of the street? I raise the recruiting trumpet for the interpreters."

This type of interpretation of knowledge in regard to medical and sanitary sciences requires special qualifications and special training. This fact has been recognized by experienced health administrators, and an attempt has been made by the American Public Health Association to draw up suitable qualifications for health educators.[1] (See Appendix.)

The health educator must select the proper educational material that should be presented to each particular group in the community.

[1] *Educational Qualifications of Health Educators.* Committee on Professional Education of the American Public Health Association. Oct. 1943.

Each group should be approached in a different way. For example, a list of influential and responsible citizens should be selected. They are reached best by personal contact through the health officer or members of his staff. This selected group should have a thorough knowledge of the objectives, activities and achievements of the department. Sometimes this result can be accomplished best by a personal letter from the health officer from time to time.

**Health Advisory Committee.** A useful device is the advisory committee of the health department. The members are chosen by the health officer from business clubs, social organizations, church societies, women's clubs, etc. The committee has no official status. It meets at regular intervals to advise the health officer in relation to general policies, and serves as a very effective agency in interpreting the work of the department to the community. Similar results may be secured through addresses and informal talks by the health officer to men's luncheon clubs, women's clubs, professional associations, etc.

**Local Public Officials.** Local public officials are a special group which should be continuously informed of the activities of the health department. In the end, the local governing body will be responsible for the necessary official action which determines the budget of the department, and will pass on the effectiveness of the service and necessity for its continuance. The persons comprising this group, therefore, should be thoroughly familiar with the activities of the health department.

**Medical and Allied Groups.** The health officer should make it his special duty to keep the local medical, dental and allied professions informed as to the policies and program of the health department. These professions should be the most effective and important allies of the departmental program. The department's activities should have their official sponsorship. The medical and dental societies should be requested to select a *public health advisory committee*. The health officer should keep in close contact with this committee, and it, in turn, will interpret the activities of the health department to the general profession. The health department may build up goodwill by rendering actual service to physicians and allied groups through consultations in communicable disease control, diagnostic laboratory service, through arrangements for postgraduate teaching in prenatal work, in diagnosis of tuberculosis, diagnosis and treatment of venereal disease, or other clinical aspects of disease that relate to preventive medicine, and by other means.

The educational authorities in the community, such as the school committee, the school principals and also the teachers, should be thoroughly familiar with the work of the health department, and be in sympathy with its purposes. This is best accomplished through personal contacts on the part of the various members of the health department staff with the educational department.

All members of the staff should use every available opportunity in their contacts with the public to build up goodwill for the department through actual services, cheerfully and courteously rendered. Not only the thing accomplished, but the manner of the doing, determines the effectiveness of public health work. Well conceived organization, well trained personnel, and efficient service are not enough. The health officer must realize that, under our social system, results are often obtained, programs approved, and budgets passed on a personal basis. He must not only do good work for the community, but also win its sincere confidence and good will. The health officer should train his personnel to understand that educational work is of major importance in every contact with the people.

**Budget.** The budgetary allotment for health education activities, as well as the personnel required in different types of health organization, have been discussed in the appropriate place and need not be repeated here. The actual direct costs of the health education work are small. Three to five per cent of the total budget is usually allotted to this activity. These funds are expended for educational materials, printing and publishing, postage, etc., and for salary of personnel.

## REFERENCES

1. *Principles and Practice in Health Education.* Report of Health Education Conference at Sayville. 1930. American Child Health Association, 450 Seventh Avenue, New York City. 1931.
2. Turner, C. E. *Principles of Health Education.* D. C. Heath and Company, Boston. 1939. (Second edition.)
3. Rose, Mary S. *Teaching Nutrition to Boys and Girls.* The Macmillan Company. 1932.
4. Pfaffman, Mary, and Stern, Frances. *Food and Your Body: Talks with Children.* M. Barrows Co., Boston. 1932.
5. *Parent Education.* A publication of The White House Conference. The Century Company, New York. 1931.
6. Hiscock, I. V. *Ways to Community Health Education.* The Commonwealth Fund, New York. 1939.
7. Tolleris, B. K. *Annual Reports: How to Plan and Write Them.* National Publicity Council, New York. 1946.
8. Lamkin, N. B. *Health Education in Rural Schools and Communities.* A. S. Barnes and Co., New York. 1946.
9. Gillett, L. H. *Nutrition in Public Health.* W. B. Saunders Co., Philadelphia. 1946.
10. Strain, F. B. *Teen Days: A Book for Boys and Girls.* D. Appleton-Century Co., New York. 1947.
11. Diehl, H. S. *Textbook of Healthful Living.* McGraw-Hill Book Company, New York. 1945. (Third edition.)
12. Bauer, W. W. and Hull, T. G. *Health Education of the Public.* W. B. Saunders Company. Philadelphia. 1942.

13. Nyswander, D. B. *Solving School Health Problems.* Commonwealth Fund, New York. 1942.
  Of special value are the publications of:
  The United States Public Health Service.
  The Children's Bureau.
  The United States Department of Agriculture: charts, motion pictures, and bulletins in nutrition, dairy sanitation, food sanitation, and the like.
  The National Tuberculosis Association, 50 West 50th Street, New York City.
  The American Social Hygiene Association, 50 West 50th Street, New York City.
  Metropolitan Insurance Company of New York.
  John Hancock Life Insurance Company of Boston.
  American Medical Association: pamphlets, charts, posters, and "Hygeia," a magazine devoted to popular health education, 535 North Dearborn Street, Chicago, Illinois.

# CHAPTER XXV

## MENTAL HYGIENE

THERE is no more difficult subject for the health officer to face than that of mental hygiene. He is urged to consider ways and means whereby the technics of mental hygiene can be so systematized that they can be interrelated with other official public health activities. He realizes that the results of any activities that he may initiate along these lines will probably not be concrete or measurable. Most health departments are loath to experiment with new and untried administrative methods, since each new effort cuts into the budget and may thus curtail other activities of proved effectiveness.

Thus, the more conservative health officer is deterred by the very magnitude and complexity of the task and prefers to await future developments and better methodology, rather than run the risk of expending time and effort in fruitless endeavor. He realizes that the knowledge of effective preventive measures in the field of mental hygiene is extremely limited and the tools with which one has to work are, as yet, highly inadequate.

The very term "mental hygiene" is perhaps an unfortunate and confusing one. The scope of interest that is usually included in any discussion of the field of mental hygiene comprises two fairly distinct and somewhat unrelated elements. Mental hygiene is frequently defined as the subject which is concerned with the *prevention of mental disease* and the *promotion of mental health.*

The promotion of mental health represents, in great part, those efforts that are made to adjust the individual to his environment and to prevent failures of adaptation to community life. Measures are taken to aid individuals in correcting or ameliorating mental maladjustments which distort life, impair happiness and efficiency, and which sometimes may even develop into tragic situations. However, the mental hygienist, in his efforts to correct these difficulties, must not delude himself into thinking that the measures that may be taken toward promotion of mental health will result in the prevention of mental disease or defectiveness. Most authorities agree that we have no concrete evidence that any efforts or methods that have been developed to promote mental health have kept a single person out of a hospital for the insane. These efforts have been highly productive in promotion of happiness and contentment and, in many instances, have had a direct effect in improvement of physical health, but reliable evidence is lacking that they have lessened significantly the incidence of the major psychoses.

For the most part, we must confess that we do not know either the direct or indirect causes of mental disorder or defectiveness. As is the case in cancer, we must await further accretion of knowledge of vital processes before we can hope to understand the primary causes of a great proportion of the cases of major psychoses that develop in a community. Possibly this knowledge will come from the field of fundamental physiology or perhaps—more basic and elementary still—from the fields of physics or chemistry.

It is a truism of public health practice that preventive measures can be applied best where primary causal relations are best understood. When basic causal factors are not well understood, any measures that may be taken represent, for the most part, efforts toward amelioration of the ill effects produced by the condition, rather than actual prevention.

Thus, in discussing mental hygiene we are, in reality, discussing two separate aspects of the subject:

a. Measures which relate to the preventable causes or amelioration of the results of mental disorder or mental deficiency.

b. Measures which relate to promotion of mental health of those in the community who have difficulty in adjusting themselves to their environment.

These two different aspects of mental hygiene are related to some degree. Both are community responsibilities, which are allied from the administrative point of view, since the official activities in both fields will become, in some part at least, the responsibility of a single governmental department.

## PREVENTION OF MENTAL DISEASE

Under this title we shall discuss those measures which relate to the preventable causes or the amelioration of the results of mental disorder or mental deficiency.

In any discussion of this subject it is important to emphasize the fact that *insanity* is essentially not a medical, but a legal term. Insanity refers to persons who have mental disease of such a degree that they require legal commitment to an institution, or are legally incapacitated from carrying on their affairs.

**Prevalence of Mental Disease and Mental Deficiency.** At any given time there are about five persons per thousand of population in any community who have mental disorder of such degree as to make hospital commitment an advantageous procedure.

The prevalence of mental disorder in the community is probably much greater than this figure would indicate. Freeman and his associates [1] have made an epidemiological study of mental disease in a section of Baltimore. They found eight persons per 1,000 of the population over 15 years of age to have a definite psychosis. From 2 per cent to 3 per cent of the people of the area had a definite personality disorder. This incidence was lower in Negroes than in whites. Contrary to general opinion, the rate of mental disorder was much higher (six times) in homes of lowest economic status than in homes of the better classes.

There is little or no evidence that insanity is increasing. General paresis and other forms of cerebral syphilis have declined rapidly, due to earlier recognition and better therapy of syphilis. Because of our aging population, cerebral arteriosclerosis is on the increase. The apparent increase in insanity in some parts of the nation is due to better recognition of the various abnormal mental conditions. More adequate hospitalization facilities may also have influenced the apparent increase of mental disease.

The term "mental defective" is a matter of definition. It has been estimated that approximately three persons per thousand in an average community are mentally defective, but many of these persons are quite capable, under suitable supervision, of maintaining a productive and happy existence. Approximately one mental defective per thousand population in the United States requires some form of institutional care.

It is frequently stated that mental defectiveness produces more degeneracy, pauperism and crime than any other single condition. This is probably an over-statement, but certainly the cost to society of mental deficiency is tremendous. Some authorities believe that mental defectiveness is increasing more rapidly than the increase in our population. Others believe that the apparent increase is due to a better understanding and more frequent recognition of the condition. The major menace to the community occurs not from imbeciles, but from the higher grades of mentally defective women and girls of childbearing age. Due to their lack of restraint, they frequently act as a source of distribution of venereal disease. Not infrequently these women have children who are mentally defective also, so that the chain goes on unbroken.

**Hospitalization for Mental Disease.** It is frequently stated that one person out of every 22 in the population will be institutionalized at one time or another during his life, because of mental illness. More than 50 per cent of all hospital beds in the nation are assigned for care of mental disease. The Bureau of the Census estimated [2] that at the end of 1943 there were 574,735 patients in mental hospitals in the United States. The turnover is larger than one realizes, for there were 268,958 admis-

[1] Freeman, A. W. and Cohen, B. M.: "Preliminary Observations on the Epidemiology of Mental Disease." *Am. J. of Pub. Health.* 1939, 29:633.
[2] Bureau of the Census, U. S. Dept. of Commerce: *Patients in Mental Institutions, 1943.* Government Printing Office, Washington, D. C. 1946.

sions and 267,237 discharges during the year; 19.2% of these patients were discharged as dead. Seventy-three per cent—196,893—were first admissions.

The commonest diagnoses for admission to state hospitals for the permanent care of psychiatric patients were:

1. Dementia praecox ............................... 22.3%
2. Cerebral arteriosclerosis .......................... 12.7%
3. Manic-depressive psychoses ........................ 11.1%
4. Senile psychoses ................................. 9.8%
5. General pareses ................................. 6.2%
6. Alcoholism ...................................... 4.7%

The number of patients with mental disease, in hospitals, varies greatly in different states: from 2 per thousand population in some states to 5 per thousand in Massachusetts and New York.

The actual number of patients in mental hospitals is, of course, no real index as to the prevalence of mental disease. This is a social and economic matter. Increase in hospitalization occurs when beds become available. As our population ages, there will be a greater demand for beds for senile dementia, and as the nation becomes urbanized, the opportunities for care of patients with mental disease in the home become limited. Thus we can anticipate an increased demand for hospitalization of mental patients in the future. The decline in hospitalization in New York State has been brought about by the release of patients to their homes under a parole system, with provision for supervision of these patients by social workers and other hospital personnel.

But increase or decrease of hospitalization does not necessarily mean an increase or decrease in disease prevalence.

**Preventive Measures.** Those in charge of state budgets insist that the prevention of mental disease be promoted actively, because of the great cost to the state for custodial care of these people. We have no available means that offer any promise of success in this field.

Reduction in hospitalization of mental disease for many years to come must be on a basis of improved social and administrative procedures in caring for these persons, rather than in actual prevention of illness.

It is difficult to institute measures for prevention of mental disease and mental deficiency unless one can give proper weight to the various causes of these conditions. Due to limitation of our present knowledge, this is impossible. A few of the causes are clear-cut and, to some degree, preventable; others are not.

*Hereditary Influences.* We have too little information to state categorically that heredity plays a definite role as a causative factor in mental disease. A person undoubtedly inherits his general psychological make-up from his ancestors, just as he inherits their physical characteristics; and, to some degree, therefore, psychopathic tendencies may be said to be transmitted from parent to child.

Munro,[3] in a study of consanguinity and mental disorder, found a definite and specific familial incidence of mental disease. This incidence decreases in an orderly way with decreasing degree of relationship to the patient. Abnormalities of personality, hypochondriasis, chronic alcoholism, paranoid and eccentric traits are particularly common in families of schizophrenics, where the parents are consanguineous. He suggests that the patient's brothers and sisters carry the recessive genetic factor. He also believes that there is some evidence that incomplete dominant factors determine manic-depressive psychosis. Certain types of mental deficiency undoubtedly are unit characteristics which may be transmitted from parent to offspring as a recessive character, following the laws of Mendel. This is particularly true of the higher grades of mental deficiency. Heredity usually plays no part in the etiology of the lower grades of mental defectiveness. This condition is often due to prenatal or birth injury, or other similar cause.

Many authorities are of the firm opinion that the progeny of the higher grades of mental defectives are almost sure to become a burden on society, and that the state obviously must take the necessary steps to prevent procreation by this group of individuals. This has been accomplished to some degree by segregation, or by sterilization. Legal restriction preventing marriage of the insane, mental defectives and epileptics has been of some value in preventing procreation, but, on the whole, has been unsuccessful.

Sterilization has been the subject of an enormous amount of discussion. The moralist questions the right of the state over the individual in such fundamental matters. Whatever the theory may be, practical expediency would seem to demand that mentally defective people shall not be permitted to have children. Sterilization is a simple, safe and sure method of bringing about this result with very little inconvenience to the individual. The procedure might readily be subjected to abuse and must be safeguarded by administrative machinery which protects the right of the individual while it promotes the interest of the state. Various administrative devices have been formulated to this end in a considerable number of states. The commonest method vests the final decision in regard to advisability of sterilization of an individual upon a board of experts appointed by the governor and selected for their knowledge of sociology and the principles of public welfare. Often the state health officer is a member of this board. Sterilization is being utilized more and more by the various states, particularly for those mental defectives who show criminal tendencies.

Sterilization or segregation of mental defectives as a means of eventual reduction of the proportionate numbers of these persons in society is based on the hypothesis that the condition is, in a major portion of cases, a recessive, inherited characteristic. The hypothesis itself is question-

[3] Munro, T. A.: "Consanguinity and Mental Disorder." *Jour. Mental Sc.* 84:708, 1938.

able; but even if it is correct, the statisticians tell us that if society were able to prevent all known mental defectives from having progeny by whatever means, it would be necessary to carry out these procedures through a great many generations before an appreciable result could be secured. If the methods used were completely effective, perhaps the year 2500 would begin to show a definite result from the continuous sterilization program.

*Specific Disease.* There are many specific diseases in which the infective agent has a special predilection for the brain as part of the pathological process of the disease. Mental disease may result from these specific infections or pathological conditions. Syphilis is the most outstanding example of such a condition. Included in this general category are pellagra and other types of hypo-vitaminoses, typhoid fever, malaria, erysipelas, encephalitis, septicemia, cerebrospinal meningitis, and particularly fetal injury due to virus infections of the mother during pregnancy. Prevention of these types of mental disease is centered in prevention of the initial condition. The most concrete results in prevention of any type of mental disease have been achieved through prevention of syphilis, or more productive still, through adequate treatment of early syphilis.

*Head Injury.* Head injury is a factor in causation of mental disease and particularly mental deficiency. Injury of the baby at birth is not an uncommon direct cause of low-grade defectiveness. Preventive measures obviously should be directed at better prenatal care and better obstetrical practice.

*Morphinism, Alcoholism, etc.* Morphinism or other drug addiction, together with alcoholism, are causal factors which are responsible for the commitment of a certain proportion of individuals with mental disorder to a state institution. Measures that have been adopted by the government to prevent mental disease due to these specific poisons have not been highly effective. Many authorities believe that drug or alcoholic addiction is itself a symptom of a personality disorder, rather than a primary cause of the psychosis.

*Industrial Intoxications.* Absorption of certain poisons by inhalation or otherwise that may occur in association with some of the newer industrial processes has resulted, in certain instances, in mental disease. The serious situation produced by the absorption of tetraethyl lead is a striking illustration of this danger. Preventive measures are obviously dependent upon better knowledge of the toxicology of industrial processes and introduction of proper safeguards to prevent a repetition of this type of accident.

In the small number of instances that we have mentioned above, there exist opportunities for actual prevention of mental disease and deficiency. Further than this we cannot go at present. We must await more knowledge as to causal factors before we can undertake measures which may be aimed toward prevention of mental disorder, but which may shoot wide of the mark.

**Readjustment of the Convalescent from Mental Disorder to Home Conditions.** Formerly, a person who was once committed to a hospital for the insane was always regarded by the society to which he might return as an insane person. A great advance has been made in this respect in recent years. The public has been educated to realize that mental disease is often curable and the patient may return to a useful place in the community.

In ten years' time, out of each 100 persons who have been discharged from the New York State mental hospitals, 55 will be living in the community, 23 will have died, and 22 will again be residents of a mental hospital. Forty-two of the fifty-five will have lived continuously in the community during the ten-year period without serious recurrence of mental illness. The readjustment of the convalescent from sheltered hospital conditions to the home situation, and the gradual resumption by him of the burden of life requires skillful guidance. The mental hospitals have adopted a technic which is quite similar to the plan followed by tuberculosis sanatoria. The psychiatric social worker is utilized to visit convalescents in their homes at regular intervals in order to assist them in their readjustment to home conditions. These convalescent patients also return to an outpatient consultation clinic of the hospital from time to time for advice and aid.

## PROMOTION OF MENTAL HEALTH

The second portion of the mental hygiene program deals with the promotion of the mental health of the community. This result is secured in a positive way through promotion of facilities for healthful recreation and enjoyment of life. Any and all factors that tend to lessen the burden of mental worry and strain, and that make life more fruitful and agreeable, aid in the promotion of the general level of mental health. In addition, certain definite steps may be taken in order that we may recognize, and often prevent, mental maladjustment of the individual. In certain instances where maladjustment has actually occurred, suitable corrective measures may be instituted successfully.

Cobb [4] has pointed out, in a very interesting little book, *Borderlines of Psychiatry,* that there are six or more million persons who are partially incapacitated because of psychoneurosis. Furthermore, he emphasizes that every person is subject to emotional disorders at some time during life, just as everyone is susceptible to communicable disease. Every man, and particularly the group that have difficulty in interpersonal relationships, is helped through a community-wide plan for mental hygiene.

[4] Cobb, Stanley: *Borderlines of Psychiatry.* Cambridge, Mass., Harvard University Press. 1943.

The methods that are adopted depend for their success upon an understanding of the real causes of maladjustment.

We are accustomed to think of mental maladjustment in terms of the complex, difficult case that requires long continued psychiatric analysis and supervision by a competent psychiatrist. But there are many minor problems in mental hygiene that are intimately connected with the whole problem of living, and which are not solely the province of the psychiatrist. They can be handled best by the informed person who has first-hand knowledge of the intimate life of the people concerned and who has their respect and confidence. Thus, aid in adjustment of human behavior need not be confined to a limited group of specialists. The simple general principles of mental hygiene should be part of the fund of human knowledge, practiced by everyone who has to deal with people. The key persons in the community who will have most influence, and will also have most opportunity to aid individuals with mental maladjustment, are the physicians in private practice and the public health nurses. There are a few simple principles which must be remembered:

1. Individuals in need of assistance in making difficult adjustments rarely understand the situation or know how to take proper steps without the help of those possessing some psychiatric knowledge.

2. The causes of most maladjustments arise in the early years of childhood. Best results are obtained if the condition is recognized in early childhood and corrected at that time. Thus, a consulting child psychiatrist who can train the public health nurses to recognize and handle mental maladjustment when and where they find it, is an invaluable aid in any health service.

3. The first step in aiding an individual is to determine his inherent capacity to make an adjustment to his own environment.

4. Having done this, one must then aid the individual to find the level at which he can live most successfully. When this has been done, certain logical steps follow, namely:

   a. Cultivate a frank emotional attitude.
   b. Teach the person to deal with actualities so that he does not evade difficulties or transform them into false situations.
   c. Aid the individual in the cultivation of an objective view of life.
   d. Attempt to distribute his interests through a wide and varied range of activities.

It is clear that all these various steps may be taken by a public health nurse or social worker who has had proper training in mental hygiene, who knows and understands the individual and the family, and who can help them solve their particular situation. Most important of all is the understanding of the family physician.

The physician who has had a good training in psychiatry will apply this knowledge in everyday practice. A program which incorporates the principles of mental hygiene as an integral part of medical care is of tremendous help to patients.

## FUNCTIONS OF GOVERNMENT IN A MENTAL HYGIENE PROGRAM

**State Functions.** The major burden of the cost of mental disease falls on the state. Practically every state in the Union has now assumed the function of the medical care and hospitalization of the mentally diseased and incompetent. At the present time the great proportion of persons with actual mental disease are under treatment in public institutions, or are under parole or observation by these institutions. From an administrative point of view these state mental hospitals and schools are the logical places from which any and all official preventive measures should originate. One hardly need state that any program of this type will not be successful unless these institutions are adequately staffed by well qualified psychiatrists.

Some state hospitals for the insane are still the haven of the medically incompetent, but the improvement in this situation has been marked in recent years.

**Mental Hygiene Clinics.** The essential feature of the preventive program is the mental hygiene clinic, which may be staffed by physicians from the mental hospital, with a suitable corps of psychiatric social workers. The clinics may be held at the hospital itself, or may be extended to strategic points of the area which the hospital serves. The psychiatric social workers see new patients in the clinic and follow the discharged patients from the hospital to their homes in order to aid them in their readjustment to community life.

**Education.** Another function of the state program is the education of the public in relation to mental disease; its causes, methods of prevention and cure. In some areas this part of the program has been carried out very successfully in recent years and has resulted in a completely changed attitude on the part of the general public toward mental disease. One of the most important phases of the educational program is the training of medical students, interns and physicians in the recognition, differential diagnosis, treatment and prevention of mental disease.

**Federal Governmental Functions.** The functions of the Federal Government in the mental hygiene field are largely consultative and investigative. The United States Public Health Service has a special division of mental hygiene. Its officers advise the various states in relation to their mental hygiene programs. In addition, the division has studies under way in relation to methodology and procedure.

This division also has direct charge of two federal hospitals for drug addicts, a large hospital for the insane from the merchant marine, and, as an accessory duty, the division has charge of the medical care of federal prisoners.

**Local Governmental Functions in Relation to Promotion of Mental Health.** *Department of Public Education.* Special classes for mentally retarded children are gradually increasing in popularity and effectiveness in public school systems. In addition, authorities believe that school systems should maintain proper facilities for the study of children that are experiencing special difficulties, in order that proper readjustment can be made. The results have been so encouraging that this phase of the work should receive an increasing amount of attention.

Educators recommend that every university should possess a department of mental hygiene as part of the student health service. The work should be under the charge of a well trained psychiatrist, who should be available at all times for consultation with university students who are suffering from maladjustment.

*Voluntary Associations.* The unofficial mental hygiene association has a definite and valuable part to play in the community mental hygiene program. Its chief functions are:

1. To make studies as to the cause and methods of prevention of mental disorder. The society may aid in the determination of actual prevalence of the disease in the state or local community.

2. To stimulate interest on the part of the government, the medical profession, and the public at large in the proper care of the mentally diseased and defective.

3. To carry out a program of popular education concerning suitable methods that may be utilized for the promotion of mental health.

4. To serve as a clearing house of information concerning the most effective administrative methods in the care of and prevention of mental disease and deficiency and in the promotion of mental health.


## THE HEALTH DEPARTMENT AND THE MENTAL HYGIENE PROGRAM

The mental hospital of the state should serve as a nucleus for the whole state program in mental hygiene. In almost all the states the function of hospitalization of the insane and the mentally defective has been assigned to a separate department of mental disease. In some states this department is given a more comprehensive and suitable name, the Department of Mental Hygiene.

**The Local Health Departments.** The major portion of work in promotion of mental health in the local health department is a function of the Division of Child Hygiene and of the public health nurse. To perform her work properly, every public health nurse should have special training in the fundamental principles of mental hygiene. This training enables her to incorporate mental hygiene as an integral part of public health nursing. It trains the nurse also to recognize mental hygiene problems in the individual or family when they arise. She will recognize mental deficiency and major psychoses, will understand and have sympathy for minor mental problems, and will know when to utilize the services of a specialist or a mental hygiene clinic. This training also will enable the public health nurse to realize her own limitations. Detailed case work in mental hygiene by the public health nurse is impossible. She should not attempt to handle the major psychoses and psychoneuroses, the difficult behavior problems of childhood, alcoholism or drug addiction, or such conditions as insomnia, emotional outbursts of adults, etc., without the aid of a psychiatrist.

The nurse must understand how to deal with apprehension, worry, undue fear, or over-solicitude. She should not simply write in her record "unco-operative," but should find out why the patient acts as he does, and what she can do about it. Temper tantrums, food fads, nail biting, thumb sucking, and a score of other minor difficulties of childhood often can and should be handled adequately by the understanding public health nurse. In a word, the public health nurse should be trained to understand people, as well as disease, and to deal with the common mental hygiene problems as part of her daily activities in her contacts with the community.

In those cities that have well developed welfare and public health departments, there sometimes occurs confusion as to whether mental hygiene is a function of the public health nurse or the social worker. Both will be called upon to meet adjustments of personality difficulties and habit training. At times, overlapping of activities of the social worker and the nurse will occur. Job finding, actual relief, or long time adjustment of the psychoneurotic or chronically maladjusted child, which usually involves complete change of environment—all these are the function of the social worker. The care of the more serious maladjustments requiring long time observation or a continuous plan of rehabilitation involving economic and social readjustment is also the function of the social worker, and does not fall within the province of the public health nurse. In general, the nurse should limit her activities to:

1. Recognition of mental hygiene problems when they arise.

2. Handling of simple short-time problems when they occur, especially among children, and particularly those problems which are associated with the general problems of physical hygiene. She should be familiar with the use of psychiatric technic in her approach to problems of physical illness, and should utilize her knowledge to spread sound mental hygiene information in the same manner as she inculcates knowledge in regard to other matters pertaining to personal hygiene.

Many health departments have employed a child psychiatrist to aid in the solution of mental hygiene problems that are encountered in the well child conferences and in the nurse's field work. The child psychiatrist will be most effective if he serves as a consultant, taking up the various cases as they arise with the well baby clinic physicians and the public health nurses. He will hold group discussions with the public health personnel and show them how these individual problems of mental maladjustment may be solved.

**The Health Officer.** The health officer who is alive to the needs of his community will find that the whole broad field of mental hygiene touches and, in fact, invades his more specific activities and functions at every point. He may not have the direct responsibility for the development of the mental hygiene program, but he should be familiar with the differential diagnosis, and the methods of care of mental disease and deficiency. Many phases of his general program will have a direct effect in the prevention of mental disease, as, for example, adequate venereal disease clinic service. He should also be familiar with the principles and the methods of promotion of mental health, and should aid his staff of public health nurses in dealing with and in solving the special mental hygiene problems that arise in connection with their everyday work.

## ORGANIZATION OF A MENTAL HYGIENE SERVICE

**The State.** The most satisfactory arrangement is the allocation of all state functions in relation to mental hygiene, including hospitalization, to a state "Department of Mental Hygiene." The major activity of this division and the great proportion of the budget will be concerned with the hospitalization of mental disease and deficiency.

The National Committee for Mental Hygiene has estimated [5] that the following facilities are required for an adequate community mental hygiene program in the United States:

| | |
|---|---|
| Mental hospitals | 1 bed per 150 population |
| Institutions for mental defectives | 1 bed per 1,000 population |
| Community mental hygiene clinics | 1 psychiatrist per 100,000 population |
| School psychiatrists | 1 psychiatrist per 40,000 school children |
| Hospital ex-patients, and the mentally retarded in the community | 1 psychiatrist per 150,000 population |
| Counselling for control of crime and delinquency | 1 psychiatrist per 250,000 population |

The state hospitals are not merely treatment centers, but are the basis of the whole mental hygiene program.

This state department will organize *mental hygiene clinic service,* using each mental hospital and training school as a center. These clinics may be held at the hospital itself or may be distributed in various strategic centers in the areas served by the state hospital. They are staffed by experts from state hospitals. Attached to the mental hygiene clinic service are the psychiatric social workers. The clinic has the responsibility for

[5] Interstate and Foreign Commerce Committee, U. S. House of Representatives. Hearing on H. R. 2550. 1945.

the follow-up of persons who are paroled from the institution. Experience indicates that there should be approximately four visits a year to the clinic by each person on parole. The psychiatric social worker will make an average of three home visits per annum to each person on parole. The list of paroled persons will number from 5 to 10 per cent of the total number in the institutions.

Since a large proportion of the mentally defective persons in the state will not be institutionalized, the state department of mental hygiene should maintain as complete a registration as possible of all mental defectives within the state.

*The psychopathic hospital* is an important and integral part of the state hospitalization program. The psychopathic hospital deals with the acute, early, usually curable forms of mental disturbances. Usually its patients are not subjected to legal commitment, though they are sometimes committed for a short period. Stay in the psychopathic hospital is limited—usually for a two weeks' period—for the purpose of observation and diagnosis. The patient is then legally committed to a mental disease hospital, if necessary.

**Local Organization.** *Psychiatric Service. Public Schools.* In addition to special classes for mentally retarded children, a modern public educational system includes a psychiatric service to deal with behavior problems and maladjustments among the children of the public schools. This program is developed by the department of education, with the advice of the state department of mental hygiene.

*Psychiatric Service. Juvenile Courts.* Those responsible for the establishment of juvenile courts in various parts of the United States have developed the far-sighted policy of psychiatric service for youthful offenders. Those persons who have been most interested in this type of work feel that the results have at least been informative and of some utility. The plan is still in its infancy, but is certain to be more and more effective as new information is obtained and better methods are developed.

*Psychiatric Service. Adult Criminal Courts.* In a few instances, psychiatric service has been developed for selected persons passing through the criminal courts. The method offers promise of increasing usefulness as knowledge grows in relation to this most complex and difficult subject.

*Preschool and Child Guidance Clinics.* In a few cities, preschool and child guidance clinics have been established, usually under the sponsorship of unofficial agencies. These clinics deal with problems of conduct and personality. The work is very time-consuming and expensive. Full study and treatment of a case may require weeks and months.

The essential point that must be stressed in development of all the various local psychiatric services is that each and all of them should be an integral part of the whole state program of mental hygiene. The state department of mental hygiene should be fully cognizant of all proposed local developments, whether under official or voluntary agencies. Local bodies of any sort, whether they be the juvenile court, educational de-partment or voluntary association, should seek freely the advice and counsel of the state department and should develop their own local pro-gram—not as a separate entity, but as an integral part of the whole plan.

*The Health Department.* Under present conditions and with our pres-ent knowledge, local health departments—municipal or county—should not organize a separate division of mental hygiene. As has been stated above, the chief mental hygiene activities of the local health department centers in the Division of Child Hygiene. The foundation for success of this program rests in the selection of a child psychiatrist to aid the nurses in handling this very difficult group of children. The mental hy-gienist will do no case work himself, except as a special demonstration, but through consultations and group conferences, he gives continuous training to the public health nursing staff in relation to the mental hy-giene problems in the field. Small health departments with a few nurses may not be able to obtain the services of a child psychiatrist. The state health department through its advisory public health nursing service may fulfill this function of training and advising local public health nurses in mental hygiene technic.

*Health Centers.* A few municipalities have been so fortunate as to develop Health Centers. The conception of the Health Center requires that all the health and welfare work for the district will radiate from the unit. The voluntary as well as the official agencies should be in touch with the Health Center, if not actually housed there, and thus the Health Center serves as a clearing house of information as well as a center of clinic activities.

The Health Center should serve as a clearing house for the mental hygiene problems of the district, as well as the distributing point of the mental hygiene educational program. The development of a *Habit Clinic,* conducted in connection with the other child hygiene clinics, would serve a useful purpose. Such a clinic would have a dual value, in that it would serve to re-educate the maladjusted children of the district, and also would be most useful to teach and demonstrate methods of promo-tion of mental health to the public health nurses and other field work-ers of health and welfare that are connected with the unit.

## REFERENCES

1. Bassett, Clara. *Mental Hygiene in the Community.* The Macmillan Com-pany, New York. 1934.
2. Thom, Douglas A. *Normal Youth and Its Every Day Problems.* D. Appleton and Co., New York. 1932.
3. Berry, P. J. and Gordon, R. G. *The Mental Defective: A Problem in Social Inefficiency.* McGraw-Hill Book Co., New York. 1931.
4. Brown, S. *Training of the High Grade Mental Defective for Community Life.* Mental Hygiene. 1932, Vol. 16, p. 440.

5. Symonds, P. M. *Mental Hygiene of the School Child*. The Macmillan Company, New York. 1934.

6. Gesell, A. *The Guidance of Mental Growth in Infant and Child*. The Macmillan Company, New York. 1930.

7. *Mental Hygiene*. Quarterly Journal. Nat. Com. for Ment. Hyg. New York.

8. Cobb, Stanley. *Borderlines of Psychiatry*. Harvard University Press, Cambridge, Mass. 1943.

9. Fry, C. C. *Mental Health in College*. Commonwealth Fund, New York City. 1942.

10. Crutcher, Hester. *Foster Home Care for Mental Patients*. Commonwealth Fund, New York City. 1944.

11. Lennox, William G. *Science and Seizures: New Light on Epilepsy and Migraine*. Harper and Brothers, New York. 1941.

The special pamphlets, brochures and other publications of the National Committee for Mental Hygiene, New York City, are particularly valuable and authoritative.

# CHAPTER XXVI

## INDUSTRIAL HYGIENE

In previous chapters we have discussed the administrative measures relating to general sanitation, hygiene, and prevention of illness which pertain to the whole population. Special groups of the population have been given special consideration; for example, school children, infants and pregnant mothers. The most important group of the population, from the economic point of view at least, is the wage earner. Over one fourth of the whole population spends over one fourth of its time at work. More than 20 million people in the United States are employed in manufacturing, mechanical, or mining industries. The workers are subjected to special hazards during this work period. For example, silica dust is such an integral part of industry that over 500,000 workers are exposed to it in the course of their daily duties. Iron and steel workers have a much higher fatality rate from pneumonia than any other similar age group in the nation. Thus the health of the wage earner is worthy of special consideration. All necessary measures for the protection of life and the promotion of health of the individual at work may be considered as the special field of industrial hygiene. It must be remembered that efforts toward the promotion of the health of the worker must have a profound effect upon the health and welfare of the whole community. Only a few years ago, industrial illness and accident were the major causes of loss of time from work. Unnecessary industrial hazards, and carelessness on the part of the workmen, caused untold loss of life, permanent disability, and family misery and poverty.

Industrial hygiene has become a very broad and important field and an obvious function of government. Public health officials have not given the subject the consideration that it deserves.

The reasons for the delay in the development of industrial hygiene as part of the public health program in the United States are fairly clear. Only very recently have we become an industrial nation. Agricultural pursuits predominate in many of the states at the present time, and in these states industrial hygiene is not, as yet, a factor of great importance. We have been and are still a heterogeneous population that has grown rapidly. Each person has been interested in his own welfare, and has felt little responsibility for his fellows or his community. It has been a policy of each man for himself.

It must be confessed that health officials, with very few exceptions, did not take the lead in the development of industrial hygiene. The impetus has come in great part from the workers themselves, and, to a lesser degree, from industry.

As industry has developed, State Bureaus of Labor and Industry have been formed. They have interested themselves in the welfare of the workers, and have naturally included health protection in their activities. To some degree, industry itself has voluntarily assumed responsibility for the protection of life, prevention of illness, and promotion of hygiene of its own employees.

The great diversity in the degree of development of industrial hygiene in different parts of the country is due to the fact that we are not a national entity, but a federation of different states. Each state is autonomous and sovereign within its own borders. The Federal Government has limited powers and functions. Thus, adjoining states may have entirely different regulations and different organization in dealing with the whole field of industrial hygiene.

Industrial development in the United States began with the introduction of the textile industry in the early years of the last century. It resulted in the exploitation of child labor. Initiation of industrial hygiene measures may be said to have begun with the first child labor laws of Pennsylvania in 1848. Massachusetts adopted laws in 1877 concerning fire protection in factories, and safeguards for industrial machinery. These laws also instituted certain requirements for removal of dust, and for proper lighting, heating and ventilation of factories. New York passed its first laws to regulate employment of women and children in manufacturing establishments in 1886.

At the end of the century industrial hygiene was making progress. Nearly half the states had regulations for prevention of accidents in mines. Most of the states had passed some legislation relating to female and child labor. Legislation concerning sanitation of working conditions, including proper ventilation and illumination of factories and work shops, had been passed in more than one half of the states. Regulations concerning factory inspection had been adopted in fourteen states.

Federal legislation moved more rapidly than that of most of the states. By 1890 there were numerous provisions for the advancement of hygienic working conditions of federal employees, as well as regulations concerning safety appliances on interstate railroads. By 1910 laws were in force also concerning prevention of hazards and providing for inspection of coal mines, and prohibiting the manufacture of matches from white phosphorus, as well as many other regulations.

About the year 1910 marked the initiation of *workmen's compensation* in the United States. It was adopted by New York in that year, and within the next ten years practically every state that had any industrial problems at all had adopted some form of workmen's compensation.

California in 1911 first required reporting of occupational disease. Physicians were required to report these conditions to the State Department of Labor or the State Board of Health. As a direct result of *workmen's compensation laws* there has been a tremendous development in industrial sanitation and an improvement in the methods of medical supervision of industrial workers.

The large insurance companies, particularly those that deal in industrial group insurance, have done more to improve the health of the industrial worker than any single agency, governmental or otherwise. This aid has been given both directly to the industry itself, through expert advice, and indirectly to the worker by the simple method of raising group premiums in hazardous industries. The industry is compelled to protect the worker by suitable means in order to lower its insurance premiums.

The American Association of Industrial Physicians was formed in 1916. It has been an active force in the development of the medical and surgical care of the sick or injured industrial worker.

The State Health Department of Massachusetts was the first to recognize the special responsibility of the State Health Department for the prevention of illness and protection of health of the industrial worker. Dr. W. C. Hanson of the Massachusetts Health Department made a study of the dusty trades in 1905 and demonstrated the many avoidable factors and processes in the leading industries that were injurious to the health of the workers. In 1912 the activities of the Massachusetts State Health Department in relation to industrial hygiene were transferred to the State Department of Labor.

**Occupational Disease Laws.** Workmen's compensation related at first to occupational injury. Compensation for occupational disease was not initiated until 1919 when Wisconsin and California enacted such laws. The movement grew rapidly, so that by 1945 almost every state had some form of *occupational disease legislation*. From the first there has been confusion concerning the definition of an occupational disease. The Connecticut Compensation Act of 1927 states: "An occupational disease shall mean a disease peculiar to the occupation in which the employee was engaged and due to causes in excess of ordinary hazards of employment as such." A New York court decision considers an occupational disease as one which results from the nature of the employment. It is a natural incident to a peculiar occupation. This hazard is attached to that occupation and is in excess of the hazard attending employment in general.

These definitions have required interpretation, and most states have formed a schedule of occupational diseases that are compensable. The occupational disease compensation law of Maryland, for example, lists thirty-four diseases that are reportable and compensable.[1]

## DIVISIONS OF INDUSTRIAL HYGIENE

The various activities that are included in the whole scope of an industrial hygiene program are difficult to define and delimit. The health department must attempt to protect the health of all individuals in the community at all times. Procedures directed toward the whole community protect the worker both at his home and at work; but the wage earner is subjected to special hazards which are a direct result of his occupation. These should receive special consideration.

The various activities of an industrial hygiene program may be roughly grouped as follows:

1. Measures taken toward the prevention of industrial accidents.

2. Measures taken to prevent diseases due to specific poisons that may be used in industrial processes. Included in this general category are measures taken to prevent diseases due to harmful dusts.

3. Promotion of a hygienic working environment, with abatement of all conditions that may be injurious to the workers. Many industries may possess all necessary safety appliances, and use no poisonous processes, but the work may be injurious to the employees because of unsanitary working conditions. Examples that may be cited are overcrowding,

---

[1] 1. Anthrax
2. Lead poisoning or its sequelae
3. Zinc poisoning or its sequelae
4. Mercury poisoning or its sequelae
5. Phosphorus poisoning or its sequelae
6. Arsenic poisoning or its sequelae
7. Poisoning by wood alcohol
8. Poisoning by benzol or nitro-, hydro-, hydroxy-, and amino-derivatives of benzene (dinitro-benzol, analin, and others) or its sequelae
9. Poisoning by carbon bisulphide or its sequelae, or any sulphide
10. Poisoning by nitrous fumes or its sequelae
11. Poisoning by nickel carbonyl or its sequelae
12. Dope poisoning (poisoning by tetrachlormethane or any substances used as or in conjunction with a solvent for acetate of cellulose or nitrocellulose, or its sequelae)
13. Poisoning by formaldehyde and its preparations
14. Hydrocyanic acid poisoning
15. Chlorine poisoning
16. Ammonia poisoning
17. Cadmium poisoning
18. Manganese poisoning
19. Chrome ulceration or dermatitis or their sequelae

20. Epitheliomatous cancer or ulceration of the skin or the corneal surface of the eye, due to pitch, tar, bitumen, mineral oil, or paraffin, or any compound, product or residue of any of these substances
21. Glanders
22. Compressed air illness or its sequelae
23. Miners' diseases, including only cellulitis, bursitis, ankylostomiasis, tenosynovitis and nystagmus
24. Cataract in glassworkers
25. Radium poisoning or disability due to radioactive properties of substances or to roentgen rays (x-rays)
26. Poisoning from methyl chloride or other halogenated hydro-carbons
27. Carbon monoxide poisoning
28. Poisoning by sulphuric, hydro-chloric or hydro-fluoric acid
29. Respiratory, gastro-intestinal or physiological nerve and eye disorders due to contact with petroleum products and their fumes
30. Disability arising from blisters or abrasions
31. Disability arising from bursitis or synovitis
32. Dermatitis (venenata)
33. Silicosis
34. Asbestosis

poor lighting, poor ventilation, various conditions that are productive of over-fatigue, as well as many other unhygienic working conditions.

4. Promotion of the general health of the worker. This part of the program has grown tremendously in recent years. In some of the larger industries the workers are given a complete medical examination on employment, and at certain periods thereafter. Continuous medical and nursing service is furnished. This medical service is not simply an emergency clinic, but provides aid for correction of physical defects, and promotes the general well being of the employees through recreational facilities and by many other means. The purpose of this work is preventive in nature. The function of the emergency dispensary is primarily to treat minor injury in order to prevent infection or serious after-effects. The pre-employment examination is used to be sure that no employee will be assigned to work that would in any way be a tax on his physical capacity. Routine re-examinations are conducted at suitable intervals to detect minor physical defects in their early stages, and thus enable the worker to obtain early and proper medical or surgical attention. Some industries employ public health nurses as home visitors to aid and advise the worker and his family in the home in case of serious illness or disability.

5. All well planned industrial hygiene programs should place special emphasis upon health education of the worker. This information should relate not only to the specific hazards of the particular industry in which the individual is at work, but should include general information concerning individual hygiene and the promotion of community health.

An industrial hygiene program is a co-operative project of industry, labor and government. Certain activities are the direct responsibility of industry; others of government. Labor itself must be informed of each step of the program, approve of the whole plan, and aid in its execution.

An outline for a suitable industrial hygiene program has been prepared by the Division of Industrial Hygiene of the United States Public Health Service.[2] The plan is flexible, practical, and is sound economically. It is presented herewith in summary form:

*Types of Services:*

1. Medical (physicians, dentists, nurses).
2. Engineering (industrial hygiene engineers, chemists).
3. Safety (safety engineers, first-aid crews, shop safety committees).
4. Welfare (trained welfare workers, or personnel managers, welfare committees, recreation committees, etc.).

## THE MEDICAL SERVICE

*Personnel:*

1. Physicians: One or more well-qualified physicians to provide full-time service in the plant. The chief physician is the medical director.

[2] *Outline of an Industrial Hygiene Program.* Supplement No. 171 to the Public Health Reports. 1943.

Small plants (500 employees or less) may combine to employ one or more physicians or to secure the services of a group of physicians in the community on a rotating service plan.

2. Nurses: One or more full-time or part-time registered nurses who work under the supervision of the physician.

3. Other assistants, such as dentists, technicians, clerks, as determined by the medical director.

*The Dispensary:*

Each plant should have a dispensary. The following conditions should be considered:

1. Space: Is there room enough?
2. Location: Is it located properly?
3. Beds: For sick or injured workers, chiefly for emergency.
4. Ambulance service.
5. Equipment and supplies.

*Duties of the Medical Service:*

1. Emergency medical care of all employees who are injured or become ill on the job.

2. Continued treatment of employees suffering from occupational diseases or accidents.

3. Regular inspection of health and accident hazards in the shops in co-operation with the safety department, engineering department, or other units, for the prevention of occupational disabilities.

4. Annual periodic examination of all employees and executives with a view to helping them improve and maintain health through the discovery and correction of ailments.

5. Monthly physical examination, including laboratory tests, of workers who are exposed to special hazards.

6. Maintenance and analysis of sickness records, and tabulation of these records monthly.

7. Co-operation with the personnel department in the proper job-placement of new workers.

8. Make sure that employees returning to work after an absence due to illness or injury are capable of working safely and efficiently.

9. Promotion of a health education program.

10. Make detailed plans for handling large numbers of seriously injured workers in the event of disaster.

11. Co-operation with all other services in the plant which relate to the health of the workers, such as the food service, the welfare service, safety program, and recreational committees.

## THE ENGINEERING AND SAFETY SERVICE

The Engineering and Safety Service is responsible for the detection and removal or control of environmental conditions in the plant which endanger health and safety.

*Personnel:*

1. The industrial hygiene engineer. Very few plants have industrial hygiene engineers with the combined knowledge of the control of occupational diseases and occupational accidents, including practical experience in the maintenance of production. Since this is true, and since it is seldom necessary for a plant to have the full-time services of an industrial hygiene engineer, it is suggested that plants utilize the services of governmental industrial hygiene bureaus (Federal, state, and local) to obtain impartial surveys and expert consultation. The engineers from these bureaus can make detailed surveys, work out the steps to be taken, and instruct plant engineers as to their application.

2. Safety engineers are trained to identify conditions or practices that might result in accidental injuries to workers. They also conduct safety education programs and organize and direct safety committees.

3. The safety committees. There should be separate shop safety committees, under a central safety committee, in large plants. The plant physician should be a member of the central safety committee. Safety committees investigate accidents, make recommendations for accident prevention, formulate safety rules and regulations for the plant, and see that recommendations and rules are complied with.

4. Every plant should have at least one first-aid or stretcher crew, composed of interested employees. The crew may be trained by the medical service, a trained safety engineer, or a first-aid teacher with a Red Cross certificate. The first-aid crew works under the supervision of the medical service and the safety committee.

*Engineering Control:*

In every modern industry there are one or more conditions peculiar to the particular processes and operations which are potential threats to the health and safety of the workers. These are called occupational hazards; most of them can be eliminated or reduced to harmless limits by engineering methods. Further protection of the worker must sometimes be provided by supplying approved devices and clothing. The most important occupational hazards are:

1. Exposure to poisonous fumes, dust, and gases.
2. Excessive noise.
3. Poor illumination.
4. Excessive heat, cold, or humidity.
5. Contact with chemicals and other substances which produce skin diseases.
6. Operations which may result in accidental injuries, as burns, cuts, crushing, wounds, etc.
7. Overcrowding in the workroom.
8. Poor ventilation in the workroom.
9. Poor housekeeping.

*Control Methods:*

Good housekeeping is rule 1–A for the control of occupational hazards. This is everybody's job. It means simply maintaining an orderly, workmanlike shop, indoors and out.

*Control of Poisonous Fumes, Gases or Dusts:*

This is a job for experts. Industrial hygiene engineers must design specific measures for each hazardous operation. In general, these measures involve various types of ventilation; personal protective equipment and clothing for the workers; alterations in processes, materials used, or location of the operation.

*Sanitary Facilities:*

These need no discussion. They comprise the following elements:

1. Lockers and dressing rooms.

2. Wash rooms. Toilets and shower baths, with adequate drinking fountains.

3. Cafeteria or lunch room.

*The Safety Program:*

1. Every operation must be designed so it can be done safely.

2. All moving parts likely to injure the worker must be guarded.

3. In certain operations, workers need safety shoes, safety goggles, etc. Women workers should have hair nets and practical work clothes.

4. Daily inspections of all operations by the safety engineer, to identify unsafe practices and conditions.

5. Frequent meetings of the safety committees.

6. Investigations of accidents to determine causes and prevent future accidents.

7. Safety meetings for all personnel at regular intervals.

8. Enforcement of safety regulations by foremen, with the full support of the safety committees.

9. Training each new worker to do his job the safe way.

## WELFARE SERVICES

*Medical Care for Nonoccupational Disability:*

Nine in every ten absences because of sickness are the result of diseases and accidents that are not directly related to the occupation.

The commonest causes of absenteeism are shown in Fig. 26. Graph 1 represents the actual days lost from various illnesses, and Graph 2 represents the causes of absence because of illness. The average time lost per illness was approximately 8 days.

A few large industries have already developed excellent services for the care of employees and their families, including medical, dental, surgical, nursing, and hospital care. On the whole, however, plant medical services have not yet broadened their scope to include this general medical care. Most industries do not believe that this is their function. In isolated communities with inadequate medical facilities, it may be necessary to extend the scope of the plant's emergency medical service for general illnesses.

*The Preplacement Examination:*

Modern industries have adopted the preplacement examination as an effective tool for placing all workers in jobs which they can do safely and efficiently without endangering themselves and their fellow workers.

The objective of the preplacement examination is to utilize every available worker. In no instance should it be interpreted as a means of rejec-

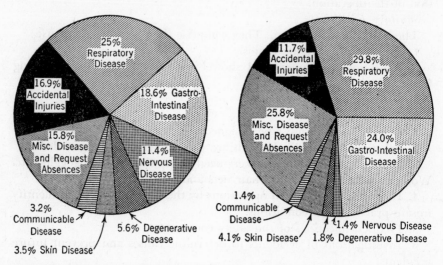

FIG. 26. *Causes of Lost Time among Industrial Workers.* Graph 1—Cause of 40,942 days lost time (severity). Graph 2—Cause of 5,402 absences (frequency). Source: McGee, L. C. and Creger, J. D.: "Gastrointestinal Disease among Industrial Workers," *J. A. M. A.,* 120:1367, 1942.

tion of handicapped persons. Many industries with realistic personnel policies nowadays reject less than 1 per cent of applicants.

The preplacement examination includes:

1. Complete medical and occupational history.
2. Complete physical examination.
3. Test of eyesight.
4. Blood pressure reading.
5. Laboratory analysis of urine.
6. Blood count.
7. Blood test for syphilis.
8. X-ray picture of the chest to detect tuberculosis, especially of applicants whose physical examination suggests the possibility of tuberculosis.

One-eyed workers, and many applicants with handicaps such as hernia, high blood pressure, defective vision or hearing, and crippling conditions may be employed and placed by the physician and employment office at jobs they can do efficiently and safely. Applicants found infected with syphilis may be employed, providing: (1) Their disease is in a non-infectious stage; (2) they have no other disqualifying complications; and (3) they remain under treatment.

*Special Problems:*

Attention should be given to the special needs of the workers. Included in this category are:

1. Maintenance of health under the special strain of night work and rotating shifts in a 24-hour industry.

2. Better nutrition in the workers.

3. Personal and family problems which cause worry and emotional difficulty.

*Health and Safety Education for Workers:*

An overall program should be organized to give all employees in the plant the information and training they need to protect themselves and to co-operate intelligently with the health and welfare services. This program should be inclusive and continuous. If well planned, it can be made most effective and interesting.

## FUNCTIONS OF INDUSTRY IN AN INDUSTRIAL HYGIENE PROGRAM

The scope and value of this health promotion service to the health of the worker and to the community at large is well illustrated by a report of the Industrial Management Council of the City of Rochester, New York, for 1938. Of the 81 industries in the city that reported to the Council, 61, employing 38,000 people, had some form of health promotion service.

|  | Full time | Part time | On call | Total |
|---|---|---|---|---|
| Physicians employed .... | 6 | 26 | 40 | 72 |
| Nurses employed ....... | 43 | 1 | — | 44 |
| First-aid workers ....... | — | — | — | 91 |
| Pre-employment physical examinations ............ | | | | 9,605 |
| Re-examinations ............................. | | | | 5,107 |
| Number of persons cared for in dispensary ......... | | | | 303,718 |
| Number of persons receiving first aid ............. | | | | 66,027 |
| Calls at plant dispensary for check: | | | | |
| By physician ................................ | | | | 42,237 |
| By nurse ................................... | | | | 196,547 |
| Number of home visits by nurses ................. | | | | 20,555 |

This very large amount of medical and nursing care in the prevention of illness and the promotion of health has an undoubted, though un-measurable, effect upon the health of the whole community.

This type of health promotion service by industry has one great defect: its usefulness has been limited in great part to larger industries, employing 250 or more people. Now over half our industrial workers are employed in smaller industries, with less than 250 employees. The solution should not be a difficult one.

**Industrial Health Plans for Small Industries.** The smaller industries, with less than 250 employees, obviously cannot carry out, in the same way, the comprehensive industrial health plans that have been so successful in the larger industries. A very satisfactory method of solving this problem is the co-operative health service programs that have been organized successfully in several areas.[3] The Industrial Hygiene Division of the United States Public Health Service, the National Association of Manufacturers,[4] and particularly the Health Advisory Council of the U. S. Chamber of Commerce,[5] have been active in promoting this type of organization. The reader who is interested in the details of this type of service is urged to write to the above organizations for suggestions.

## FUNCTIONS OF GOVERNMENT IN AN INDUSTRIAL HYGIENE PROGRAM

The functions of government in an industrial health program are, in the main:

1. Adequate reporting of industrial disease.
2. Protective legislation.
3. Factory inspection.
4. Studies and research in regard to the effect of various industrial processes upon the health of workers, including industrial poisons, dusty trades, etc.
5. Advisory and consultative service to industry and labor in regard to health matters.
6. Health education.

**Reporting.** The Department of Health has developed the machinery for reporting communicable disease, and thus it is a simple matter to educate and instruct the physicians in each community to report all occupational disease that may be encountered by them through the usual channels.

**Protective legislation** has been a very important factor in the promotion of the health of the individual worker. It progresses very slowly; in fact, legislation often lags far behind our newer knowledge of the dangers that are inherent in certain industrial processes. In some instances protective legislation has not provided for the suitable application of known methods for protection of the workers. Some of the legislation has been poorly conceived, and has worked a handicap on both industry and labor. Nevertheless, it has been, and still is a very potent force in the prevention of

[3] "Small Plants Health Service Successful." Brief report in *Industrial Medicine.* 1946, Vol. 15, p. 114.
[4] "Who's Too Small for a Health Program?" National Association of Manufacturers, 14 West 49th Street, New York, N. Y.
[5] "Medical Service for Workers in Smaller Plants." Health Advisory Council of the Chamber of Commerce of the United States. Washington, D. C. 1944.

industrial disease and accident. Not only must the legislation state clearly what an occupational disease is, but provision must be made for an impartial medical board which shall determine whether or not a claimant is suffering from an occupational disease, and also the extent of disability that has been produced.

**The Industrial Medical Board.** The Industrial Medical Board should be competent, impartial, and have no political affiliations. The members —preferably three in number—should be given suitable terms of office and suitable compensation. They represent the state, and should be appointed by the Governor, preferably from a list of names that may be submitted by impartial persons, such as deans of the medical schools within the state, and the president of the State Medical Society. Criteria for membership should be: extensive knowledge and experience in the diagnosis and treatment of occupational disease. In some states the medical board serves only in the capacity of advisor to the administrative agency of the Bureau of Industrial Hygiene; in other states its findings are final.

The functions of the medical board are:

1. To advise the administrative agency (or determine for it) whether or not the claimant is suffering from the occupational disease for which compensation is claimed.

2. To determine the degree of disability caused by the occupational disease.

**Factory inspection** by duly authorized governmental sanitary agents is a fundamental part of an industrial hygiene program. Too often the factory inspectors have not been well qualified men, and have simply carried out a routine job. The inspector must be familiar, not only with the principles of illumination, ventilation and general sanitation, but must know the details of the various industrial processes and be familiar with the substances used in industry that may produce disease in, or injury to, the worker. He must be constantly on the alert for dangers inherent in new industrial processes, and should study the medical statistics of his factories as an epidemiologist studies communicable disease incidence in his community.

**Government Investigation.** Government should be active in the study and investigation of industrial processes that may be injurious to workmen. It stands on a middle, neutral ground. It is anxious to promote and aid industry in every possible way, but cannot permit the development of industrial processes that will cause injury or illness to the workers. New industrial processes are being developed continually; new untried substances are being employed. The pharmacological reactions of many of these new substances have never been tested. Frequently, the use of these new substances has resulted in disaster to the workers. It is the function of government, by investigation and studies, to prevent these untoward events.

**Advisory Service.**  In addition to factory inspection and research service, the government should furnish an advisory and consultative service to industry in relation to its special problems in hygiene and sanitation. Industry should not feel that the state is simply an inhibitive or punitive agency, but rather that it is making every attempt to aid industry in solving its problems, to the advantage of the industry, as well as for the promotion of the health and welfare of the worker. In other words, the industrial hygiene program of the state should be a constructive and helpful one, rather than a policy of inhibition which exercises a domineering spirit in the carrying out of police powers.

**Health Education.**  The state should do everything in its power to aid industry and labor in the development of its joint program of health education of the workers. The state can be of great aid along these lines, as it has special facilities and an experienced personnel that may be utilized to great advantage.

## ORGANIZATION

It will be noted that in the above discussion of the functions of government in an industrial hygiene program we have not specified just what governmental agency or bureau should carry out these functions. Though the functions of government are fairly definite, we have, as yet, developed no general policy throughout the various states as to administrative procedure. The activities have been divided, in the main, by state governments, between the State Department of Health and the Department of Labor and Industry. Most local health departments have no special program for the protection of the industrial worker, other than their general community health activities.

Mountin [6] in 1943 reviewed the distribution of industrial health services by various state agencies. The work was divided between the Departments of Health, Labor and Industry, Industrial Accident Boards, Workmen's Compensation Commissions, and other bureaus. The major health protection activities were assigned to the State Health Department. Approximate annual expenditures were about $4,500,000. With a labor force (1940) of about 53,000,000 workers, this represents 9 cents per capita per annum (exclusive of expenditures for Workman's Compensation). Greatest expenditures occurred in the wealthier, highly industrialized states, although West Virginia, because of its large outlay for the protection of coal miners, ranked high with a per capita expenditure of 48 cents. Almost every state had some form of official organization for the protection of the health of the worker.

In 1946, the only states without industrial hygiene services were North and South Dakota, Nebraska, Arizona, New Mexico and Nevada. None of these states have extensive industrial developments.

[6] Mountin, J. W. and Flook, E.: "Distribution of Health Services in the Structure of State Government." *Pub Health Rep.* 1943, Vol. 58, p. 33.

One thing is clear. Industrial hygiene is a specialized service, requiring expert knowledge. We can be sure that the various phases of the program cannot be carried out effectively by the smaller health department, or by local boards of health of the county or city. Basically, industrial hygiene is a state function. Large municipalities, with a big industrial population and with more or less autonomy as granted in their charter, may organize a division of industrial hygiene on a similar basis to that of the state; but leadership must come from the state, and major industrial hygiene activities will fall within the province of state government.

Some authorities believe that it is most desirable to assign all matters relating to the prevention and control of occupation disease and accident to one Board of Industrial Hygiene. Such a board, with proper personnel, could unify the activities of various state departments and eliminate duplication of supervision, inspection, and control that undoubtedly would result if the activities and responsibilities were divided.

Should such a Board of Industrial Hygiene be a division of the State Department of Health? This is not feasible because the Health Department is not a suitable agency to maintain factory inspections and enforce the Workmen's Compensation Act.

Should the Board of Industrial Hygiene be allocated to the Department of Labor? This is not a satisfactory arrangement because the Department of Labor has no suitable machinery for effecting proper reporting of occupational diseases, nor does this Department have the laboratory facilities or medical and laboratory personnel to conduct the necessary investigations in regard to industrial processes that may produce health hazards.

It is the opinion of the author that the work should not be organized as a Board of Industrial Hygiene but should be organized as a joint co-operative project of two state departments, namely, the Department of Public Health and the Department of Labor and Industry. It may be administered on lines familiar to the co-operative school hygiene programs of the State Departments of Education and of Public Health. The functions of government are clearly marked. Certain duties and activities may be allocated to the State Department of Public Health; others to the State Department of Labor.

**Reporting of Industrial Diseases.** One factor in intelligent handling of industrial disease is adequate reporting of these diseases as they occur. The situation is closely analogous to the reporting of communicable disease. The state health department already has the proper machinery set up for reporting disease to the state by practicing physicians, and thus it becomes the obvious agency to carry out this activity. A long list of specific conditions has been prepared by some states. This list has included diseases due to many of the industrial poisons. It includes silicosis and other diseases due to dusty trades, caisson disease, diseases due to exposure, excessive heat, etc. Such a comprehensive list is unsatisfactory, since the average practicing physician will be confused with its very complexity, and since also new processes are being introduced continuously which may produce conditions that are not included on the list. One policy might be adopted which would make reportable *all pathological conditions* that were due directly to the person's occupation. A more practical, but less informative, method would be to require the reporting of all diseases or conditions compensable under the Workmen's Compensation Act of that particular State. (See the list incorporated in the Compensation Law of Maryland, page 333.)

All morbidity and particularly all mortality certificates should state very clearly and in detail the actual occupation of the persons concerned. The certificate should not give the occupation of a person merely as laborer, mill worker, or mechanic, but should state exactly just what procedure was followed, and what process was used by the worker.

**Factory Inspection.** It is not reasonable to have two separate groups of state factory inspectors, one from the Department of Labor to determine hours of labor and industrial safeguards, another group from the Department of Health to determine questions of proper ventilation, illumination, dust hazards and general sanitation. It is much more logical to allocate all activities relating to enforcement of *state laws and regulations* concerning employment, including health and sanitary regulations, to the Department of Labor and Industry.

Activities relating to the last three items of the industrial health program, namely, research and investigation, expert health advisory service, and health education, can best be carried out by the health department.

A separate division of industrial hygiene in the health department of any industrial state is highly advantageous. It would not be an expensive division to maintain, for it would consist essentially of a small expert personnel which would be required to carry out the special functions already indicated, namely:

1. The development of proper machinery for reporting of occupational disease.

2. Study of industrial hazards and problems, together with analysis of data from reports of industrial disease prevalence.

3. Aid and advice to industry and labor in solving each particular industrial hygiene problem.

4. Aid to industry and labor in developing programs of health education among the workers.

**Federal Government.** The Division of Industrial Hygiene is organized in the United States Public Health Service. It has played a very important part in the development of industrial hygiene work in the United States since its initiation in 1914. Its chief activities have been:

1. Aid to States in the organizations of this industrial hygiene program.

2. Investigation throughout the United States in all matters that concern the health protection of the worker.

3. Aid to other national bureaus and departments, such as the Department of Labor and the Bureau of Mines, in the solution of special problems in industrial hygiene.

The Division undoubtedly will continue to play an invaluable part in the development of health promotion and protection of the worker in industry throughout the nation.

**Rehabilitation.** World War II brought out as never before the importance of rehabilitation for those young men who were handicapped by the war and unable to resume their normal places in the world because of physical or emotional disability. We discovered that we had a few facilities for this important work, and no very clear understanding of the best methods which should be followed.

Sheltered work shops had been sponsored in the past by private philanthropy, and to a limited degree through public support, but they had not met with wide success. One great deterrent, particularly during the depression period, was that the handicapped person who received special training could not secure a position through normal commercial channels. Employers were loath to take a handicapped person because he was certain to do substandard work, and more important, workmen's compensation laws applied to these people as well as to normal employees, and thus the industry might assume an unwarranted employee risk.

Evidence is accumulating that the well-trained handicapped person is a good investment as an employee. Fifty-one per cent of a group of 300 persons studied[7] had a better accident record than normal controls; 49 per cent had a better absentee record; 58 per cent had a better productivity record; and 95 per cent as good or better efficiency rating than their fellow employees.

Rehabilitation is an individual matter, and thus becomes an expensive procedure. It cannot be carried out on a mass basis. It requires:

1. Job analysis. This includes a study of the physical demands of the job, and the environmental conditions to which the worker must be subjected.

2. Worker analysis. An appraisal of the worker as to his capacities and the conditions to which he can be exposed with safety.

3. Selective placement. This represents a careful matching of the physical demands of the job to the capacities of the handicapped person.

4. Training. On-the-job training is perhaps the best method.

5. Supervision. The foreman should understand fully the problems of the disabled person, and should give adequate supervision.

6. Follow up. Management should follow up all placements of handicapped persons to be certain that no mistakes have been made. Job modification and possible transfer to other departments may be required.

7. Evaluation. A record of the experiences of the industry with handi-

---

[7] *Desirability of Employing Disabled American Veterans.* National Service Headquarters, 1701 Eighteenth St., N. W., Washington, D. C. 1945.

capped workers, and an evaluation of their capacities and performance are essential parts of the program. Factors to be emphasized are: productive capacity, absenteeism, efficiency, and proneness to accident.

It is now clear that a community-wide program for rehabilitation of persons who are disabled by accident or illness is a wise and profitable community measure. It is necessary to combine a suitable plan for training of the patient with intelligent selective placement in a job for which the individual has capacity and interest.

This will make it possible to employ otherwise derelict persons, enabling them to enjoy security and to contribute to the welfare of their families and that of the community.

The needs for the immediate future in the field of industrial health have been summarized by Dr. L. D. Bristol when he was Health Director of one of the largest industries in America. They are:

1. Greater emphasis upon active promotion of the health of the industrial worker. Occupational disease must be controlled, and industrial accidents must continue to be curtailed. But the next important step is the organization of a general, comprehensive health promotion program for the worker.

2. More general and effective teaching of industrial hygiene should be given in medical schools and in postgraduate schools of public health. Trained and qualified leaders in this field are all too few.

3. The development of a system of appraisal of industrial health and safety activities, in order to measure the quality and effectiveness of various procedures. Dr. Bristol has been a leader in this field, and has worked out a schedule whereby the quantity and quality of the work of medical departments of industry may be surveyed and evaluated.

## REFERENCES

1. Clark, W. I. and Drinker, P. *Industrial Medicine*. Doubleday, Doran, New York. 1935.
2. Lanza, A. J. and Goldberg, J. A. *Industrial Hygiene*. Oxford University Press, New York. 1939.
3. Sappington, C. O. *Essentials of Industrial Health*. J. B. Lippincott Company, Philadelphia. 1943.
4. McCord, C. P. *Industrial Hygiene for Engineers and Managers*. Harper and Brothers, New York. 1931.
5. National Institute of Health. *Official Manual of Industrial Hygiene*. W. B. Saunders Co., Philadelphia. 1943.
6. Woodward, L. C. and Rennie, T. A. C. *Jobs and the Man. A Guide for Employers, etc., in Dealing with Workers*. Thomas, Springfield. 1945.
7. Hamilton, Alice. *Exploring the Dangerous Trades*. Little, Brown and Co., Boston. 1943.
8. Poole, F. E. *Industrial Physical Examinations. Objectives and Methods*. J.A.M.A. 1947, Vol. 133, p. 91.

# CHAPTER XXVII

## NUTRITION

THE scope of modern public health service is much broader than mere supervision of community sanitation and control of communicable disease. The health officer must attempt to maintain the general level of health of the mass of the people entrusted to his care at an optimum point. We now recognize that suitable nutritional standards play a very important part in growth and development of the child, in prevention of disease in the individual, and in the building and maintenance of adequate community health standards. Thus every public health administrator must be familiar with the general principles of the whole field of nutrition.

The health officer should have a knowledge of those food requirements which:

1. Are necessary to maintain life.

2. Represent optimum conditions for production of the greatest vigor and stamina.

It is his duty also to study actual diseases which are a result of poor nutrition; those definite clinical entities that may be produced by a faulty dietary.

The health officer must be familiar with normal dietary requirements for the adult and the growing child, and must know also whether or not the community under his jurisdiction has the facilities for supplying their needs. He must know his community, its resources, its distribution facilities, its dietary habits and faults, and must endeavor through education and other means to provide an adequate and suitable nutrition for his people.

It is obvious that if the food supply of any community is not adequate in all directions, nutritional disturbances are inevitable. Inadequate food supply may be due to lack of purchasing power, lack of transportation and distribution facilities, or to dietary ignorance. Equable distribution of food in the United States has been greatly improved in recent years through the development of cold storage and, particularly, cold storage transportation, as well as through perfection of the wholesale and retail distribution methods for fruits and vegetables. In fact, the development of cold storage alone has revolutionized our dietary habits in recent years, to the great nutritional benefit of a large element of the population. Through this development, an adequate food supply containing all the necessary elements has become available to most of the people at all seasons and at a moderate cost. Other methods of food preservation, such as canning, have added greatly to the national dietary.

It must be remembered that it is perfectly possible to have secured an adequate, even optimal, food supply for a community, and yet nutritional disturbances will develop in some of the members of the community because those individuals may have been deprived of their per capita share of certain essential food elements.

The American dietary is composed in the main of:

|  | Per Cent Caloric Value |
| --- | --- |
| Cereals, about | 35 |
| Meat and meat products, eggs and fish, about | 25 |
| Milk | 15 |
| Sugar | 13 |
| Vegetables | 5 |
| Fats | 4 |
| Fruits | 3 |

From these data we may conclude that the national food supply cannot be considered as optimal, but is relatively adequate. The chief weakness in the national supply is lack of sufficient milk and milk products. Some sections of the nation are adequately supplied with these foods, but in many large sections, particularly in the southern part of the United States, the amount of milk consumed is wholly inadequate.

**Normal Food Requirements.** Gillett has suggested that the family food budget be divided into fifths: one fifth for vegetables and fruits, one fifth or more for milk and cheese, one fifth or less for meat, fish and eggs, one fifth or more for bread and cereals, and one fifth or less for sugars, fats, and other groceries and food adjuncts. Whatever the level of food expenditure, at least as much should be spent for milk (including cream and cheese) as for meats, poultry, and fish, and as much should be spent for fruits and vegetables as for meat, poultry, and fish.

It is not pertinent to this text to give a complete review of normal food requirements. A brief summary of the general principles of nutrition is essential, however, in a discussion of administrative procedures which relate to provision for a suitable community supply of essential food elements.

Food requirements for a community may be divided into:

*a.* The indispensable or structural group.
*b.* Supplementary group.

The indispensable [1] group of foods in any satisfactory dietary consists of a liberal amount of milk (the equivalent of a quart a day per child

[1] The term "indispensable foods" is not exact, for it is possible to obtain growth in children and to maintain health at all ages without the use of milk. It is very difficult,

and one pint per adult) together with a group of vegetables and fruits, the whole supplying a requisite amount of amino acids, vitamins, minerals and roughage. The function of this indispensable or structural group is the maintenance of growth and the metabolism of tissues.

The supplementary group of foods maintain heat and provide for the output of muscular work. They include cereals, legumes, meat and meat products, eggs, tubers, sugar, vegetable oils, etc.

Nutritional disturbances are dependent upon deficiencies in quality and quantity of food. Individuals may be underfed, but much more often are misfed. In practically no portion of the United States is the purchasing power of the people so low or the distribution of food so inadequate that any individual need lack actual caloric requirements.

But there is a vast difference between caloric and protein requirements that are necessary to maintain life for a long period, and an optimum intake, *e.g.,* a dietary that will be utilized with greatest advantage to growth, development and health. It is well recognized that a great variety of dietary customs and habits may provide sufficient calories as well as sufficient protein to maintain life. Thus, the Indian on the Paraguay River may exist on meat alone; the Eskimo may consume a diet which preponderates in fat; the Oriental will subsist on a diet, the main constituent of which is rice; the African will live almost wholly on yams; and a Central American will get his protein and his calories from a dietary of black beans. Basically, all these diets contain a daily quota of at least 2,500 calories and at least 40 grams of protein. This is about all they have in common; yet they are the customary and almost exclusive foods of masses of people.

Thus it is evident that man can subsist under an unfavorable dietary regimen. But the health administrator is not particularly interested in mere subsistence. In addition to meeting the relatively simple requirement that everyone shall have "enough to eat," he must plan his activities so that an optimum dietary may be available. Furthermore, he must know when his community is on a nutritional basis which represents dangerous ground, due to lack of certain individual essential food elements, such as vitamins and minerals.

**Calories and Fats.** The National Research Council [2] has recommended 2,500 calories daily for a man in sedentary life. Women require slightly less; growing boys and girls a great deal more. From 20 per cent to 25 per cent of the calories should be in the form of fat. There is no evidence that animal fats are superior to vegetable fats, and they are more expensive. Some fats are of greater value than others because of their content

---

however, to arrange a suitable dietary without an adequate milk supply. Gamble prefers the term "structural" food elements.

[2] "Recommended Dietary Allowances," National Research Council Reprint and Circular Series No. 122, August 1945. All subsequent dietary recommendations in this chapter are based on the reports of the National Research Council.

of fat-soluble vitamin A—*e.g.*, butter. Most of the calories in the dietary are obtained, of course, from carbohydrate foods.

**Proteins.** The specific need of protein nutrition is for the amino acids of which proteins are made. Different proteins vary in their content of the essential amino acids.

Beefsteak will probably remain the preferred food of the athlete, but there is little evidence that animal protein is highly superior to vegetable protein in its nutritive values. Stare and Thorn[3] suggest that the amount of protein in the diet of an active laborer may be safely reduced to 50 grams a day, of which as little as 5 grams may be in the form of animal protein.

**Amino Acids.** Studies on young adults have indicated that at least eight amino acids are required to maintain nitrogen equilibrium in man. The exact requirements of each of these essential amino acids is unknown. The National Research Council's Food and Nutrition Board[4] recommends a daily allowance of 70 grams of protein of animal and vegetable origin. It is believed that this amount will suffice to supply the protein requirements of the average adult in health.

Protein starvation of the body may be disastrous. It results in the body drawing upon its own body proteins for metabolic needs. In cases of impaired gastro-intestinal function, in injury to tissues by burns or trauma, or in bone fractures, additional nitrogen losses occur, which require special supplementation of essential amino acids. There is convincing evidence also that adequate intake and utilization of dietary protein is essential for antibody formation. Impairment of this mechanism is one of the serious consequences of protein deficiency.

## VITAMINS

**Vitamin A.** We shall not discuss the mass of experimental work that has been done on this essential food element. The vitamin has been isolated in practically pure form $(C_{20}H_{29}OH)$ and is a water insoluble unsaturated alcohol. Xerophthalmia and night blindness are produced by a severe degree of deficiency of this vitamin, but the marked manifestations of vitamin A deficiency are seldom encountered. It is of great interest because a lack of vitamin A is of such primary importance in its effect upon the general health and length of life in a community. It is of special importance in promoting growth of the child and adolescent. A lack of this vitamin produces a lowered resistance to certain infections. It is stored in the body, particularly in the liver, and a high intake results in a reserve supply. Experimental results suggest strongly that an amount of vitamin A which will sustain good health in the adult may be insuffi-

[3] Stare, F. J. and Thorn, G. W.: "Some Medical Aspects of Protein Foods." *Am. J. Pub. Health.* 1943, Vol. 33, p. 1444.
[4] "Recommended Dietary Allowances," National Research Council Reprint and Circular Series No. 122, August 1945.

cient to supply the additional nutritional requirements of reproduction and lactation. Thus pregnant and lactating mothers should be supplied with an abundant amount of this vitamin. There is strong suggestive evidence that low intake of vitamin A increases susceptibility to the development of pulmonary tuberculosis in the adolescent period. A high intake of this vitamin is important for the growing child, particularly during the adolescent years. Recommended daily requirements are:

> 1,500 I. U. for infants.
> 2,000–4,500 I. U. for children.
> 5,000 I. U. for adults.
> 6,000 I. U. for pregnant and lactating mothers.

The chief sources of vitamin A in the dietary are leafy and yellow root vegetables, both canned and freshly cooked; whole milk and cream, butter, egg yolk, and fish liver oils. Ordinary cooking does not destroy this vitamin, as it is relatively heat stable.

Carotene is a precursor, or provitamin, of vitamin A, and is the substance out of which the body can manufacture this vitamin. It is present in abundance in carrots, sweet potatoes, and other yellow root vegetables. Carotene crystals are commercially prepared and are available at low cost.

The health officer can readily translate these simple facts in relation to vitamin A into a practical working program. For example, he will not be interested solely in the *safety* of the milk supply, but will stimulate the *consumption* of an adequate supply of milk. His program will place particular emphasis upon the importance of foods containing vitamin A in the dietary of pregnant and nursing mothers. The educational work in the community will stress continually the importance of milk and yellow root vegetables in the dietary of the growing child. In rural areas the health officer should co-operate with the farm and home demonstration agents from the department of agriculture in stimulating the development of household gardens, and in securing an adequate and safe supply of milk and milk products.

**Vitamin B Complex.** The following factors have been established as distinct components of the original water soluble vitamin B:

1. Thiamin.
2. Riboflavin.
3. Niacin.

In addition, there are several less well understood components, such as $B_4$, a thermolabile substance, absence of which causes paralysis in certain experimental animals; factor W, known to be essential to growth; $B_6$ (or H), the absence of which produces dermatitis in rats. $B_6$ has been synthesized and is a derivative of the nitrogen base pyridine. Only the first three will be discussed.

1. $B_1$, *or thiamin,* is a chemically pure substance that has been isolated and synthesized. The lack of vitamin $B_1$ in the dietary results in certain *physiological* manifestations, such as anorexia, failure of normal growth,

gastro-intestinal upsets and neuro-muscular disturbances. These vague disturbances may occur, particularly in children, without recognition as to their cause, and often are not associated, in the mind of the physician, with any vitamin deficiency. The pathology of vitamin $B_1$ deficiency is represented by definite characteristic changes involving the nervous system, called beriberi. This disease is most frequent in the tropics, but is also encountered in Labrador and other parts of the world. The disease is characterized by polyneuritis. It seems probable that alcoholic neuritis is not due to intoxication by alcohol itself, but to a deprivation of vitamin $B_1$.

2. *Riboflavin* has been isolated and synthesized. It is essential for certain oxidation reduction processes constantly going on in body cells. It promotes growth and vigor. A characteristic symptom of riboflavin deficiency is the presence of deep fissures at the angles of the mouth that are so commonly seen in tenant farmers in certain rural sections of the southern states.

3. *Niacin or nicotinic acid* has been isolated and synthesized. It is the active agent of the original pellagra-preventive factor first postulated by Goldberger in 1927. (Pellagra was thought to be a contagious disease when Goldberger was assigned by the United States Public Health Service to work on it. He noted in a psychopathic hospital that none of the staff had it, but the patients did, and that the chief difference in the two groups was their diet.) Many of the patients in mental institutions in the southeastern United States made complete recoveries when their dietary deficiencies were corrected. The physiological signs of lack of riboflavin and nicotinic acid are vague, and are more commonly encountered in children. They include failure to gain in weight and develop normally, disturbances of digestion, loss of appetite, chronic constipation, general weakness, mental apathy and lack of energy. As the condition slowly progresses, the characteristic clinical manifestations of *pellagra* finally appear, with marked gastro-intestinal disturbance, typical skin lesions, emaciation, mental disturbance, etc. Typical pellagra is thus the last chapter of a long story, the late stages of a slowly progressive malnutrition.

Beriberi is rare in the United States, but pellagra is very common in certain sections of the country. In addition to the large number of frank clinical cases of pellagra, whole masses of people have an inadequate intake of niacin and are "pre-pellagrins." They do not manifest typical signs of pellagra, but do suffer from an inadequate vitamin intake, and always improve when this element is added to their diet.

Nutritionists report that a patient with cheilitis will recover when riboflavin alone is added to the diet, but may relapse. With the addition of B complex to a well-balanced diet, the patient will get well and stay well. Similarly, pellagrins can make an initial recovery with niacin alone, but will relapse shortly and require B complex (yeast) and a balanced diet for full recovery.

Recommended daily requirements for thiamin are:

0.4 mg. for infants.

1.2 mg. for adults.

Recommended daily requirements for riboflavin are:

1.5 mg. for children up to 10 years.

2 mg. for adults.

The economic condition of the people plays an important part in correction of vitamin B deficiency. All the components of the vitamin B complex are found in many protein foods such as meat, in certain vegetables, such as cabbage and tomatoes, and in some fruits, such as bananas. It is particularly abundant in the germ cell of seeds. Whole wheat flour and "unmilled" rice will supply ample $B_1$ and their use will correct a $B_1$ vitamin deficiency, but these products do not keep well on storage and may be difficult to secure.

**Whole Wheat Bread.** The U. S. Department of Agriculture has shown that whole wheat bread, in practically all categories, is superior as a food to enriched bread. Essential food elements are removed from the whole wheat flour by refining processes. We cannot return them all, for we do not know what they are. Many people have prejudices against whole grain bread. Thus the nutritional educational program in the schools should emphasize the importance of this food. This is particularly true in zones where milk, milk products, and meat are not readily available.

Vitamin B complex deficiency in the southern United States is related to the poor economic status of certain groups of people, but is more closely related to poor food habits.

As Sebrell[5] has pointed out, such things as freight rates, the price of cotton or of tobacco, the production of turpentine, and many other factors over which the health officer has no control, have a profound influence on the incidence of pellagra.

Control of vitamin B deficiency is theoretically simple. It is secured by addition to the diet of meat, whole wheat bread, whole grain cereals and milk, as well as a large variety of other foods. It often requires an intensive educational program, however, to change dietary habits of a whole mass of the population so that they will add the necessary food ingredients to their diet. Furthermore, the dietary changes will come about very slowly. One great advantage of a school lunch program is that it teaches the children the value of a well-balanced varied diet. In times of emergency, as, for example, during the great Mississippi flood, it was necessary for the health department to supplement the dietary of masses of people by addition of substances rich in vitamin B, such as dried milk and canned tomatoes. In addition, dried brewers' yeast, which is very rich in vitamin B, was freely distributed to the homeless and disturbed population as a therapeutic measure.

[5] Sebrell, W. H.: *The Nature of Nutritional Diseases Occurring in the South.* Annual Conference of Milbank Memorial Fund, March, 1939.

**Vitamin C,** or ascorbic acid, has been isolated and synthesized, $C_6H_8O_6$. This food essential was the earliest known of all vitamin requirements. It is easily destroyed by heat. For example, pasteurization of milk at 145° for 30 minutes destroys some of the vitamin C in the milk. Storage in the body is not prolonged, and failure to provide vitamin C in the diet results in disaster. Absence of vitamin C produces definite and characteristic symptoms which soon develop into the typical

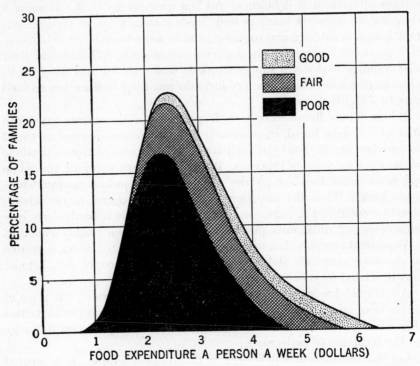

FIG. 27. *North American families:* Chart illustrating the influence of economic factors, and also of intelligent planning, upon family nutrition. It is interesting to note that a family with a large income may be poorly fed, whereas a mother with much smaller food budget sometimes provides her family with a wholly satisfactory diet. (From Stiebling, H. K. and Phipard, E. F. *Diets of Families of Employed Wage Earners and Clerical Workers in Cities.* U. S. Dept. Agriculture, Circular 507. Washington, D. C., 1939.

picture of *scurvy.* The general knowledge concerning this disease and the methods used for its prevention is now so widespread that the severe form of clinical scurvy has almost completely disappeared from the face of the earth. Sub-clinical scurvy is still highly prevalent, and frequently goes unrecognized. Spongy gums, which bleed easily on moderate pressure, are thought to indicate a mild deficiency of this vitamin.

Many fruits and vegetables, both fresh and properly cooked, contain vitamin C in abundance. Fresh fruits, such as oranges and tomatoes, are very high in vitamin C content. Potatoes are an abundant source of vitamin C that has not been widely utilized. An illustration of faulty utilization of readily available essential foods was the discovery by the State Health Officer of widespread vitamin C deficiency in northern Maine, in a county which produces more potatoes than any other single section of the nation. The essential food element was easily available, but was not used. The normal requirements are 60 mg. per day for children up to 10 years of age. Adults require about 75 mg. daily. Pregnant and lactating women require twice this amount.

**Vitamin D.** A pure crystalline form of vitamin D has been isolated from tuna fish oil, and several sterols having vitamin D activity have been synthesized. Lack of vitamin D produces a disturbance of the calcium-phosphorus metabolism. Thus, an adequate supply of the vitamin is essential for normal growth and development. This is not strictly a dietary deficiency since essentially the same beneficial effects can be secured through sunlight as through addition of vitamin D to the diet.

Cream and eggs contain vitamin D to a considerable extent. Cod liver oil contains large amounts of this vitamin, and has almost become a standard article in the dietary of the average growing child during the winter months in the northern climates. The use of viosterol or ergosterol is a most effective method of supplying vitamin D, but it is not a perfect substitute for cod liver oil.

The normal daily requirements for infants and children are 400–800 International units. A good grade of cod liver oil will contain ample vitamin D for a child if one tablespoonful is given daily. It must be borne in mind that excessive overdoses of vitamin D may be dangerous.

Exposure of the bare skin to direct sunlight is the most satisfactory source of vitamin D.

**Vitamin E** is the antisterility vitamin. It is probably an alpha tocopherol. ($C_{29}H_{50}O_2$.) Its importance in human metabolism has not been definitely established as yet.

Vitamin E deficiency has not the same practical importance as the other vitamins, because it is widely distributed in so many foods, and because so small an amount is required by the body for normal metabolism. Vitamin E is found in meat, in fatty foods, as well as in green vegetables and seeds of all types.

**Mineral Salts.** There are many gaps in our knowledge in relation to the body requirements for the various mineral elements. "Salt sickness" of cattle, seen in Florida, has been shown to be a cobalt deficiency. The question naturally arises as to whether humans can develop deficiencies of "trace" elements in different parts of the country where the essential element may be entirely absent. Iodine deficiency is an example.

*Calcium and Phosphorus.* The metabolism of these two minerals is closely interrelated. The body may receive an adequate supply of these elements, yet be unable to utilize them properly because of lack of vitamin D. They are essential for the normal development and growth of the child, and both of them may be obtained from milk. Many other foods contain calcium and phosphorus, such as cereals, vegetables and nuts; but small children do not utilize these elements readily from sources other than milk. The minimum daily intake for normal metabolism is:

Calcium: .023 gm. daily per kilo of body weight, or about 1.0 gm. per day. Lactating mothers require 2 gm. per day.

Phosphorus: .034 gm. daily per kilo of body weight.

These elements are stored by the body and may be utilized as required. Excess intake results in no injury.

Phosphorus is usually acquired abundantly in any dietary containing meat, fish, eggs, whole grain cereals, milk and milk products and some vegetables, such as potatoes. The best source of calcium is milk.

*Iron and Copper.* Iron is essential for the formation of hemoglobin. An intake of 12 mg. per day is recommended. Exclusive milk feeding will produce anemia, but iron may be added in early infancy in the form of egg yolk. The factors concerned with the utilization of iron are not fully known, and the body's method of storing it is not completely understood.

Copper is also essential in hemoglobin formation. Apparently, this element enables the body to utilize iron. The body requirements of copper are very small. Iron is abundantly supplied by meat, whole wheat cereals, eggs and many vegetables.

*Manganese, Fluorine, Silicon.* Manganese is essential to metabolism. Fluorine, silicon and other elements are found in the body in minute amounts. Whether or not they are essential to normal metabolism is not known. Certainly, all these elements are supplied in any ordinary mixed diet.

*Iodine* is an excellent example of an essential food element which may be the only factor lacking in an otherwise adequate diet, yet the absence of which may lead to serious consequences. Iodine is needed by the body in very minute amounts, yet it is essential for normal body metabolism. It is required for the manufacture of thyroxin, the internal secretion of the thyroid, and possibly for other purposes. It is effective when administered in any form and in any manner. It is well conserved by the body, for a six months' requirement may be given in two weeks. Any excess that is ingested is excreted. Fifty milligrams a year are sufficient for normal thyroid secretion of an adult.

Iodine deficiency occurs in large areas of the United States and is a matter of primary public health importance. Iodine is found in quite sufficient amount in most of the surface waters and in the soil of the Atlantic Coast, but the surface waters and the soils of the Great Lakes region, as well as many other areas of the United States, contain little or no iodine.

This element is found in abundance in sea water and all sea food, and in vegetables that are grown in soil which contains iodine.

Public health officials have met the iodine deficiency situation in various ways:

1. By the addition of suitable amounts of iodine to municipal water supplies.

2. By the use of iodized salt. Potassium iodide is added to table salt in the proportion of one part to five thousand. The average person consumes 3.5 kilograms of table salt per annum, and thus an ample iodine supply is secured.

3. By prophylactic iodine tablets given to school children. (Iodine deficiency is particularly important in the adolescent period.) A total of 2 grams of sodium iodide, usually given over a two-weeks' period, are supplied twice yearly. This method has been used with success in regions where goiter is very prevalent.

4. By the use of green vegetables which have been grown in a soil in which the iodine content is high, such as green beans, spinach, lettuce, etc.

5. Refrigeration has made seafoods containing iodine more widely available.

**Fluorine.** Fluorine has been thought of as a harmful rather than a useful element, because if it is found in water supplies in excessive amounts, it will produce "mottled" enamel in the teeth and even injure tooth structure.

Evidence is accumulating that a certain minimum level of intake may be beneficial in retarding dental caries. Dean [6] found that there was three times as much dental caries in children of Quincy, Illinois, as in Galesburg. The first city had 0.2 part per million of flourine in the water supply; the second city, 1.8 parts per million.

A few communities have attempted a long-time study of the value of adding fluorine to the water supply (1 part per million) in caries prevention. Suitable control cities will be observed.

## MALNUTRITION

The health administrator must recognize that malnutrition is a relative term. His object is to produce conditions whereby every adult, and particularly every child, will have the optimum opportunity to develop the maximum of health. He must recognize that malnutrition may occur in the presence of an abundance of essential food elements. These elements must not only be available, but must be properly utilized. Among contributing factors which may lead to malnutrition may be mentioned:

1. Physical defects, such as diseased tonsils and adenoids, bad teeth or sub-acute infections of various types.

[6] Dean, H. T., Jay, Philip, Arnold, F. A., McClure, F. J. and Elvove, Elias: "Domestic Water and Dental Caries, Including Certain Epidemiological Aspects of Oral L. Acidophilus." *Pub. Health Rep.* 1939, Vol. 54, p. 862. See also Arnold, F. A., Dean, H. T. and Elvove, E.: "Domestic Water and Dental Caries," *Pub. Health Rep.* 1942, Vol. 57, p. 773.

2. Wrong food or poor eating habits. These factors may influence metabolism in adults, as well as in children.

3. Poor health habits, such as lack of sunshine and fresh air, lack of exercise and play, lack of rest and sleep, etc.

**Signs of Malnutrition.** It is important to remember that a child may not be underweight, and still be malnourished. The weight chart or even the growth curve cannot be relied upon as the sole index of normal metabolism. Poor posture, flabby muscles, listlessness, pallor, poor appetite and poor digestion, poor elimination, irritability, inactivity, mental dullness, —all these and many more may be signs of malnutrition.

**Educational Measures.** A continuous program should be developed both for adults and children in relation to:

    *a.* Symptoms of malnutrition and its ill effects.
    *b.* Chief causes of malnutrition.
    *c.* The methods of prevention of malnutrition.

Programs of this sort that are suitable for all age groups and for all stations of life have been very effectively developed by many health organizations. They are the best example that we have of the value of a simple specific educational technic that has undoubtedly influenced the health of great masses of people.

The health officer cannot buy suitable food and give it to every person in his jurisdiction as the farmer feeds his flocks and herds. Through a great variety of methods he can be sure that abundant and essential food elements are available in suitable form, and can then teach his people the advantage and necessity of utilizing these elements. He must first be sure of his community food resources. There are certain guiding principles in studying the nutrition of whole populations. Two parts are necessary to any nutrition survey:

    1. Dietary assays.
    2. Assessment of the state of nutrition of a sample of the population.

Four types of dietary assays may be employed, all of which have some value:

    1. A statistical record of the food resources of a country.
    2. Determination of dietaries of institutions.
    3. Dietary assays of sample families. These are taken on the basis of weekly food purchases (or food consumption in a farming country).
    4. Dietary assays of sample individuals.

**Summer Camps for Children.** Summer camps are usually organized by voluntary agencies for the under-privileged children of the community. They should have the active support of the health department. They are often organized as tuberculosis preventoria, but have only an indirect effect in preventing tuberculosis. They should be recognized and valued for what they really are—namely, malnutrition camps. Their chief function is storage of abundant amounts of vitamin A for utilization during the winter, and teaching children better food and health habits. A rapid gain in weight of these malnourished children is often brought about in these summer camps.

**Emergency Rations.** The distribution of food in times of emergency is usually administered by the Department of Public Welfare. The Health Department is often called upon for advice in these matters and should take an active interest in the proper planning of emergency rations. Each emergency, whether due to floods, drought, tornado, temporary economic distress or other disaster, is an individual situation which requires its own solution, and no general rules for emergency relief can be developed. Often misunderstandings occur as to just what the minimum food requirements of emergency rations are. Two points of view may be developed:

1. Minimum caloric requirements for a mass of people.
2. Minimum food elements which will provide proper body nutrition. A community may exist for a considerable period if only the former are provided, particularly if reserves have been abundant. In emergencies, rural communities are frequently able to supplement minimum caloric requirements with vitamins A and C through a supply of wild greens of various types that are not available to city populations.

People deprived of essential vitamins may show extraordinary resourcefulness in supplying them. When the Greeks were required to emigrate from Asia Minor after the World War in 1919, they were dumped on the beaches of Macedonia and given scanty corn rations for food. They spread some of the corn on blankets and wet it down, so that it sprouted and grew. This supplied an ample source of vitamin C.

If the emergency is continued over a period of more than a month or two, emergency rations must include not only necessary caloric requirements, but also essential food elements. The three major plans that have been developed in "feeding the multitude" are:

1. Community kitchens.
2. Furnishings of food to the family through commissaries or otherwise.
3. Supplementing the family budget for purchase of food.

*Community Kitchens.* The first plan has its particular place in disasters that are of temporary duration. It is also of great value in supplying food to migratory populations, as, for example, the migratory field laborers of the west and south. The method is relatively inexpensive and is most effective in supplying necessary food elements, if conducted with expert knowledge and judgment. It is not a suitable method of continuous family relief.

*Furnishing Food to the Family.* The second plan has been widely used and theoretically is sound, since an adequate, well balanced dietary can be supplied at low cost to meet the needs of each particular family. Where racial groups are mixed, as in a large city, with a great variety of food habits and customs, this method will not be successful unless very wisely administered. The tendency has always been for the administrator to develop a dietary that is too standardized and inflexible, often entirely unsuited to the various racial groups.

*Supplementing the Family Budget for Food Purchases.* Experienced social welfare workers believe that this plan is the best, since it retains family integrity, and allows the various racial groups to choose their food according to their own taste and habit. It will not be successful unless accompanied by expert advice and supervision in regard to food purchases.

### THE PLACE OF THE NUTRITIONIST IN THE PUBLIC HEALTH PROGRAM

The nutritionist has been given almost no part in the development of official public health programs in the United States. The reasons for this lack of foresight are obvious. Clear-cut, clinically defined disease entities which are produced by faulty diet do not play a significant role in the mortality and morbidity statistics of the United States. Beriberi, scurvy, pellagra, night blindness, nutritional edema, and other readily recognized clinical conditions that are produced by food deficiencies are not encountered frequently in our medical clinics. This group of diseases has relatively little public health importance in most parts of the United States.

Thus, it is not surprising that the leaders in the field of public health have been tardy in recognition of the important part that the promotion of sound nutrition must play in the protection of the health of the individual and of the community. Only recently has it been realized that food deficiencies may not be obvious and glaringly apparent but, rather, are insidious in onset and often concealed in a maze of sub-clinical, indeterminate, confusing symptoms. We are beginning to learn, however, that the effects of malnutrition upon great numbers of our people are very real, and play an important part in the production of illness and disability, retarding the development of unsuspected numbers of children and checking their full degree of physical and mental growth.

The subject requires the careful attention of public health officials because of the fact that infants and young children are most seriously affected by nutritional deficiencies. Thus the important issue in relation to nutrition that health department executives in the United States must face, is the necessity for adequate provision of optimum food requirements for each individual in the community during the period of growth and development, and the dispersion of knowledge to the community concerning suitable utilization of proper food elements.

We are a most fortunate nation in one respect. Faulty nutrition in the United States is not due to a basic lack of essential nutritional elements, nor to faulty distribution, storage, and refrigeration of food.[7]

The essential food elements are abundant and easily procured. Poor

---

[7] One exception to this rule is the natural iodine deficiency of a large zone in the north central states.

nutrition is due, in great part, to a failure to utilize properly these read-ily obtainable foods. It is true that this failure is due in some degree to a low purchasing power of a certain proportion of families in some sec-tions of the country. In general, however, improper nutrition is due to a lack of knowledge and understanding of the simple elementary prin-ciples of proper food requirements for the body.

This limitation of knowledge is not confined to the parents and their children. School teachers, public health nurses, and health officers are often unaware of the importance of a sound nutritional regimen.

Staff members of the voluntary health and welfare agencies that are vitally interested in promoting the health of children in their various communities frequently do not realize their responsibilities or oppor-tunities in this field. The hiatus in knowledge on the part both of those who desire to teach and aid, and of those who are the recipients of this assistance, is three-fold in nature:

1. Lack of an elementary knowledge of the basic principles of the nor-mal food requirements of the body.

2. A failure to grasp the importance of the influence of proper nutri-tion upon normal development and optimum growth.

3. Failure to recognize nutritional deficiency when it exists.

Most authorities have accepted as an established principle of gov-ernment in relation to the public health, the tenet that it is the function of the official health service to act, not simply as a police agency in the protection of the community against an invasion of infectious disease, but also to do everything in its power to promote individual and com-munity health.

If this principle is accepted we must, of necessity, agree that the promo-tion of a proper nutritional status in the individual and the community is an important governmental function.

How can this desirable condition be achieved? Is it solely a public health function? If the poor nutrition of any individual is due to the low purchasing power of the family, the matter becomes at once a pub-lic welfare function. If it is wholly due to lack of knowledge, and if best results are to be obtained by instruction of the children, then the whole subject should be assigned to the department of education.

Experience in this field has shown us that no single agency should be asked to carry the complete responsibility. Rather, a co-ordinated plan should be developed in which the various official and non-official agen-cies participate. The initiative should come from the state health depart-ment. The local health department will give leadership and direct serv-ice in the local communities, and the state should furnish advisory serv-ice and assistance to local communities.

What is the purpose of a community nutrition service? What are its aims and how may they be accomplished? What personnel should be em-ployed, and how shall the workers be utilized to greatest advantage?

What part should the nutritionist play in the organization and development of this program?

The purposes of a community nutrition service are threefold: (1) recognition of nutritional defects when they occur, and in as early a stage as possible; (2) correction of nutritional defects when they have been discovered; and (3) promotion of normal nutrition in the community so that nutritional defects may be prevented.

**Recognition of Nutritional Defects When They Occur.** It would seem feasible to employ the same type of organization that is now utilized in detecting other physical defects in the community. The medical examinations in well-baby clinics, preschool clinics and school health programs, examinations for summer camp admissions, etc., seem to be the most suitable means for the determination of the degree of nutritional deficiency in the individual and in the community as a whole.

The difficulty is that we have been too optimistic about our ability to recognize malnutrition when we see it. What are our objective criteria? What do we mean by the terms "well-nourished," "mal-nourished"?

Obvious advanced stages of malnutrition are detected with ease, but these are not the conditions we are looking for. Derryberry has made an interesting study which was reported in the Public Health Reports, February 18, 1938, entitled "Reliability of Medical Judgments of Malnutrition."

The basis of his test was a single examination: six pediatricians examined each of 108 boys. Five pediatricians examined each of 113 girls. The rating bases were *excellent, good, fair,* and *poor.* A sample of the results is given below:

| Physician | No. Boys Rated Poor | Physician | No. Girls Rated Poor |
|-----------|--------------------|-----------|---------------------|
| A | 2 | G | 26 |
| B | 6 | H | 31 |
| C | 7 | I | 31 |
| D | 10 | J | 32 |
| E | 12 | K | 32 |
| F | 15 | | |

Only one boy was rated poor by all six physicians. Of 25 rated poor by at least one physician, only three were so rated by as many as four physicians. Two boys received every rating in the scale.

Sixty-three of the 113 girls were rated poor by at least one of the five physicians. Only six of these 63 were rated poor by all five. Two girls received every rating in the scale.

One must conclude that the rating of nutritional status of a child from a single physical examination, even though the work is done by a trained pediatrician, is dependent upon which examiner makes the rating. In other words, this method of examination does not utilize any exact objective criteria for the determination of the nutritional status of the child.

Shall we give up the whole business as futile? What objective criteria may be utilized? What indices may be used? Research is hard at work on this problem, with encouraging results. There are various possibilities for the development of simple diagnostic technics along the following lines:

1. The use of the X-ray of certain of the bones to determine asymptomatic deficiency states; frank rickets and scurvy are readily detected by this means.

2. The use of the photometer in the detection of latent avitaminosis A.

3. Chemical tests for determination of vitamin A. One difficulty here is that this vitamin is stored in the tissues, so that the vitamin circulating in the blood stream may not be an accurate index of deficiency.

4. Hematological tests for determination of nutritional anemia.

5. Titration of ascorbic acid as a test for latent avitaminosis C.

6. Chemical tests for determination of vitamin $B_1$.

7. Quantitative determination of plasma proteins in relation to nutritional edema.

All these objective tests are of research value, but as yet no simple field technic has emerged, no single test or combination of tests has been formulated that can be utilized with confidence and ease in order to determine the exact degrees of malnutrition in any given population of children. What ready means are available by which we may recognize nutritional deficiencies when they occur, particularly during the early stages?

The use of height and weight charts has been largely abandoned as a simple measure of normal growth and development. These criteria may have been discarded because we did not interpret our results properly. One must acknowledge, of course, that any single observation of any type, simple or complex, is of little value for purposes of objective determination of the exact nutritional condition of the child. But if we continue to watch the growth of the child, and make repeated observations on height and weight, we have a fairly satisfactory index of normal or retarded development of the child.

There is another method of determining whether a child is malnourished or not; namely, the collection and proper evaluation of the dietary history. Some authorities claim that this technic is valueless, and insist that it is necessary to spend days with the child to obtain accurate information. However, those who have had experience in this field believe that the method has great value if properly done. There are two parts to the technic: the collection of data, and the evaluation of the information. Each is equally important. Poorly taken, these records are valueless. When taken by a person with judgment, tact, and experience, they may be quite accurate. The Bowes and Church charts are valuable aids in evaluating dietary histories. (See reference No. 6.)

An excellent plan is to develop a combined organization of field nutritionist and pediatrician of the health department, whereby the nutrition of the children in the community may be determined by:

*a.* Objective determination of dietary deficiency states,

*b.* Analysis of the dietary intake of child.

One must remember that extraneous factors may influence a child's nutritional status. A child may be obviously malnourished yet the dietary analysis will show ample intake. Physical examination demonstrates no fault in food assimilation, no diabetes, no chronic infection. The field nurse discovers that the child is hyper-active, and does not get the normal amount of rest. Further study shows that this is a compensatory reaction against conflict in the home. Forcing food may be good temporary therapy for this child, but the basic requirement is relief of the essential causal factor of the malnutrition. Rest, regular life, and tranquillity are essential, rather than more food. In other words, one is faced with a problem in mental hygiene rather than in nutrition.

Even though methods may soon evolve which will make our selection and classification of malnourished states much more objective, it would probably not be feasible to set up an organization which will do all these tests on every child in school. It would be a difficult task to analyze and appraise the dietary of every one of the million-odd school children of a large city.

Until the test for determination of malnutrition is as simple as the Schick test or the tuberculin test, one cannot expect to determine the exact degree of malnutrition in every child.

But the method of random sampling is still effective. The dietary assay technic can be carried out to such a degree that we can at least detect the general dietary deficiencies of any given group.

**Correction of Defects.** The correction of nutritional defects requires a well planned system of instruction which must be conducted on an individual basis. The nutritionist should plan and organize this type of instruction, but she will do little individual teaching. The major portion of this work will be assigned to public health nurses, since the public health nurse is the person who is in closest touch with home conditions and is most familiar with the family life of the community. The nutritionist instructs the nurses, and the nurses in turn instruct the families.

Some of the various activities for correction of nutritional defects that may be undertaken by the public health nurse, with the aid and guidance of the nutritionist, may be mentioned:

1. Corrections of improper food habits in individual children.

2. Interviews with parent and child concerning proper food requirements to meet the needs of the malnourished child.

3. Details of arrangement of special diets for certain types of patients.

4. Instruction to mothers concerning special feeding problems of infants.

5. Individual instruction to undernourished expectant mothers and to nursing mothers.

*Community Clinical Services for Correction of Nutritional Defects.*
The clinic services for the correction of nutritional defects have long
since become an accepted community responsibility. Hospital outpatient
departments and dispensaries have organized special diet instruction
clinics for special types of patients. Prenatal, well baby, and child health
clinics have given particular attention to problems of nutritional deficiency. The community nutritionist may be of great value to the community by aiding in the organization of such services, if they do not
already exist, and may assist effectively in perfection of the technic of
those nutrition clinic services that have already been established.

*Direct Aid.* Individual instruction is the paramount element in the
plan for correction of nutritional defects. The program is not completely
effective, however, without the addition of another indispensable factor,
namely, direct aid. Some provision must be made whereby the essential
food elements may be supplied to those children in the community with
nutritional defects, whose parents are so poor that they cannot provide
their children with the necessities of life. This need has been met in
many communities through voluntary agencies. It is an obvious responsibility of the department of public welfare. The community nutritionist
may be of invaluable aid to the department of public welfare, through
wise planning and guidance in relation to the necessary aid that must be
given to those persons in the community who suffer from nutritional deficiencies and are in such unfortunate circumstances that they cannot provide for their own needs.

**The Promotion of Normal Nutrition in the Community.** This is the
largest task, the most difficult, and the least spectacular. Those responsible for its execution must not only possess clear insight concerning the
theoretical aspects of their subject and the objectives of their work, but
must also have an imaginative mind and a tenacity of purpose that will
surmount all obstacles. The program must be developed on a continuous and long-time basis. The results will not be immediately measurable
or even demonstrable in any concrete and specific manner.

It is true that our present knowledge concerning the factors that will
produce optimal conditions for normal growth and development has advanced to the point where we can be sure that if certain broad principles
of nutrition are followed, then certain definite results will be obtained.

But human beings are not rats or guinea-pigs. We have no feasible
methods whereby we can demonstrate a human nutritional experiment
to the community. We cannot carry out a well controlled dietary experiment on a large number of subjects and prove to all the people that
one type of diet leads to good health, another to disaster. Progress will
be slow, for the dietary habits and traditions of a people are the most resistant to change of any native quality or characteristic.

The program for promotion of good nutrition is divided into two parts:
community education and direct aid to the needy.

A broad educational program in the principles of a proper dietary regimen is the keystone of a sound and healthy nutritional status of the whole community. Complete success will not be achieved, however, unless the educational work is supplemented, in varying degree, by proper provision, through organized community effort, for the actual supply of necessary food elements to those in need.

*Community Education.* The educational work in nutrition may be carried out in great part through group teaching. This is in contrast to the program for correction of nutritional defects, which must be individualized. A few of the various methods of group teaching that have proved successful may be mentioned: (1) parent meetings; (2) diet demonstrations; (3) radio addresses and other types of public lectures; (4) teachers' meetings; (5) prenatal dietary instruction to special groups; (6) courses of instruction for public health nurses; (7) school-wide nutrition projects; and (8) instruction through newspapers, pamphlets and posters. All of these various activities may be planned and organized by the community nutritionist. Much of the effective teaching will be carried out by her. For example, the school-wide projects are planned by the nutritionist in conjunction with the department of education. The materials for teaching the children, the exhibits, diet demonstrations and the like, are prepared by her for the teachers, but the actual instruction of the children is, of course, the responsibility of the individual teacher.

The community nutritionist can multiply her efforts tenfold if she adheres to the principle that she cannot devote her time to individual instruction.

Family budgeting, personal and family nutritional problems of the community are her responsibility, it is true, but this type of work is best carried out by the public health nurses who are assigned to the various districts. The nurse knows the various families and is familiar with individual problems. Thus, she is the best person to give direct service. The nutritionist should serve as consultant to the nurses. As an instructive exercise, the nutritionist may actually go with a nurse into a home to solve some especially difficult nutritional problem. One cannot emphasize too strongly, however, that she will dissipate her energies and limit her usefulness, if her own personal activities are developed on an individualized basis.

**Direct Aid.** As we have already stated, no program for promotion of normal nutrition on a community-wide basis is complete without some provision for the actual supplementing of the diets of needy persons with the essential food elements. This need has been met effectively and spontaneously in most communities through voluntary agencies. No appeal to the generosity of mankind is greater than the wail of a hungry child. Perhaps the most serious nutritional need in the community that has not been met effectively is the provision of proper and sufficient food for the pregnant mother who does not have the means to purchase enough food for herself and her unborn child. One effort to meet the nutritional requirements of the poor that has been carried out effectively in most communities is the school program of supplementary milk furnished to young children through various agencies in many parts of the United States.

This supplementation of the family dietary of the needy is a direct governmental responsibility which is usually assigned to the department of public welfare. There is no other activity of the community nutritionist that is of such obvious and demonstrable value to the community as the technical aid that she may give to the department of public welfare in the planning of the supplementary diets for the recipients of public aid.

### THE NUTRITIONIST IN THE STATE AND LOCAL HEALTH DEPARTMENT PROGRAM

We have considered in some detail the functions of a community nutrition service and indicated the part that the nutritionist may play in organization of the program. We must recognize that, from the very nature of her work, her functions will be, in great part, educational and consultative. She will render little direct personal service. How can the nutritionist best fit into the present organization of state and local health services?

*The State Health Department* should assume the leadership in promotion of nutritional service for the community. A well qualified nutritionist should be attached to the state health department staff. She may be assigned either to the division having responsibility for local health service development, or to the division of child hygiene. In one state, at least, the nutritionist is attached to the division of health education, a very logical arrangement.

The state nutritionist should be an outstanding leader in her field. Her functions are educational and advisory. She works through the local health departments and also through her colleagues on the state staff. Her major activities will include:

1. Aid to local health departments, and local welfare departments also, in formulation of their plans for an adequate nutritional program.

2. Preparation of popular educational material for general use throughout the state. This will include press releases, pamphlets, radio talks, material to be used for instruction in public schools, exhibits of all sorts, as well as other dignified and effective publicity.

3. Education of the state personnel, and particularly the local health department personnel, concerning the technic of their nutritional activities. Both group classes and individual conferences are effective methods of instruction of local health department personnel. The personnel of local voluntary agencies may well be included in these instructive exercises.

**The Local Health Program.** Every local health department should have the benefit of the advice of a trained and competent nutritionist. Here direct service is given and direct results are obtained. Where possible, the nutritionist should be a full-time employee of the local health department. She should possess the necessary technical and personal qualifications so that she can carry out effective work. In addition, she should be a good teacher and should also have had social service experience. Her various duties and activities may well include the following projects:

1. Preparation of the educational material for the community at large, including talks to parent education groups, women's clubs and other organizations that are interested in public health affairs.

2. Organization of the nutritional work in the public schools, including: conferences with the teachers concerning the content of their teaching material that may relate to nutrition; education of the children through the school lunch program; mid-morning supplementary food for undernourished children; and parent conferences. (Certain school children will be found, on school medical examination, to be definitely undernourished. The nutritionist may set aside certain hours at the school for consultation with the parents of those children who require special attention.)

3. Guidance of personnel. One of the major functions of the community nutritionist is the training and guidance of the local health department personnel. Most of the details of activity that are planned by the nutritionist will be carried out by the public health nurses. Thus the nutritionist should train the staff nurses in:

  *a.* The principles of normal nutrition;
  *b.* The recognition of nutritional defects which may occur;
  *c.* The principles of family budgeting;
  *d.* The requirements for special diets;
  *e.* Prenatal food requirements;
  *f.* The methods of correction of faulty food habits;
  *g.* Elements of infant feeding.

Through organized, systematic courses of instruction with weekly or monthly conferences and frequent individual interviews, the staff nurse will become an effective force in promotion of the nutritional status of the community.

4. Participation in maternal hygiene and prenatal programs.

5. The dental hygiene program will perforce include nutrition work as one of its most important constituents.

**Nutrition Clinics.** Three types of nutrition clinics are frequently developed:

1. Clinics in conjunction with the general child hygiene clinics and well baby service. This plan is well suited to the "Health Center" development in some of the larger cities.

2. Clinics for special instruction of parents of malnourished children.

3. Therapeutic nutritional clinics, usually attached to and sponsored by a larger hospital or outpatient dispensary.

**Nutrition Camps.** A few official health departments sponsor summer nutrition camps. Usually, however, these camps are under the auspices of voluntary health agencies. The effectiveness of these nutrition camps can be greatly augmented if the regimen is carried out under the supervision of a competent nutritionist.

**Organization of a Nutrition Service.** Larger municipal health departments cannot afford to be without the services of a full-time nutritionist. In general, a reasonable distribution of personnel would be one nutritionist for each twenty-five to thirty public health nurses; or, if considered in relation to population, one nutritionist per 100,000 to 200,000 inhabitants. She is of general aid to all divisions, but is most frequently attached to the division of child hygiene. In communities smaller than 100,000 two plans have been followed.

In one plan, nutritional advice and assistance have been supplied to the local health department through the state health department. The state nutritionist spends a certain proportion of her time with each of the various local health departments, guiding and assisting the local personnel in formulation of their programs.

In the second plan, some smaller communities have secured the services of a full-time nutritionist through the co-operative utilization of her time by both official and non-official agencies. The department of public welfare seeks her guidance in its work relating to proper nutritional supervision of the indigent. Voluntary agencies utilize her services for supervision of summer camps and other nutritional activities. The department of education may share in the program, and, in some instances, the local hospital may employ her on a part-time basis to organize the therapeutic food clinics for out-patients. All the various organizations share in the cost of the nutrition work. The administrative difficulties encountered in this loosely-knit type of organization are obvious, but not insurmountable.

In one small city the local branch of the American Red Cross took as its responsibility the cost of supplying the city with a competent nutritionist. This local branch did not utilize the nutritionist's services directly, but assigned her to the various organizations that required her services. This is an excellent temporary arrangement, but does not place the responsibility for the service where it belongs, namely, upon the official health and welfare agencies.

Many authorities on government believe that an ideal arrangement for smaller communities would be the allocation to a single governmental agency of all governmental functions relating to public health and public welfare, under a single administrative head. Under such a plan of organization, the nutritionist would be employed as a full-time member of the department of health and welfare, and would be fully occupied with the multitude of official duties that would come within her scope in two related fields, namely, the promotion of the public health and of the public welfare. A plan of this type would have obvious advantages and should result in effective permanent work.

Some communities do not appreciate the value of a full-time, well qualified nutritionist as an integral part of the public health and public welfare service. It may be necessary, in the initiation of this type of work, for various interested voluntary organizations to try many different plans of sponsorship in development of this new type of activity.

These plans should be demonstrations only. When the nutritionist has proved her worth to the community, the responsibility for the continuation of the service should be transferred to the official health and welfare departments, and the nutritionist should be given official recognition and a permanent position in the governmental organization.

## REFERENCES

1. Sherman, H. C. *Chemistry of Foods and Nutrition.* Seventh edition. The Macmillan Company. 1946.
2. McCollum, E. V. *New Knowledge of Nutrition.* Fifth edition. The Macmillan Company. 1939.
3. Rose, M. S. *Foundations of Nutrition.* Third edition. The Macmillan Company. 1938.
4. Oleson, R. *Distribution of Endemic Goitre in the United States as Shown by Thyroid Surveys.* U.S.P.H. Reports. 1929, No. 44, p. 1463.
5. Kimball, O. P. *The Prevention of Goitre in Detroit and Cleveland.* J.A.M.A. 1931, Vol. 97, p. 1877.
6. Bowes, A. D. and Church, C. F. *Food Values of Portions Commonly Used.* Pub. by Anna D. Bowes, Philadelphia. 1946. Sixth edition and subsequent editions.
7. Stiebeling, H. K. and Phipard, E. F. *Diets of Families of Employed Wage Earners and Clerical Workers in Cities.* U. S. Dept. of Agriculture. Circular No. 507. Washington, D. C. 1939.
8. Getting, V. A. *Fluorine and Dental Caries.* New Eng. Jour. Med. 1946, Vol. 234, p. 757.
9. *Food and Life.* U. S. Dept of Agriculture Year Book. 1939.
10. Jolliffe, Norman. *Preventive Medicine in Modern Practice.* Chapter on Nutrition. New York Academy of Medicine. Paul B. Hoeber, Inc., New York. 1942.
11. *Inadequate Diets and Nutritional Deficiencies in the United States.* Publication of National Research Council. Bulletin No. 109. Nov. 1943.
12. Gillett, L. H. *Nutrition in Public Health.* W. B. Saunders Company, Philadelphia. 1946.
13. *Medical Evaluation of Nutritional Status.* Series of reprints by the Milbank Memorial Fund, 40 Wall Street, New York City, beginning in 1940.

See also the many publications of the Milbank Memorial Fund on the various phases of nutrition.

# CHAPTER XXVIII

## ADULT HYGIENE

THE function of the health department is the prevention of disease, the prolongation of life and the promotion of physical health and efficiency of the whole community. Health officials point with great pride to the reduction of mortality and the increase in life expectancy in all parts of the United States in recent years. An analysis of the data shows that striking results in the reduction of death and the prevention of illness have been obtained almost exclusively in the younger age periods. Public health programs have had little or no effect upon the older age groups. In fact, there has been little increase in life expectation after the age of 50 years. In certain specific instances, quite contrary conditions have been observed. Deaths from some of the diseases of later adult life, as, for example, cancer and heart disease, have shown a steady increase year after year.

Part of this increase in the death toll of certain specific diseases in later life may be due, in reality, to better diagnosis. In part, it is due to a change in the age distribution of the population. As we have shown in the frontispiece, our population is aging. There are many more elderly people in the United States than there were 25 years ago, and thus the deaths from degenerative diseases have increased. There is a good deal of question as to whether this increase is real or only apparent. Whatever the facts, whether or not these specific death rates are increasing or remaining stationary, nevertheless these debilitating and destructive diseases of adult life which cut short the natural life span of threescore and ten represent a challenge to health officials.

Our lack of success in this field may be due to the fact that little has been done by health departments in the promotion of adult hygiene. Many health officials believe that little can be done. We do not have sufficient knowledge concerning the etiology of chronic nephritis, or chronic rheumatism or cancer, for example, to warrant the development of extensive community programs for the prevention of these diseases. Furthermore, health departments have not attempted to organize extensive programs of adult health education, because the health officer has believed that the results would not be commensurate with the efforts expended. Health education must be imparted to the early age groups, and during the formative period. The adult mind is crystallized, habits

371

are formed, prejudices are established. The adult may be interested in community sanitation, and the prevention of illness in his children, but is not receptive to instruction concerning matters of personal hygiene that may influence his own fixed habits, or mode of life.

A great many physicians feel that adult hygiene will prove a most unfruitful field of work. They believe that after a person has reached adulthood, any measures that may be sponsored by health officials in the effort to prevent or postpone the degenerative diseases of late adult life will be of little avail. A man's pattern of life is formed by the time he has reached 25 years of age. His mental attitudes have become fixed, his habits formed and his physical make-up established. The probable cause of his eventual decline and the duration of his span of life have been determined by hereditary influences and by the vicissitudes of infancy, childhood and adolescence. The type of vital organs that he may possess and their potential reserve powers, his heart, his arteries, his brain, his glands of internal secretion, his muscular co-ordination and his adjustment to life have all been determined, and little can be done to change them.

If this is true, then an adult hygiene program should concentrate on prevention of accidents, the lowering of hazards that are a concomitant of industrial life, and the promotion of environmental sanitation. Emphasis in health education should be shifted to child hygiene, the promotion of health education in the schools, the promotion of health measures in infancy and childhood, and the prevention of the acute communicable diseases. The essential thing is that a person should be subjected to favorable influences during the developmental period of his life.

Thoughtful physicians have not been willing to urge their clientele to come for a careful annual routine physical check-up, if they feel perfectly well. These physicians believe that such a procedure is a waste of time, money and effort, and gives a sense of false security. Even if degenerative changes are found, it is seldom possible to check their further development, nor can the physician institute measures which would be of any particular aid in prolonging life or preventing premature death. This rather conservative, but very logical, attitude of many physicians must receive due consideration, for there is a great deal of truth in the statement that routine annual physical check-up, as ordinarily carried out, offers little of value to the patient.

It is probably true that, with our present knowledge, or lack of knowledge, our efforts towards prolongation of life in the older age groups will not be so strikingly effective as have been the results obtained in the younger age groups. Nevertheless, a great deal can be accomplished through organized community effort in promotion of health and efficiency in adult life. Results will come by the process of attrition, by attack on specific conditions through means which offer some hope of success, and by enlargement of the program as new scientific knowledge is gained in relation to those conditions about which we now have little applicable information.

Geriatrics. Geriatrics is a new word that has been coined to emphasize the increasing importance of promoting the health of the person past middle life. In simplest terms, it is that part of medical science which deals with the process of growing old. It is interested largely in individuals over 40 years of age, rather than in the young adult, and is concerned with the prevention of illness and promotion of health in these age groups.

It may be said that the aging process begins as soon as a man reaches maturity, and thus geriatrics, if it is to prevent the degenerative processes, must begin its influence at 30 years or even earlier. This is true, since the genesis of much of chronic illness occurs in early adulthood. Oftentimes, a preventable illness of early childhood is a direct cause of premature old age.

Prevalence of Chronic Disease in the United States. Certain data have become available through extensive community-wide surveys [1] which give us an accurate index of the importance of chronic disease in the nation. Fig. 28 from the National Institute of Health survey gives the estimated prevalence of the seventeen most common chronic diseases in the United States in 1937.

We have been accustomed to evaluate the extent and distribution of chronic illness in the community on the basis of *mortality returns*. Heart disease leads as a cause of death, with cancer in second place; thus it is reasoned that the prevention of cancer and heart disease are the most important unsolved problems of geriatrics. Furthermore, these deaths occur in the later decades of life, and therefore special attention must be given to individuals past 50 years.

These graphs indicate that we must modify our ideas on these points. The most important disabling chronic disease is rheumatism. The highest peak of chronic disease incidence with permanent impairment occurs in the age group of 35 to 44 years (20 per cent of the total). See Fig. 29.

Rheumatism. Throughout the greater part of the United States, chronic arthritis is the most disabling of all the ills of mankind. The disease has not received the recognition that it warrants, because it does not cause death. In fact, there was no general conception of its real prevalence until the house-to-house canvass of Lombard in Massachusetts revealed the high prevalence of chronic arthritis and the degree of disability and loss of efficiency because of this disease. Since we know so little concerning the etiology and methods of prevention of chronic ar-

---

[1] National Health Survey, 1935–1936: *The Magnitude of the Chronic Disease Problem in the United States*. Bulletin 6, Sickness and Medical Care Series. National Institute of Health, U. S. Public Health Service, Washington, D. C. 1938 (rev. 1939).

thritis, it is obviously impossible at the present time to incorporate a program of prevention of chronic rheumatism in health department practice. The disease is mentioned at this point to indicate one of the great unsolved public health problems that must await further increment to scientific knowledge before we can even hope, by community effort, to bring about a reduction of its ill effects upon the people. We

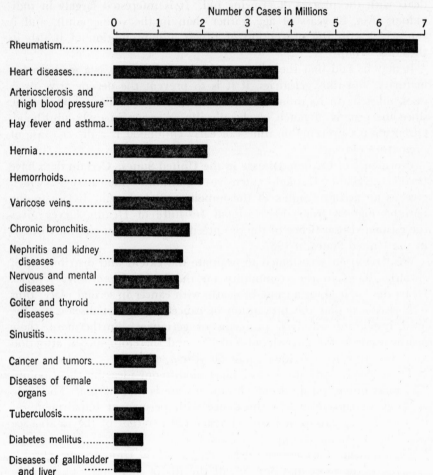

FIG. 28. *Estimated Prevalence of Specified Chronic Diseases in the United States (1937)*. Source: National Health Survey, U.S.P.H. Service, 1937.

must confess that, at present, this most disabling disease of adult life is quite beyond our control.

But this is not a good reason for abandoning the whole subject as hopeless. Research as to the causes of rheumatism must be pushed actively. Better methods for the care of these patients will yield effective results in the prevention of complete disability. Epidemiologic studies of the various types of rheumatism are an important activity of the

health services of the future. Rehabilitation of the chronic rheumatic
is also a most important community function.

At the present time, it seems most appropriate to allot a few beds in
each of many research centers for the study of rheumatism, rather than
to establish large state-supported institutions for the treatment of these
diseases. As our knowledge increases, it may become feasible to develop
extensive government-supported special hospitals for the care of chronic
rheumatism and other degenerative diseases.

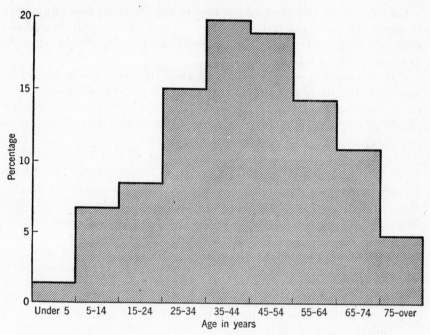

Fig. 29. *Percentage Distributions of Persons in the U. S. with Chronic Disease or
Permanent Impairment, according to age groups.* Estimated 1937. Source: *National
Health Survey,* U.S.P.H. Service, 1937.

**Diabetes.** Crude death rates from diabetes have continued to rise in
every state in recent years, in spite of improved therapeutic technics.
However, where adjustments are made for the increasing proportion of
persons in the older age groups, these apparent increases in the diabetic
death rate disappear. At present there is a marked concentration of
diabetic deaths in old, obese women.

The diabetic frequently dies of diabetic coma, gangrene, or pulmonary
tuberculosis. Each of these complications is preventable, if the patient is
carefully handled, and they should be attacked vigorously. Thus, though
we have little knowledge that can be incorporated in a community program which will aid directly in the prevention of diabetes, we have
very definite means which will aid in prolongation of life of persons
suffering from this disease. If present information is intelligently applied,

the diabetic may live a long and useful life. The important factors which will bring about this striking innovation in control of diabetes are:

   *a.* The diagnosis of the disease should be made early in its course.
   *b.* The patient should understand his condition, and particularly his limitations and handicaps.
   *c.* Treatment should be readily available, under expert medical supervision.

*Case Finding.* The prognosis is best in the incipient case of diabetes in which the condition is discovered early, and the carefully treated patient will live the longest. Thus, a continuous search should be made in the community for the diabetics.

Early diagnosis is essentially the responsibility of the family physician. Since heredity plays a part in diabetes, the family doctor should search for the disease among the relatives of his diabetic patients. A diabetic should never marry a diabetic, because, if some other fatal disease does not intervene, all the children will have diabetes.

Diabetes usually begins between the ages of 45 and 65 years. Thus, closer attention should be paid to people in these groups. The disease is more common in women than in men. The Jewish diabetic death rate is more than twice the rate in Gentiles. Obese people are much more likely to develop the disease than thin people. These epidemiological features of diabetes make a community case-finding program more simple and more effective.

The functions of the health department in control of diabetes are:

   *a.* General dissemination of information concerning the early symptoms of the disease, so that the patient will seek medical advice early in the course of his illness.
   *b.* Provision by the community of readily available clinic service for those who cannot afford to pay for expert and continuous medical supervision. Insulin treatment is expensive. In many instances it must be continued throughout life. Usually, clinic service for the indigent can be provided in connection with the general hospital outpatient service of the community.
   *c.* Insulin should be readily available to every diabetic. Some communities have made provision for free distribution of insulin to indigent patients through local health department channels. In a few states, insulin is distributed by the state health department laboratories in the same manner as any other biological product, such as diphtheria antitoxin. It is sold at cost, or is given free to indigents, the distribution being handled by the local health officials.

Hospitalization facilities for the care of diabetic accidents, such as diabetic coma or other serious complications of this disease, are essential component parts of a complete community program for the control of this disease.

**Cancer.** The problem of reducing the high cancer death rate has been a baffling one to the health officer.

Cancer is now the second most common cause of death, and is responsible for approximately 10 per cent of all deaths in the United States. The advancing crude death rate from cancer is undoubtedly due in great part to our aging population.

**Encouraging Trends in Cancer Mortality.**[2] The Metropolitan Life Insurance Company has pointed out that the outlook for the control of cancer is definitely promising. There is evidence that cancer patients are seeking medical care earlier in the course of the disease and that their chances of survival have improved materially. Encouraging, too, are the facts regarding the trend of the cancer death rate among the many millions of Metropolitan industrial policyholders, who are a representative sample of the urban populations of the United States and Canada. Among white female policyholders (ages 1–74), the death rate from cancer, adjusted to discount the effect of the aging of the group, has been quite generally downward for about a third of a century; among insured white males, the mortality from the disease until very recently had been increasing, although at a diminishing rate; but in the past few years it has also tended downward.

Even more impressive are the facts regarding specific sites, or locations, of the disease. The age-adjusted death rate from cancer of the skin, for example, has been declining for about 25 years, during which period the mortality among white policyholders has been cut in half. Almost as marked a decrease is recorded for cancers of the buccal cavity, where the relative decline seems to have been accelerated in the past decade. Far more important, in terms of the number of lives involved, has been the long-term decline in the mortality from cancer of the female genital organs, the leading site of the disease among women. The death rate from cancer of these organs has decreased by almost one fifth among white women in the past third of a century.

The favorable experience for the sites just mentioned is presumably the combined result of a decrease in the incidence of the disease and a reduction in its fatality because of modern therapy—surgical and radiological. The mortality from cancers of the stomach and liver has also shown a marked decline, but it is likely that a considerable part of this decrease is spurious. These organs are frequently the site of secondary cancer involvement, and as reporting has improved in accuracy, the primary site, such as the breast, has been recorded more often on the death certificate. Similarly, because of more accurate diagnosis, it is probable that an increasing number of deaths, instead of being attrib-

[2] Metropolitan Life Insurance Company: *Encouraging Trends in Cancer Mortality.* Statistical Bulletin, Vol. 26, No. 7, p. 1.

uted to cancers of the stomach and liver, have been reported as due to cancer of the intestines. Thus the upward trend in the death rate from cancer of the breast and from cancers of the peritoneum, intestines, and rectum which was noted until recently, undoubtedly has been the result, in part or in whole, of better diagnosis and reporting. In the past few years, however, even these sites have shown a slight decrease in mortality. What gives added significance to this improvement is the fact that, at the same time, cancers of the stomach and liver have recorded relative decreases.

The death rates from cancers of the bladder and of the prostate, which for many years had moved steadily upward among white males, have also in recent years shown a slight downward tendency.

The only important site to record an uninterrupted rise in mortality is the lung and pleura, and even here the rate of increase is slowing down. The striking increases in death rate for this site must be interpreted with caution, however, inasmuch as many cases which would have gone unrecognized years ago are being correctly diagnosed and reported, as hospitalization, operation, and autopsy become more common.

*Cancer Control Programs.* We know that certain types of cancer can be checked and life prolonged, or even sometimes the sufferer may be cured of cancer if the diagnosis of the condition is made in its early stages, and if proper surgical or other measures are employed. Thus the essentials of any community plan for cancer alleviation are:

a. A dissemination of information to all the people concerning the early symptoms of the disease.
b. Provision for early diagnosis by competent specialists.
c. Adequate facilities for treatment.

*Health Education.* The function of the health department is to disseminate freely throughout its jurisdiction a thorough knowledge as to early warning signs of cancer. For example, every woman in the community of whatever age, should know that if she has a lump in her breast, no matter how small it may be, or how free from pain, nevertheless she should seek competent medical advice at once. Educational material, if properly presented, may be supplied without the danger of developing a cancer phobia. These matters should be common knowledge, just as is the knowledge concerning the value of antitoxin for diphtheria.

*Cancer Clinics.* The community should provide readily available facilities for expert diagnosis of the disease. The New York City Cancer Committee in 1946 evolved a plan of sponsorship of cancer clinics within the metropolitan area, in a number of the larger and well-equipped hospitals. The plan of organization of these clinics was based on the very successful Strang Cancer Prevention Clinic [3] at Memorial Hospital in New York.

The plan of operation of these clinics requires skilled diagnostic services, with all facilities for very careful examination of the patient. The general examination is supplemented by special tests when they are indicated.

Patients who come to the clinic are presumably normal people. They may have come of their own volition, or be referred by their physician. If any abnormality is found in the individual, he is referred to his family physician, who is given a complete report of the clinic findings. The cost of the maintenance of this type of service is nominal, and has been met at the Strang Clinic by the fees charged to the patient for the service.

Those who are interested in the details of organization of a cancer clinic are referred to The New York City Cancer Committee, 130 East 66 Street, New York, or to the Strang Cancer Prevention Clinic, Memorial Hospital, 444 East 68 Street, New York City.

*Biopsy Service.* Free pathological diagnostic service has been provided by several state health departments as part of the free laboratory diagnostic procedure of the department.

Should the health department supply actual treatment facilities for cancer, with provision for hospitalization, surgical intervention, radium and other necessary therapeutic measures? This is a debatable question. Certainly, it is a very expensive program. Nevertheless, this obligation has been assumed by the health departments of a few of the larger cities and states.

The Massachusetts plan for the control of cancer is one of the most comprehensive, and is divided into three parts:

*Education.* An intensive educational campaign, "cancer week," inaugurated the service. Well advertised local meetings were held in various centers throughout the state. Prominent speakers were presented, the meetings were well sponsored, and the attendance was large. Radio broadcasts were used extensively, as well as local newspaper articles, editorials and other well known methods of publicity. This initial publicity was supplemented by a continuous plan of education of the people in relation to cancer. A great variety of methods has been employed. The newspaper articles seem to have produced the most satisfactory results.

The elements of the educational program are:

1. The material should be addressed to those age groups which will benefit most by the knowledge.

[3] This splendid pioneer clinic is a real tribute to the enthusiasm and organizing talents of Dr. Elise L'Esperance, who founded it in memory of her mother, and carried it through the trial period on her own resources.

2. Individuals should be taught to recognize such abnormalities as pre-cancerous lesions and conditions producing chronic irritation, and to take measures to effect their removal.

3. A person in the cancer age group should present himself to his physician for check-up if he notices that he is not in his normal state of health, or if he has any unusual symptoms.

*Tumor Diagnostic Service.* A tumor diagnostic service is conducted which furnishes any physician in the state, at no cost, a pathological report on the nature of specimens suspected of being cancerous.

*Diagnostic cancer clinics* are permanently located in convenient geographic centers in the state. These clinics are organized by a cancer committee of the local medical society. The diagnosticians of the clinic are selected by the local medical society, with the approval of the state health department, and serve without pay. A radiologist, a surgeon, and a pathologist are present at each clinic. The clinics are usually organized in connection with a local hospital and are for the purpose of diagnosis only. The follow-up social service work is an important feature of the clinic service. Each clinic receives a subsidy from the state for general expenses, for social service and clerical work. The diagnostician gives his time to the clinic. Usually the clinic meets regularly once a fortnight or oftener, if necessary. A well planned clinic will see at least 400 patients a year. The great value of the clinics is that they have developed a better diagnostic acumen in the medical profession at large and have aroused a public interest in and awareness of the early symptoms of the disease.

*A state cancer hospital* was established at Pondville, with some 200 beds and with all necessary diagnostic and therapeutic facilities, including an ample supply of radium. The hospital has a very large outpatient clinic, which gives diagnostic service, and also follows those patients who have been discharged from the hospital. Patients pay for the actual hospital care, if they are able; otherwise, the expenses of hospital care are reimbursed to the state by the local community in which the indigent patient has an established residence.

The hospital has met a real need in the state and has been very successful. The state cancer service is expensive, but has been effective, and the program has met with popular approval.

*Appraisal of the Value of a Cancer Control Program.* Eight years after the cancer control work was begun in Massachusetts, an appraisal was made of its various components. It was found that the community-wide lecture campaign caused a short flurry of increased visits to physicians' offices for consultation, but these results were of temporary value. The average period between onset of symptoms and time of seeking medical advice in 1926 was six months. After eight years' intensive education, this period was still six months. This certainly was discouraging. One point was encouraging, however. Physicians were giving their patients exact diagnosis and adequate therapy much earlier than ever before.

Thus, the key to a good cancer control program is the family physician, who will give continuous education to his own community and, through his own efforts, plan for early exact diagnosis of his patients and make provision for their early treatment. The health department should aid and supplement the work of the practicing physicians in every possible way. Co-operative teamwork of the local medical profession and the local health service seems to offer greatest promise of results in the cancer control program.

**Mental Disease.** The role of the health department in a mental hygiene program has been considered in a previous chapter. Certain phases of this program may be considered as an integral part of a comprehensive adult hygiene project. The cost of hospitalization of mental disease is one of the largest items in the budget of any state. Any plan that would prevent the occurrence of even a small fraction of these disorders would represent an enormous saving of state money. But there exists little concrete information concerning suitable methods for prevention of mental disease. One thing can be done. A well developed plan for the prevention and for the proper treatment of syphilis will certainly effect a reduction of mental disorders due to this disease. It goes without saying that every local health department should establish an effective anti-venereal disease program.

In addition, a few states have established mental hygiene clinics which are sponsored by the Department of Public Health or the State Bureau of Mental Disease. These clinics are scattered and few in number and are still in the developmental stage, so that we have had no opportunity to determine whether or not the mental hygiene clinic is an effective and practical technic which should be adopted as an integral part of official public health practice.

**Heart Disease, Cardio-renal Disease, Arteriosclerosis.** Heart disease is far in the lead as a cause of death in the United States, and is increasing yearly. Most striking is the augmentation of coronary disease, which has increased markedly as a cause of death during the past 25 years. This increase may be due in part to the aging of the population, but the marked increment is more probably due to improvement in diagnosis. Deaths from this disease are twice as common in men as in women. It is primarily a disease of men from 45 to 65 years.

Factors that seem to predispose to coronary disease are heredity, obesity, arterial hypertension, diabetes, sedentary occupation, worry, fatigue, and perhaps excessive use of tobacco.

We do not know the primary causes of coronary disease, and thus measures that might be employed by the community in attempting control of this disease would be premature. But the disease has a striking epidemiology, which gives some clues as to possible preventive measures. The health department should study the epidemiology of all cardiac diseases as assiduously as it studies other major causes of community illness. The preventive measures in all heart diseases are personalized—an integral part of physician-patient relationship; a matter of understanding and confidence. The community does have its definite part to play in gaining an understanding of the nature of these diseases.

Syphilis is not a common cause of coronary occlusion but is an important cause of heart disease.

As our population continues to age, it is almost inevitable that the crude death rate from diseases of the heart will increase, but there is no reason why one should be disturbed or alarmed about this perfectly normal and inevitable situation. In some cities and states, voluntary agencies have been organized for the prevention of heart disease. Their efforts have been diffuse and the results have not been measurable. The reason is, obviously, that we possess so many theories and so few facts in relation to the etiology and methods of prevention of this general group of degenerative diseases; at least, facts that can be incorporated or translated into an effective practicable community health program.

We do know that life can be prolonged and made more efficient for some of those persons having these conditions, with less of suffering and distress, if the diagnosis is made early in the course of the disease and if the patient understands his limitations and is under suitable medical supervision.

As in cancer, the keystone of any program for the control of heart disease is the practicing physician. It does not seem probable that extensive popular educational campaigns by the Health Department will do any particular permanent good.

But if medical students are well trained in the incorporation of the principles of preventive medicine in their clinical practice, and if they apply these principles when they go into practice, then a good program will get under way.

Early recognition of heart disease, skillful handling of the patient, sound advice as to the regulation of life, and teaching the patient to recognize his limitations will undoubtedly promote the health and prolong the life of the patient with cardiac disease. But this is the function of the private physician and is not the province of the official or voluntary health agency.

Dublin [4] has pointed out that the community has a role to play in the control of heart disease. The major obligations of the community in relation to cardiovascular disease are:

1. Provision of facilities for the detection of incipient heart disease.

2. Provision for convalescent care. Dublin suggests that the utilization of facilities formerly employed in sanatorium care of tuberculosis would be a sensible procedure.

3. Utilization of public health nurses for home nursing care.

[4] Dublin, L. I.: "Heart Disease and Public Health." *American Heart Journal.* 1942, Vol. 23, p. 16.

4. Provision for domiciliary care by physicians in chronic cardiac disease. Many of these people are elderly, many are poor—thus part of the cost of their care must be provided from public funds. The Social Security Act, providing for sickness benefits and for old age benefits to those who have retired, is an important measure in prolonging the life of the cardiovascular patient.

**The Periodic Health Examination.** A community-wide policy of annual physical examinations of presumably healthy persons who have passed their fortieth birthday has been advocated for many years. It has been claimed that this procedure is the solution for the great problem of the prevention of degenerative disease. This type of procedure has been highly successful in child care, and is now almost a universal practice in good pediatrics.

In theory at least, it should be possible, by a careful annual check-up, to detect degenerative disease in its incipiency. It is obvious that early recognition is a very important factor in the control of a degenerative disease. Even though we do not know the cause of essential hypertension, nor are there any specific methods that can be employed in the prevention of coronary disease, nevertheless early recognition should aid the physician in guiding his patient so that the patient's life can be more satisfactory, with a minimum of suffering and discomfort, and a maximum of adjustment and content.

The American Medical Association has formulated suitable schedules and physical evaluation forms for annual physical examinations of adults, and the New York County Medical Society[5] has compiled excellent instructions to physicians for this type of health service.

**Purpose of the Periodic Health Examination.** This movement has attempted to make preventive medicine operative. In many segments of the community and under particular conditions, the periodic health examination has proved applicable and useful. Thus, in industry and in certain business undertakings, the periodic health examination of individuals has been practiced to the benefit of business and industry as well as those examined. But with the population at large, the periodic health examination has not proved acceptable, since only a very small percentage of the population has ever been persuaded that it is beneficial to submit to an examination while in an apparent state of health, in order to determine whether anything is wrong or anything might be improved upon. There are at least four major reasons why the public has never favored the periodic health examination idea. One is that the medical profession itself has not seriously accepted or developed the technic of the periodic health examination; two, the public itself has not been adequately educated on this score. A third factor may be the

---

[5] *Health Examinations. A Manual for the General Practitioner.* Special Committee on Preventive Medicine, Medical Society of the County of New York. Published by Mead Johnson and Company, 1947.

confusion that has surrounded the periodic health examination in that it has been presented as promising what it could not always achieve, namely, the early discovery of disease. A fourth reason is that complete health examination has been a very expensive procedure, which could not be paid for by the average man, if conducted annually.

The periodic health examination must be understood for what it is and what it will accomplish. It is most useful in those persons who are in middle life and past middle age. It is a service that must be individualized. It does not lend itself to mass production methods, but must be a conference between patient and a physician in whom the patient has complete confidence. Its purpose is, in part, to detect incipient disease. But far more important is the opportunity it affords to give counsel concerning adjustment of the patient's mode of life, so that he can face the inroads of the aging process adequately and intelligently. The procedure is, basically, the function of the family physician.

The purpose of regular examinations, to be more specific, is fourfold. First is the analysis of the health status of the patient and the probable effects of his previous life on physical and mental health. Second is the extension of hygienic advice. Third, in this connection, is a determination of the capacities and limitations in the individual's occupation. Fourth is the prompt correction of remedial defects, including the application of such control therapy as may be indicated.

The effectiveness of such examinations depends upon the comprehensiveness of the data obtained, and upon the wisdom of the medical adviser. It is here that individual physicians in private practice can render the greatest aid to the preventive medicine of the future.

The intervals at which inventories should be held depend upon the age of patients and on other individual or local circumstances. Infants require relatively frequent examinations, while one check a year is adequate for apparently well young adults. For persons over 45, two inventories per year are probably desirable. The pediatrician can usually assume that children beyond the first few years are well unless they announce otherwise, whereas the geriatrician cannot be so sure of the insidious phenomena with which he is dealing.

Both laymen and practitioners have been slow to recognize the need for periodic examinations in practice, though they have rarely opposed them in principle.[6] Both groups have been conditioned by the tradition that medical attention is required only when there is conscious illness. Periodic examinations also acquired a poor reputation because they were often badly done. They were frequently hurried, superficial, and—as in industrial or school practice—of a routine nature. Yet the essence of such checks is individualization. The past and present history

[6] There have been exceptions, as in Dr. Logan Clendenning's *The Human Body*. See also "The Potentialities and Limitations of Individual Preventive Medicine," *Philadelphia Medicine*, Vol. 37, No. 4 (June 13, 1942) by Iago Galdston, M.D.

of the individual, laboratory data, and special functional tests are of importance to the physical examination.

All this is necessarily expensive and time-consuming, which increased the laymen's disinclination to bother with the whole business. No doubt individuals are also loath to submit to these procedures for a variety of personal reasons such as dislike for the impersonal attitude assumed by some specialists, awe for the technical paraphernalia employed, and a vague fear of possible findings.

It has been suggested that instead of "periodic examination" the term "health inventory" be employed. This word suggests to laymen a relatively careful and deliberate procedure, and their response to its use has already been encouraging. Basically, however, the need for such inventories must be conveyed to laymen through all possible means of health education. Essential to this newer type of preventive medicine is lay education.

**Preventive Practice by Private Physicians.** The private practitioner is, of course, in a position to educate his patients on this score. His frequent failure to do so many be ascribed in part to a reluctance to urge an apparent extension of his own services, but is primarily a result of his background. Trained to seek out and treat disease, he finds it difficult to shift the emphasis of his service. The remedy here clearly lies in placing a greater emphasis upon the teaching of preventive medicine in the medical schools. This applies not only to undergraduate training, but also to post-graduate courses.

**The Health Department and the Periodic Physical Examination.** Health departments have been urged to establish clinic services for periodic health examinations of adults in the community health center. The proposal is to organize this service along the same general lines as the well child clinics.

The administrative difficulties of this plan are so overwhelming that few health officers have been willing to enter this field of preventive medicine. As noted above, a few health departments have experimented with cancer prevention clinics. These, in essence, if properly conducted, are true geriatric services, since a thorough physical examination would reveal early physical defects other than cancer.

There is a general feeling that the individual should not receive this service free, but should pay for it. It is the established custom for all health department services to be given without cost.

As pointed out in the chapter on comprehensive medical care (see page 566), the average individual will not pay for an annual physical examination on a fee-for-service basis. If a system of prepayment for medical care is developed, these annual physical check-ups will be included as an essential part of this service, and it has been found that under these circumstances, the purpose of the periodic physical examination will be served.

The solution of these problems is not simple. It seems probable that this unsolved administrative dilemma in preventive medicine will occupy the best talent in the field of public health administration during the coming generation.

**Accidents.** Accidents cause a large toll of preventable injury and death in any community—particularly in a highly industrialized community. Most important are:

> *a.* Industrial accidents.
> *b.* Accidents in the home, such as falls, burns, carbon monoxide poisoning, etc.
> *c.* Automobile accidents.

*Industrial Accidents.* The health department may aid in prevention of industrial accidents through:

> *a.* Insistence upon installation of industrial safeguards in industrial hazards of all types.
> *b.* Aid in "Safety First" education of all industrial employees. (See chapter on Industrial Hygiene.)

*Home Accidents.* Many accidents in the home will be prevented if the health department takes an active part in the dissemination of general information concerning the common cause of these accidents and the simple methods of prevention. A program of education of adults and children through the schools, the newspapers and other sources of information has been shown repeatedly to yield measurable results in the actual reduction of suffering and death from home accidents.

*Traffic Accidents.* The health department should take an active part, in co-operation with the Highway Department, in the regulation of automobile traffic so that the rising toll of injury and death from automobile accidents may be curtailed. It is the function of the health department through the school health service to aid in the instruction of children in regard to traffic regulations in order to teach them the necessary precautions that are required in prevention of injury from this important source.[7]

**General Health Education.** It is the duty of the health department to disseminate information in relation to all the various matters that pertain to proper living. It must be confessed that much of this information will not be utilized. One can have little expectation that proper personal hygiene and health habits can be developed in the adults of the community by general educational measures. As stated previously, health education must be largely accomplished in childhood during the habit-forming period.

---

[7] It is interesting to note that automobile accidents now occupy the place formerly held by typhoid fever as a cause of death. Forty years ago the specific death rate for typhoid fever was 25 ± per 100,000, with no deaths from automobile accidents. Today these rates are exactly reversed.

## REFERENCES

1. *A Manual of Suggestions for the Conduct of Periodic Examinations of Apparently Healthy Persons.* Published by the American Medical Association.

2. Bigelow, G. H. and Lombard, H. L. *Cancer and Other Chronic Diseases in Massachusetts.* Pub. by Houghton Mifflin Company. 1933. (See particularly valuable and comprehensive bibliography.)

3. Hedley, O. F. *An Analysis of 5116 Deaths Reported as Due to Coronary Occlusion.* U.S.P.H. Reports. 1939, Vol. 54, p. 972.

4. MacDonald, E. J. *The Evolution of Cancer Control in Massachusetts.* Women's Medical Journal. September, 1938.

5. *Public Health Laws and Policies in Massachusetts.* Document No. 1200 of the Legislature of the Commonwealth of Massachusetts. 1936.

6. Boas, E. P. *The Unseen Plague: Chronic Disease.* J. J. Augustin, New York. 1940.

7. Roemer, M. I. *A Program for Preventive Medicine for the Individual.* Milbank Memorial Fund Quarterly. 1945, Vol. 23, p. 209.

8. Dorn, H. F. *Illness from Cancer in the United States.* Reprint No. 2537 from the Public Health Reports. 1944.

9. *Cancer Control.* Committee on Publications, 483 Beacon Street, Boston, Mass. 1943.

10. Levin, M. L. *The Epidemiology of Cancer from the Viewpoint of the Health Officer.* Am. Jour. Pub. Health. 1944, Vol. 34, p. 611. (Contains a good bibliography.)

11. *Medicine in Modern Practice.* New York Academy of Medicine. Paul B. Hoeber, Inc., New York. 1942.

12. Dublin, L. I. and Lotka, A. J. *Twenty-five Years of Health Progress.* Metropolitan Life Insurance Company, New York. 1937.

13. Smillie, W. G. *Preventive Medicine and Public Health.* The Macmillan Company, New York. 1946.

14. Publications of the American Heart Association, 1790 Broadway, New York City.

15. Publications of the American Society for the Control of Cancer, 350 Fifth Avenue, New York City.

See also current publications, as for example:

*The Journal of Gerontology.*

*Cancer Research.*

*Vital Statistics of the U. S. Bureau of the Census.*

Reports of the Metropolitan Life Insurance Company, the National Institute of Health, and others.

# PART IV

# ORGANIZATION OF PUBLIC HEALTH PROGRAMS

Part IV

ORGANIZATION OF CRIME—PRISONS, TREATMENT, ETC.

# CHAPTER XXIX

## MUNICIPAL HEALTH ADMINISTRATION

MUNICIPALITIES are secondary governmental units incorporated within the larger primary governmental unit,—the state. The state is the sovereign power. Municipalities are granted certain prerogatives, usually by special charter from the state. These charters vary greatly as to powers and functions. In some instances the city may be given almost complete autonomy. New York City is an example. The practice of public health as a municipal function shows almost as many variations in the different cities in the United States as there are cities. The population of a city may be a few thousand or many millions. The city may be a residential suburb, or it may be almost completely industrialized. There is also a great variation in the per capita wealth of cities, in distribution of racial groups, as well as in the types of municipal organization.

It is obviously impossible, therefore, to set up exact criteria in relation to municipal health department administration that would be applicable or suitable for all cities in the United States. Theoretically, we should be able to outline a health program, enumerate the personnel required, state in detail the duties and activities of each person and propose a suitable detailed budget. Such a plan would have little practical usefulness in any given situation. The most practicable method of approach is to state certain principles of health department organization, define a program within broad limitations, cite examples of successful health programs, and suggest the lines of probable future development. We shall discuss first the functions of a municipal health department, and then consider the formation of a suitable organization to carry out these functions.

### FUNCTIONS OF A MUNICIPAL HEALTH DEPARTMENT

The city health department is a primary unit of health service. The state renders advisory service with some degree of supervision, and may actually take charge of a situation in an emergency. The city health department renders actual personal service to its people. Certain functions and activities are accepted as good health department practice—applicable to all municipalities, large or small.

Established functions of a local health service are:

1. Vital Statistics.

2. Communicable Disease Control, including tuberculosis and venereal disease.

391

3. Child Hygiene in all its phases, including prenatal and maternity work, infant and preschool hygiene, school hygiene, etc.

4. Sanitation, including general sanitation, food and milk control, and all allied subjects.

5. Public Health Laboratory.

6. Health Education.

In addition to the generally accepted functions of a local health service, there are other community needs that are becoming more and more apparent as a public health responsibility, and thus logically a function of an official health department. Among these functions may be mentioned the following:

A. The whole field of adult health promotion. Included in this category are:

1. Efforts toward the promotion of the health of persons with cardiac disease.

2. Amelioration and rehabilitation of individuals suffering from rheumatism.

3. Efforts toward cancer control.

4. Protection of the health of the industrial worker.

5. Mental hygiene in all its aspects.

6. Prevention of injuries and deaths from accidents.

B. In addition, the health department may be charged with the duty of caring for the sick poor in their homes or in institutions.

C. A few health departments have also been empowered to administer public clinics and hospitals for all ages and all groups of the population.

Administrative procedures have not been worked out in many communities to provide for these various functions. Some forward-looking health departments, however, have attempted to meet the most obvious community needs in an acceptable way, drawing upon past experience to guide them in initiating the new administrative technics which must be devised to meet new conditions, or new public requirements.

We shall not attempt in this text to indicate all the possible ways that a local health officer may meet his particular community needs. Each administrator must use his own initiative and judgment in reaching his own solutions.

We have attempted to point out the broad scope of a local health service, and to indicate the probable lines of future development. But the construction of an exact administrative pattern, or the projection of a plan to meet all contingencies, in each local community, is not feasible.

Certain well-established functions of a local health service may be presented in some detail.

**Vital Statistics.** The recording of births and deaths has only recently been considered a health department function. We now realize that vital statistics, if properly interpreted, are a real index of the success of the health program. It is essential that this governmental function be incorporated in health department practice. Births are reported directly to the health department on standard forms, by the persons responsible for the delivery of the child,—physician, midwife or lying-in hospital. The report should be made within ten days of the birth. The original certificates are sent to the state; duplicate certificates are kept in fireproof vaults, properly filed, and are constantly consulted. They are a permanent record and are of immeasurable value.

Deaths are reported to the health department immediately, usually before a burial permit may be granted. The certificate is signed by the physician who attended the last illness and should be properly filled out as to cause of death in accordance with the international classification. The original birth and death certificates are forwarded to the state health department. Duplicates are kept in the health department files.

In smaller health departments, the division of vital statistics may also keep the morbidity records for the division of communicable disease. In this instance, the division will have charge of all statistical data, the making of charts, spot maps and graphs, the records of all sorts, such as clinic service records, immunization records, records of medical examination of school children, etc. The analysis of all the statistical data and the compilation of material for the annual reports and for other purposes are functions of the division of vital statistics.

**Communicable Disease Control.** The specific administrative methods for control of the various communicable diseases have been discussed in detail in previous chapters. The major activities of this division in any city health department are related to the communicable diseases of childhood, such as diphtheria, scarlet fever, measles, whooping cough, etc. Many city health departments assume only the simple functions of isolation, quarantine and release of cases. These activities are carried out by a sanitary inspector or a public health nurse. This is an antiquated practice. Each visit to a case of communicable disease should be an instructional visit. It is the function of the health department to aid practicing physicians in early and exact diagnosis, and to determine, if possible, the source of infection. It should also teach each family the essentials in prevention of cross infection in the family, as well as the methods of protection of the public. There must be an especially close relationship between the divisions of communicable disease and of school hygiene, as well as an integration with the public health laboratory service of the city.

It is a function of the municipality to make suitable provision for hospitalization of communicable disease. In general, hospitalization is resorted to only when the patient cannot receive satisfactory care at home, or cannot be properly isolated under home conditions. In certain diseases, hospitalization is of definite value in preventing the spread of the infection, notably in typhoid fever and, to a lesser degree, tuberculosis. Hospitalization seems to play little part in prevention of the spread of diphtheria, scarlet fever, measles, poliomyelitis, cerebrospinal fever and many other diseases. Thus, hospitalization for communicable disease is in great part not strictly a preventive, but rather an alleviatory procedure. It is undoubtedly a factor in reduction of the mortality, if not the morbidity, that is produced by these diseases. Many health officers question whether or not hospitalization for communicable disease is a primary function of the city health department. If we accept the criterion that the health department should do all in its power, not only in the prevention of disease, but also in the prolongation of life and prevention of suffering and death, then hospitalization for communicable disease, including tuberculosis, falls within the scope of the city health department.

It is the function of this division to stimulate in every way the standard immunization procedures, particularly for smallpox and diphtheria. The department must keep abreast of the times concerning new, practicable, specific preventive measures that may be discovered, and should be alert to use them. For example, the use of suitable procedures in the preven tion or abortion of measles may be attempted.

Should the health department give free immunization for prevention of diphtheria or smallpox to all children who apply, or only to those families that are too poor to afford a family physician? This question has caused endless controversy. The obvious answer is that the practicing physician should protect (as a routine measure) all those children who are under his care. Until this becomes a common practice, the munici-pality is compelled to protect itself from invasion of infection by offering to immunize all the children who have not been protected by their family physicians. It is the duty of the health department to do everything in its power to secure community immunity by every possible means, and to educate the people as to the value of the various immunization pro-cedures. In a few cities the health departments have given up free im-munization clinics, and have paid private physicians a small fee for each immunization of the indigent in their private practice.

Another function of this division is to provide a readily available supply of biological products for treatment of needy cases of communicable disease. This again is primarily a function of public welfare rather than a preventive method, but immediate necessity knows no rule nor law. These cases are often urgent emergencies, so that it is the most satisfactory policy to administer the distribution of biological products, such as diph-theria antitoxin, through the communicable disease division of the health department.

The division keeps careful continuous records of all the reportable diseases: an active file of all current cases under observation, and a closed file of discharged cases. It collects and analyzes the epidemiological data in relation to sources of infection, keeps a cross index of contact infec-tions, and a current file of carriers.

*Tuberculosis Control.* It is the function of the health department to reduce tuberculosis morbidity and mortality. Details concerning the required activities have been discussed in a previous chapter. The major activities are centered around case finding, domiciliary care and hospitalization. The latter occupies so much attention and requires so much money that the former activities are often neglected. The domiciliary program is essentially:

a. Early diagnosis—secured by educational methods and diagnostic facilities.
b. Continuous follow-up service in the homes, usually by public health nurses.
c. Observation and control of contacts, particularly the younger children in the home.

Standard practices may be divided into four groups:

a. Case finding.
b. Clinic service.
c. Field nursing.
d. Institutional care.

An active service would be organized on approximately the following scale:

a. Facilities should be provided for 1,500 clinic visits for each 100 annual deaths from pulmonary tuberculosis in the community.
b. The file of active cases should be equal to at least 5 cases per annual death.
c. Case finding work should uncover at least two new cases each year per annual death.
d. An average of at least three clinic visits annually should be made for each person registered in the clinic. One fourth of these cases should be in the incipient stage.
e. An average of three contacts should be examined for each new case found.
f. At least fifty nursing visits should be made to homes for each annual death. A fourth of these visits should be to post-sanatorium cases.
g. Provision should be made for at least one hospital bed (occupied 300 days) per annual death from the disease. Many communities have supplied two beds for tuberculosis per annual death. Twenty-five per cent of hospitalization should be for incipient cases.

These criteria represent quantity and not quality of service. They give some index of the relative importance of the various activities, as well as an index of the emphasis that has been placed on each by the active municipal health departments of the United States. They are approximate only, and should be modified to meet local conditions and special needs.

*Prevention of Gonorrhea and Syphilis.* The attempted control of gonorrhea and syphilis is a definite, but very baffling, function of the municipality, particularly the smaller city. In so far as possible, these diseases should be handled in just the same manner as other communicable disease. Isolation of the patient is seldom feasible and defeats its own purpose. It is used only for intractable, vicious, nonco-operative patients, and as a last resort. Reporting of these diseases to the health department by physicians has become of increasing value. Usually, the physicians report to the health department by some key number, giving name and identification only if the patient refuses treatment and becomes a menace to the community. The health department can be of great service to those individuals who neglect their treatment, by a tactful follow-up plan which reminds the patients that continued treatment is essential to their health as well as a matter of community benefit.

Educational methods aimed toward the prevention of syphilis and gonorrhea are utilized as actively as possible. They undoubtedly have some value. Treatment of cases of the disease is primarily the function of the practicing physician. Many cities, through the state health department, supply arsenicals, heavy metals, and antibiotics as well, to the physicians, either free or at cost. The health department may establish clinics for the adequate treatment of the indigent. This is a special problem, as these diseases are in great part "class diseases" accompanying poverty and ignorance, and the treatment is prolonged and expensive. Organization of public venereal disease clinics is not practicable in small cities (less than 50,000 population). In many cities, the venereal disease clinics are organized as an integral part of the local hospital outpatient services. The clinics are supervised by the health department and sometimes given a subsidy, but their administration is the sole responsibility of the hospital. This plan assures high quality of the therapeutic service, but frequently the most important part of the clinic service, namely the epidemiological work, is neglected by the hospital. Standard practice requires facilities for about 750 registrants per 100,000 population, with an average of at least 15 visits per annum for each case of syphilis that is accepted in the clinic. The service is of little public health value, if it is organized simply as a treatment clinic. Best results are secured through follow-up of the cases, determination of sources of infection, the returning of lapsed cases for treatment, and the bringing in of the immediate contacts to the clinic for examination. If the simple epidemiological principles that are utilized in other contact infections are applied in the administration of venereal disease control programs, excellent results will be obtained. The important thing to remember is that early diagnosis and prompt treatment are our most successful measures in venereal disease control. The actual number of infectious cases of syphilis in the community at any one time is quite small. One should concentrate on finding them and bringing them under treatment.

**Child Hygiene.** Activities in this division are usually divided into four groups:

    *a.* Prenatal and maternity service.

    *b.* Infant hygiene—from birth through one year of life.

    *c.* Preschool hygiene—from one to five years, inclusive.

    *d.* School hygiene—from six years to adult life.

Everyone will agree that the municipality has a special responsibility in the safeguarding of its children, protecting them from illness, and preparing them for a productive, healthful and useful life. Health departments have met their share of this responsibility. In some instances they have carried out activities that more properly are the responsibility of the parent and the practicing physician. These activities should be considered as temporary, and the functions should be released to the private physicians as soon as physicians are willing to assume them.

A good example is prenatal and postnatal care. The physician or hospital that delivers the mother should have the responsibility for medical phases of prenatal and postnatal care. This plan has not always been followed. To meet a real need, prenatal and postnatal services have been developed for the poor by voluntary agencies in many cities. A few health departments have organized prenatal clinics. Most health officers believe that this clinic service is not a function of the health department. The public health nurses of the department may be of great aid in education of prospective mothers as to proper prenatal procedures, and may also aid the obstetrician or lying-in hospital by adequate prenatal and postnatal nursing service. It is the personal opinion of the author that the health department should not develop its own prenatal clinics, but should encourage the private physicians and hospitals to offer this service. The health department may aid these agencies through its nursing service and through its educational work.

The supervision of midwives, through licensing, instruction and inspection is a health department function, as is also the inspection and licensing of lying-in hospitals.

*Infant hygiene* is a development of recent years and has met a real need. The clinical phases of this activity are a function of the practicing physician rather than the official health department, and the responsibility for this type of service is gradually being assumed by the progressive physicians. Until such time as this work can be allocated to the physicians where it really belongs, it will probably be carried as part of municipal health department practice. Since a small proportion of the population is too poor to afford the services of a physician, the maintenance of a well baby clinic for indigent families will probably continue to be a necessary function of the health department.

A well-organized service for the supervision of well babies requires health department facilities for at least 1,200 well baby clinic visits per

1,000 live births, with an average of four visits a year per child registered. This requirement should decrease greatly as practicing physicians gradually assume this activity.

The field nursing service in child hygiene is a useful and valuable health department activity. At least 30 per cent of all live births will be registered for field nursing service, and an average of four visits per annum should be made to each baby registered. An additional activity is the supervision of baby boarding homes; monthly inspection, usually by the public health nurse, is required.

*Preschool Hygiene*—ages 1 to 5 years, inclusive. The clinic service for children of this age group is just as important a function of the health department as the infant hygiene service.

The great proportion of this work should be carried on by the private physicians, but provision should be made for children whose parents are too poor to pay for this care. This is the age period of communicable disease, and all possible methods should be employed to protect these children from the ravages of these diseases. Dental hygiene should receive its greatest impetus in the preschool age group, and mental hygiene makes some of its most important contributions to children under 6 years of age.

Proper nutrition of the preschool child will have a profound effect upon his growth, his physical and mental vigor.

Physical defects that are discovered at this period of life can frequently be checked in their incipiency. More and more, health departments are placing emphasis on a well-planned well-child program for children of the preschool age group. This is a sound policy. It has been adopted in many cities and has met a real need. This activity should gradually be transferred to practicing physicians. Nursing service consists of instructional visits to the parents and is very valuable. The nurse knows community resources, and can help the family in the proper utilization of community facilities.

*School Hygiene.* Care of the health of the school child is an obvious municipal function and is a joint responsibility of the Departments of Education and Health. The educational features of the program should be allotted to the former bureau. The medical and nursing services are a health department function. Standard practice requires morning inspection, weighing and measuring once a month, usually by the teacher, nursing inspection for detection of minor infections of the skin and scalp at least once a year, and annual sanitary inspection of the school buildings. All the school children should be given a careful physical examination at least three times during school life. An opportune time to examine the children is when they are in the first, fourth and ninth grades. The correction of defects of school children that are found on physical examination is not a function of the health department. Some health departments provide facilities for dental service to the younger children

—preventive dentistry—and a few arrange for postural clinics under medical and nursing guidance. Home visits by school nurses are a very effective procedure.

Health education in the schools is essentially a pedagogical function and is not a direct health department function. The department may aid in instruction of teachers, may supply materials for teaching, etc. A general discussion of the functions and organizations of a school health service has been presented in a previous chapter, and need not be elaborated further here.

**Sanitation.** The ideas concerning the functions and scope of activities of the city health department in relation to sanitation have changed greatly in recent years. Several major activities that formerly were part of health department practice have been abandoned or transferred to other municipal departments. For example, the practice of fumigation and terminal disinfection has been given up entirely. Garbage and waste disposal has been transferred to the department of public works. Supervision of the esthetic side of city cleanliness, such as rubbish collection, disposal of dead animals and removal of nuisances is not a real function of the health department and should be transferred to another department. Other municipal activities which are related to health protection, but are not a direct health department responsibility are: control of smoke, accident prevention, supervision of recreational facilities of the city, and many others. The control of housing, and particularly prevention of overcrowding, the control of vermin and fly breeding and the control of mosquito breeding are more definitely related to prevention of illness and are frequently made a part of health department activity.

Certain functions of city government are practically always allotted to the health department.

*Milk Sanitation.* It is the function of the health department to insure an adequate safe milk supply for the city. Carefully drawn municipal regulations are invaluable in this respect. The "Standard Milk Ordinance," which has been sponsored by the United States Public Health Service, has been widely adopted as a practical and workable technic. Eventually, there should be a nation-wide acceptance of uniform milk standards. A careful check is made on all pasteurization plants and on the facilities for distribution of milk. The trend is to consider dairy inspection as a joint responsibility of the *state* departments of agriculture and health, rather than a municipal function. There should be uniform state-wide regulations for all dairies within the state and reciprocal arrangements with other states wherever milk is shipped from one state to another.

The city health department has an additional check on all milk supplies through frequent sampling and suitable laboratory testing. A routine of one laboratory test of each dealer's milk each month is a usual practice. Where no state-wide uniform dairy inspection exists, the health department may be compelled to assume the responsibility for dairy inspection of the milk shipped into the city.

*Inspection of the cleanliness and the sanitary facilities of food handling establishments* is a health department function. This includes instruction of food handlers in methods of maintaining general cleanliness. Medical examination of food handlers as a routine by the city health department is not a feasible procedure. Some cities require that all food handlers shall have at least one stool and urine examination for the typhoid carrier state, as well as examination for carriers of *Endamoeba histolytica*. The value of such a procedure is questionable. The health department has charge of enforcement of city regulations concerning the proper cleanly sanitary preparation, storage and marketing of food, particularly of meat and meat products, fish, shellfish and all other foods of this type. Uniform state regulations in regard to all these matters would greatly simplify the administration of regulations relating to food sanitation.

*Supervision of the safety and sanitary quality of the city water supply* is an important health department function. Administrative matters relating to the water supply system are not directly within its province. The health department also has supervision over the sewage disposal system of the city. The safety of the disposal system should be tested by frequent bacteriological and chemical tests. The sanitary inspection service also enforces the regulations of the city concerning individual sewage disposal installations, such as septic tanks, privies, etc. Inspection of ventilation and illumination of public buildings, housing inspection, and enforcement of rules and regulations in regard to industrial hygiene and many other activities are carried out by the sanitary inspection division of the health department.

Sanitary water supply and sewage disposal systems are of wide importance, far beyond the boundaries of the city which they serve. The principle has been clearly recognized, and state governments are gradually assuming more responsibility for the development and for the control of effective water supply and sewage disposal systems throughout the state. Because of interstate relationships, the national government has greatly aided the states in these matters.

**Laboratories.** The city health department provides laboratory facilities for two major purposes:

*a.* A laboratory check on the safety and quality of the water supply, and the milk supply, as well as other foods.

*b.* A diagnostic laboratory service for the division of communicable disease.

A small laboratory is not a practical or economical unit. A city with a population of 50,000 or more may organize a laboratory for simple diagnostic tests. The more complicated and difficult procedures, as well as those laboratory procedures that are best done on a large scale, should be handled by a large, central, preferably a state, laboratory.

An active laboratory will do at least 6,000 annual laboratory examinations per 100,000 population. This should include daily bacteriological examination of the water; at least 60 bacteriological tests of pasteurized milk, and 200 tests of raw milk for each 100,000 gallons of milk consumed.

In some cities, a joint or combined municipal laboratory is established in a hospital, which does all the clinical laboratory tests that are required, and also carries out the public health laboratory work. These laboratory activities may be supported on a co-operative basis, or the city may purchase its laboratory services under contract. This type of organization is fraught with administrative difficulties, but it must be admitted that a single community laboratory, carrying out all necessary laboratory functions, is an ideal plan, at least in theory.

**Popular Health Instruction.** Health education is a primary function of the city health department that is frequently neglected. The technic of health instruction has been discussed in a previous chapter. All members of the department should do everything in their power to acquaint the public with the health problems of the city and the suitable methods for their solution. Popular health instruction should be carried on in a dignified, sensible manner. This is an essential point in holding the respect of the medical profession in the city and in winning the confidence and support of the people.

*Industrial Hygiene.* It is the function of the health department to make and enforce regulations to prevent industrial accidents, to promote industrial safeguards and also to supervise the health of the workers in the dangerous trades. These activities are often incorporated in the sanitary inspection division.

*Adult Hygiene.* The development by health departments of clinic services for the early diagnosis of cancer, heart disease, and other degenerative diseases, is in its initial stages. If a comprehensive plan of prepayment for medical care is organized in the community, then it is obvious that the periodic physical examination of the presumably well adult would become an integral part of the plan. In this case, the health department would limit its facilities for the early detection of degenerative disease to the indigent and needy person.

The great field of rehabilitation of individuals who have some permanent physical or mental handicap is as yet largely unexplored by public health administrators. In many communities, voluntary agencies have promoted rehabilitation facilities, with some success. Notable is the work of the National Tuberculosis Association, the National Society for the Prevention of Blindness, and others.

**Organization of Cancer Clinics.** Dr. Elise L'Esperance of Memorial Hospital in New York has been a pioneer in the organization of clinics for the early detection of cancer. The Strang Cancer Prevention Clinic, which was established under her personal auspices, demonstrated that there was a real public demand for this type of health service.

The principles of organization are that persons in adult life who are presumably well, may secure a comprehensive physical examination for the purpose of detecting early manifestations of degenerative diseases, and also may obtain advice in regard to the proper regulation of life so that, in so far as possible, degenerative diseases may be avoided, ameliorated, or postponed. The service is primarily for the early detection of cancer, but obviously the physical examination, if well done, will detect other degenerative diseases as well.

Most of the clinics of this type, that have followed the general plan of the Strang Clinic, have been established in well-equipped hospitals where diagnostic facilities are readily obtainable, and a varied group of consultants are available; but it is possible for a health department to establish this type of clinic in a health center if suitable diagnostic facilities are at hand.

The clinic should be open to any individual, apparently well, who wishes to have a thorough physical examination, as a precaution against the development of cancer. It has been customary to request the applicant to pay for the actual cost of these examinations. If any abnormal condition is found, the patient is not treated, but is referred to his own physician, to whom is sent a full statement of the findings of the clinic.

The clinic should be organized as a part of a medical or public health facility, since the equipment and personnel are required for part time only—perhaps two afternoons a week. Thus the nurses, social service workers, secretarial aid, the x-ray technician, and the other facilities that are needed for the clinic may be assigned to it from the general services. The key to success is the physician in charge, who should be skilled in all phases of the detection of early cancer, and thoroughly interested in this type of preventive medicine. He should serve on a part-time basis, but should be well paid for his work.

## ORGANIZATION OF MUNICIPAL HEALTH DEPARTMENT

We have discussed in some detail the functions of a city health department. Let us now consider how the department should be organized to render the proper services most economically and effectively. A brief review of general municipal organization is necessary.

There are two common types of municipal government: the mayor and council plan, and the city manager plan. Many modifications and variations of these two types exist. A minor plan is the commission form of city government. The commissioners are elected by popular vote, one for each major activity of city government. They serve as a committee of the whole in determining the general administrative policies of the city. Obviously, this is not a cohesive organization and cannot function effectively because of the lack of unified centralized responsibility.

**Mayor and City Council.** The mayor is the chief executive, elected by popular vote for a term of years. The legislative body formerly consisted of two chambers: the board of aldermen and the common council. This plan has been abandoned in most cities for the more workable system of a single common council. The members of this body are elected by popu-

SUITABLE PLAN FOR ORGANIZATION OF A HEALTH DEPARTMENT

IN A SMALL CITY (75,000 to 100,000)

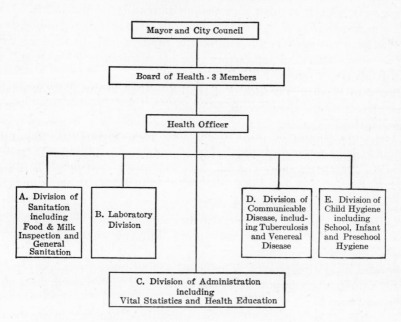

Each division has a full-time director.     The Health Officer assumes direct charge of Division C.

FIG. 30. *Suitable Plan for the Organization of a Health Department in a Small City.*

lar vote for a term of years, with overlapping terms of office. The chief functions of the council are:

*Advisory* to the executive. It determines the general policies in regard to management of the city government.

*Legislative.* It makes the regulations and ordinances of the city.

*Semi-judicial.* The council may hold public hearings in regard to certain matters relating to city policies.

*Fiscal.* It passes the city budget.

*Approval of Appointments.* The council approves the appointments of the executive. In many cities appointments are subject to civil service regulations as well.

**City Manager Plan.** The city manager plan has been found to be particularly well suited for the smaller cities of 50,000 to 100,000 population. A small city council is elected by popular vote. This body then selects a trained, experienced administrator as business manager of the city. The city manager is vested with executive powers and is charged with administration of city affairs. He is responsible to the city council and serves for a term of years, or at the pleasure of the council. He selects all the city personnel, with approval of the council, and manages the general affairs of the city.

Under either the mayor and council plan, or city manager plan, the city government is divided into various bureaus or departments. The different functions of city government are allocated to the various bureaus.

The health department is one of the fundamental divisions of city government. The most satisfactory type of organization is the board of health plan.

**Board of Health.** The Board of Health consists of three or five members, chosen by the chief executive of the city for a term of three to five years, with overlapping terms of office. The position is honorary, with no salary. Members should be representative citizens, interested in public affairs and familiar with the general principles of public health. Some of the members should be physicians. The major functions of the board are:

1. Selection of the health officer.

2. Determination of the general policies of the department. This includes approval of the budget and of appointments of the personnel by the health officer.

3. Semi-legislative powers. The board should make rules and regulations, which, when approved by the mayor and city council, have the effect of law.

4. Semi-judicial powers. The board may hold hearings in regard to certain matters pertaining to health affairs of the city.

The Board of Health meets at regular (monthly) intervals, or during emergencies at the call of the health officer. The health officer serves as a secretary of the board and is a member *ex officio*.

**Advisory Boards of Health.** In many communities the Board of Health has *advisory powers only*. The health officer is selected directly by the Mayor, and not by the Board of Health, and is a member of the mayor's cabinet. This plan has certain advantages, in that the chief executive can co-ordinate all municipal functions by the direct allocation of responsibility to each of his departmental or division heads. The plan has the great disadvantage that the position of health officer may become subject to political preferment, since the incumbent serves "at the pleasure" of the executive officer.

Many students of public administration object to the organization theory of administrative boards that are inserted between the chief administrative officer and his divisional directors. This certainly would not be an effective administrative procedure in the organization of a large private business, and the plan does not look well on an organization chart. But the community at large has continued to adhere to the plan of administrative boards in local departments of *education* and *public health,* although they have been eliminated in almost all other governmental divisions. The reasons for the retention of this policy are obvious, and the author believes that they are sound, despite the cumbersome nature of this type of organization.

**Health Officer.** The health officer is the executive of the health department. He should have administrative ability, as well as scientific training. The health officer should serve full-time, should be a physician and should have at least one year's formal training in public health, or its equivalent.[1]

It may not always seem feasible for cities with a population of less than 50,000 to employ a full-time qualified medical health officer. In such a case, it is not a wise policy to employ a part-time medical executive. A better plan is to form a joint city-county health department, for which a qualified full-time health officer may be employed to serve both the city and the surrounding contiguous territory. (See Chapter XXX, on Rural Health Administration.)

The health officer is appointed for a term of three to five years by the board of health. He may be appointed directly by the mayor or city manager.

The chief functions of the health officer are:

1. Organization and administration of all the activities of the health department. He should carry out the policies of the department in accordance with the general plan as determined by the board of health.

2. Selection of the personnel—with the approval of the board of health and in accordance with the general regulations of city government.

3. Preparation of the budget and responsibility for expenditures within its provisions.

4. Interpretation of the activities of the health department to the mayor and city council, and to the public at large.

5. Specific activities. In most health departments, except those of very large cities, the health officer himself carries on certain specific activities in addition to his general administrative duties, such as health education, communicable disease control, epidemiology, child health service, certain medical services, etc.

**The Public Health Council.** Health officers have found a public health council to be a very useful and effective body. It consists of from fifteen to twenty influential and representative citizens who are interested in public health or some of its phases. They may be selected by the health officer from social, professional and business organizations, and have no official status. The council may meet quarterly or on special call of the health officer. It acts in advisory capacity and serves to interpret the activi-

---

[1] Qualifications for health officers as recommended by the American Public Health Association will be found in the Appendix.

ties of the health department to the public, and to aid in carrying out the department's program in the most effective manner.[2]

**Divisions of the Health Department.** The organization should be as simple as is consistent with good administration. The number of divisions will vary somewhat in accordance with the size of the city. Even in very large cities there should be no more than ten divisions. The organization should be on a functional basis, in so far as possible. Basic divisions of activity are:

1. Administration.
2. Vital statistics.
3. Sanitation.
4. Communicable disease control, including tuberculosis and venereal disease.
5. Child hygiene, including all phases of this activity.
6. Public health nursing.
7. Public health laboratories.
8. Health instruction.

Various divisions of activity may be combined; for example, health instruction and also vital statistics may be included under the division of administration; the laboratory may be carried under the division of communicable disease control; public health nursing may be developed with the division of child hygiene. In very large organizations, subdivisions of various basic functional divisions may be required. For example, the division of sanitation may have subdivisions of:

*a.* General sanitary inspection.
*b.* Milk control.
*c.* Food control.
*d.* Industrial hygiene.

However the department may be organized, each division should have a full-time director, selected by the health officer and responsible to him for the activities of the division. Each division should be assigned certain definite functions with as little overlapping responsibility as possible.

**Staff Meetings.** The health officer should hold regular—usually weekly —meetings of the executive staff to discuss general policies of the department, to correlate the work of all divisions, and to iron out difficulties and misunderstandings. Each divisional director should be permitted to make the plans for his own department, in so far as they are in accordance with the general policies, and should have administrative charge of all the details within his province, including the handling of his personnel.

**Divisional Organization.** *Administration.* In all instances the health officer himself should have direct charge of this division and should employ the necessary clerical staff to conduct the ordinary business and

---

[2] See discussion of The Public Health Council, page 510.

carry on necessary correspondence. In some large cities a special executive, under supervision of the health officer, is given direct charge of detailed administrative procedures, such as control of purchases, of supplies, the pay roll, etc.

Popular health instruction is frequently placed under the direct supervision of the health officer and is not organized as a separate division with its own director. This important phase of work is a special responsibility which requires close attention. Very often the individual who is given direct charge of this activity is a person trained in the technic of mass education and is attached to the health officer's personal staff.

*Vital Statistics.* In large cities vital statistics should be organized as a separate division with a trained director and a competent staff. In smaller cities this activity may readily be amalgamated with the division of administration. The necessary clerical staff, trained in statistical methods, compiles, files and tabulates the data. Interpretation of the data is the important feature of vital statistics practice. If the health officer has no trained person on his staff who can do this work for him, it should come under his immediate supervision.

An alternative plan in smaller cities is to place vital statistics under the division of communicable disease. This plan has many advantages. The tabulation and recording of morbidity data may be included in the vital statistics activities. This gives an opportunity to check the morbidity against the mortality data. In such an organization, the director of the division of communicable disease would analyze and interpret all the vital statistics data, as well as the morbidity data, and would have direct charge of all vital statistics activities.

*Sanitation* is always organized as a separate division of activity, even in the smaller cities. In large cities there may be several subdivisions of work, each with its sub-director, as already noted. It is most important that the director of this division should be thoroughly trained in sanitary science and familiar with all the problems that arise in connection with environmental hygiene. Lack of appreciation of the importance of employing a trained man for this position is one of the weakest points in our health organization in the United States.

All matters related to or allied with general sanitation should be administered by this division. The possible exception is the laboratory work of the division. It is not good administrative practice to form two laboratories, one for sanitation and one for communicable disease. A better plan is to organize a separate division of laboratories which will serve all divisions of the health department.

*Control of communicable disease* is one of the major activities of the health department and is usually organized as a separate division with its own director. In the smaller cities, the health officer may assume direct charge of this activity. The director of this service must be a physician, competent in the diagnosis and methods of control of all types of communicable disease. The activities of this division are divided into three main groups:

a. General infectious disease control.
b. Control of tuberculosis.
c. Control of venereal disease.

In each of these subdivisions the type of activity is threefold:

a. Epidemiological.
b. Clinical, including provision for diagnosis and hospitalization if necessary.
c. Nursing supervision.

*General Infectious Disease Control.* The director of the division usually has personal responsibility for the control of general infectious diseases. In large cities he may have from one to several full-time medical assistants who aid in the diagnosis of communicable disease. Hospitalization for contagious disease may also be administered by this division. If the specialized plan of public health nursing is followed, communicable disease nurses are assigned to this division. Their activities are supervised by the director of communicable disease, and their nursing technic is supervised by the director of public health nurses.

a. *Tuberculosis.* The clinic service is organized by the division. The clinics are usually staffed by physicians who are expert in the diagnosis of tuberculosis and are employed part-time. The hospitalization of tuberculosis is also organized under this division. In some instances the municipal diagnostic clinics are staffed by personnel from the tuberculosis hospital. Field nursing service in tuberculosis may be specialized. It is organized on the same basis as other communicable disease nursing.

b. *Venereal Disease.* As in tuberculosis control, the clinic service is organized by the division of communicable disease, and staffed by part-time experts in the diagnosis and treatment of syphilis and gonorrhea. Nursing service for the clinics and for the follow-up work may be organized on a specialized nursing basis or under the generalized plan. The personnel required for tuberculosis and venereal disease clinics and the details of organization of these special services have been discussed in previous chapters.

*Child Hygiene.* The organization of the activities relating to child hygiene depends in part upon whether or not the city health department has charge of the school health service. An ideal arrangement is a division with a full-time medical director who has had special training in child hygiene. The major activities of the nursing service are centered in this division, so that public health nursing is often organized as a subdivision of child hygiene. When the specialized nursing plan is followed, the infant hygiene nurses and the school nurses are assigned to the division. Their general activities are supervised by the director of child hygiene and the details of their nursing technic are supervised by the director of nurses.

Many of the child hygiene activities in the city, such as prenatal work, postpartum visiting and instructional nursing visits to infants, may be carried out by volunteer organizations, such as the Visiting Nurse Association. If the work is well done, it is often advisable for the health department to subsidize the voluntary organizations, and assign certain definite activities to them. This subsidy represents purchase of services, and is sound administrative practice.

Well baby clinics may be organized by the division. The clinical staff is usually on a part-time basis—pediatricians who have special interest in child hygiene activities. The preschool clinics are organized on the same basis as the well baby clinics. Often no distinction is made between the two types of clinic; simply, the work in the later age periods is less intensive.

*School Hygiene Program.* This activity is organized by the Division of Child Hygiene. In large cities it may be a subdivision of work with its own director. In some cities the Department of Education has entire charge of the program. The "summer round-up" program of preparation of children about to enter school is a part of the general school hygiene program. The clinical activities of the whole school hygiene program are usually conducted by part-time physicians who aid the director of the division of child hygiene in the physical examination of the school children. If the specialized nursing service plan is followed, the school nurses are assigned to the division, and work under the director of the division. When the nurse devotes all her time to the school nursing program, fairly adequate service can be developed with one nurse to each 2,000 school children.

*Public Health Nursing.* A discussion of the advantages and disadvantages of the general plan of public health nursing as compared with the specialized plan has been given in a previous chapter. The general tendency, particularly in smaller cities, is to organize the nursing service on the generalized plan. Each nurse is assigned a geographic area. She carries on all types of public health nursing in her district. Reasonably adequate service requires one nurse per 2,000 population, if bedside nursing (morbidity service) is included, or one nurse per 5,000 population, if the nurse limits her activities to public health affairs. The nurse who is carrying on a generalized program will do various types of work which are related to the activities of various divisions of the health department, such as communicable disease control, tuberculosis visiting work, venereal disease follow-up, infant and preschool work, school nursing, nutritional work, etc. When the generalized plan is followed, therefore, it is essential to develop a special division of public health nursing with a director. The director should be a well qualified public health nurse with administrative ability. She should have the same status as other divisional directors. She must be in close touch with the other divisional directors, must be familiar with their plans, and must develop a nursing program that is in harmony with the work of the functional divisions.

If the specialized plan of nursing is followed, it is also a good administrative policy to develop a division of public health nursing with its own director. The director will supervise the technic of the field nurses, and will assign her personnel to the various functional divisions as required.

Even in the smaller cities where only five or six nurses are employed, one of the nurses should be selected as supervisor. She will be held responsible for the technical performance of the nursing activities. In smaller cities the public health nursing activities are frequently organized under the division of child hygiene, with a supervisor of nurses who is directly responsible to the director of this division.

*Laboratories.* The organization of the public health laboratory service is somewhat similar to public health nursing in that the activities relate to several divisions, and the service rendered is on a technical rather than on a functional basis. Though the laboratory serves several divisions, it should be organized—at least in large cities—as a separate division with its own director. The organization of the laboratory, as well as its detailed activities, have been discussed in a previous chapter. The essential feature of the organization is that the director shall be well trained in public health laboratory methods and interpretation, and shall have administrative ability. The director should be in close contact with other divisional directors and should develop his activities so that the laboratory will be of greatest service to them, and to the city as a whole. If possible, the laboratory should be under the same roof as the other divisions, and not in a distant public building or hospital.

In smaller organizations, it may be necessary to organize the laboratory under the division of communicable disease. The actual work is done by technicians. The director of communicable disease supervises the laboratory technic and interprets the laboratory results.

A few smaller cities have attempted to organize a joint clinical-public health laboratory, usually through co-operation with the local hospital. This is not a satisfactory plan from the administrative point of view because of the dual responsibility of the laboratory director. Frequently this plan has failed. It is a better arrangement for the health department to purchase laboratory service from the clinical laboratory of the local hospital than to attempt the formation of a joint laboratory. None of these makeshift arrangements is very satisfactory. Many health authorities believe that it is better to have no laboratory service at all than to develop a poor laboratory that gives unsatisfactory and unreliable results. It certainly is the obligation of the health department to provide rapid, accurate diagnostic laboratory services for the community. The state-subsidized branch laboratory plan is the most effective system that has been devised.

**Cost of Municipal Health Work.** A figure that is frequently set for an adequate public health program for a city is two dollars per capita per annum. This is exclusive of hospitalization for tuberculosis, care of the sick poor, or allied services and activities sometimes carried by the health department, such as garbage disposal, etc. The expenditures for health work by the average city in the United States is much lower than this figure—approximating a median of perhaps one dollar per capita. Since the great proportion of health officers will be working under average conditions, it seems best to arrange the budget on the basis of this latter figure. It is realized that the program will not be ideal, nor in fact, adequate, but it does serve the purpose of meeting actual conditions. It must be recognized that many functions which are logically the responsibility of the official health agency are carried out successfully by voluntary agencies, at no direct cost to the taxpayer. These activities may gradually be assumed by the health department. At the same time the health department may be carrying on activities which are not its true function. These may gradually be transferred to other bureaus of the city government, or in the case of many clinical activities, may be returned to the private practicing physician where they rightfully belong.

Those public health activities which are carried on by voluntary agencies can be correlated with the health department program in a very satisfactory way, and at no direct cost to the taxpayer, if the health officer (or his representative) serves on the executive committee of the voluntary agencies and aids in the determination of their general policies.

Allocation of departmental funds to the various divisions of activity is a difficult matter. There is no standard practice, since the health problems are so varied in the different cities and in different geographic areas of the United States. Furthermore, it may be wise for the health officer to direct special attention toward certain activities for a temporary period, to the relative neglect of other important functions. As a general guide the following distribution of funds may serve a useful purpose.

|  | Proportion of Total Funds, Per Cent |
|---|---|
| 1. Administration | 10 |
| 2. Vital Statistics | 5 |
| 3. Communicable Disease Control exclusive of hospitalization | 15 |
| 4. Sanitation | 10 |
| 5. Child Hygiene | 15 |
| 6. Public Health Nursing | 35 |
| 7. Laboratories | 5 |
| 8. Public Health Education | 3 |
| 9. Contingent Fund | 2 |

If, for example, the city has a population of 100,000 with a budget of $1.00 per capita, each of the above percentages can be translated directly into thousand dollar units. Thus, ten thousand dollars annually would be allotted to administration, five thousand dollars to laboratory work. Even if the municipal appropriation for health work is only 50 cents per capita, the same general distribution of funds to the various bureaus would be followed. Certain activities might be curtailed more than others. The most elastic portion of the budget centers around child hygiene and public health nursing.

The allotment given above is a very rough guide, but it illustrates the relative emphasis that has been placed on various activities by experienced administrators of municipal public health affairs.

Tuberculosis and communicable disease hospitalization has not been included in the above budget. These activities should always be segregated as they are not entirely public health functions. Standard practice requires two hospital beds per annual death from tuberculosis in the city. A city of 100,000 for example, with 50 deaths from tuberculosis a year should maintain at least 100 hospital beds which would cost a minimum of $1,200 per bed per year, or a total of $120,000. This item, together with an additional expenditure of $15,000 to $20,000 for hospitalization of diphtheria, scarlet fever and other communicable diseases, represents a total which is equal to the cost of all other health department activities. Some of the costs for hospitalization will, of course, be paid by the patients' families, so that the entire cost of these items is not met by taxation.

## HEALTH CENTERS

Health centers are being developed more and more in the large cities. This plan is the most significant development of the century in municipal health practice. It represents in reality a decentralization of the health services, which are brought directly to the people. The health center becomes a community center. It plays as important a part in the life of the people of the district and serves as essential a need as do the public schools. The reason for this is that the orientation of health work has changed. It is no longer a police function controlled from a central office by a series of official push buttons, but has become an educational force which reaches into the home and affects the family life of every resident of the city.

The health centers are located in strategic points in the municipality and furnish housing, not only for official health activities, but also for the various voluntary agencies in the city that are actually engaged in public health work and allied activities. Quarters for the official personnel, such as public health nurses and sanitary inspectors for the district, are located in the center, as well as the necessary facilities for clinic services, such as well baby clinics, tuberculosis clinics, immunization clinics, dental hygiene clinics, etc.

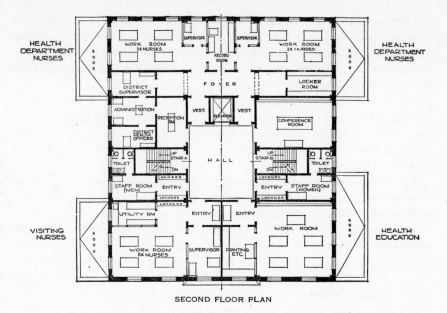

SECOND FLOOR PLAN

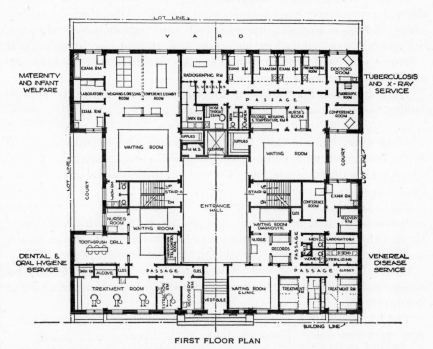

FIRST FLOOR PLAN

FIG. 31. *Health Center Design.* First floor: Maternity and Infant Welfare; Dental and Oral Hygiene; Venereal Disease Service; Tuberculosis and X-Ray. Second floor: administration, including health officer and health department nurses, and bedside nursing service. Note the space devoted to health education. (From *District Health Development in New York City.* 1939. E. A. Salmon, Consultant.)

Centers of this type can give adequate service to a limited zone only. The area assigned to a health center should not be greater than it can encompass. In Boston each health center serves about 60,000 persons, but in the more densely populated New York health districts, from 200,-000 to 300,000 people are assigned to one center.

The key to efficient development of health centers lies in the selection of well trained administrators as District Health Officers. The administration of the health activities at the center must be the direct responsibility of the District Health Officer—with certain exceptions which we shall describe:

The central bureaus of the health department will continue to be organized on a functional basis, of course, but the work in any given field will be administered in the district by the District Health Officer.

For example, the tuberculosis control services of the city are planned, organized and directed by the director of the division of tuberculosis control of the central bureau, but the activities of the tuberculosis service of any given district are the direct administrative responsibility of the District Health Officer.

In some cities, certain functions of the health department have remained centralized. For example, vital statistics, laboratories, epidemiology, industrial hygiene, supervision of water supply, sewage disposal, and general food sanitation, including milk control, are functions that cannot readily be decentralized and may be conducted best from the central health department office.

Those functions that represent *direct service* to the individual and his family, however, can best be decentralized in a large city, if they are to be of real benefit to the community. Noteworthy in this respect are all the various activities in child health promotion. This includes all school health work, well baby clinic service, dental hygiene, promotion of good nutrition, mental hygiene, etc. Control of the communicable diseases of childhood is included in this category.

Public health nursing is the most obvious service that requires decentralization. In fact, many cities that do not have health centers have divided the city into nursing zones, and have arranged for nurses' offices so that each nurse will have permanent headquarters in her zone.

Venereal disease clinic work, tuberculosis clinic activities, health education, and certain sanitary inspection activities, lend themselves well to decentralization.

The transition from a central health department of a large city, organized on a functional (vertical) basis, to a decentralized (horizontal) health district plan is fraught with serious administrative difficulty. The director of a functional division of venereal disease control is perfectly willing to have a well-equipped venereal disease clinic established in a health district, but he wishes to draw a circle around that clinic as his complete province, over which he must have absolute administrative control. If this should occur with each one of the divisional activities of the health center, then the District Health Officer would become nothing but a superintendent of a building and his chief concern would be the secretarial and janitorial work. The administrative intricacies that must be worked out in order to make the health center plan function effectively require consummate administrative tact and skill and a sincere desire on the part of all participants to make the plan really work. There should be a two-way administrative path between director and personnel whereby every person on the staff not only has his definite tasks to which he is assigned, but also may have the opportunity to suggest new and better methods of accomplishment.

The Commissioner of Health should take charge of the district health centers himself, and the District Health Officers should be responsible directly to him. In a very large city, there may be a Deputy Health Commissioner whose sole activity is the administration of health centers. Policies in regard to the details of allocation of functions to the health centers are worked out by the Commissioner and his cabinet. Each director of the seven or eight major functional divisions of the health department should be present at these conferences. Once the policies for the district health work have been determined and all conflicting interests reconciled, then the plan of work may be presented to the District Health Officers for execution. Each District Health Officer is responsible to the Health Commissioner or his Deputy for the conduct of the work, and not to the various directors of the functional divisions. For example, the director of the public health nursing division of the city will determine uniform nursing procedures for the whole city and will select, train, and supervise all the public health nurses. The supervisor of nurses within a given district will be responsible to the director of nurses for the quality of nursing service that is given. But all plans and programs for nursing service within the district will be worked out by the District Health Officer in conjunction with the nursing supervisor of his district, and in accordance with the master plan established for the whole city by the Commissioner of Health.

In some cities, divisional directors of functional services have resisted the decentralization plan and have felt that the district health units have stripped them of their authority and efficiency. Such is not the case. As a matter of fact, the plan gives the functional divisional director the time and opportunity to plan his broad general policies, yet relieves him of the many tedious details of petty administrative procedures. The divisional director makes the broad general plans; the District Health Officer executes them.

**Modified Health Center Plans.** It is generally conceded that the health center plan is applicable only to the very large cities with a population of 300,000 or more. But the smaller cities can adopt a modified health center plan with great benefit. The city may be divided into health districts, and the nursing services as well as all the well baby clinic services may readily be housed in suitable but inexpensive quarters in the center of each district. One city has utilized the public schools as health centers. In this city, public health nursing is on the generalized plan, but because of the importance of school nursing service, the nurse was given quarters in the school. Since the nursing work was generalized, the infant welfare clinic service was also established adjacent to the nurse's room in the school building and later the prenatal clinic was likewise established there.

The Visiting Nurse Associations, from the very first, decentralized their work and housed each nurse in her district. The reason for this was that the visiting nurses gave direct service to the people. Health departments may follow this example and adhere to the general principle that whenever direct services are to be given the center of the activity should be brought as closely and as conveniently as possible to the groups of people that are to be aided and protected thereby.

## PUBLIC HEALTH AND PUBLIC WELFARE

It must be recognized that many of the smaller cities (50,000 population or less) cannot afford to pay for the services of a full-time, well trained, experienced director of public welfare, and also a full-time, well qualified health officer.

Students of municipal government have asked the logical question: "Since public health and public welfare are such closely related functions of government, would it not be both economical and effective to fuse these two types of activity into one division of 'Public Health and Welfare,' and select one well paid executive to direct the work?"

The modern trend in public health administration is to devote more and more attention to *promotion of health*. The correction of physical defects of childhood, the improvement in nutrition, the hospitalization of communicable disease, including tuberculosis, many phases of public health nursing work, as well as many other like activities, have been developed by health officers as an integral part of the public health program; but, in reality, these functions are closely related to the realm of public welfare. Public health and public welfare have become so closely interrelated that we have no exact criteria as to just where a public health function ends and a welfare function begins.

A few cities have attempted to combine the governmental functions relating to the care of the indigent, sick, aged and infirm with the public health function of the city. The results, on the whole, have not been very satisfactory. The needs of the welfare division are so obvious and the necessity so immediate, that frequently a top-heavy welfare program is developed to the disadvantage of the far more important, but less evident, necessity for public health activities.

The success of such a plan depends, in great part, upon the selection

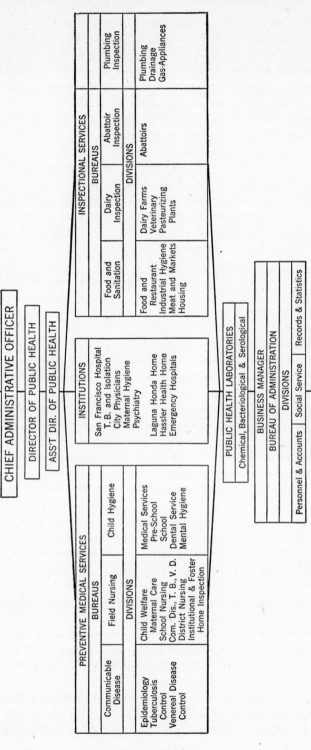

Fig. 32. *Organization Chart of the Department of Health of San Francisco,* August 1, 1943.

of the director of the service. He should have a medical degree, supplemented by suitable public health training. He should also be trained
and experienced in the broad field of sociology.

The promotion of the public health under such a program should be
the major, dominant and compelling force of the department. Public
welfare should not be the major function, but should be correlated with
the requirements of the public health needs of the community.

**Medical Care of the Indigent.** In some cities, the health department
is asked to assume the administration of all medical functions of the
municipality. Under these circumstances, the Department of Public
Welfare administers direct relief, social assistance, old age pensions,
protection of widows and orphans, and the like; but all medical, nursing,
and hospital administration is assigned to the department of public
health. The organization chart of the Department of Public Health of
San Francisco is a good example of this type of administrative plan.
(See Fig. 32.)

It will be noted that the health officer has divided the work into three
major sections:

1. Preventive Medical Services.
2. Inspectional Services.
3. Institutional section.

All the municipal hospitals are assigned to the Institutional Section.
This section has a full-time, well qualified administrative officer in charge,
who is responsible to the Director of the Health Department.

One real disadvantage of this type of organization is that the Hospital
Division absorbs so overwhelming a proportion of the total health department budget that other equally important activities of the Department may be overshadowed and receive less appreciation and perhaps
less consideration than they warrant.

In certain cities the domiciliary medical care of the sick poor is assigned to the Department of Health, chiefly because of the fact that it
is the only municipal department with physicians on its payroll. Often
the work of the health department physicians who care for the sick poor
is not closely co-ordinated with the outpatient services, nor with the ward
service of the municipal hospital. This results in little but detriment
to the patient.

Hydrick has suggested that in densely populated areas, there should
be one central Department of Medicine and Hygiene, with a strong, well-
trained medical director. There should be two distinct divisions of
activity, organized on a functional basis, with a qualified director in
charge of each. One division should be Public Medicine, and the other
Public Hygiene.

All community medical and nursing services, including hospitalization, should be administered under the Medical Division of this department, and all hygiene activities, including sanitation and health educa-

tion, should be carried out by the Division of Hygiene. Each Division should have its own specially trained personnel. Any and all community services requiring physicians or nurses would be assigned to the Medical Division. This would include all immunization procedures, prenatal and well baby clinics, and school medical service, as well as the administration of municipal hospitals and the bedside care of the sick poor.

## RELATIONSHIP OF THE CITY TO THE STATE HEALTH DEPARTMENT

The city health department should look to the state for advice and for leadership in public health affairs. The city forwards all vital statistics data to the state and gives information in relation to the prevalence of communicable disease. The state in turn renders valuable aid, particularly to the smaller cities and along those technical lines that cannot be developed satisfactorily by the city itself on a small scale. For example, the state can give expert advice on the sanitary engineering features of water supply and sewage disposal, furnish certain types of laboratory service, aid in tuberculosis hospitalization, and give advice on other technical and administrative matters.

## COMBINED CITY–COUNTY HEALTH DEPARTMENTS

The value of the combined plan of the city-county health department has been discussed in another chapter. It is a logical development. The rural areas in the environs of a city represent in reality a social unit and a population zone that is closely allied to the incorporated city by bonds of common interest. Often the municipality has too small a population to warrant the development of an adequate health program, with full-time health officer and other personnel. When the rural area surrounding the city is included in a health department organization, a very satisfactory program may be established which will be of mutual advantage to the municipality and the county. The city or incorporated towns included in such a health unit should always pay more per capita for the service than the rural area since they derive special benefits and receive additional service.

## APPRAISAL OF HEALTH ACTIVITIES

**History.** Dr. Charles V. Chapin,[3] health officer of Providence for over 40 years, had more influence on the advancement of sound municipal health practice in the United States than any other one man. He had a keenly analytical mind which cut through loose thinking, pretense and complacency. Whatever he did, he had a good reason for doing. If his results were unsatisfactory, he was the first to say so and to change the method of the work. His own chief critic, he subjected every practice to logical analytical

[3] Chapin, C. V.: "A Report on State Public Health Work Based on a Survey of State Boards of Health." Published by American Medical Association. 1915 (out of print).

processes. He is largely responsible for initiation of the appraisal of health activities in the United States.

In 1915, Dr. Chapin was asked to make a survey of the state health departments. This was the first comprehensive analysis of health activities in this country. It was published by the American Medical Association and is now out of print. It created a good deal of consternation in some of the more complacent state health departments, but eventually did a great deal of good. The Committee on Administrative Practice of the American Public Health Association, in 1921, sponsored a survey of health activities in all cities of over 100,000 population in the United States, 83 in number. The results were published in Bulletin No. 136 of the U. S. Public Health Service. In 1924, the U. S. Public Health Service made a survey of the 100 largest cities in the United States according to a comprehensive schedule. Bulletin No. 164 gives a report of the results, and contains a summary of health activities in each city, with a brief appraisal of the effectiveness of the health work, together with suggestions for betterment. This report was compiled in co-operation with the American Public Health Association.

The Committee on Administrative Practice of the American Public Health Association then developed a standard appraisal form for health work in municipalities. This schedule of appraisal was used extensively for several years, for the improvement of health work. Each year a contest was held, and the cities in each category that had the highest appraisal scores were suitably rewarded.

The annual health conservation contests between municipalities served a useful purpose during the pioneer stages of the development of local health administration. They were particularly valuable to health officers in demonstrating the deficiencies of the local health program to the fiscal authorities.

This type of appraisal was superseded by the "Evaluation Schedule" of the American Public Health Association. This schedule is based on the health conservation plan, and is intended to be used by health officers for the analysis and appraisal of community health programs.

The Association furnishes also a "Guide to the Evaluation Schedule." Each year the data that are obtained from the Evaluation Schedules are summarized in a booklet called "Health Practice Indices." [4] For example, in 1945 this booklet presented, in 71 line charts, the health practices of 243 local communities in the United States and Canada during 1943–44. These data, analyzed on the basis of median and quartile distribution of various types of activity, are of great value to the local health administrator in planning his own program. Graph 33,

[4] Health Practice Indices 1943–44. A collection of charts showing the range of accomplishments in various fields of community health service. Prepared by the Subcommittee on State and Local Health Administration for the Committee on Administrative Practice of the American Public Health Association, 1790 Broadway, New York, New York. 1945.

taken from "Health Practice Indices," gives the local health department expense per capita for 1944.

No suitable appraisal form has been devised for state health depart-

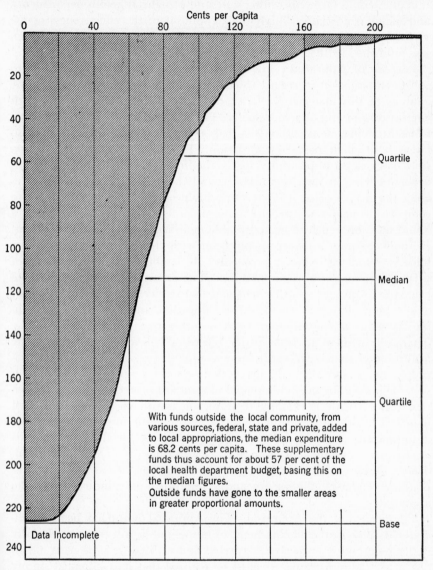

FIG. 33. *Cents Per Capita from All Sources Spent by Health Department.* Source: American Public Health Association "Health Practice Indices 1943–44."

ment practice. As noted above, the first state survey was made in 1915 by Dr. Chapin. The Conference of State and Provincial Health Authorities of North America, in 1925, requested that a survey be made of the organization, activities, personnel, salaries, and expenditures of the various state health departments. This was done by the International Health Division of the Rockefeller Foundation and published by the U. S. Public Health Service as Bulletin No. 184. This report is simply a compilation of essential facts concerning state and provincial health departments, and includes no critical analysis or appraisal of the effectiveness of the various programs. A revision of Bulletin No. 184, as a second edition, was published in 1932, with a third edition in 1943.[5]

**Purpose of Appraisal.** The primary purpose of the appraisal is to collect information in regard to current administrative practice, and by analysis of this material to derive certain concrete standards of health administration and of achievement. The material can be made available to health department officials for their information and utilization, in so far as it fits their particular situation. The appraisal has great utility, since it gives an opportunity for methodical self-analysis by the health department of its own organization and methods of procedure. It enables the health officer to determine his progress from year to year; to compare his achievements with those of previous years; and serves as a sound basis on which to make suitable modifications in future programs. He may compare his own organization with that of other cities of the same size and with similar problems. He is able to judge the value of progressive, successful, new methods. The appraisal gives him concrete evidence to present to other agencies in the city that are doing health work—both official, as the Board of Education, and unofficial—concerning the value of co-ordination of all health activities. It encourages the health department to keep better records. The appraisal enables the health officer to make a readily understandable presentation of his activities to the governing body in order to secure proper legislation or a suitable budget for the development of standard procedures or new activities. It is particularly valuable in aiding the health officer to secure a well balanced health program for his city. By providing minimum standards as to quantity of service for various phases of public health work, a basis is provided for judgment as to adequacy in quantity of the service rendered. Quality of service is largely dependent on fitness and integrity of those rendering the service and is indicated only indirectly by the appraisal.

**Significance of the Appraisal.** The Appraisal Form has been of undoubted value in the advancement of municipal health practice. If fully understood and if properly interpreted and utilized, it is of great aid to any health administrator. It must be realized that it is intended simply as a relative measure of health activity of a community. It serves an excellent purpose as a means of self-analysis and self-criticism of effi-

---

[5] Mountin, J. W. and Flook, Evelyn: *Distribution of Health Services in the Structure of State Government.* Public Health Bulletin No. 184 (third edition). U. S. Government Printing Office, Washington, D. C. 1943.

ciency of the program. Its obvious defect is that, in great part, it is a measure of *quantity,* rather than *quality,* of work.

Health officers should be warned particularly against the tendency to become so involved in the intricacies of scoring and numerical application of procedures that they obfuscate the real purpose and value of the appraisal.

Everyone recognizes that it is impossible to place an absolute *numerical value* on most phases of health work, or to gauge the effectiveness of health service on a mathematical basis. The scoring system is simply a mechanical device, like a graph or chart, which enables the observer to picture the whole situation. One cannot weigh enthusiasm, devotion, intelligence and diplomacy of the personnel. No score is given to the qualities of administrative acumen or scientific accuracy of members of the department. One public health laboratory may do 5,000 examinations poorly and get a good score. Another laboratory may do half as many examinations and do them well; yet the appraisal form will give the higher rating for the poor work. It is, in fact, impossible to give an accurate numerical valuation which will represent true quality of service. Many services may be of little value, or no value at all, because of a poorly planned program or untrained personnel. For example, the number of nursing visits that are made is not important. Rather one would wish to know the actual content of each nursing visit. What good does each nursing visit do? And what is the cost?

### Appraisal of Public Health Nursing

The National Organization for Public Health Nursing has developed an appraisal form for public health nursing services in local communities. The schedules include all the nursing services of a community, including industrial nursing and also hourly bedside nursing care. A staff of experts is available at the National Headquarters to make appraisals of community nursing services on request, and to aid departments of public health in the organization of nursing programs.

**Summary.** The health officer should recognize the inherent value of the appraisal form, but should not take the numerical valuation of the various schedules too seriously. He should recognize that the appraisal form *per se* does not emphasize the most important factors in good health work; namely, quality of service, qualifications of personnel, economy of operation and suitability of programs to meet particular situations.

The schedule of the appraisal form should not be the index by means of which the health officer determines his future problems. Rather, the health department should use the appraisal form primarily as a means to measure progress from year to year. But the health officer must use his own judgment as to the relative importance of various departmental activities that may be required to meet the needs of his particular situation. His effort is directed toward accomplishing the greatest real service that he can, with the resources that are available to him. New activities should be developed along those lines that are of greatest importance to his particular community, and not in accordance with a standardized schedule.

## REFERENCES

1. Hiscock, I. V. *Community Health Organization*. The Commonwealth Fund, New York City. Third edition. 1939.
2. Geiger, J. C. *Health Officer's Manual*. W. B. Saunders Company. 1939.
3. Tobey, J. A. *Public Health Law*. The Williams and Wilkins Company, Baltimore. 1939.
4. Picken, R. M. F. *Public Health Administration*. Printed by Local Government Finance, University of Wales, England. May, 1939.
5. Stern, B. J. *Medical Services by Government*. The Commonwealth Fund, New York City. 1946.
6. Mustard, H. S. *Government in Public Health*. The Commonwealth Fund, New York City. 1945.
7. *Health Practice Indices*. American Public Health Association, 1790 Broadway, New York City. 1946 and subsequent editions.
8. *Public Health Centers*. *Architectural Record's* Building Type Study No. 67. Publication of U.S.P.H. Service.
9. *Health Center Districts. New York*. Handbook of Statistical Reference Data. Neighborhood Health Development, Inc., 137 Centre Street, New York City. 1944.
10. Mustard, H. S. *An Introduction to Public Health*. The Macmillan Company. Second edition. 1944.

# CHAPTER XXX

## RURAL HEALTH ADMINISTRATION

THE administrative problems of the small city, town and the country districts, which relate to public health, are quite different from those of the larger cities. By and large, a city of fifty thousand population or more should organize its own health department. But a very great proportion of the population in the United States lives in cities of less than fifty thousand population. The federal census limits the rural area to cities, towns and villages of less than 10,000 population, but for purposes of public health administration, all cities with a population of 50,000 or less, with adjacent communities, scattered villages and isolated farm houses will be included as rural population.

### HISTORY OF THE DEVELOPMENT OF RURAL HEALTH ADMINISTRATION IN THE UNITED STATES

The establishment of local boards of health represents the first official attempt to attack rural health problems in America. These boards have been in existence for more than one hundred years and in some rural areas they still function in very much the same manner as they have through the generations. The first local boards of health were established in Massachusetts in 1797. Connecticut followed in 1805. In New England and some of the northern and eastern states the township has been the unit of local government; in the southern and western states, the larger, more populous county is almost universally the unit of local government.

The state is, of course, the sovereign power, but from the first, the state has granted very broad powers to local boards of health of both towns and counties. In actual practice, however, the functions of these boards have been limited to control of communicable disease and abatement of nuisances. Because of the miasmatic theory of contagion, the latter was a natural corollary of the former. The real intention of the board of health in abatement of nuisances was to check epidemics of disease.

During the past fifty years municipal health activities have advanced rapidly and effectively; meanwhile rural health administration remained stationary for generation after generation.

District Health Officer Plan. An attempt toward the improvement in rural health service was made by some of the states through the district health plan. The district health officer system was developed most extensively in Massachusetts and New York, though various modifications of the plan have been tried in several other states, as, for example, Maine, Florida and Pennsylvania. Where this plan is followed, the state is divided into arbitrary units of territory by the state health department. A district health officer is selected by the state health officer for each jurisdiction. He becomes, in fact, a deputy state health officer for his territory, is paid by the state and is responsible to the state health officer. His duties are to represent the state health department in his territory and to advise with and supplement the work of the local health departments.

This type of organization has rendered valuable service in the control of communicable disease, and particularly in epidemiological investigation. The district health officer becomes an expert in accurate and early diagnosis of communicable disease, is familiar with state law and procedures and is called on constantly by local boards of health for solution of difficult problems. He is in close touch with the state health department and can inform the central organization of pending outbreaks or of potential danger. Usually his territory is very large, covering an area of several thousand square miles and giving service to populations of more than a hundred thousand. This plan does not give well-rounded adequate health service, but has the great advantage that the work is centralized and co-ordinated. The district health officers usually are well trained and highly qualified men. They work under a uniform plan, cover a large territory, and carry on a heavy schedule of work.

**Public Health Nursing.** Various voluntary organizations, notably the Red Cross and the Tuberculosis Associations, have established public health nursing centers in rural areas. Usually this has been a specialized service, covering a limited field. The results have been excellent. The service has been stimulated by the central organization, but paid for as a rule by local voluntary subscription. The quality of the service varies, because of inadequate supervision and lack of a centralized unified plan. Often the work is not correlated with the other public health activities, official and unofficial, of the community. The major defect of the service is that it lacks stability and continuity because it is dependent upon voluntary contributions.

Local government units, towns, villages and particularly departments of education have employed public health nurses for special service, particularly for school nursing, and maternal and infant hygiene programs. This service tends to be more stable than that of the voluntary organizations, but otherwise it has the same defects. In fact, the program is often less intelligently planned, and the selection of personnel and supervision of activities are less satisfactory than the systems of voluntary public health nursing service.

In Pennsylvania and to a lesser degree in some other states the State Health Department has furnished health service for the entire rural area of the state. In Pennsylvania the state appoints and pays a part-time medical director for each county, furnishes public health nurses, school medical inspectors, sanitary inspectors and other special services and organizes local public health clinics for more than three million rural people. The whole organization is directed and paid for by the State Health Department. Each division of the state organization directs its own type of activity in each of the various rural areas.

Some state health departments have attempted to meet the needs in the rural areas by assigning various specialists to visit the rural field at irregular intervals, and to aid and advise local health departments in the control of tuberculosis, in devising maternal and infant health programs, organizing clinics for toxoid administration, in improvement of milk sanitation, etc. Often the result is a sporadic "campaign" of activity, which is of some educational value, but of little or no permanent benefit.

## COUNTY HEALTH DEPARTMENT

**Historical.** In 1911 a devastating epidemic of typhoid fever occurred in Yakima County, Washington. Dr. L. L. Lumsden of the United States Public Health Service was assigned to study the epidemic. He recommended to the county authorities that the best method for preventing the repetition of such a disaster would be the organization of a county health department, supported by county funds, with a full-time physician in charge. As a direct result of this recommendation, the first county health unit in the United States was established.[1] Meanwhile, the Rockefeller Sanitary Commission had been conducting a campaign for the control of hookworm disease in the southern states. The commission found that the campaign for treatment of cases and education of the people was of great value in alleviating suffering in any area, but that permanent results leading to improvement of sanitary conditions and eventual prevention of infection could not be obtained unless there remained in the area a small, permanent nucleus with a continuous, comprehensive program of gradual sanitary betterment. In order to assure stability and continuity, it was obvious that such an organization must have official sponsorship and local support. The Rockefeller Foundation, therefore, developed the policy of stimulation of the organization of county health service with full-time personnel by temporary grants toward the development of county health units. Aid was not given directly to the county government, but through the State Health Department. The State Department of Health in turn assumed all responsibility

[1] Jefferson County, Kentucky (1908), and Guilford County, North Carolina (1911); both claim priority in the establishment of full-time county health unit service. See Freeman, A. W.: "Rural Health Organization in the United States." *Southern Med. Jour.* 1934, Vol. 27, p. 517.

for the development and supervision of the service and also gave a subsidy to the county for the health unit work. A very similar plan of federal aid in establishment of county health units was developed by the United States Public Health Service under Dr. Lumsden.

From the very first, the method proved effective and met with popular approval and support. There was an experimental period of about five years during which a great variety of types of organization, of administrative methods, and of personnel were tried. The method of trial and error was followed, mistakes were made and rectified, and a satisfactory workable plan was finally developed which was of almost universal application. From 1918 on, the growth of county health units has been rapid. In that year there were some thirty county health units with full-time personnel in the United States.

By 1940, the principle had been adopted in 1,381 counties in the United States, and a large proportion of the rural population in the country had secured a public health service with full-time personnel under the county or district plan. Every state in the Union except two sparsely settled western states and three small New England states had established full time rural health service, and several states had health units in every county in the state. Not only had the quantity of work increased enormously, but the quality of service had improved to such a degree that many rural areas were given just as adequate health supervision as were the large municipalities.

**Organization.** The organization of county health department service is based on the county as a unit of government. This has the advantage that the county is an accepted administrative unit with all the various established departments of governmental activity: education, police, the judiciary, public welfare, roads, agriculture, etc. It is also the taxing unit and, to a lesser degree, a political and social unit.

Any city in the county with a population of 50,000 or more may have its own health department; though it is often more practicable to include all cities and towns of whatever size under the unified county health service.[2]

In a county having a population of 25,000 or less, it has not been found feasible to organize standard county health unit service for reasons that will become apparent. Even in counties with a population of 25,000 to 30,000 people, but with a large, sparsely settled area and a total annual income of less than $10,000,000 ($300.00 per capita) a standard county health unit is not a feasible organization unless a substantial subsidy is received from the state.

The essential principles in the organization of a county health unit are:

---

[2] Birmingham, Alabama, for example, is a city of over 300,000 people. The city has no autonomous health organization, but its organization is a part of the Jefferson County Health Unit.

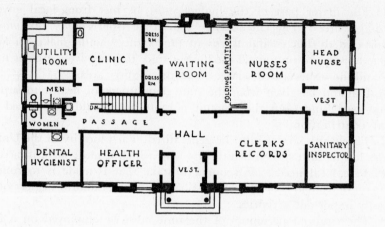

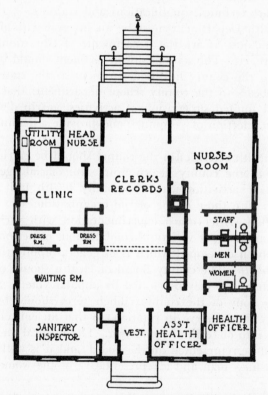

FIG. 34. *Health Center Design.* Ground Floor Plans of County Health Center Buildings at Ayer, Massachusetts, and Blountville, Tennessee. These health centers were planned and constructed by the Commonwealth Fund of New York, as demonstrations. (Published through courtesy of the Commonwealth Fund.)

429

1. The major part of the budget must be met from local governmental sources. The chief source should be from *county tax money*. Incorporated villages and towns in the county should make an additional appropriation toward the budget since they receive a greater number and more specialized services than the country areas.

Aid should be given from the state department of health to supplement local funds, but the amount of state aid should not exceed the local contribution.

2. The health service must be generalized. Each locality in the United States has its own special health problems which it must solve in accordance with local needs. A frequent mistake that is made is to concentrate on one obvious or interesting phase of activity and to neglect other equally important activities.

3. The essential personnel of the unit must be employed on a full-time basis, and should not carry on any other type of work. They must possess necessary technical qualifications and training.

4. The Health Department must be an integral part of the governmental services, just as are the departments of education, justice, police, agriculture, etc. The state health department should bear the same relationship to the county health department as the state department of education bears to the county school department; that is, the state should have a limited supervision of activities, aid in development of technic and in selection of personnel, and provide a definite permanent subsidy.

5. All the health activities in the county should be carried out under the direction of the county health unit. Non-official agencies should either fuse their activities with the county health unit or correlate their activities with those of the official organization.

**Standard Plan.** After much experimentation with various types of organizations and a great variety of combinations of personnel, a standard plan has been developed which is of general application.

*Board of Health.* The county Board of Health should consist of five to seven members and may be elected by popular vote or appointed by the governing body of the county. Their term should be for 3 to 5 years and they should serve in rotation, so that an entirely new board would not go into office in any one year. The medical and dental professions should be represented on the board, and it is well to include a prominent business man and a representative of the women's organizations.

The Board of Health is responsible to the county governing body for the development and conduct of the program of the Health Department. The Board of Health selects the health officer. He is responsible to the Board for the activities of the Health Department, serves as secretary of the Board, and is a member *ex-officio*. The health officer selects the personnel of the unit.

*Advisory Committee.* In addition to the Board of Health, many health officers organize an advisory public health committee. This committee may have fifteen or twenty members who are selected by the health officer. They are chosen as representatives of important organizations in the county, such as churches, clubs, women's organizations, representative medical men, business men, etc. The committee has no legal standing. It usually meets quarterly and serves as a very valuable agent in interpreting the work of the Health Department to the public at large.

*Personnel.* The personnel required to carry out the elements of a rounded health program must include the following:

*a. Health Officer.* He should be a physician, qualified by training and experience to meet demands of his office. It is generally agreed that he should possess the equivalent of one year's theoretical training in a school of public health.

*b. Public Health Nurses. At least 2.* Each nurse should be a graduate of a recognized training school, with special training and experience in public health nursing.

*c. Sanitary Officer.* The qualifications for sanitary officers have been set forth by the Committee on Professional Education of the American Public Health Association. (See Appendix.)

*d. Clerk.* The essential qualifications for the clerk are that she should have reasonable training in office methods, but more important than professional qualifications, she should be a local, well-known and highly respected person who has a wide familiarity with the social fabric of the county. The other personnel are field workers. The clerk is the office representative of the unit and is an invaluable asset in translating the desires of the people to the health officer and in interpreting the purposes of the department to the practicing physicians and to the people.

A diagram for the organization of a typical county health unit is given in Fig. 35.

A minimum personnel of five persons cannot, of course, give a complete health service to thirty thousand people. As the work becomes established and grows in popularity, it is anticipated that additional personnel will be added. Generally recognized standards for adequate service require additional nurses up to one nurse for every 5,000 population, and additional sanitary inspectors up to one for every 15,000 population. Medical and dental services for the administration of school health work, well baby clinics, etc., may be purchased on a unit-of-work, or on a part-time salary basis.

*Typical Budget.* A typical budget for a minimum standard unit may be planned as follows:

At least half the budget should be met from official county funds. Outside contributing agencies, such as the United States Public Health Service, may give financial aid in order to develop, consolidate and establish the work. These funds should be given through the State Health Department and not directly to the county. The state should contribute a permanent subsidy of one fourth the total budget or more, depending upon local circumstances.

The very poor sections of a state need health service more than the wealthier rural areas, and can least afford to pay for it. Thus, the state

ORGANIZATION OF A TYPICAL COUNTY HEALTH UNIT

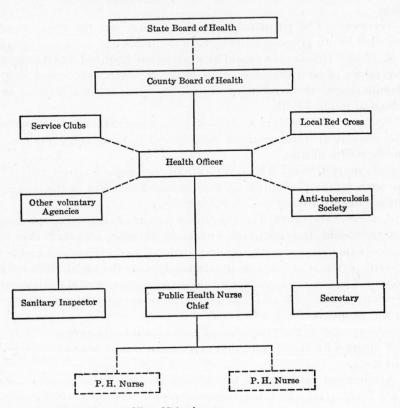

Service is built up by adding additional nurses.

FIG. 35. *Diagram of a Typical County Health Unit Organization.*

subsidy should not be on a uniform per capita or per county basis, but should be allocated in accordance with need. In some instances, over half the budget for county health work may be supplied from state and federal sources. (See chapter on the Social Security Act.)

*Basic Activities.* The basic activities of the County Health Department are:

1. Vital Statistics.
2. Communicable Disease Control.
3. Maternal and Infant Hygiene.

4. School Hygiene.

5. Sanitation.

6. Public Health Education.

**Functions and Duties.** *Board of Health.* The Board of Health usually holds monthly meetings. The appointment is honorary and no compensation is received. The Board has no executive duties. Among its chief activities are:

1. It receives the reports of the health officer and supervises the work of the department.

2. It determines the general policies of the unit.

3. It makes such health rules and regulations as may be necessary, so long as they do not conflict with the state law.

4. It selects the health officer after consulting with the State Health Department.

*Health Officer.* 1. The health officer is the executive for the Board of Health, and administers the work of the department, planning and co-ordinating the activities of each of its members. He selects the personnel, after consulting with his Board of Health and with the State Health Department. The various members of the unit are responsible to him for performance of their duties. In addition to the administrative work, the health officer has his own definite field activities.

2. Communicable disease control and epidemiological investigations. The health officer must be an expert in the diagnosis of contagious disease. He should be available to all the physicians in the county for consultation service in diagnosis of suspected communicable disease. He should be familiar with field epidemiological methods and, in conjunction with the state epidemiologist, should work out the details of any epidemics that may occur in his territory. He is directly responsible also for the enforcement of all regulations of the Board of Health in relation to contagious disease control.

3. Physical examination of school children. In the smaller counties, the health officer will make all physical examinations of school children. This work is usually planned for the fall and winter months. If there are five thousand children of school age who are examined carefully twice during primary school life, there would be about one thousand examinations to be made each year, not including the check-up examinations of defective children that had been discovered on previous examinations.

In larger counties, the health department may employ some of the physicians of the county on a part-time basis to aid in the medical examination of the school children.

4. Physical examinations in connection with the maternal and infant hygiene programs. The field of maternity and infancy is the special province of the nurse. She organizes the clinics and carries out the major part of the work. The health officer may make the physical examinations

of well babies in the preschool clinics and also may make certain selected prenatal examinations. In many of the large counties, the practicing physicians aid in the physical examinations in the clinics, sometimes on a pay basis, sometimes as volunteers.

5. The tuberculosis clinics are organized and conducted by the health officer with assistance from the state department. One or two clinics a month are sufficient for the average county.

6. Medical prophylactic work.

*a. Typhoid Vaccination.* In those areas where the endemic typhoid fever rate is high (200 per 100,000 population more or less), it will be profitable to organize typhoid vaccination clinics. Most health departments have found from long experience that the actual vaccination cannot be delegated to the nurse, but should be done by the health officer. The clinics should be planned for the early summer period. Strategic spots are chosen such as a country school house, or other community center, and a regular schedule is worked out. Each center should have at least fifty patients. Babies under two years and people over sixty may be excluded, as well as individuals who have had typhoid fever. The vaccine is given in divided doses at three periods, one week apart. A one hour period should be allotted to each center; from 50 to 100 people can be vaccinated in that time. The vaccination should be free and no distinction made because of economic or social status. It should never be compulsory.

As the typhoid fever rate for the country drops year by year, the typhoid vaccination service can be curtailed, until only those few spots of high endemicity are covered each year by vaccination campaigns.

*b. Smallpox Vaccination.* The health officer should be prepared to give smallpox vaccination at any time, to anyone in the county who may request it. Parents should be urged to have their babies vaccinated during the first year of life and again on entering school. Smallpox vaccinations may be done at the well baby clinics, preschool clinics, in the school, or at the office of the health department. They should not be done by the nurse.

*c. Diphtheria Toxoid.* Prevention of diphtheria should be stressed for children in the early age periods. Parents should be urged to have their babies immunized during the first year of life. They should be done by the health officer, or by practicing physicians in their offices as part of the normal procedures of medical practice. Frequently physicians keep a card index of the babies they have delivered, and at the end of 6 months they send the parents a note that the baby should be brought in for diphtheria immunization. Those parents who are unable to pay for this service may bring their babies to a health department immunization clinic. The immunization may be done in the well baby clinics, preschool clinics or in the first two or three years of the primary schools. From an administrative point of view, Schick tests are not necessary, either as a preliminary measure or as a means of determining the effect of the immunization. (See Chapter IV.)

The important goal for the health officer is immunization of at least 30 per cent of all infants during the first year of life, and at least 50 per cent immunization before the age of 6 years. If he maintains this standard, diphtheria may invade the community, but will not extend to epidemic proportions.

*d. Venereal Disease Clinics.* One period a week should be set aside by the health officer for diagnosis of venereal disease and for the treatment of indigent cases. The number will not be large, but some provision must be made for the care of these patients. Only those cases are given free treatment that have been referred to the health officer by practicing physicians. In the larger counties this work can be done by practicing physicians who are employed on a part time basis or per treatment basis by the health department. This work is best organized in conjunction with the outpatient service of the community hospital.

In many county health departments, there is developing a tendency to set aside certain funds from the budget for medical treatment phases of the public health program, and to employ the practicing physicians of the county to do this type of work for the health department.

*Laboratory Examinations.* The small county health department should not attempt to do laboratory work. The smallest successful diagnostic laboratory unit must have a personnel of at least three persons: director, technician and helper. Many simpler types of organization have been attempted, but have failed. The health officer has no time to supervise the work. A single technician can give a limited service only, and this proves expensive. Co-operative laboratory service has been attempted, the health department combining with the local hospital to give a joint diagnostic and clinical laboratory service. This causes administrative difficulties, due to the divided responsibility. There is a definite trend to develop community health centers, with a community-subsidized hospital, and unit administration of all local medical, nursing and health protection services that are provided by the community. It would be possible under these conditions to organize an effective laboratory which would serve the needs of the hospital as well as the health department. (See section on Medical Care.)

If the area contains 50,000 population or more, a local laboratory service may be attempted. A much more satisfactory arrangement is the development and full utilization of state laboratory service, with the extension of the state laboratory work to branch or district laboratories.

*Public Health Education.* One of the chief activities of the health officer is health education. He uses every means at his command to interpret the work of the department to the people. This is a function of all members of the department, but each one carries it out in a different way. The health officer reaches the people through addresses to various organizations, churches, schools, men's clubs, and women's social organizations, through motion pictures, articles in the local newspapers, radio, and other means of publicity. He co-operates with the county superintendent of education in planning the system of health instruction in the public schools, and aids the county public school teachers in developing better methods of teaching health lessons.

*The Public Health Nurse.* The rural health nurse has a varied and interesting task. It is impossible to give more than an outline of her activities and duties. In the smaller units, she must give a service to 2,000 or 3,000 homes scattered over a wide area, whereas her sister nurse in the city will serve only a thousand readily accessible homes. Thus the work of the county nurse tends to become diversified and unless she concentrates on special problems, her efforts may be so scattered as to be wasted.

*a. Prenatal Work.* Prenatal clinics will probably not be feasible. The nurse works through the practicing physicians, encouraging them to use her to follow their cases in private practice, and aiding the doctors and the prospective mothers in making preparation for the baby. In a county of 25,000 people, the nurse would have about 250 prenatal cases in her files each year, so that an intensive service cannot be given.

*b. Supervision of Midwives.* The supervision of the activities of midwives is a function of the public health nurse. In some of the southern states this is a real responsibility. Most of the midwives are Negroes with little education and very little training.

*c. Infant Hygiene.* Well baby clinics can be organized in the larger centers of population. A regular schedule is arranged by the nurse with the health officer. He gives the physical examinations. There is a tendency toward development of this type of work through the family physician rather than in formal clinics.

*d. Preschool Work.* Organization of the preschool work is one of the functions of the public health nurse. It is an extension of the infant hygiene activities, and the present trend is to fuse the infant and preschool work, so that a continuous program may be planned for each child, and the rural mother can bring several of her children to the clinic on a single visit, rather than make a separate visit for each child.

Large counties with several market centers can be reached effectively by the establishment of *Health Stations* in each of three or four communities. The headquarters of the county health work are in the county seat, and as a general rule, all the staff work out from the center. A health station consists of two or three modestly equipped rooms in a centrally located building of the village, where the nurse can meet her clientele, where well baby clinics are held, supplies stored, and committee meetings held. The health department staff should establish a definite schedule, when each of its members will be at the health stations at a certain time. The work should be planned so that the health station is open at least two afternoons a week, and definite programs are assigned to the allotted periods.

*e. School Hygiene.* The most important activity of the public health nurse in the school hygiene program is the follow-up of physical defects in order that corrections may be secured. Many health officers insist that the nurse accompany them during the physical examinations of the school children. This is often a waste of time. The health officer should make the examinations and fill out the records. The nurse should go over these records of the physical defects with the health officer and expend her time in visiting the parents and arranging means for the correction of defects that may have been found.

*f. Communicable Disease.* The county health nurse has a limited amount of work in connection with communicable disease control. She will have from twenty-five to fifty cases of tuberculosis on her files that should be visited once a month, if possible, as well as arrested cases of tuberculosis that should be visited at longer intervals. Cases of typhoid fever treated in the home should be visited frequently. Control of the minor diseases of childhood, such as pediculosis, scabies and impetigo are time-consuming and troublesome duties of the public health nurse. When cases of diphtheria and scarlet fever are treated in the home, the nurse may make two instructional visits, to aid the mother in the proper care of the patient, and particularly to give instruction concerning precautions to be taken to prevent the spread of the infection.

*g. Public Health Education.* The nurse's function as a public health educator is equally as important and fruitful as the health officer's, but is carried out on quite different lines. She seldom gives addresses or public talks, but works through the home and the schools. She arranges conferences with groups of mothers or prospective mothers, plans "little mothers" classes, sends personal letters to pregnant women, and to parents who should have their children's defects corrected, and uses her imagination and ingenuity in a hundred ways in raising the standards of personal hygiene and public health of the community.

The most important principle of administration in relation to the county nurse is that she is not an assistant to the health officer, but has a more or less independent program with special functions and duties that are her peculiar sphere. Her activities complement the other activities of the unit. Working alone, her efforts would accomplish little; without her work the health activities of the department would be sadly ineffective and lop-sided.

*Sanitary Officer.* The activities of the sanitary officer will vary, to some degree, in accordance with the type of population and general economic status of the county. In general, he is concerned with all those activities which relate to environmental sanitation. One of the defects of our present system has been the low standards of training of the sanitary inspection personnel. This condition is gradually improving.

(A discussion of the training and qualifications of the sanitary officer will be found in the Appendix.)

*a. Sewage Disposal.* Each home in the area should have some form of sanitary disposal of human waste. Most of the towns of one thousand population or more will have a municipal water carriage system. This system will have been constructed with the approval of the State Health Department and requires only supervision of proper maintenance by the sanitary officer. The village and country homes must have some type of individual disposal system. The sanitary officer must be familiar with the various types of septic tanks and sanitary toilets that are suitable for rural homes, and must actively urge their installation in all homes that are not provided with proper facilities. He must be familiar with details of construction, and with costs of installation and maintenance. In many areas the chief activity of the sanitary officer is the supervision of the installation and maintenance of sanitary pit privies.

*b. Water Supplies.* The larger towns usually have a municipal water supply which has been installed under the supervision of the State Health Department. The sanitary officer has a direct responsibility for proper maintenance of these systems. He must make an inspection of each system at frequent intervals. If a system of chlorination of the water supply is used, the plant and records should be inspected at frequent intervals (once a week). Laboratory samples of these municipal water supplies are sent to the State Laboratory by the sanitary officer at suitable intervals.

The sanitary officer has a special responsibility for the safety of individual water supplies to which the public has access. This includes the water supplies of country schools, tourist camps and roadside stands, etc.

In addition, the sanitary officer should be familiar with all the various types of proper construction for wells and should urge the scattered country home owners to improve their private water supply, so that there is no danger of contamination of their drinking water.

*c. Food.* The sanitary officer has charge of the sanitary condition of food handling establishments in the county. This includes restaurants and other public eating places, such as roadside stands; meat markets and shops handling other perishable food, slaughter houses, etc. Milk sanitation is an important activity of all rural health departments, and the sanitary officer must be familiar with the details and the technic of proper production of milk and milk products.

The Board of Health establishes certain rules and regulations in regard to all matters relating to the proper handling of food, and it is the duty of the sanitary officer to enforce these regulations and to aid the proprietors in meeting the requirement of the Health Department. Food handlers should be taught the simple principles of food sanitation.

*d. Mosquito Eradication.* Where malaria is prevalent, the sanitary officer must be familiar with the breeding habits of the anopheles vector, and, after consultation with the State Health Department, he must be ready to recommend the most feasible method of mosquito control in the infected area. He must be familiar with the elementary principles of control of mosquitoes by various types of drainage, as well as the costs of installation and maintenance, and must aid the landowner by advice and counsel in carrying out mosquito control projects.

*e. Nuisance Abatement.* A miscellaneous group of activities is included under nuisance abatement. Many of them have little or no relationship to disease prevention, having been carried down from the period of the "miasmatic theory" of disease. Formerly it was thought that bad odors from decaying vegetation, dead animals, sewer gas, etc. produced diphtheria, typhoid fever, malaria and other diseases. It has remained as a duty of the sanitary officer to assume responsibility for the abatement of these nuisances, and will probably remain a part of his activities for years to come.

*f. Health Education.* The sanitary officer has his own peculiar function as a health educator. He is closer to the people than any member of the department. He knows their more intimate prejudices and personal peculiarities. Thus his work has the great advantage of individual personal contact and he reaches the key men in the community, who, in turn, influence the public opinion of their own group. The sanitary officer seldom gives public addresses, or writes public health articles, but nevertheless his influence in the community may be very effective and far-reaching.

*Secretary.* The secretary is the representative of the department in the office. The others are field workers, and spend only a small proportion of their time in office work. She is always there.

*a. Office Business.* All office business is in her hands. She makes all appointments and keeps the schedules of clinic services. She carries on the routine office correspondence and keeps the accounts. All the files of the office records are her responsibility.

*b. Vital Statistics and Reporting of Communicable Disease.* Local registrars of births and deaths report directly to the secretary. She makes a copy of each record and forwards the original to the State Health Registrar. The physicians report all cases of communicable disease to the secretary by telephone or otherwise. She forwards a summary of these data to the State Health Department and keeps suitable record of the cases as well as a check on isolation and quarantine for these diseases.

*c. Maps, charts and graphs* of the activities of the health department as well as the maintenance of continuous spot maps of important infectious disease in the area are the province of the secretary.

*d. Supplies.* The secretary has entire responsibility for all supplies. These include:

Containers for laboratory specimens that are to be distributed to physicians and used for shipment of cultures, etc. to the central laboratory.

A suitable stock of smallpox vaccine, anti-diphtheria serum, and other biological products that are necessary for the work of the unit and for the prevention of disease in the county. The state laboratory furnishes her with a duplicate of all the laboratory findings in communicable disease for the county, and these are properly checked and filed.

The clinic cards, school examination cards, records of defects that have been discovered in children, and records of the correction of defects serve to keep the secretary busy in her particular sphere of work in the unit.

*e. Health Education.* Since the secretary is always in the office and is in continuous touch with the physicians and with the various people who visit the unit for one purpose or another, she has an unusual opportunity to interpret the work of the Health Department to the people, and to win their confidence and support.

The important feature of county health department organization is that each individual has his own definite and more or less independent program and responsibilities. The work is not planned from day to day or week to week, but from year to year.

At the beginning of each year, the health officer, in conference with his whole group, plans the work for the year and lays out certain objectives. Then each member of the group plans his own program, so that it fits in with the departmental unified plan. The duties and responsibilities of each one of the personnel are clearly defined and from this point on each member of the unit is individually responsible for his own share of the program. Weekly meetings of the department are held to determine the progress that is being made and to make any necessary alterations in the plan for the year's work.

*Voluntary Organizations.* There are many voluntary organizations in the county that are interested in public health and welfare. Chief of these are the local Tuberculosis Association, the Red Cross, Parent-Teachers Associations, men's service clubs, church societies, women's clubs and many others. Their activities should dovetail with those of the official health service, with no conflict and no misunderstanding. If feasible, the health department should be represented on the executive boards of the major voluntary organizations.

In general, these organizations should not supplant any of the functions of the official body, but rather supplement its activities. Their greatest usefulness is in the general field of remedial service, as, for example, the summer camp for under-nourished children, the extra expense for an out-door sleeping tent for care of tuberculosis in the home, the purchase of spectacles for children with defective eyesight, the cost of special orthopedic appliances for crippled children. These, and a thousand other needs, are a very effective and happy outlet for the energies of the voluntary groups, which can be a tremendous asset to the health department in protecting the people, and advancing the health standards of the community.

**Where Is the Standard Health Unit Not Feasible?** In those small counties where the population is 15,000 or less, or even in counties with a population up to 25,000 but with a per capita income of $300 per annum or less, it has not been found feasible to establish a health department with even a minimum standard personnel. The same is true in those states (as in New England) where the unit of government is the township rather than the county.

Various expedients and modifications of the standard plan have been tried to meet the needs of these smaller governmental units.

*Sanitary Officer Only.* In areas where sanitary problems loom very large, some states have encouraged the employment in the smaller counties of a sanitary officer only. Such a plan results in rapid advances in environmental sanitation—particularly in construction of sanitary privies, but other public health activities are neglected. It is a good introductory service, useful and necessary. In some instances, it has led to the establishment of a complete program.

*Public Health Nurse Only.* Many counties have employed a public health nurse as the sole health worker in the county. Excellent results have been accomplished, but the program is always limited in its scope, and important phases of health work are omitted entirely. It is not a good introductory service, for experience has shown that it is often more difficult to develop a full program following a single nurse than following a single sanitary officer.

*Sanitary Officer and Public Health Nurse.* A few counties have employed a sanitary officer and public health nurse. In some instances, supervision of the work is provided for through a district health officer who is paid by the state and who has a jurisdiction of several counties. This plan more closely approximates adequate health service than almost any other and is a fairly good substitute for county health departments in the sparsely settled areas.

### DISTRICT HEALTH UNITS

A much more satisfactory plan of health administration for the more sparsely settled rural areas than the three plans already mentioned is the "health district." The general public health program for the district is very similar to that of the standard health unit, and the administrative machinery is set up along similar lines.

The local governmental units (counties as a rule) that are concerned, pool their interests and financial resources. The units should be contiguous. An ideal health district should consist of a population of about fifty thousand persons and an area not to exceed one thousand square miles, with a ready means of communication.

The plan has many administrative pitfalls. The area may be so great, and communication so poor, that a single medical officer cannot render effective service. Each governmental unit concerned is jealous of its own

prerogatives and autonomy. In many instances a single unit will with-
draw its support on some slight pretext and thus endanger the whole
project. Thus the district plan requires strong support and close supervision by the central (state) organization. The key positions, and particularly the health officer, must be supported, in great part, by state subsidy.
Funds from local sources should not be disbursed directly by the county,
but should be paid into the common fund. The district board of health
should be made up of representatives from each of the counties and
should have the power to determine general policies. It should also have
a strong voice in the selection of the district health officer, even though
the funds for his support are supplied entirely from state sources. The
health officer should have the power of selection of all personnel. For
example, a nurse who is assigned by the district health officer to a certain
county is not the exclusive civil servant of that county and should not be
subject to appointment or removal by the county in which she serves.
Furthermore, the district health officer should be free to shift his personnel in an emergency. All health work of the district should be cleared
through the central office of the health officer and all the work of the
district should be co-ordinated by him.

A diagram of this type of unit is given in Fig. 36. The district is
made up of the following units:

|  | Area | Population |
|---|---|---|
| County A .............. | 440 sq. miles | 14,823 |
| County B .............. | 537 " " | 26,320 |
| County C .............. | 428 " " | 12,642 |
| Total | 1,405 sq. miles | 53,785 |

The district health officer is located in County B. The personnel consists of:

1. Central office.
   District medical health officer.
   Supervising nurse.
   1 sanitary officer assigned to work in Counties A and C.
   2 clerks.
2. Branch offices.
   3 nurses and one sanitary officer assigned to County B.
   2 nurses assigned to County A.
   2 nurses assigned to County C.

The major weakness of this organization is lack of sufficient medical
service. The efficiency of this health district could be greatly augmented
if sufficient funds were added to the budget to pay for the part-time
medical and dental services in each of the counties. This work should
be done by the local physicians and dentists, who are selected for the work
by the District Health Officer in conjunction with the public health committee of the District Medical Society. These physicians would conduct

the school medical examinations, the well baby clinics, the immunization clinics, and the like. This work would be organized by the District Health Officer and the physicians would be paid for their assistance, preferably on a per-hour basis.

If sufficient subsidies can be secured from state and federal sources to initiate and establish this type of district health organization in those sparsely settled rural areas that are without suitable health protection, it seems highly probable that in due time, each of the local units will

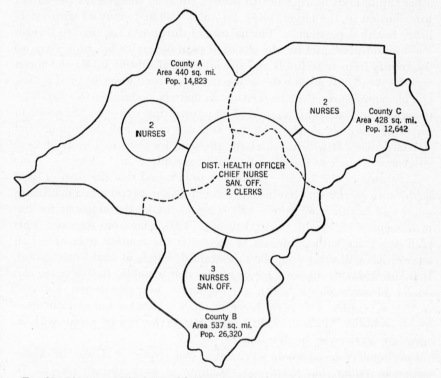

Fig. 36. *Diagram of District Health Unit Organization.* One medical officer has charge of the health work of three counties. The total area of the district is about 1400 square miles and the total population 50,000.

assume more and more local financial responsibility for the conduct of the work, and that, eventually, rural health organization will reach the same state of development and receive the same local support as municipal health organization.

In the New England States, particularly Massachusetts, where the small, intensely individualistic township is the unit of government, a determined effort has been made to unite twelve to twenty townships into a health district, and to carry out an adequate health program along accepted lines. Each township certified the health officer as its agent, delegated certain powers to him, and contributed to the budget in proportion to its population or other mutually agreeable method of allocation of funds. The state and voluntary agencies have given substantial subsidies toward the units. It must be agreed that no more difficult problem in health administration can be found in the United States.

*Increased State Subsidy.* A further modification of the standard plan has been developed for the smaller and poorer counties in Alabama, Tennessee and some of the other states. The county which desires adequate health service, but cannot afford it, has been asked to contribute a per capita tax toward a health budget equal to the average per capita contribution of the larger, more favorably situated counties with established health departments. The balance of the budget required to furnish a minimum personnel for the standard plan of service has been given to the county from state funds and special Federal subsidy under the Social Security Act. This is not a departure from our usual governmental policy, but has ample precedent in relation to matters pertaining to education, to agriculture, etc. This method of administration will solve the problem for those counties that are almost, but not quite, able to support the standard plan. It will not solve the problem for the small units of local government, such as the New England township.

*Expansion of the Service.* It must be understood that the plan of local health unit service that has been presented does not represent a maximum quality of health work which will bring about ideal conditions for improvement of the health of rural people. This is far from the case. This plan of service with minimum personnel is the *smallest* unit of health service that will meet even the minimum demands of health protection. It is ridiculous to suppose, for example, that a public health nurse can render adequate public health nursing service to a population of 10,000 to 15,000 people. The plan, however, does serve as a foundation upon which to build. Without it, little effective service can be given; with it, adequate service can be developed.

Development of adequate service does not require a change in organization or policy, but simply an extension of work and an increase in personnel along established lines, following the skeleton of the structure that has already formulated the basic requirements of a sound administration.

No one can guess what the rural people will eventually demand as an adequate and satisfactory public health service. Authorities have estimated that an expenditure of $1.50 per capita per year should eventually represent a logical expenditure for an official rural health protection program. But the demands for other facilities of public betterment, such as the development of improved schools and improved roads at public expense during the past fifty years, have been much more extensive than the most foresighted leaders ever anticipated. It is impossible to estimate how extensive will be the demand for health protection, what directions it will take, or how rapidly it will grow. It is safe to say that the development of health protection for the rural areas cannot lag behind the municipal development, as it has in the past, but must go hand in hand with the progress that is made in the larger centers of population.

**A Plan for Local Health Units for the Nation.** Dr. Haven Emerson,[3] Chairman of the Subcommittee on Local Health Units of the Committee on Administrative Practice of the American Public Health Association, published in 1945 a comprehensive plan for health units for the entire nation.

The report is based upon the thesis that an effective administrative unit for local health services requires a population of 50,000 or more persons. It suggests, as a base line, a per capita expenditure of $1 for local health work.

The report notes that there are 38,000 local jurisdictions of civil government in the 48 states. This includes the 3,070 counties. A great many of these local governmental units do not have sufficient population or funds to organize and support their own local health services on an adequate basis.

The report considers each state separately, and suggests the reorganization of local health departments in order to give complete and comprehensive health services, under full-time personnel, to the entire United States.

At the time of the report—1945—it had become apparent that the county health unit was not the complete answer to satisfactory rural health administration for all parts of the country. More than one half of the counties of the nation were organized on a full-time health service basis, but over 40,000,000 people of the United States were still without the benefits of a good local health department. In some instances, no health work was organized because the county had too small a population; in other areas, the township was the unit of local self-government, rather than the county. In certain states, legal obstacles prevented the establishment of full-time local health departments on a county basis. The great benefits of full-time local health services had been demonstrated, but the nation-wide realization of these benefits was being greatly delayed. It seemed probable that future advances along county health unit lines would be slow.

The report proposed to cut straight through administrative, obstacles, in order to secure maximum nation-wide benefit. It recommended the reorganization of local health services for the nation into 1,197 units of health jurisdiction. The make-up of each unit was to be based on such factors as: population, area in square miles, per capita wealth, number of hospital beds per 1,000 population, and number of persons in the area per practicing physician. The plan was approved, in principle, by nearly all the state health officers.

[3] Emerson, Haven: *Local Health Units for the Nation.* New York, The Commonwealth Fund, 1945.

A comparison of the personnel required by this comprehensive plan, as compared with existing personnel and expenditures (as of 1942) showed that a smaller number of full-time health officers would be required, even though the new plan covered the whole nation, whereas existing plans gave services to only 75 per cent of the population. The per capita expenditure would be increased from an average of 61 cents per capita to 97 cents. The big increase in personnel would occur in increased nursing services, increased full-time trained personnel in health education, increased clerical staff, and increased professionally trained sanitary personnel.

This report contains a mass of detailed information on local health administration in the United States, and should be carefully studied by all those who are interested in the subject.

The plan is ideal in its concepts, but will encounter great practical difficulties. Foremost perhaps is the unwillingness of local communities to surrender their local autonomy. The plan—to be successful—must be subsidized very heavily by the various state departments of health, with assistance from Federal grants-in-aid.

The local communities will not take the same interest in a type of health work that is largely state-supported, as compared with a health department that is an integral part of local self-government, and which is supported from local tax funds. One by one, the traditional time-honored principles of small town—"local community"—democratic self-government must be sacrificed in the interests of efficiency, economy, and better systems of government administration for community welfare.

The one-room county school, the county road, the covered bridge, the almshouse, and the part-time local health service—all served their time and useful place, but they are not suitable under the changed community economy. It seems quite probable that the county as a unit of self-government will develop more and more limitations as time passes, and as our mode of community life is modified.

## REFERENCES

1. Freeman, A. W. *A Study of Rural Public Health Service.* The Commonwealth Fund, New York City. 1933.
2. *Public Health in New York State.* Report of the State Health Commission to Gov. F. D. Roosevelt. Publication of the New York State Health Department. 1930.
3. Hamilton, John H. and Milam, D. F. *Twenty Years of County Health Work in North Carolina.* South. Med. J. 1934, Vol. 27, p. 875.
4. Barnes, M. E. *The Strength and Weaknesses of County Health Organization.* Amer. J. Pub. Health. 1929, Vol. 19, p. 731.
5. Mustard, H. S. *Rural Health Practice.* The Commonwealth Fund, New York City. 1936.
6. Emerson, Haven. *Local Health Units for the Nation.* The Commonwealth Fund, New York City. 1945.

7. *A 50-Bed Rural Hospital and Health Center.* Hospital Facilities Section, U.S.P.H. Service. J. Amer. Hosp. Ass'n. July, 1945.
8. *Proceedings of the National Conference on Local Health Units.* The University of Michigan School of Public Health. September 9–13, 1946. Pub. by American Public Health Association, 1790 Broadway, New York City.

See also the publications of the Committee on Administrative Practice of the American Public Health Association, 1790 Broadway, New York City, and the *Public Health Reports* of the United States Public Health Service, Washington, D. C. on rural health administration.

# CHAPTER XXXI

## STATE HEALTH ADMINISTRATION

THE function of a state health department is to preserve the health of all the people within its borders. As has been noted previously, the state is the *sovereign power* in our governmental system, and not the Federal Government, as is so often thought. This is a point which requires reiteration, since the erroneous idea that the Federal Government is the sovereign power has led to many serious mistakes in governmental planning concerning health affairs, as well as in other phases of governmental activity. It is also important to remember that the counties, municipalities, townships or other governmental units do not possess autonomy, other than the authority and powers which are specifically granted to them by the state. The state may, and frequently does, delegate certain functions and authority to other governmental units. This authority may be withdrawn. For example, if a health department of a city does not function properly, the state health department may intervene, and carry on all health affairs in the city.

It is impossible to give even an outline of state health organization within the United States. There are forty-eight separate, autonomous, sovereign governmental units. Each has developed along different lines to suit individual needs and local conditions. No two states have exactly the same organization. Furthermore, it is not possible to lay down specific, or even general principles, of state health administration that would be suited to all the various states. There is a great variation in the states in area, density of population, wealth, type of industry, climate, racial grouping, specific health problems, traditions and customs and other factors which may affect administrative procedures. A health organization which would be suitable for Nevada, for example, with a small population and an enormous area, would be entirely unsuitable for Connecticut, with over two million population, highly industrialized, and all living within a short half day's journey from the state capitol.

Furthermore, our ideas in regard to the scope of health activities is constantly changing and enlarging. Scientific research is continually developing new methods for the prevention of disease; administrators are forging ahead in methods of practical application of these new discoveries. Thus it would not be proper to lay down any standard form of health organization or administration for any state. One can simply outline the important functions of a state in preserving the health of its people, in so far as we now understand the application of general public health

448

principles. We shall cite examples of various successful public health practices in different states, and point out the probable lines of future development. We shall not attempt to develop standardized criteria as to suitable budget, proper number of personnel, or range of activities. It is generally recognized that standardization is dangerous, for it leads inevitably to stagnation. Imagination is an essential qualification in any administration, and imagination should be used in the development of a health program rather than the more customary method of adopting the principle of the children's game called "Follow the Leader."

## DEVELOPMENT OF STATE HEALTH DEPARTMENTS

Public health work as a separate function of state government is a relatively recent development in the United States. Lemuel Shattuck in 1849 made a sanitary survey of Massachusetts. In his report he made a strong recommendation to the state legislature for the establishment of a state department of public health. As an eventual result of this survey the first state health department in the United States was established in Massachusetts in 1869. The need for this type of organization was so apparent that within the next ten years, eighteen states had followed the precedent of Massachusetts. By 1900 twenty more states followed suit, and finally in 1913 every state and territory had established some form of state health organization.

An outline map [1] of the United States giving the date of establishment of each state health department is shown on page 16.

No state health organization is as yet functioning perfectly, and no standards of practice have met the approval of any large group of health administrators. Thus, any suggestions that are made in this text as to the functions and organization of a state health service should not be considered as an ideal plan, or even an advantageous one for any given situation, but simply represent the consensus of sincere and thoughtful men who have stumbled along their way, and have finally developed a workable machinery which is meeting the particular needs for their particular situation at the present time. Any comparisons that may be made of one state organization with another do not represent criticism of either organization. Each health officer meets his special problems in the most expedient way. He may recognize fully that it is not the ideal way, but he also recognizes that all progress in a democratic form of government is a result of compromise; some working arrangement which strikes a balance between the ideal and the everyday practical facts of life.

### STATE BOARD OF HEALTH

The Governor is the executive officer of the state. He is responsible to the people for the conduct of state government, and is thus directly re-

[1] *Health Departments of States and Provinces of the United States and Canada.* Bulletin No. 184. U.S.P.H. Service. 1932 (Revised).

sponsible for the health activities of the state. The state government is usually divided into various bureaus or departments on a more or less functional basis. The health service is generally considered as a major function of state government and the state health department is almost universally organized as a separate and distinct division of activity. (Exceptions to this rule will be discussed later.)

The Governor may select a Commissioner of Health, as a member of his cabinet, and delegate to him the executive functions of the health department. A much more satisfactory type of organization from many points of view is the *State Board of Health*.

**Functions of the State Board of Health.** *Advisory.* The chief function of the State Board of Health is to advise the health officer on the general policies of the health department.

*Legislative Powers.* The Board may make sanitary rules and regulations, which, when approved by the Governor and the legislative body, have the force of law.

*Selection of Personnel.* The Board should select the health officer and should aid and advise him in the selection of important members of his personnel.

*Approve Budgets.* The review and approval of the annual budget of the department for presentation to the Governor is one of the important functions of the Board.

*Quasi-Judicial Powers.* In a large proportion of the states, the Board has the right to hold hearings in relation to violation of the sanitary code.

*Interpretation of Activities.* In addition to these specific functions, the Board interprets the activities of the health department to the executive and legislative bodies, and to the people at large. It also serves as a buffer between the health department personnel and activities, and rapid unfavorable political upheavals in state government, thus maintaining stability in the department and continuity of program.

**Qualifications of Members.** The most essential qualification for membership on the State Board of Health is that the member shall be a representative, public-spirited citizen, who is interested in, and familiar with public health affairs. Many states have designated specific qualifications for membership on the State Board of Health; for example, the requirement that a certain number of the Board must be physicians, or sanitarians, or engineers, pharmacists, educators, veterinarians, etc. Eleven states require that all members of the Board must be physicians. These specific designations for membership which are written into the law are of questionable value. It is much more important that the members shall be representative and intelligent persons who have a real interest in, and knowledge of, public affairs.

**Compensation.** The position should be an honorary one, the members serving without compensation. They may receive reimbursement for actual expenses, with, perhaps, a modest per diem honorarium.

**Organization.**[2] For purposes of greatest efficiency, a Board should consist of five, or at most seven, persons. They should be appointed by the Governor (with the consent of the Senate) for a term of five years, with overlapping terms, so that the terms of not more than two members expire each year. This plan gives continuity to the health program, since a majority of the Board is always familiar with its activities.

Regular quarterly meetings of the Board are usually sufficient, with specially called meetings in time of emergency.

The health officer is usually a member of the Board *ex-officio* and acts as its secretary.

**Executive Officer.** *Qualifications.* The state health officer should be the recognized leader in public health affairs in the state. He should be selected on the basis of suitable qualifications, most important of which are:

a. A thorough general knowledge of sanitary science and preventive medicine.

b. Proved executive ability.

c. Experience in developing public health programs.

It is not possible for the executive officer to possess expert knowledge in all the details of public health technic, such as statistical methods, laboratory procedures, etc. It is essential that he have a general knowledge of technical subjects, and be able to direct and correlate the activities of the department in a unified program. Thus, administrative ability and experience are most important qualifications.

Experience has shown that it is a sound policy to select a medically trained man for the health executive. The health officer deals so largely with the physicians of the state, and is so dependent upon them for the success of his program, that it is essential for him to hold their respect and to win their co-operation.

*Selection of the Health Officer.* In about one half of the states the health officer is selected directly by the Governor. In most of the remaining states he is selected by the State Board of Health, as already indicated. The latter is the better policy. In many states, the term of the Governor is for two years only. Bitter experience has repeatedly shown that an excellent, well-formulated health program can be wrecked by political upheavals. These have resulted in frequent changes in state health executives, each time a new governor has been elected. The consequence is a lack of continuity in development of the health program, with no security of tenure of office, a disturbed morale of the personnel, and inefficient service.[3]

[2] A great variety of methods has been devised for selection of the members of the State Boards of Health. For details see United States Public Health Service Bulletin No. 184, third edition, 1943.

[3] Nineteen different appointments as State Board of Health Executive were made in South Dakota in the 50 years from 1890 to 1940. During the same period, Minnesota and Connecticut each had only four different Health Officers. See Paterson, R. G.:

The health officer should be selected with great care by the Board of Health for a definite term of years—five years' time is sufficient to enable satisfactory program development, without danger of stagnation or bureaucracy. The selection should be made on as broad a basis as possible, in order to secure the best available man. It is a mistake to require that the selection be limited to individuals residing within the state. The New Mexico regulations for selection of the state health officer are admirable in this respect. This state requires only the broad general qualifications that "the state health officer shall be a person trained and experienced in sanitary science and public health administration." This is an almost perfect basis for selection.

The state health officer should devote his full time to his executive duties, and should receive a salary commensurate with his training and ability. The salary scale for state health officers varies greatly in the different states. Though salary is not a major consideration, it is obvious that no properly qualified man can be induced, nor should he be asked, to assume the responsibilities of this office unless he receives compensation which gives due recognition to his special qualifications.

In addition to the salary, a definite sum should be allocated for the use of the health officer, and certain key men in the department, for the purpose of attending important national public health meetings, such as the annual Surgeon General's Conference of State Health Officers, the American Public Health Association annual meeting, and others.

*Important Duties of the State Health Officer.* Some of the important duties of the state health officer are:

*a. Organization of the state health department.* The health officer has executive direction of all health activities. He is directly responsible to the State Board of Health for the proper functioning of the whole department.

*b. Selection of personnel.* The State Board may advise him in the selection of divisional directors and other key personnel, but the executive officer should have responsibility for employing and discharging the personnel of the department (within the limits of the Civil Service regulations).

*c. Preparation of the annual budget of the department* (with the approval of the State Board of Health) for presentation to the Governor.

*d. Supervision of disbursement of allocated funds,* including the regulation of salaries of the personnel. The funds may be disbursed by voucher through the state treasurer; supplies may be purchased through the state purchasing agent, or through other commissions.

*e. Serve as secretary to the State Board of Health* and prepare the agenda for the regular meetings.

---

*Historical Directory of State Health Departments in the United States of America,* published 1939 by the Ohio Public Health Association.

*f. Specific duties.* In many of the smaller states the health officer assumes direction of some essential division of activity, such as vital statistics, public health education, etc.

In addition to these specific duties, the health officer serves as a leader in interpreting the activities of the health department to the legislative body, to special groups, and to the public at large.

## FUNCTIONS OF THE STATE HEALTH DEPARTMENT

**Minimum Functions.** The desirable minimum functions of a state health service have been formulated by the American Public Health Association.[4] They are in brief:

1. Study of state health problems and planning for their solution as may be necessary.

2. Co-ordination and technical supervision of local health activities.

3. Financial aid to local health departments as required.

4. Enactment of regulations dealing with sanitation, disease control, and public health, which have the force of law throughout the state.

5. Establishment and enforcement of minimum standards of performance of work of health departments, particularly in communities receiving state aid for public health.

6. Maintenance of a central laboratory, and where necessary branch laboratories, for the standard functions of diagnostic, sanitary, and chemical examinations; production or procurement of therapeutic and prophylactic preparations, and their free distribution for public health purposes; establishment of standards for the conduct of diagnostic laboratories throughout the state; laboratory research into the causes and means of control of preventable diseases.

7. Collection, tabulation, and publication of vital statistics for each important political or health administrative unit of the state and for the state as a whole.

8. Collection and distribution of information concerning preventable diseases throughout the state.

9. Maintenance of safe quality of water supplies and controlling the character of the disposal of human waste for all communities of the state.

10. Establishment and enforcement of minimum sanitary standards for milk supplies.

11. Provision for services to aid industry in the study and control of health hazards due to occupation.

12. Prescription of qualifications for certain public health personnel.

13. Formulation of plans in co-operation with other appropriate agencies for the prompt mobilization of services to meet the health needs.

The Association states that, as a general principle, the local community

[4] "Desirable Minimum Functions and Organization Principles for Health Activities." An official declaration of the American Public Health Association, adopted 1940 and supplemented 1941 and 1943.

should assume primary responsibility for the conduct of the health program, since the "major part of direct service to people can be most efficiently and economically rendered on a community basis." But it is indispensable to good health administration that authority should be vested in the state department of health to make sure, for the state as a whole, that an adequate health service is provided to all the people, and to make suitable provision that the health of people in certain local communities will not be jeopardized by inertia or incompetence of the local authorities.

Furthermore, it is the duty of the state to give leadership and guidance to local communities in planning for health activities, and under certain situations it may be necessary for the state to aid in the selection of personnel and to give substantial financial assistance to local communities for the furtherance of their public health work. It is the opinion of the author, an opinion which is not shared by many other experienced public health officials in this field, that the state should not furnish more than one half the funds for local community health services. There may be exceptions to this rule, of course. But as a general rule, the local community will not take a sincere interest in the work, if it is too heavily subsidized by the state. The local community will feel that the old, simple adage, "the purse determines policy" still holds, and that the subsidized health work is in reality a state health department activity, rather than a local community responsibility.

## STATE HEALTH DEPARTMENT IS A TECHNICAL BUREAU

The function of a state health department is that of a scientific technical bureau for the prevention of disease and the promotion of the health of all the people. Such a department should serve the following purposes: [5]

1. *An advisory body.* The preservation of the public health is today a specialized service requiring technical training. So numerous are its branches that it cannot be expected that any individual can be adequately trained in the diverse fields embraced by this work, nor can it be expected that the separate municipalities can afford the services of such diverse personnel. It is therefore advisable that the state should maintain a highly trained scientific staff whose function it shall be to advise with the boards of health of the cities and towns. This is the prime purpose of the state health department.

2. *A correlating agency with power over intercommunity problems.* Many health problems of the present day cannot be confined to a single

[5] This statement of the functions of a State Health Department is taken almost verbatim from the Report of the Massachusetts Special Commission to Study and Investigate Public Health Laws and Policies, 1936 (House Document No. 1200). Since the author was Chairman of the committee which wrote this particular section of the report, he feels justified in using this material, and expresses his gratitude to his fellow members of the committee for permitting him to do so.

community, owing to social and economic conditions and particularly to development of rapid transportation. It is inevitable, therefore, that conditions will arise that may be a serious problem for a neighboring municipality yet of no concern to the community of origin. Thus the local board of health may fail to observe reasonable precautions in the handling of a case of typhoid in a home where meals are served to automobile travellers that may not jeopardize its own community, yet may menace the lives of those from other communities who may dine at this house. The neglect of food manufacturing establishments that sell their products principally in the neighboring towns may impose upon these latter a hazard against which they have little protection. It is desirable, therefore, that the state agency should have some authority to deal with these intercommunity health problems.

3. *Establishment of minimal standards.* In order to afford some guarantee of adequacy in local health administration and to maintain a minimum standard of health protection, it is essential that the state should have authority in all vital matters, and especially in those that may not be confined in their effects to a single community, to establish and to insist upon the enforcement of certain minimum standards of health practice in all communities within the state. Such standards should apply to all articles of food, to control of communicable diseases, to adequacy of essential services, and even to the technical qualification of those carrying on official public health activities. It is equally essential, however, that the local communities should have power, if they so desire, to enforce standards more stringent than the minimum standards that are established by the state.

4. *An agency offering certain specialized direct services.* Direct services of the health department should emanate from the smallest possible political unit that is consistent with efficiency and economy, inasmuch as the smaller the unit, the closer the contact with those receiving the service. It is inevitable, however, that certain services, because of their technical nature, cannot be made available even by the health departments of some of the large cities. Thus the manufacture and distribution of biologic products is too technical a procedure to be carried out economically by a municipality. It is therefore in the interest of both efficiency and economy that the state rather than the municipalities should render certain of these direct services. The decision as to the types of services to be rendered in individual communities is dependent on many variable factors, including the size, location, economic status and type of health problems of each community.

5. *Dissemination of information.* Public health succeeds or fails according to the extent to which it succeeds in educating the public as to its aims and methods. While it is true that no other form of popular education can surpass that carried on through personal contacts, as for example by the public health nurse, it is none the less essential that there should

be a central state agency around which much of the educational program may be built. This is a phase of public health that will assume greater importance in future years as greater emphasis is given to the problems of personal health.

6. *Research.* Progress in public health, as in other fields of human endeavor, is dependent upon study and research. Few would challenge this statement, and yet there are many who have maintained that research is the function of educational institutions and not of governmental agencies. It is fair to say that in the field of public health there are many important problems that cannot be studied effectively other than by official health departments, and that progress along certain lines must wait upon the initiative of these departments. Many of the outstanding achievements of the past in the public health field have emanated from careful observations by health department personnel. Some of these achievements have been of life-saving value, others have added to the better enjoyment of life, and still others have served the important purpose of eliminating unnecessary health expenditure. All, however, have contributed to the community well-being and represented a real return on the community investment. In order that progress may be made in the future, it is essential that facilities be provided to health departments so that they may conduct studies of new methods for the prevention of disease and the preservation of health.

**Aid to Local Health Organizations.** The chief activity of the state health department is one of advice and aid to the local health organizations, which in turn render direct service to the people. The state should give a few direct services. (Public health laboratory service is one of the major exceptions to this rule.) The state may conduct demonstration clinics with the aim eventually to turn over services of proved value to local health departments.

A local health service is one which is conducted and financed wholly or in part by a governmental division smaller than a state. These units of government are the counties, townships and municipalities. In most states, the counties are the only units of government that exist on a *state-wide basis,* and that possess the power to collect taxes and make appropriations for public purposes. In New England and a few other states a much smaller unit of government, the township, is the primary taxing and disbursing body, while the county government is rudimentary. In addition to counties and townships, incorporated cities or municipalities exist within the larger units of government. These municipalities are granted more or less autonomy by the state, the exact degree of which is determined in each separate instance by special charter. Thus, in developing a state-wide program of local health work, the state health officer must deal with county government or township government, and in addition, with municipal governments, which may be incorporated within the larger jurisdictions.

We are at present passing through a transitional stage in state health organization. The logical course is to develop each local governmental health service in the state to a point where the state will act only in an advisory and correlative capacity, with a purely nominal supervision of local programs. This stage has been reached in the case of many of the large cities. Many local jurisdictions, however, particularly in the rural areas, possess little or no local health organization or personnel. In these areas the health service is sadly deficient. State health administrators have realized this deficiency, so that in recent years a very large proportion of the efforts of many state health departments has been devoted to the development of efficient local health departments, especially in the smaller cities and rural areas.

**Technical Service.** There are certain specific activities which, because of their very nature, can best be carried out by the state health department itself.

*a. Continuous Services.*
1. Compilation and interpretation of vital statistics.
2. Preparation of biological products for free distribution.
3. Laboratory diagnostic service in communicable disease control.

*b. Intermittent services* rendered by the state to local communities.
This is usually expert technical consultation service.
1. Expert sanitary engineering advice rendered to municipalities in relation to public water supplies and sewage disposal plants.
2. Expert advice in relation to local enforcement in infractions of the sanitary code.
3. Assistance in times of disaster, or in times of special need.
4. Laboratory analysis, chemical and bacteriological, of public water supplies.

**Temporary Activities.** Certain activities have been assumed by the state health department during the developmental stage and before concrete, clear-cut administrative methods have been devised for integration of the activity in the local health department practice. For example, state health departments have carried out local diphtheria toxoid programs, have organized child hygiene clinics, industrial hygiene clinics, mental hygiene clinics, child guidance clinics, etc., for a temporary period in local communities. This is, of course, a health education procedure, and is intended to interest the local community in its own health problems to such an extent that the community will itself assume the responsibility.

**Relationship of the State and Municipal Health Departments.** In general, the state renders only advisory service to municipalities, and concentrates most of its direct activities in the more sparsely settled rural areas that do not have the facilities or leadership to solve their own problems. The state may aid directly in developing new or special municipal health activities, such as tuberculosis clinics, child hygiene programs, etc. It usually offers free diagnostic laboratory service to all municipalities, including distribution of certain biological products, and may assist with epidemiological investigations in case of emergency. The state has direct responsibility for the supervision of all municipal water supplies, and also for sewage disposal plants. It may aid in the hospitalization of tuberculosis, particularly in the smaller cities. The state conducts the hospital, and the municipalities pay for the actual care of their own municipal patients. Some states subsidize special services within the municipalities, such as venereal disease clinics, aid in public health education methods, etc.

**Relationship of the State to County Health Departments.** The relationship of the state to county health departments is in the developmental stage in most of the United States. Eventually, county health service will be on more or less the same basis as municipal health service, with adequate local financial support and interest, with competent personnel, and with well-planned and organized programs. The present stage of development has made it necessary for states to place special emphasis on, and give special consideration to, the organization of county health units and other types of full-time rural health organizations. The organization and growth of county health departments with full-time personnel in the United States in recent years has been phenomenal, but as yet is far from adequate to meet the needs of the rural population. This subject has been discussed in detail in another chapter.

The state usually gives the county health unit a definite subsidy of one half or more of the total budget of the unit, aids in the selection of personnel, and advises in the formulation of the program. In the early stages at least, the state maintains a direct supervision of the health unit activities. It does not give direct service, but aids and instructs the local full-time personnel in carrying out their own activities.

## ORGANIZATION OF THE STATE HEALTH DEPARTMENT

The state department of health is usually organized on the basis of divisions which are determined on a more or less clear-cut functional basis. The most important division administratively is the *division of local health service.*

The direct supervision of this activity should be in the hands of the health officer himself, or, in the larger states, a separate division may be formed with its own director. The director of the division of local health service should be deputy state health officer. He should have under his immediate supervision, or subject to his orders, various types of personnel that are qualified to aid and advise in the several types of activity of local health service, such as public health nurses, sanitarians, etc. In the larger states it is often necessary to divide the state on a geographic basis, with an assistant state director of local health work for each geographic division. One district director of local health service cannot supervise adequately more than 20 county health units.

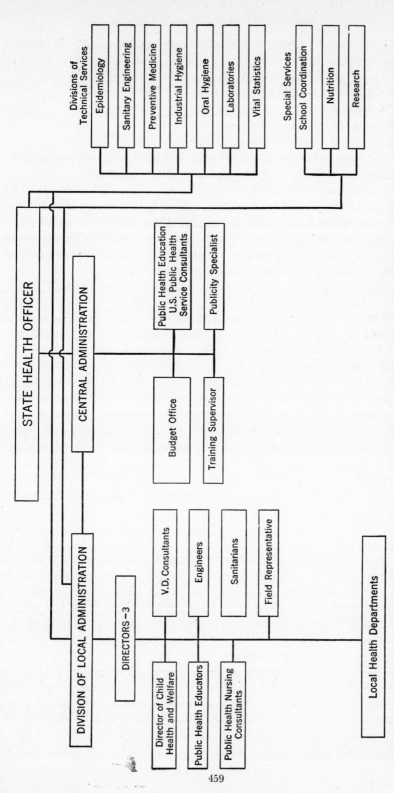

Fig. 37. *Organization Chart of the North Carolina State Board of Health.* Source: Reynolds, C. V., State Health Officer, *Reorganization of the State Board of Health,* September 1, 1943.

459

This type of state health organization may be illustrated by a chart of the organization of the North Carolina State Health Department. The health department has four divisions:

1. Division of Central Administration.
2. Division of Local Administration.
3. Division of Technical Services.
4. Division of Special Services.

The latter may be considered a small division for experimentation in administrative technics and development of new methods.

At the present time many counties have no organized health work. In others, the work is conducted by a part-time health officer. In these instances the state may be compelled to give direct service in case of emergency, such as during epidemics, and may also conduct demonstration health activities for the purpose of encouraging local support toward eventual establishment of an adequate local service.

As already noted (see chapter on Rural Health Organization), it has not been feasible to establish an adequate health service with full-time personnel in a county with less than 25,000 population, or in poor counties with even a larger population. Many counties in the United States have less than the necessary minimum of population and wealth for this type of health organization.

Some states have met the difficulty by granting additional subsidy to the poorer and smaller counties. Other states have attempted to organize a co-operative health unit, in which two or more counties have co-operated in the formation of a local health unit, with full-time personnel. This latter plan has not been very successful because of local jealousies and the desire of county governments for complete autonomy. In some instances, the director of the co-operative unit is paid by state funds. The remainder of the personnel is paid from local sources, but is subject to his orders, and a common budget for all activities is sponsored by all the counties. This rather complicated plan has obvious advantages as well as defects.

**District Plan.** Under this plan of organization, the state is divided into large geographic areas. A full-time district health officer, paid by the state, has charge of each district. In reality, he is a deputy state health officer for the area. He advises and assists the local public health personnel in all health matters. The local officials retain their autonomy, the state officer acting chiefly in a consultative capacity. Several of the more populous states, notably New York and Massachusetts, have utilized this general plan of organization.

The method is very effective as an epidemiological service. One great advantage of the district plan is that the district health officer is usually a well-trained, efficient man who can carry through an emergency situation. The general tendency has been to supplant gradually this type of organization by full-time county health units.

A few states have assumed direct responsibility for all public health activities outside incorporated municipalities. This is essentially the plan in Pennsylvania and Delaware, and might have certain advantages in large, sparsely settled states, such as Nevada and Wyoming.

**Technical Functions.** In addition to the major activities which relate to development of local health service, there are certain technical functions which are common to every state health department. Each may be organized as a separate division of activity, or, in the smaller states, two or more functions may be developed by a single division. In the large state organizations, there may be subdivisions of activity in relation to a single function, each subdivision having its own director. The major technical functions are concerned with:

1. Vital Statistics.
2. Communicable Disease Control.
3. Sanitation.
4. Public Health Laboratories.
5. Public Health Education.
6. Child Hygiene.
7. Public Health Nursing.
8. Industrial Hygiene.
9. Oral Hygiene.

Other functions are sometimes assigned to the state department of health. A few miscellaneous functions of state government that are only indirectly related to public health affairs are also occasionally incorporated in the activities of the state health department, as, for example, plumbing inspection, barber shop inspection, and particularly the examining and licensing of physicians, of dentists, public health nurses, morticians, plumbers, etc. Adult hygiene is sometimes organized as a special service.

There is great variation in type of organization in the different states in carrying out these technical functions. We shall outline a simple form of organization, giving examples of variations that may seem important.

**Central Administration.** Usually, the health officer has direct supervision over the Division of Central Administration. This division has the responsibility for all accounting and personnel, leaves of absence, vacations, payment of salaries, purchase of supplies, preparation of the budget, etc. In a few states this division has its own director, who is not a physician, but a person trained in accounting and business methods.

In many of the smaller states, vital statistics is not a separate division of activity, but is directed by the health officer and fused with the Division of Central Administration.

Frequently, Public Health Education is not a separate division, with its own director, but its activities are carried out under the immediate direction of the state health officer.

The development of local health service may either be under the direct supervision of the health officer and incorporated in the division of cen-

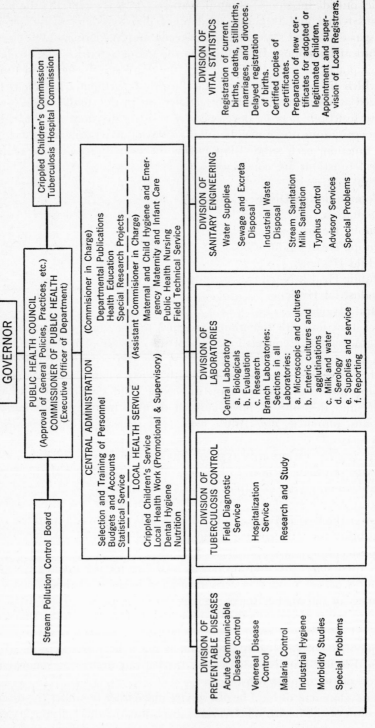

FIG. 38. *Organization Chart of the Tennessee Department of Public Health.*

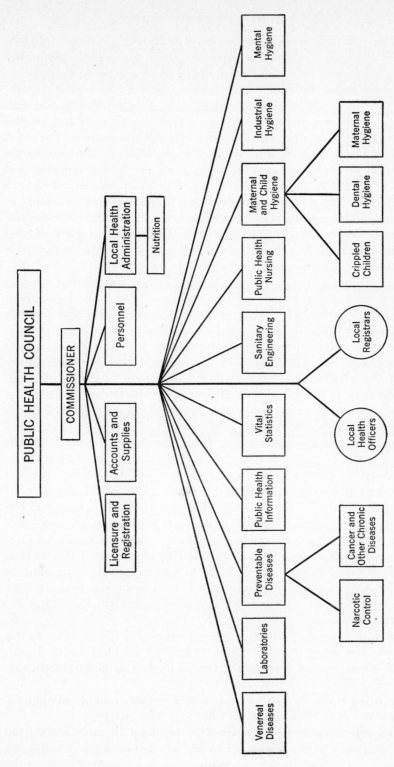

FIG. 39. *Organization Chart of the Connecticut State Department of Health.*

tral administration, or may be carried as a separate division of activity under the direction of the deputy health officer. The organization of this special division of activity has been discussed in a previous chapter.

**Vital Statistics.** This is an important technical service rendered to the state as a whole. It includes the registration of births, deaths and marriages, as well as other essential data. Actual compilation and analysis of the data are technical, but not extremely difficult matters. The interpretation of the findings, however, is very important in determining the soundness of procedure and the progress of the health program, and serves as an aid in planning future activities of the whole state health department. The director of the division is one of the key members of the staff. In the smaller states, the health officer himself, or the director of communicable disease, may serve as analyst and interpreter of vital statistical data. In this case the division is organized simply with a technical staff to make the proper records and compilations.

Local registrars are selected by the state department of vital statistics through local health department channels, usually with one registrar for each voting district. The local registrars are paid on a fee basis for each certificate, by the local government—municipality, county or township.

The work in the central office of the division of vital statistics requires approximately one statistical clerk for each 150,000 population of the state. The allotment for supplies and particularly for postage for this division must be liberal. A fair allotment for the Department of Vital Statistics should be from 5 per cent to 10 per cent of the total state health department budget.

**Communicable Disease Control.** This important activity is usually organized as a separate division. The relative emphasis that the state health department must place on the work of this division is dependent upon the effectiveness of local health services throughout the state. If they are well organized, the division simply acts in an advisory and correlative manner. If local health services are inadequate, the state division has a heavy burden in checking and running down local epidemics, such as smallpox or typhoid fever. In periods of emergency this division may be required to take actual charge of a local epidemic situation. In addition, there are special problems in control of diseases having a high local endemicity, such as diphtheria, trachoma, malaria, hookworm disease and others.

Morbidity reports of all reportable communicable disease come to this division. Usually, physicians report directly to the local health departments. These, in turn, forward the reports to the Communicable Disease Division of the State Department of Health.

The division has its own director, with a suitable number of epidemiologists and clerical personnel to carry out its activities.

Diagnostic laboratory service may be organized in this division, but since laboratory service is required by several other divisions of the health department, it is better to organize the whole laboratory service in a separate division.

*Tuberculosis Control.* This activity is often organized as a separate division, because of the great importance of this work, and particularly when the state health department has charge of the hospitalization program for tuberculosis. A more logical arrangement is to incorporate the work as a Subdivision of Tuberculosis in the Division of Communicable Disease. The chief function of the state in tuberculosis control work is to provide hospitalization facilities for those areas of the state without local hospitals, and to stimulate and aid local tuberculosis prevention programs. The state may aid in the establishment of local clinics, by subsidy, through demonstration clinic service, or otherwise.

*Venereal Disease Control.* The state aids in diagnosis of venereal disease through development of adequate free laboratory facilities. The state may aid in the development of local venereal disease control programs, and may assist in the establishment of local clinics by subsidy or otherwise. Many states have supplied anti-syphilitic remedies free, or at cost, to local clinics and to physicians. Some few states have organized and supported financially, free diagnostic and treatment clinics. The state frequently supplies an educational stimulus to the people through lecture and pamphlet service.

Venereal disease control activities should not be organized as a separate division, but as part of the Division of Communicable Disease Control. In the larger states, a subdivision for this service may be formed with its own director and budget; administratively, it should be a subdivision and not a major activity.

The expenditures for the Division of Communicable Disease Control vary greatly, depending upon the system of organization in the various states. If the state health department has an extensive tuberculosis hospitalization program, this activity alone may absorb more funds than all the rest of the state health activities combined.

If we include in this division only those activities commonly allotted to it and do not include tuberculosis hospitalization, the expenditures for the work will represent from 10 per cent or less of the total state health appropriation. Ample funds are required in this division for travel, and an item for purchase of biological products may be included in the division budget. It is also wise to provide a contingent fund for emergencies in relation to the activities of this division.

**Public Health Laboratories.** A good state public health laboratory service is a great asset to the whole health department. It is a real aid to physicians through furnishing diagnostic criteria for their patients, and has served as an important factor in winning the co-operation of physicians toward carrying out the whole state health program.

The director of the laboratory service must be well qualified in all technical procedures, and must have administrative ability as well. The work should be organized as a separate division of activity and should include the laboratory work of all divisions of the state health department. Its largest activity will be concerned with diagnostic procedures for the Division of Communicable Disease, but it should also do the laboratory work for the Division of Sanitation, food and drug analysis, laboratory studies for the Division of Industrial Hygiene, etc.

Some states, for the sake of economy, have developed their laboratory service in the State University. This plan has many administrative difficulties. The laboratory should be under the direct auspices of the state health department and should be housed with the other divisions as an integral part of the state health department.

The actual procedures of a state laboratory have already been discussed. (See chapter on Public Health Laboratories.) The scope of its work and organization of the service depend upon the total population of the state, the area, transportation facilities for laboratory specimens, etc. It is not feasible, for example, for small states—one million or less population—to manufacture any but the most simple biological products. They should not attempt to produce diphtheria antitoxin, tetanus anti-sera, etc., which are only manufactured successfully on a large scale.

In order to insure satisfactory diagnostic services in communicable disease, where speed of diagnosis is an important factor, the laboratory must be readily accessible. Thus, branch laboratory systems have been developed in many larger states. These are miniatures of the central laboratory. They work under its direction and carry out many of the same laboratory procedures as the larger laboratory. They are particularly valuable where rapid diagnosis is important.

Another plan which serves to distribute laboratory service is called the "approved laboratory" system. The state develops standards of technic for local laboratories. It then holds annual inspections and gives certificates of approval. In some instances the local laboratories receive a small subsidy from the state.

*Distribution of Biological Products.* These products are usually distributed through the division of communicable disease control, but may be prepared by the division of laboratories. As a general rule, prophylactic materials such as typhoid vaccine, diphtheria toxoid, silver nitrate ampules, etc., are distributed free of charge. Therapeutic products, such as diphtheria antitoxin, insulin, etc., are distributed at cost, and free to indigents. The distribution is not direct, but through local health department channels.

No fees are charged for diagnostic laboratory tests, as a rule, nor for analysis of public or semi-private water supplies. The state cannot attempt to do water analysis of private water supplies.

*Special Laboratory Work.* The laboratory may carry out a great variety of tests, including analyses of foods and drugs, laboratory activities for the department of industrial hygiene, studies of water, sewage, stream pollution, oyster and shell fish sanitation, swimming pool and bathing beach sanitation, and many other tests. In general, the field studies should be done by the division in charge of each separate activity, and the laboratory procedures should be carried out by the Division of Laboratories and the results reported to the division concerned.

The appropriation for public health laboratory services may vary in the different states between 5 per cent and 35 per cent of the total budget, with a mean of about 15 per cent. One cannot compare the expenditures of one state with another, as the same activities are not always included in the data presented. When biologicals are manufactured and distributed free of charge, the actual saving to the citizens may be greater than the entire cost of the whole laboratory service. A fair apportionment for laboratory service for the average state is 15 per cent to 20 per cent of the total appropriation.

It is not possible to make an estimate of the efficiency of laboratory service on the basis of per-specimen cost of examinations, since per-specimen cost depends so much on the type of examinations. It is frequently stated that a well-organized state laboratory will do at least one examination for every ten persons in the state annually at a cost not to exceed thirty-five cents per specimen examined. These figures are not an accurate index of completeness or efficiency of state laboratory service. A detailed analysis of the quality of the service and the various types of activity that the laboratory undertakes is necessary to determine whether or not the laboratory is actually giving an efficient service.

**Division of Public Health Engineering.** This division has a broad scope of activities and is one of the most effective and important divisions in the state. Activities of this division include a study of all problems relating to public and semi-public water supplies and sewage disposal plants. Included also are stream pollution, the sanitation of public bathing beaches, swimming pools and the disposal of human waste in individual homes.

Sanitation of food, including preparation, shipping, storage and marketing, sanitation of restaurants and other public eating places, sanitation of public meeting places, hotels, theaters, etc., all come within the province of this division. In some states, milk sanitation, shell fish sanitation, sanitary features of malaria control, etc., are special and important problems.

As in other state activities, the extent of the work of this division depends upon the degree of development of adequate local health service. Where municipalities and counties have a well-developed sanitary service with competent personnel, the state service is advisory, with correlation and integration of local activities. Where local sanitary service is inadequate, the state personnel must often actually carry out the necessary protective measures.

This division has the responsibility for the proper supervision of all

the municipal water supply and sewage disposal plants in the state. All
plans of municipalities for installation of new equipment or modification of old must be submitted to the state sanitation division for approval.
The plants are inspected when necessary, and chemical and bacteriological
tests of these supplies are made at regular intervals.

Many of the other sanitary functions mentioned above are concerned
with matters that are primarily of local significance. Usually, the procedures can be handled readily by local inspectors, with the aid and back-
ing of the state department.

Milk sanitation is state-wide in scope. A uniform state-wide milk sanitation code is advisable. Local inspectors may enforce local pasteurization and marketing regulations, but dairy inspection is best carried out
on a state-wide basis by the state department of health, the state department of agriculture, or better, by co-operative arrangement. State-wide
dairy inspection insures uniformity, and prevents duplication of inspections which are the bane of the dairy farmer's existence.

*Personnel.* Every state should have as the director of this division a
well qualified, experienced public health engineer. In the larger states
he will require several assistant engineers to cover the whole field of work.
The number of other personnel for the division will depend upon the
special needs and sanitary problems of the state. The average state with
a fairly well developed local sanitary service, and no special sanitary problems, such as malaria, would plan to expend about 10 per cent of the
total state appropriation on sanitation.

**Public Health Education.** The scope of activities of this division has
already been defined. (See chapter on Public Health Education.) The
work of the division is so important that the health officer frequently
assumes direct responsibility for these activities. Some of the larger
states have formed a separate division for this work, with its own director.

If local health departments are well developed, the chief function of
the division is to aid them in their programs, supply them with ideas
and materials. The state is the central depot for exhibit material, lecture material, lantern slides, posters, and moving picture films, which
are loaned free of charge and are circulated about the state.

The division has charge of the annual report, the preparation of educational material on various subjects for each of the other divisions, and
all radio broadcast programs for the state health department. The division arranges schedules for lecture service, prepares newspaper releases,
and has general charge of all other publicity material of the health department.

The work of this department is bungled more often than that of any
other. The reason is that one rarely finds a person with a medical or
other scientific training who has ability along publicity lines. The director of the work must be primarily a publicist. He must have an understanding of public relations, a flair for journalism, and an ability to

present scientific facts in a popular and appealing way. In reviewing the best public health educational material that has been prepared by the various states, one almost invariably finds that the most effective work is done in those states that employ a person to direct the work of this division who is thoroughly familiar with the technic of mass education and appeal.

It is generally conceded that the work of this division can be carried out effectively at a cost not to exceed 3 per cent to 5 per cent of the total state health budget.

**Child Hygiene.** The development of child hygiene as a separate division of state activity is a relatively recent movement. In 1915, only a half dozen states devoted special attention to this subject. Voluntary agencies had long realized that the subject had been neglected, and they are largely responsible for its development in local and state governments. Following the passage of the Shepard-Towner Act in 1921, federal subsidy for state and local maternal and child welfare activities became available. During the following ten years child hygiene service of some type became established in every state. When the federal subsidy terminated in 1930, these activities were thoroughly incorporated in state health department practice. This activity received new stimulus under the Social Security Act. The Children's Bureau utilized its funds effectively in aiding the various states to formulate sound local child hygiene programs. Its great contribution was the assistance given in obtaining good personnel and in giving aid for special training of key persons in the different state divisions of child hygiene.

The chief activities of the state division of child hygiene are:

*a.* Maternity and prenatal work.
*b.* Infant hygiene.
*c.* Preschool hygiene.
*d.* School hygiene.
*e.* Care of crippled and handicapped children is often a state health department responsibility.

*Maternity and Prenatal Work.* The state does not render direct service, but gives aid and advice to local health departments in developing their programs. Some states do send, on request, monthly prenatal letters to expectant mothers.

The state regulates the practice of midwifery and, in some instances, develops systems of instruction and local supervision.

Lying-in hospitals are licensed by some state health departments. Almost all states have a uniform regulation in relation to prevention of ophthalmia neonatorum, with free distribution of silver nitrate ampules and compulsory use of silver nitrate in the eyes of all the new born.

*Infant Hygiene.* The chief state function is to aid in forwarding local programs. The state may conduct demonstration clinics for a temporary period and, in some instances, states have subsidized local clinics. Education in the whole field of child hygiene is one of the very important phases of a state-wide health education program.

**The E.M.I.C. Program.** During the years of World War II the Federal Government provided for maternity and infant care of soldiers' families under an emergency maternity and infant care program. The funds for payment of this service were administered through state governments, which in turn distributed the funds to local health departments. This plan is described in some detail in the chapter on child hygiene. There was at first a great deal of confusion in the administration of the program. Many physicians refused to participate in the plan.

Each mother chose her own physician, who was paid on a uniform basis, with special additional payments, when required, for special services. It was the first time, in most states, that physicians received payment for medical care through official sources. Furthermore, certain minimum standards of prenatal and postnatal care were set. Physicians resented this encroachment by government on medical practice at first, but gradually accepted the plan. Many mothers realized for the first time what adequate prenatal and postnatal care really should be.

*Preschool Hygiene.* The procedures in relation to preschool hygiene are similar to those followed in infant hygiene. There is a tendency to place less emphasis on the distinction between infant and preschool hygiene. Rather, the program is a continuous one throughout early childhood, though less intensive after the second year of life. Special emphasis is placed on prevention of contagious diseases of childhood, and on correction of remediable defects. The state health department should stress diphtheria immunization and smallpox prevention through educational methods, and by actual assistance to local health departments. Most states have some system of free distribution of immunizing agents, particularly diphtheria toxoid and smallpox vaccine.

A program for the stimulation of correction of defects has been developed in many states. The major items are correction of orthopedic defects and dental hygiene. Following the Social Security Act, actual correctional service has been given by the state, through the organization of dental hygiene clinics and orthopedic clinics, as well as tonsil and adenoid clinics. The organization of these special correctional clinic services is discussed in the chapter on the Social Security Act.

*School Hygiene.* As already noted, state-wide school hygiene programs in many states are under the direction of the State Department of Education. Nearly half the states have some form of compulsory school health examinations. In the great proportion of these states, this activity is carried out by local school or health agencies, with the aid of, or actual supervision by, state agencies. In a few states the State Department of Health and the Department of Education have a joint responsibility for the school health program. Theoretically, this is the best plan, but it leads to divided responsibility and many administrative difficulties. The most successful plan, from an administrative point of view, places the school medical and nursing service under the direction of a well-organized local health department, with supervision of this program by the state health department. Health instruction in the schools should be the province of the Department of Education.

**Public Health Nursing.** The proper organization of a state public health nursing service is a subject concerning which there is a good deal of controversy. The functions of this service are well defined, namely,

a. To aid and advise local health agencies in the development of their public health nursing programs.

b. To maintain proper standards of public health nursing throughout the state:

(1) By determination of eligibility requirements for public health nurses throughout the state.

(2) By aiding in the selection of local personnel.

(3) Through organization of a plan for continuous education of the nurses actually in the field.

It is a general principle that the state itself should not give actual public health nursing service; though a few of the states, and also the Western Provinces of Canada, which have very large areas with a widely scattered population, have found it advantageous to provide nursing service, at state expense, to these outlying districts. These nurses work under pioneer conditions and are sometimes called upon to perform duties requiring great courage and self-reliance.

The personnel required in a state health department to carry out a successful program depends upon many factors, such as: area of the state, density of population, and degree of development of local nursing service. An average state with a population of about a million people would require a director of the nursing service, an assistant in the central office, and perhaps three or four regional or district supervisors distributed in the various areas throughout the state.

*Organization.* A number of the state health officers have organized the state nursing program as a special division of activity. Since the activities of the public health nurse relate in great part to maternity and child hygiene, most of the remainder of the states have organized public health nursing as a section of the division of child hygiene. There is a director of child hygiene, usually a physician, who has charge of all activities, with an assistant director, always a nurse, who conducts the nursing program. The National Organization for Public Health Nursing objects to this arrangement. This organization takes the stand that public health nursing is an essential technic, and should be a separate division of activity. The division should have its own director, who should have the same recognition and status as other divisional directors.

If the public health nursing is combined with the division of child hygiene, and this is the commonest type of organization at present, a suitable professional personnel for a Division of Child Hygiene of an average state with about one million population would be:

  a. Director of Child Hygiene and Public Health Nursing—a physician.
  b. Nutritionist—advisory.
  c. Dental Hygienist—advisory.
  d. Assistant Director in charge of public health nursing—a nurse. Other nursing personnel as outlined above.

Approximately 15 per cent of the state health appropriation is usually devoted to the Division of Child Hygiene and Public Health Nursing. In case two separate divisions are formed, there may be an equal apportionment of this fund between the two divisions.

There is a general tendency to consider all child hygiene work, and public health nursing as well, not as special technics of state health service, but rather as advisory functions of the state health department in development of local health activities. In this case, it would be a logical administrative procedure to include child hygiene and public health nursing as subdivisions or as an integral part of the major division of Local Health Service.

**Oral Hygiene.** The review of physical examinations of one million young men who were drafted into the military services for World War II revealed that the most prevalent defect of young Americans was faulty teeth. Furthermore, there had been no apparent improvement in the teeth of this group of men over the teeth of their fathers who were examined a generation previously for World War I. This situation obviously warranted special consideration of the whole field of oral hygiene. The United States Public Health Service added consultant dentists to its personnel, giving them the same rank and status as physicians. These men aided the various states in the formulation of dental hygiene programs.

In some states, a special division of dental hygiene was organized in the state department of health, with a dentist in charge who had had special training in the field of oral hygiene. Other states have organized their state-wide dental hygiene programs under the general supervision of the department of child health.

**Food and Drugs.** The enforcement of the food and drug laws of the state is a responsibility of the health department in a few states. Usually, a separate division for these activities is not formed. Milk sanitation, shell fish sanitation, general food sanitation, etc., are the province of the Division of Public Health Engineering. The necessary laboratory tests are done by the Public Health Laboratory Division.

**Industrial Hygiene.** The phenomenal growth of industrial hygiene in recent years has been described in a previous chapter. The reasons are clear. The United States has had a rapid transition from an agricultural economy to a highly industrialized economy. World War II greatly accentuated this development. Many states that had had no large manufacturing interests suddenly developed factories and industrial communities, with all the special hazards and public health problems that accompany sudden population expansion, with unskilled personnel in industry, and with new manufacturing processes which had unrecognized special hazards.

The Federal Government came forward with offers of grants-in-aid to states to establish state divisions of industrial hygiene. The functions and activities of a division of industrial hygiene were determined, and proper relationships were worked out with industry and with labor. By 1945 every state had an official industrial hygiene service except North and South Dakota, New Mexico, Arizona, Nevada, Maine, and Nebraska. In most of the states, industrial hygiene divisions were centered in the state department of health. In a few states the department of labor assumed the responsibility for the activity, or in a few instances, there was joint responsibility for these state services. This plan of joint responsibility is probably the most effective.

In 1945 the various states appropriated $900,000 from state and local funds for industrial health work. In addition, approximately $600,000 was received by states from the Federal Government, for the development of industrial health work. This appropriation provided for the employment of more than 300 physicians, industrial health engineers, industrial nurses, and other personnel working toward the promotion of the health of the worker.

Much of the stimulus for this extraordinary development of industrial hygiene came from the Industrial Hygiene Division of the Bureau of State Services of the United States Public Health Service. This central staff, with its coterie of advisors and consultants, has been of great utility in outlining state programs, setting forth suitable qualifications for personnel and performance, and aiding in the solution of difficult technical problems in the field.

For the most part, industrial health services are developed most effectively on a state-wide basis. A few of the large city health departments may organize profitably a separate division of industrial hygiene, but in most states, this activity should be organized at the state level.

**Organization of a State Industrial Health Service:**

*A.* Medical Board of Industrial Compensation. It is common practice to assign administrative matters relating to industrial compensation to an impartial board of examiners. This board should be made up of competent physicians who have no political affiliation. The members should be given tenure and suitable compensation. The appointments may be made by the Governor from a list of nominees submitted by the dean of the medical department in the state universities, or by other authoritative and impartial sources. Members of the board should be of high moral caliber, disinterested, and should have had extensive experience in the diagnosis of occupational illnesses. The functions of the board of examiners in occupational disease are:

1. To advise whether or not the claimant is suffering from occupational disease for which compensation is claimed.

2. To determine the degree of disability caused by occupational disease.

The board of examiners in occupational disease may be attached administratively to the state bureau of industrial hygiene, or may be an independent body.

*B.* The Bureau of Industrial Hygiene should be an integral part of the state department of health.

The state department of labor may have factory inspectors that are concerned with the compliance of industry with state labor laws, and also may be interested in the compliance of employers with the safety provisions of the state compensation law. Thus there may be a certain overlapping of activities by various state agencies in the industrial health field, which will result in annoyance to factory managers, and confusion in state administrative procedures.

The creation by the governor of an interdepartmental health council, which is described elsewhere, should result in smoothing out interdepartmental administrative duplication.

**Mental Hygiene.** Most states have a separate Bureau of Mental Disease, sometimes called a Bureau of Mental Hygiene. Its major activities and interests are centered in hospitalization of the insane. This activity is so extensive that the expenditure for state hospitals for the insane is a very large item in any state budget. The general tendency is to develop mental hygiene as an activity of the State Bureau of Mental Diseases, using the state mental hospitals as centers and establishing mental hygiene clinics, child guidance clinics, etc., in the territory surrounding each hospital unit. The personnel of the hospitals is used in organizing and conducting the clinics.

A few state health departments have established separate divisions of mental hygiene. The chief function of the division is to stimulate, to aid and advise local agencies in developing child guidance and mental hygiene clinics.

## INCORPORATION OF THE STATE HEALTH SERVICE WITH OTHER STATE BUREAUS

A few of the smaller states, in the interests of economy and simplicity, have attempted to reorganize all state government on a functional basis, and have included state health activities under the same administration as welfare agencies. The state of Maine, for example, formed a single Bureau of Health, Welfare and Institutions. There was a commissioner for the bureau, who was appointed by the governor, with a director for each of the three services. Many health administrators believe that such an organization is not for the best interests of public health.

The point at issue is a fundamental one. Is protection of the health of the people a major or a minor function of government? No one will question the thesis that it is the duty of the state to care for the afflicted, the poor and the infirm. The hospitalization of the afflicted, the care of the widowed, the orphan, and the aged has a great emotional appeal—an obvious, concrete and immediate necessity.

A much more important duty and higher function of the state is *prevention* of illness, and the maintenance of a high standard of community health. But these functions are not so obvious or concrete, and do not have the same emotional appeal as welfare activities. Many health officers believe that if public health, a major function of government, is incorporated with the minor functions of institutional care and poor relief, there is real danger that the former function will become submerged by the latter and will not receive the consideration which it merits.

Canada has shown us the way whereby a suitable welfare program may be incorporated in a public health service in sparsely settled areas, without detriment either to the health or to the welfare service. The key to success for this program lies in the selection of a Director who is a physician with both public health training and welfare experience.

In Manitoba a joint health and welfare department has been organized to serve a large, sparsely settled province.

The Deputy Minister of Health, who corresponds to State Health Officer in the United States, is in charge of the Department. He is a physician, trained in the public health field. There are two divisions of activity: (*a*) public welfare, and (*b*) public health. The following activities are assigned to each division:

A. **Public Welfare.**

1. *Social assistance.* This service is given to unorganized territory where there is no municipal corporation. Direct aid is given to these remote people, including food, clothing, shelter, as well as medical and nursing care.
2. *Mothers' allowances.* This represents aid to widows, orphans, etc.
3. *Child care and protection.* This service includes care of neglected children and of orphans.
4. *Legal supervision* is an activity which includes the care of unmarried mothers, of delinquent children, etc.
5. *Old age pensions* and provision for the care of the blind.

B. **Public Health.**

1. *Hospitalization*
   a. Mental disease.

      *b.* General hospitalization. Subsidies to all municipal and private hospitals.

      *c.* Tuberculosis and other communicable disease hospitalization.

      *d.* Care of chronic illness. This service includes supervision of "old people's homes" and the placing of elderly people in private homes.

   2. *General Disease Prevention Program.* All the activities customarily assigned to the State Department of Public Health are carried out by this division.

The budget is divided approximately as follows:

|  | Per Cent |
|---|---|
| *A.* Division of Public Welfare | |
| 1. Social assistance | 5 |
| 2, 3, 4, and 5 (all other activities) | 21 |
| *B.* Division of Health | |
| 1. Hospitalization | |
|    *a.* Mental Diseases | 35 |
|    *b.* Hospital Subsidies for general and for communicable disease care | 26 |
| 2. General Disease Prevention | 13 |
| | 100 |

One great weakness of the program is lack of a sufficient number of public health nurses. The strength of the plan lies in its flexibility. Whenever personnel are widely scattered, each person must carry out varied tasks. Thus, a public health nurse in a remote area may be called upon to find a home for an elderly person, investigate a report of a neglected child, visit an orphan placed in a private family by the state, or do many other welfare tasks in addition to her normal public health duties.

The plan of organization that has been formulated in Manitoba is best suited to the "great open spaces" of some of our western states. It would not work successfully in a compact, heavily populated small eastern state.

## HOSPITALIZATION

Many states have developed an extensive state program of hospitalization, particularly for tuberculosis. In some instances this activity has been incorporated as one of the functions of the state health department. The hospital is considered as part of the technic of tuberculosis prevention. This is a logical procedure, but has led to administrative difficulties. Hospitalization is very expensive; the single item of hospitalization for tuberculosis may exceed the total of all other expenditures for public health by the state. In some instances, an elaborate hospitalization plan may result in curtailment of other equally important activities, and thus an excellent and beneficial single activity may react to the detriment of the whole service.

In order that a well balanced state health program may be developed, it is essential, when preparing a budget for the State Department of Public Health, to segregate all items for hospitalization, whether or not the hospitalization service is administered by the state health department.

**Medical Care.** In the chapter on The National Health Program, we discuss the proposal that the state shall be made responsible for the administration of all services that may be provided for medical, nursing, and hospital care in illness, as well as in prevention of disease, and in promotion of health.

This trend in public administration has been developing for many years in other great nations of the world, and there are some indications that a considerable proportion of the American people would be interested in the social experiment of a comprehensive plan of government-administered medical care. Under our governmental system, the state would be the basic unit of administration of medical care, with subsidy from the Federal Government to initiate the work, and to supplement the costs of medical care in the poorer areas. The local communities would have a certain limited amount of autonomy in the administration of the plan, but the state would be the central agency.

The question arises at once as to whether these state programs of medical care should be incorporated in the state department of health, or whether a separate state department of medical care should be organized. Students of public administration in the United States are divided on this point. The E.M.I.C. Plan, which was an emergency maternity service for soldiers' wives of World War II, was a medical care program that was administered through state health departments by funds provided from Federal subsidy. (See page 470.) Thus a precedent, at least, has been set.

The State of Maryland has organized a bureau of medical services in the state department of health, which is concerned with the medical care of the poor and the medically indigent. This plan reaches only a very small proportion of the total population, but does provide for a state-wide medical care plan. In other states, the medical care of the indigent is provided through the state department of public welfare.

No one can foresee the developments in this field in the near future. Farsighted young physicians who are preparing themselves for a career in public health are not only studying the established fields of epidemiology, sanitation, vital statistics, child health, and the like, but are also preparing themselves in sociology, economics, public administration, and institutional management. Administration of a state-wide program of medical care is indeed an administrative responsibility of great magnitude, and would require executive talents of high caliber. Logically the program, if adopted, should be an integral part of the state department of health, since the primary function of this department has been, and should continue to be, protection against illness and promotion of individual and public health.

**Interdepartmental Health Council.** Mountin [6] has shown in his study of the distribution of health services in the structure of state government, that there is a great dispersion of state health activities among many state agencies. Some of these activities are included in departments of welfare, social security, and emergency relief. The department of education, the department of labor, independent state hospital boards, the department of mental hygiene, and many others carry out some phase of health protection.

Dr. Mountin estimates that states expend approximately $1.90 per capita annually for all health activities, by all official state agencies. Of this total, only 18 per cent is expended by the state health department itself. The number of full-time administrative and field personnel that were employed for health work by state agencies (in 1940) was 18,737. The health departments employed 11,269, or 60 per cent of the total. Thus many state bureaus participate in health protection.

Obviously, all the varied state health activities should be consolidated. New York State resolved this matter by the administrative device of an Interdepartmental Health Council. [7] The council consists of the state commissioners of health, social welfare, mental hygiene, and education. The chairman of the New York State Health Preparedness Committee serves as an advisory member of the council. The purpose of this Council is to assure co-operation and interchange of plans within the state administration, and the co-ordination of health services that the state provides to the people in the local communities.

## SUMMARY

No single standardized plan of state health organization can be devised that will be suitable for each and every state. Public health practice by state governments has been under way for only a few years in many states, and no state has reached a stage of complete and satisfactory development. An analysis of present practice indicates that certain functions are considered as essential by all experienced administrators. The relative importance of these various essential activities has been indicated by the budgetary procedure in the various states.

An analysis of the allocation of funds by the various state health officers indicates that at the present time and under usual conditions the proportion of the budget that may be allocated to essential divisions of activity is about as follows:

[6] Mountin, J. W. and Flook, Evelyn: "Distribution of Health Services in the Structure of State Government." Chap. I: The Composite Pattern of State Health Services. *Pub. Health Rep.* 1941, Vol. 56, p. 1673.

[7] Message by Governor T. E. Dewey to the State Congress, Oct. 5, 1946.

## ALLOCATION OF THE STATE HEALTH BUDGET

| Activity | Proportion of the Budget |
|---|---|
| 1. Central Administration | about 10%–15% |
| 2. Vital Statistics | "  7%–10% |
| 3. Communicable Disease Control | "  15%–20% |
| 4. Sanitation | "  10%–15% |
| 5. Public Health Laboratories | "  15%–20% |
| 6. Public Health Education | "  3%– 5% |
| 7. Development of Local Health Service including subsidies to counties | "  15%–25% |
| 8. Child Hygiene and Public Health Nursing | "  7%–15% |

United States Public Health Service Bulletin No. 184 (1943) gives the following approximate expenditures for state health services by the various states. These do not include grants-in-aid to local health work.

|  |  | Per Capita Cost | Per Cent of Total |
|---|---|---|---|
| Central Services | | $ .08 | 15% |
| Vital Statistics | $ .01 | | |
| Health Education | .01 | | |
| Laboratories | .03 | | |
| Communicable Disease | | .245 | 46% |
| Tuberculosis | .190 | | |
| Venereal Disease | .039 | | |
| Others | .016 | | |
| Sanitation | | .125 | 23% |
| Child Health | | .047 | 9% |
| Industrial Health | | .035 | 7% |
| Total Technical Services | | $ .532 | 100% |
| Medical and Dental Care | | 1.42 | |
| Total Cost of Health Services per Capita | | $1.95 ± | |

The first step, which has now been accomplished by almost all state health departments, is the establishment of all the essential technical activities. The next step is the advancement of local health department activities to the point where they will be more or less autonomous, thus requiring only advisory and special highly technical service from the state. To accomplish this purpose, it is probable that a considerable proportion of the state health department budget must be devoted, for a period of years at least, to the direct aid and stimulation of local health service.

**Federal Subsidy.** Federal subsidy has been granted to states for the development of needed services, and for demonstrations of the value of new activities. During World War II Federal grants-in-aid to states were greatly increased, to such an extent that some states received more than half the expenditures for state health activities from the Federal Government.

Assistance was given in developing new divisions of industrial hygiene, venereal disease control, oral hygiene, cancer control, and other special services. Established divisions of the state health departments were strengthened and grants-in-aid by states to local health departments were greatly augmented.

As time passes and conditions develop, the new activities established in the state health department by Federal grants will undoubtedly demonstrate their true value, and their cost will be assumed gradually by state government. This will result in the allocation of Federal grants-in-aid largely to the development of needy local health services, and to the promotion of new state projects.

**Future Trends.** No one can predict what the future trend in state health administration will be. It probably will not follow the same trend in all states. As local health service develops and becomes more adequate and effective, state health department activities should be less extensive. The normal function of a state health department would seem to be consultative and advisory. Thus, if all the local jurisdictions had well organized and active local health departments, with trained full-time personnel and adequate local support, the state health department need consist only of a small nucleus of highly trained administrators and technical experts who would act as co-ordinators and perhaps advisers in certain of the more difficult situations that might arise. Certain activities are obviously an integral part of state health departments' practice, such as collection and analysis of vital statistics, epidemiological research, etc. Other activities are carried out best if done on a large scale, as, for example, preparation of biological products and many diagnostic laboratory tests. But the important, in fact the essential, function of a state health department is *leadership*. For a long time to come, supervision of local health activities, demonstration of good health practices, and actual direct aid to certain local health departments by subsidy or otherwise will be required of state health departments in the slow and gradual betterment of local health service.

The eventual aim of the state health department, however, is not to increase its powers and functions, but rather to build up the local health departments of the state to such a degree that they may become self-supporting, efficient, and more or less autonomous.

The reader who is particularly interested in state health activities is referred to: *Distribution of Health Services in the Structure of State Government,* by J. W. Mountin and E. Flook, U. S. Public Health Service Bulletin No. 184, Washington, D. C. 1943.

## REFERENCES

1. *Health Departments of the States and Provinces of the United States and Canada.* U.S.P.H. Service Bulletin No. 184, revised 1943 (see above).
2. Shattuck, Lemuel. *A Sanitary Survey of Massachusetts.* 1850 (out of print).

3. *Public Health Organization.* Report of Section II, Committee A. White House Conference on Child Health and Protection. 1932.

4. Maryland State Planning Commission. *Public Health Administration in Maryland.* 1938.

5. Paterson, R. G. *Historical Directory of State Health Departments in the United States of America.* Ohio Public Health Association, Columbus, Ohio. 1939.

6. Stern, B. J. *Medical Services by Government.* The Commonwealth Fund, New York City. 1946.

7. Mustard, H. S. *Government in Public Health.* The Commonwealth Fund, New York City. 1945.

See also the symposium on state health administration in the reports of the Annual Meeting of the American Public Health Association, November, 1946, in Cleveland, Ohio.

# CHAPTER XXXII

## HEALTH ADMINISTRATION IN THE FEDERAL GOVERNMENT

### INTRODUCTION

THE stranger who comes to the United States to seek information in regard to health administration has the greatest difficulty in understanding the functions and organization of the health service of the Federal Government. The whole matter may be clarified by a simple statement of the fact that is little understood, or at least often forgotten, even by ourselves: *The State is the sovereign power,* and not the Federal Government. Each state is autonomous in all the matters relating to public health within its own borders. These powers are designated to the state by the Constitution. The Federal Government possesses only those functions and powers that are specifically designated to it by the several states.

The stranger often asks for a concise summary of the public health laws and regulations of the United States. Such a presentation is not possible, for the simple reason that there are some forty-eight sovereign powers in the Federal Government, with an equal number of sanitary codes and a great diversity of public health laws and regulations.

The Constitution of the United States does not specifically delegate any public health powers to the Federal Government. Those federal laws that have been enacted which relate to public health have been passed under the general provisions which relate to:

1. The regulation of commerce with foreign nations and among the several states.

2. The levying of taxes and the promotion of general welfare.

3. The power of the President (with the consent of the Senate) to make treaties with foreign powers.

In addition, the Federal Government has, of course, the exercise of exclusive legislation in all Federal territories, such as the District of Columbia, National Parks, etc.

The major portion of the Federal health activities are conducted under the supervision of the Federal Security Agency.

**The Federal Security Agency.** The health activities of the Federal Government were rearranged and consolidated in 1946, under the administrative direction of the Federal Security Agency.

This agency was reconstituted under four main operating branches:

1. Social Security Administration.

2. Education.
3. Public Health.
4. Special Services.

The Social Security Administration supervises three important activities: (a) old age insurance, (b) unemployment assistance, and (c) the Children's Bureau.

The United States Public Health Service was assigned to the Public Health Division, and Vital Statistics, which formerly operated in the Department of Commerce, was transferred to the U. S. Public Health Service.

The Division of Food and Drugs, formerly in the Department of Agriculture, was assigned to Special Services, as was Vocational Rehabilitation.

A diagram of the organization of the Federal Security Agency as of July 17, 1946, in so far as it relates to public health administration, is given in Fig. 40.

The reorganization of the Federal Security Agency provided for uniform procedures for all state agencies that administer Federal grants-in-aid for health and welfare. Thus each state, under this plan, draws up a combined budget and proposal for all activities such as general public health, venereal disease control, tuberculosis control, child health, care of crippled children, child welfare, and other activities in which Federal aid may be secured. This combined and comprehensive budget is submitted to the Federal Security Agency as a unit, thus providing a coordinate state health program with uniform fiscal and personnel policies for all Federal aid projects.

See *Federal Security Agency: Organizational and Procedural Material.* Federal Register, Part II, Section 3, Sept. 11, 1946.

Also *Annual Report of the Federal Security Agency,* U. S. Public Health Service. U. S. Gov. Printing Office, Washington, D. C. 1945.

## THE CHILDREN'S BUREAU

The Children's Bureau was transferred from the Department of Labor to the Federal Security Agency in 1946 (with the exception of its Industrial Division). The activities of the Bureau were not modified basically by this administrative procedure, but the reorganization did serve to bring the important public health activities of the Federal Government into closer co-ordination and better working relationships.

The Social Security Act of 1935 set the pattern for the major activities of the Children's Bureau. This act provided for grants-in-aid to states by the Federal Government for the development of state and local services for

1. Maternal and child health.
2. Crippled children.
3. Child welfare.

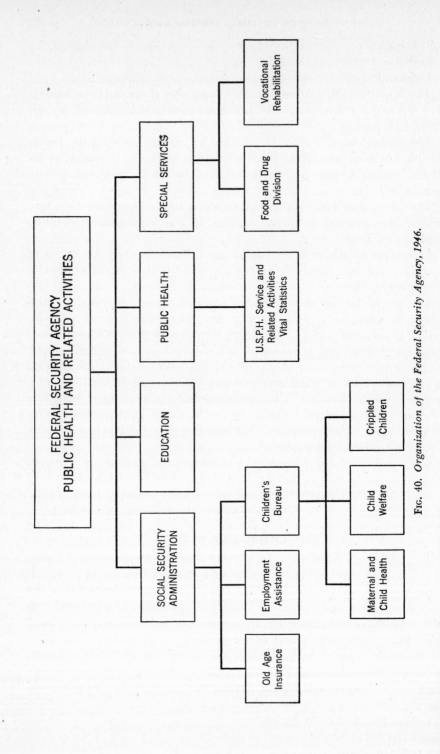

FIG. 40. *Organization of the Federal Security Agency, 1946.*

All grants-in-aid by the Children's Bureau for the development of the above services have been made to official state agencies. Usually funds for maternal and child health are allotted to the state department of public health. The state health department may use a fraction of this grant-in-aid to establish a satisfactory central child health division, but the largest portion of the grant to each state is expended in local programs for child health care. Usually the state allots the funds granted by the Children's Bureau to *official* local health agencies.

The Children's Bureau has required certain standards of training for personnel in the central state division of child health protection, and asks that suitable administrative procedures, such as periodic reports of activity and achievement, budgetary supervision, and so forth, be set up. These requirements are made in order that the Children's Bureau may be assured of satisfactory development of the program in the various states through the Federal grants-in-aid.

The initial grant-in-aid to states for children's services under Title V of the Social Security Act of 1935 has increased year by year. In 1946, the annual grants by Congress for maternal and child health services were $11,000,000: funds for services to crippled children, $7,500,000; child welfare, $3,500,000.

These child health services were in operation in all the states, including the District of Columbia, Alaska, Hawaii, Puerto Rico, and the Virgin Islands.

Grants are made by the Children's Bureau to state health departments, in the case of the maternal and child health program; to state crippled children's agencies, in the case of crippled children's programs; and to state welfare departments, in the case of the child-welfare programs. In order to obtain Federal grants, each of these state agencies must obtain the Children's Bureau's approval of its plan for providing Federally-supported services to children.

In 1946, half of the $11,000,000 granted for state maternal and child health services was matched by the states. From the matched funds, each state received an assured minimum of $35,000, and the remainder was allotted in the same proportion that the number of live births in each state bore to the live births in the United States. The unmatched portion, $5,500,000, was apportioned on the basis of a state's financial need for assistance, in providing services in accord with plans worked out with the Children's Bureau.

Similarly, half of the $7,500,000 authorized for state services for crippled children was matched by the states. From the matched funds, a minimum of $30,000 was assured to each state, and the remainder was allotted according to the need of the state, after taking into consideration the number of crippled children needing care, and the cost of providing such care.

Federal child welfare funds of $3,500,000 were allotted, which did not require specific matching by the states, but part of the cost of the services provided came from state or local funds. The Children's Bureau was directed to grant a minimum of $20,000 to each state, and to apportion the remainder according to the relation of the state's rural population to the rural population of the United States. The reason for this is that the funds were used in developing services in areas predominantly rural, and also in areas of special need.

To insure the prompt expansion of these services for children, Congress not only provided for the above authorization, but also appropriated the necessary funds for the enlarged programs for the fiscal year 1946–47.

The work of the Children's Bureau is administered through the Office of the Chief of the Children's Bureau in Washington, D. C. The major function of the Office of the Chief is to serve as a center for the development of standards of care and protection for children in the United States, that will give every child his fair and equal chance in the world. In its study of all phases of child life, the Bureau gives consideration to the physical and mental health of children, and to the social and economic factors that may affect their well being.

The functions of the Children's Bureau are outlined by Katharine F. Lenroot,[1] Chief of the Bureau, as follows:

1. To investigate and report upon all matters pertaining to the welfare of children and child life. (Act creating Children's Bureau, approved April 9, 1912.)

2. To administer grants to states under the maternal and child welfare provisions of Title V, parts 1, 2, and 3, of the Social Security Act (approved August 10, 1935, and amended in 1939 and 1946).

3. To administer funds appropriated for emergency maternity and infant care for families of enlisted men in the armed forces.

4. To co-operate with other American Republics under the program of the Interdepartmental Committee on Scientific and Cultural Co-operation.

The basic plan of administration of the Children's Bureau calls for eight regional offices, located at strategic geographic and population centers. The 1946 regional centers were in Atlanta, Dallas, San Francisco, Kansas City, New York, Washington, Chicago and Denver.

The Division of Health Services of the Bureau has a medical director in the central office, with a director in each of the regional offices; there is also a medical and technical staff in the central office to carry on the Bureau's program.

The appropriation for the Children's Bureau in 1946, exclusive of grants-in-aid to states and to "Emergency Maternity and Infant Care," was $1,132,360.

[1] Lenroot, Katharine F.: *Current Program of the U. S. Children's Bureau.* Release by the Federal Security Agency, September 1946.

**Emergency Maternity and Infant Care.** During the war years, the Federal Congress provided for maternal and infant care for wives of the four lowest pay grades of the armed forces. The Children's Bureau was asked to administer this Federal program, called the E.M.I.C. Program.

As authorized by Congress the program provided medical, nursing, and hospital maternity and infant care for wives and infants of enlisted men in the fourth, fifth, sixth, and seventh pay grades in the United States armed forces and of aviation cadets. Application for care in such cases might be granted even though not received prior to the husband's promotion, death, or discharge under honorable conditions of the enlisted man.

Under the procedure for grants to the states for maternal and child health services (Social Security Act, Title V, part 1) the Children's Bureau made grants to state health departments to provide medical, nursing, and hospital services for the wives and infants of men in the grades covered. On the basis of need, $2\frac{1}{2}$ per cent of the funds might be allotted to the states for administrative expenses. The program was in operation in all the states, the District of Columbia, Alaska, Hawaii, and Puerto Rico.

State health departments authorized care on the basis of an application signed by the wife and the attending physicians and paid for services rendered by physicians, nurses, and hospitals. Additional payments were not made by or in behalf of the wife. Services were furnished to these families without cost as benefits to which they were entitled. The program reached mothers of all races and creeds. No requirement was made regarding financial need or residence in a state.

For babies under one year of age, immunization against smallpox, diphtheria, and whooping cough was provided by the states in various ways and medical, nursing, and hospital care was made available for the baby when sick.

Wives and babies accepted for care were referred to the local health agencies for public health nursing service, health supervision, and social services that were available in the community.

The Bureau's Division of Health Services reviewed the state plans submitted for approval of the Chief of the Bureau. The division gave consultation service to state health agencies: (*a*) on handling applications for care, (*b*) on enlisting participation of physicians and hospitals, and (*c*) on stimulating increased provision of hospital beds, prenatal clinics, and child health conferences, in order to make maternity care for wives and health supervision for infants fully available to the families of enlisted men in the armed forces.

This plan caused consternation in many of the states, and the administrative difficulties that were encountered in the local communities seemed at first to be insurmountable. In many instances, the local physician, and in some cases the county and state medical societies refused to co-operate with the plan. Gradually these objections were overcome, and by the end of the war, the plan was generally accepted both by the medical profession and by the laity. In many instances, young mothers gained, for the first time, a real concept of suitable prenatal care, adequate hospital delivery, and proper postnatal care. The plan undoubtedly had an educational value of great national importance.

**Services to Crippled Children.** The services of the Children's Bureau to crippled children deserve special mention.

Grants are made to the state crippled children's agencies to enable the state to extend and improve services for crippled children. The Social Security Act as amended in 1946 authorized an annual appropriation of $7,500,000 for this purpose. The program is in operation in all the states, the District of Columbia, Alaska, Hawaii, and Puerto Rico.

The grants are used to provide medical, surgical, corrective, and other services and care for children who are crippled or who are suffering from conditions that lead to crippling, and to provide facilities for diagnosis, hospitalization, and after care of such children. Twenty states conduct programs for the care of children suffering from rheumatic fever or heart disease (1947).

The state agencies responsible for administering services for crippled children are as follows: Health departments, 30; public welfare departments, 10; crippled children's commissions, 5; departments of education, 4; state university medical schools or hospitals, 3. The state staff usually includes physicians, specialists in orthopedic and plastic surgery, orthopedic nurses, medical-social workers, and physical therapists. Local health departments, welfare departments, and school authorities co-operate with the state agency.

State plans are reviewed each year by the Division of Health Services for approval by the Chief of the Bureau. The division provides consultation service to the state agencies (a) on methods and procedures for locating crippled children, and providing services for them; (b) on standards for the selection of physicians, surgeons, and hospitals participating in the care of crippled children; and (c) on the provision of medical and social after-care services.

Each state crippled children's agency maintains a register of crippled children; nearly 405,000 were registered on December 31, 1945. Diagnosis and some treatment is provided in clinics held for crippled children, in permanent clinic centers, or at intervals, in itinerant clinics. When hospitalization and medical and surgical care are needed, the state agency assumes responsibility (a) for arranging for care at a hospital as near as possible to the child's home, and (b) for obtaining the services of the physician or surgeon. Plans are made for his subsequent care in a convalescent home, or in his own home, and for medical and public health nursing supervision, and physical therapy, to complete his physical restoration. Medical-social service is provided also to aid the children adjusting at home, at school, and in neighborhood activities. Children for whom such opportunities are appropriate, are referred for vocational training when they reach 16 years of age.

## UNITED STATES PUBLIC HEALTH SERVICE

**History.** The United States Public Health Service originated in the Marine Hospital Service which was founded in 1798. Its original function was the medical care and hospitalization of American sailors. Twenty cents was levied monthly on each sailor for his medical care, the tax being collected by the Collector of Customs. Thus, the Marine Hospital Service was founded and administered by the Department of the Treasury, because the Collector of Customs was under the Treasury Department. This arrangement was maintained for a great many years.

The Marine Hospital Service functioned effectively, and gradually passed through various stages of development. In 1878 this service was given the authority to impose quarantine measures at various ports to prevent the entry of disease from abroad into the United States. This was a natural development, as the Marine Hospital physicians were the first to see the cases of cholera, smallpox, yellow fever, or plague in the members of the crew of a ship returning from a foreign port. Formerly, quarantine of foreign vessels was a function of each of the individual states, but in 1893, the authority of the Marine Hospital Service was greatly extended in relation to quarantine, and provision was made for co-operation with state and municipal agencies. Shortly thereafter the medical examination of arriving aliens was made the duty of the Public Health Service.

Gradually, the functions and activities of the Federal Health Service were greatly enlarged to include investigations relating to the cause and prevention of diseases of man and matters pertaining thereto, and in 1912 the name was changed to the United States Public Health Service. The first research laboratory of the Service was set up in a single room in the Stapleton Hospital on Staten Island, in 1887. Congress authorized the Hygienic Laboratory in Washington in 1901. It was established for epidemiological purposes, and became the center of a wealth of fine epidemiological investigation. Power to regulate and standardize biological products was given to the laboratory in 1902. The Division of Venereal Diseases was established in 1918, and the National Leprosarium at Carville was established under United States Public Health Service auspices in 1917.

The Social Security Act of 1935 greatly extended the scope and strengthened the influence of the Public Health Service. The National Cancer Act of 1937 authorized the National Cancer Institute, and in 1939 the National Institute buildings at Bethesda, Maryland, were constructed.

On July 1, 1939, after 141 years under the administrative jurisdiction of the Department of the Treasury, the United States Public Health

Service was transferred to the Federal Security Agency, newly created by President Franklin D. Roosevelt to consolidate health, education, and welfare activities of the Federal Government.

Thus, the various major stages of development have been:

1. Hospitalization and medical relief of the merchant marine.
2. Quarantine of ships and medical inspection of arriving aliens.
3. Public health research.
4. Co-operation with state and local health authorities.

As new functions and activities have been assumed, the older functions have not been relinquished, while new and important activities are continually being added by the Federal Government.

**Organization of the United States Public Health Service.** The Public Health Service Act of 1944, Public Law 410, 78th Congress, placed the functions of the United States Public Health Service in the Federal Security Agency. As we have already noted, the Federal Security Agency was reorganized in 1946, to incorporate diverse Federal health functions under a single administration, but this reorganization made no important administrative changes in the U. S. Public Health Service, except that Vital Statistics was transferred to the Service from the Department of Commerce.

The United States Public Health Service is directed by the Surgeon General, who is chosen by the President of the United States.

The Surgeon General has a National Advisory Health Council consisting of 14 members. Ten members are chosen by the Surgeon General, each for a five-year term. The Director of the National Institute of Health, together with one member from the Army, the Navy, and the Bureau of Animal Industry, are ex-officio members of the Council. The members of the Advisory Health Council have no administrative functions, and they receive no salary. Their function is purely advisory, and the position is considered one of great honor.

The major functions of the U. S. Public Health Service are assigned to four divisions:

I. Office of the Surgeon General.
II. National Institute of Health.
III. Bureau of Medical Services.
IV. Bureau of State Services.

I. **Office of the Surgeon General.** This office is responsible for many administrative activities of the Service, including the Division of Public Health Methods and the Division of Sanitary Engineering, which considers such matters as stream pollution, water sanitation, milk sanitation, interstate vehicle sanitation, etc.

1. Division of Commissioned Officers.
2. Division of Dentistry.
3. Division of Sanitary Engineering.
4. Division of Nursing.

5. Division of Public Health Methods.
6. National Office of Vital Statistics.
7. Office of International Health Relations.
8. Office of the Executive Assistant.
9. Budget and Fiscal Office.

**II. National Institute of Health.** The National Institute of Health concerns itself primarily with research. It is located in Bethesda, Maryland. The Institute is directed by the Assistant Surgeon General, and has nine major divisions:

1. **National Cancer Institute.** This division not only conducts basic research in the field of cancer, but has other important activities as well:

   a. Grants-in-aid to private laboratories for research in cancer.
   b. Consultative services to states in setting up cancer control programs.
   c. Educational activities, including the training of physicians in the diagnosis and treatment of cancer.
   d. Radium loans to hospitals, etc.

The National Cancer Institute has a National Advisory Cancer Council, consisting of six members, that are appointed by the Surgeon General. This position as Council member is purely advisory, and carries no salary. It is a position of distinction and honor.

2. **Division of Infectious Diseases.** This division is traditionally one of the most important and active of the United States Public Health Services. It carries out laboratory and field investigations in relation to the epidemiology of a great many infectious and parasitic diseases. It has been a pioneer in the study of virus diseases and also the rickettsial infections, and has discovered the cause and worked out the epidemiology of many obscure and potentially very dangerous infections. (The Rocky Mountain Spotted Fever Laboratory at Hamilton, Montana, is a substation of this division.)

3. **Division of Physiology.** This division has a wide scope. It conducts studies in nutrition and in chemotherapy. Dental research is carried out in this division, as well as other matters relating to normal and abnormal physiology.

4. **Pathology Laboratory.** This division carries out studies in experimental pathology. It also provides pathological services to over 100 hospitals and dispensaries of the U.S.P.H. Service, to the Bureau of Prisons, to the Bureau of Indian Affairs, etc.

5. **Biologics Control Laboratory.** The enforcement of provisions of the national law for control of viruses, serums, and other biological products intended for human use, is the major function of this laboratory. The laboratory is one of the oldest and most important sections of the Institute. Its function was the chief reason for founding the old Hygienic Laboratory in 1901, which later became the National Institute of Health. This division inspects those laboratories that apply for licenses to dis-

tribute biological products through interstate channels, and carries out research in the improvement of the quality of biological products.

6. **Chemistry Laboratory.** This division, as its name implies, is concerned with the public health aspects of chemical research.

7. **Zoology Laboratory.** The Zoology Laboratory first became famous through the work of Dr. Stiles, who made the initial observations on hookworm disease in the United States. It is engaged primarily in parasitologic research, both in the laboratory and in the field.

8. **Industrial Hygiene Research Laboratory.** One of the newest of the divisions of the National Institute of Health is the laboratory for research in industrial hygiene. It conducts laboratory and field investigations in the whole broad field of the health of the worker. The work of this division promises to become one of the most important activities of the whole National Institute of Health. It carries out detailed studies on the physiologic and toxic changes in humans and animals, following their exposure to chemical and physical factors existing in industry.

9. **Division of Research Grants.** The Public Health Service Act of 1944 provided for grants-in-aid by the Federal Government for medical research to universities, to hospitals, and to suitably qualified individuals. The carrying out of this activity became the responsibility of the National Institute of Health.

A Division of Research Grants was set up, and the field of medical research was divided arbitrarily into more than twenty categories. Special Study Sections for each of these various fields were selected by the Surgeon General. The members of these Study Sections have advisory powers only, and receive no salary.

Each Study Section advises the Surgeon General on the suitability of research projects that are presented to the United States Public Health Service, with a request for a subsidy to carry out the work. This plan for nation-wide stimulation of research, with Federal grants-in-aid, has great potential value, and if wisely administered, will undoubtedly contribute markedly to the advance of medical and public health services in America.

III. **Bureau of Medical Services.** The Bureau of Medical Services has three major functions assigned to it. Each is indicated by the name of the division. They are:

1. Hospital Division.
2. Mental Hygiene Division.
3. Foreign Quarantine Division.

**Hospital Division.** The United States Public Health Service was founded originally as a Marine Hospital Service, to give medical and surgical care to American merchant seamen. This is still one of the largest activities of the Service.

The following persons are beneficiaries of the Public Health Service:

1. Persons (hereafter designated as American seamen) employed on

board in the care, preservation, or navigation of any registered, enrolled, or licensed vessel of the United States, or in the service on board of those engaged in such care, preservation, or navigation.

2. Officers and enlisted men of the Coast Guard (active and retired).

3. Officers and seamen on vessels of the Coast and Geodetic Survey.

4. Officers and crews of vessels, certain keepers and assistant keepers of the Lighthouse Service (active and retired).

5. Officers and crews of vessels of the Bureau of Fisheries.

6. Persons detained in hospitals of the Public Health Service under the immigration laws and regulations.

7. Seamen from vessels of the Army Engineer Corps and Army.

8. Seamen employed on the vessels of the Mississippi River Commission.

9. Beneficiaries of the Employees' Compensation Commission.

10. Lepers.

11. Pay patients designated as such under departmental authority, as officers and enlisted men of the United States Army and Navy, foreign seamen, etc.

12. Officers of the Public Health Service, and those employees of the Public Health Service on field duty.

13. Enrollees of the Civilian Conservation Corps.

Some twenty-six hospitals are operated by the regular staff of the service at important shipping centers, and provision is made for hospital care of sailors in some 150 ports in the United States and its insular possessions. In addition to hospital accommodations, there is an outpatient clinical service with approximately 400,000 patient visits per year.

**Other Clinical Activities of the United States Public Health Service.** The Service carries out several strictly clinical activities in addition to the marine hospital service. Among them may be included:

*a.* The National Leprosarium at Carville, Louisiana.

*b.* Freedmen's Hospital and St. Elizabeth's Hospital in Washington, D. C., are under the direction of the Surgeon General.

None of the above activities are strictly public health functions. They represent, in great part, a heritage from the period when the marine hospital service was essentially a clinical service.

**Mental Hygiene Division.** This division conducts the following activities:

1. Administration of the United States Narcotic Farms. The first farm, with a 1,000-bed capacity, and planned originally for male patients only, was located at Lexington, Kentucky. The second, of similar size, was constructed at Fort Worth, Texas, in 1937.

2. Studies of drug addiction, its treatment and rehabilitation.

3. Co-operation with states in administrative matters relating to supervision and treatment of drug addicts.

4. Furnishing of medical and psychiatric service to Federal prisoners.

5. Studies of the causes, prevalence, and means of prevention of mental and nervous diseases.

6. Co-operation with states in administrative matters in relation to the diagnosis, treatment, and rehabilitation of persons with mental disease.

**Foreign Quarantine Division.** The Federal Government administers ship and airplane quarantine in all ports of the United States and its possessions. This quarantine has two separate functions:

*a.* The prevention of entrance of disease into the United States from foreign countries.

*b.* The medical inspection of aliens who are immigrating to the United States and may become a source of infection, or, because of some physical or mental disability, may become a charge upon the state.

**Quarantine.** The diseases under Federal quarantine jurisdiction are: cholera, yellow fever, typhus fever, smallpox, leprosy, plague, and anthrax. There are three lines of defense against communicable disease:

1. Medical officers of the service are stationed abroad in many of the major ports, and working in conjunction with the consular offices, prevent diseased persons from entering ships which are bound for the United States.

2. A system of inspection is carried out, of all ships from any foreign port, at the port of entry to the United States. Both passengers and crew are inspected and the ship quarantined, if necessary.

3. A system of co-operation is organized with state and municipal health officials, particularly at ports of entry, in the follow-up work of diseases that are non-quarantinable by the Federal authorities. For example, diphtheria cases are released at the port of arrival by Federal authorities, but quarantined by the local health authorities.

Formerly all the communicable diseases mentioned above were a constant menace, but conditions have changed greatly in recent years. National quarantine has now converged on two important sources of danger—namely, ship-borne plague, and airplane-borne yellow fever and malaria.

Plague protection consists primarily in a system of inspection and de-ratization of ships, particularly those coming from known plague-infected ports. This work has been so successful, on a world-wide basis, that a survey of 4,000 ships entering United States ports showed only 8 per cent rat infestation. The inspection and rat eradication of ships is carried out by expert mobile crews that are stationed at the principal ports and may be made available quickly for the smaller ports.

Yellow fever was not considered a serious menace from about 1915 up to 1936. It did not exist in any port within 10 days' sail of the United States Coast and thus there was almost no danger of its entry. Two facts changed the status of this disease. Jungle yellow fever was discovered in South America, and airplane service developed with all South American countries. Malaria became epidemic along the coast of Brazil because of the entrance from West Africa of an important Anopheles vector, *Anopheles gambeii*. It is quite possible that this semi-domesticated mosquito may be brought to this nation by airplane traffic with West Africa. Thus a new system of national protection is required, namely:

1. De-insectization of airplanes arriving from South American and African ports.

2. Examinations, at port of entry, of all passengers arriving from South America.

3. Determination of their itinerary for nine days after their arrival in the United States.

4. Vaccination against yellow fever of all airplane personnel that travel through South American countries.

**Quarantine Stations.** The reduction in danger of invasion by pestilential disease has resulted in great restriction of detention stations, particularly in those ports where the U.S.P.H. Service has a Marine Hospital and thus potential detention facilities are always readily at hand. It now seems probable that the old type of quarantine detention station first established by Dr. John Bard in New York Harbor in 1758 has finally outlived its usefulness.

Improved technic has made possible the more rapid handling of vessels. Passenger-carrying vessels may be cleared by a system of radio pratique at some of the larger ports; and whenever possible, ships undergoing quarantine inspection and treatment are handled at the docks rather than in mid-stream, as was the common custom in former years.

**Co-ordinate Service.** This division offers an excellent example of the value of effective co-ordination of governmental services. The Division of Foreign Quarantine co-operates with:

1. The state and municipal health departments, by reporting non-quarantinable (by Federal regulation) but communicable diseases in persons arriving in the United States from foreign ports.

2. The Department of State, by detailing medical officers to consulates in certain ports in Europe, Canada, and Cuba to examine applicants for immigration visas.

3. The Department of Agriculture, by aiding in the enforcement of plant and animal quarantine measures.

4. The Bureau of Customs, by adjudication of violations of the act relating to failure of vessels to present consular bills of health to the United States Collectors of Customs.

5. The Department of Commerce, in administering quarantine procedures in regard to aircraft arriving in the United States from foreign ports.

**Medical Inspection of Immigrants.** The United States Public Health

Service makes a medical inspection of all prospective immigrants. Formerly, these examinations were made at the port of entry. This plan resulted in periods of great stress of work with resulting confusion, particularly when a large ship entered a port with large numbers of immigrants aboard. Those unfortunate immigrants that, for one reason or another, had to return to their mother country, were a frequent cause of distress to the Service, and the whole method was a constant source of friction with foreign governments and with shipping companies. A new system was evolved in 1925, whereby medical officers of the Service were assigned for work abroad at American Consulates in the principal emigration centers. Here the medical examinations can be made in a more exact and careful manner, and all necessary exclusions may occur before the immigrant crosses the sea.

IV. **Bureau of State Services.** The major function of this bureau involves the supervision of grants-in-aid to the several states for the development of state and local health services. The work of the division is divided into five parts:

1. States Relations Division.
2. Venereal Disease Division.
3. Tuberculosis Control Division.
4. Industrial Hygiene Division.
5. Hospital Facilities Division.

**States Relations Division.** Under Title VI of the Social Security Act of 1935, the U.S.P.H. Service was authorized to develop a state aid program in the promotion of a nation-wide plan for betterment of the public health. A general policy for grants-in-aid to states and territories was formulated, through a conference of the Surgeon General with the Association of State and Territorial Health Officers. A flat grant was first made to each state. Additional grants were made to certain states on the basis of special needs and special health problems. These grants were allocated in part to state health departments, to improve the quality of the central supervisory services in the state health department. But the major part of each state grant was intended to aid the state health department in its program for the development of adequate local health service, in each section of the state, particularly in the needy rural areas. The initial Federal appropriation for state aid under Title VI was $8,000,000. This annual grant has been steadily increased by Congress, year by year, as the immense value of the plan became apparent.

One important feature of Title VI of the original Social Security Act was a provision for grants-in-aid to the states for the development of training of personnel. This made it possible for each state to select and to train a better quality of personnel to carry out the increased responsibilities that were developed by Federal grants-in-aid. Thus the quality of local and state health services improved, commensurate with the increase in services that were rendered.

The value of Federal grants-in-aid in the development of local and state health services will become apparent in our consideration of these matters in their appropriate place in this text.

**Interstate Quarantine.** The Federal Health Service supplements the work of various state health organizations by a system of interstate quarantine. The Federal Government aids the states in the control of important communicable disease, through measures which may be taken to suppress interstate epidemics. Often, on request from the state health officer, the Federal Health Service has sent its personnel to an area to aid in the suppression of a serious epidemic within the confines of a single state.

The Federal Health Service has control of sanitation in interstate traffic. Supervision of the sanitary facilities of interstate vehicles is a responsibility of the Federal Government. Ships on the Great Lakes and the waterways, as well as railroad trains, are included, and special attention is given to their water supply and sewage disposal systems.

**Venereal Disease Division.** A special division of the United States Public Health Service was created in 1918 to deal with the control of venereal disease. The chief functions of this division are:

1. To investigate the cause, treatment and prevention of gonorrhea and syphilis.

2. To co-operate with state health departments in developing methods for the prevention and control of these diseases within the various states.

3. To prevent the spread of these diseases in interstate traffic.

The division was a direct outgrowth of conditions arising during the mobilization of troops for the First World War. The division has served as a stimulus for the development of effective venereal disease control programs within the different states and has called special attention to the importance of these diseases.

Surgeon General Parran gave great impetus to the work of this division through his effective campaign in public education. He placed emphasis upon:

 *a.* The economic aspects of the disease.
 *b.* The augmentation of public knowledge that scientific medicine can
    diagnose syphilis accurately and treat it effectively.

The Venereal Disease Control Act of 1938 provided ample funds for the development of syphilis control programs in the various states: $3,000,000 was allotted to states in 1939. It is an unquestioned fact that, within the space of a few years, greater advances were made throughout the nation in the control of syphilis than had been accomplished during the entire previous one hundred years.

**Tuberculosis Control Division.** In 1944, authorization was given for the establishment of a Division of Tuberculosis Control. This division was established in order to provide for:

1. Direct aid by the Federal Government to states and to local agencies for the establishment and maintenance of measures for the control of tuberculosis.

2. Research concerning better methods of tuberculosis control.

3. Development of procedures to prevent the spread of tuberculosis in interstate traffic.

**Industrial Hygiene Division.** The major purpose of this division is to aid the various states in the establishment of effective state-wide industrial hygiene services. This matter has already been discussed in previous chapters.

**Hospital Facilities Division.** The Hospital Survey and Construction Act of 1946, Public Law 725 of the 79th Congress, authorized grants to the states for surveying their hospitals and public health centers, and for planning construction of additional facilities. This division was initiated to provide for proper administration of this Act.

**Personnel of the United States Public Health Service.** The Surgeon General is in direct charge of activities. He is selected for a term of four years, and is appointed by the President, with the consent of the Senate. The Surgeon General is chosen from among the commissioned corps of the service. He may be and usually is reappointed. The Surgeons General of the United States Public Health Service, in order, have been Dr. J. M. Woodworth, 1871–1879, Dr. J. B. Hamilton, 1879–1891, Dr. Walter Wyman, 1891–1911, Dr. Rupert Blue, 1912–1920, Dr. H. S. Cumming, 1920–1936, and Dr. Thomas Parran, 1936 to date (1947).

The Surgeon General selects one Deputy Surgeon General and six Assistant Surgeon Generals from the regular corps. Each serves in his capacity for a term of four years, or at the pleasure of the Surgeon General. The Assistant Surgeon Generals are assigned as follows:

1. Director of the National Institute of Health.
2. Chief of the Bureau of State Services.
3. Chief of the Bureau of Medical Services.
4. Chief Medical Officer of the United States Coast Guard.
5. Chief Dental Officer of the Service.
6. Chief Sanitary Engineering Officer of the Service.

The Service is a semi-military organization. The commissioned staff consists of a mobile corps, made up of physicians, sanitary engineers, dentists, public health nurses, as well as other specialists in the fields of zoology, chemistry, entomology, etc. The great proportion of the professional personnel is made up of medical officers.

All commissioned officers are appointed by the President. A Reserve Corps is provided for, in order to have a suitable corps of trained men available in times of national emergency.

The routine period of service in each rank is as follows:

Assistant Surgeon, from time of first commission to completion of three years of service. Passed Assistant Surgeon from third to twelfth year of service. Surgeon, from twelfth to twentieth year of service. Senior Surgeon, from twentieth to twenty-sixth year of service. Medical Director, from twenty-sixth year of service until retired.

In general, all the appointments, retirement, pay, ranks, etc., of the personnel correspond closely to those of the United States Army and Navy, though the titles of the commissioned officers differ from those of the other military services.

**Interchange of Personnel.** Various departments and bureaus of the Federal Government have public health problems which arise in the course of their normal activities, but they do not possess trained personnel to study these problems or to direct these health activities. Under such circumstances, the Surgeon General assigns some member of his official staff for a temporary period to the department which has requested aid. This principle of lending the Service personnel to other governmental agencies for a specific project has been applied to practically all the various departments of the Federal Government.

## REFERENCES

1. Hampton, B. C. *The Public Health Service Leaves the Treasury Department.* Pub. Health Rep. 1939, Vol. 54, p. 1133.
2. Federal Security Agency: Public Health Service Reorganization Order No. 1. General Circular No. 91, Serial No. 283, Dec. 30, 1943.
3. Chart VII, Federal Security Agency, United States Public Health Service, July 1, 1946.
4. *Functional Chart, National Institute of Health.* Federal Security Agency, U. S. Pub. Health Service, Sept. 7, 1945.
5. Public Law 184—78th Congress (S. 400). An act relating to the organization and functions of the Public Health Service and for other purposes. Nov. 11, 1943.
6. Public Law 410—78th Congress (H. R. 4624). To consolidate and revise the laws relating to the Public Health Service. July 1, 1944.
7. Public Law 487—79th Congress (H. R. 4512). An act to amend the Public Health Service Act to provide for research relating to psychiatric disorders and to aid in the development of more effective methods of prevention, diagnosis, and treatment of such disorders, and for other purposes. July 3, 1946.
8. Public Law 725—79th Congress (S. 191). An act to amend the Public Health Service Act to authorize grants to the states for surveying their hospitals and public health centers and for planning construction of additional facilities, and to authorize grants to assist in such construction. August 13, 1946.

# CHAPTER XXXIII

## VOLUNTARY HEALTH ORGANIZATIONS

THE promotion of public health, the advancement of sanitation and the prevention of illness in any community is obviously a *governmental function.* As with many other duties and responsibilities, however, government, though recognizing the burden, has been slow to assume it. Socially minded persons have, in many instances, made unsuccessful efforts to stimulate an official agency to develop some health project in which they may have been interested, and, becoming impatient, have taken the much more rapid and easier method of initiating the work through voluntary unofficial organizations.

This great urge to do something for the welfare of mankind is one of the outstanding characteristics of American citizenry. It is easily explainable on the basis of the traditions of the nation and the historical development of national character. It is an admirable quality, if properly developed and well sustained. This very quality has been one of the most potent forces for advancement of public health activities in the United States. It has accomplished immeasurable good, and at times, it must be confessed, has caused almost irreparable harm. Many of the important health activities that are now incorporated in standard health department practice might not have been initiated, and certainly would not have been brought to their present state of successful operation, had it not been for the stimulus of voluntary health organizations. On the other hand, many health departments have a poorly balanced program, and have placed entirely too much emphasis on certain phases of their work, because of the pressure from voluntary organizations which have been interested in special projects.

The growth of voluntary public health agencies in the United States may be said to have been initiated with the highly effective and successful Association for the Prevention of Tuberculosis. Previous to this time many associations were established that were interested in the care of the sick, the poor, the homeless and the aged, but their activities were primarily related to welfare rather than public health. The Anti-Tuberculosis Society was organized first on a local basis in Philadelphia in 1892 and developed as a national organization in 1904. The society had a rapid growth and is well organized, with state chapters in every state in the

Union, and local chapters in thousands of villages, towns and cities throughout the United States. It has had tremendous influence on official health practice. This influence, on the whole, has been extremely beneficial.

District Nursing Associations had been organized long before this time, but it never occurred to the founders when they established district nursing that they were assuming a governmental or public health function. District nursing began in New York City in 1877 as a charitable society for the nursing care of the sick poor. The Boston District Nursing Association was founded in 1886. Its primary purpose was to give bedside nursing to the poor. There was no inkling at that time that its activities bore any direct relationship to the work of the Boston city health department. Gradually and logically the organization introduced instructional as well as curative service, so that health education became one of its major functions. The district nursing idea spread to all parts of the country and preventive work became amalgamated with curative work, so that, at the present time, most of the visiting nurses' associations which have been established as voluntary organizations in almost all the large cities of the United States, carry as large a burden of real public health work as of curative and alleviatory service.

The Red Cross is a national organization which was founded primarily for relief in case of national or local disaster,[1] including war. Gradually, the Red Cross has developed a comprehensive policy of direct, full-time, local nursing service, limiting its field, in great part, to the rural sections of the country, and giving both a public health nursing and a morbidity service.

Meanwhile, other national health organizations interested in specific fields had been established along the same general lines as the National Tuberculosis Association. The American Social Hygiene Association was established in 1905, the American Child Health Association in 1909, the National Committee for Mental Hygiene in 1909, the American Society for the Control of Cancer in 1913. The National Foundation for Infantile Paralysis is the youngest of this group.

During the same period, and later, an entirely different type of voluntary public health organization was established—the Social Foundation. These foundations are a new phenomenon in American life. Each is an incorporated, beneficent body, with a large capital fund, established by an individual or a group of persons—not for profit. The funds are expended "for the benefit of mankind." These foundations have selected the most capable leaders in the United States to serve as their advisers, and have attracted men of exceptional talents to administer their affairs. They have been interested primarily, and for the most part specifically, in the advancement of public health and public welfare. Included in this group of social foundations that have been interested in the promotion

[1] See subsequent chapter on Disaster Relief.

of public health are the Rockefeller Foundation, the Milbank Memorial Fund, the Commonwealth Fund, the Rosenwald Fund, the Cousens Fund, the Kellogg Foundation, the John and Mary Markle Foundation, the Josiah Macy, Jr. Foundation, and many others.

During this same period various other types of voluntary organizations have been formed that have interested themselves in public health and preventive medicine. Some of the large insurance companies have developed an intensive nursing morbidity service for their policy holders, together with an extensive scheme of public health education. Many of the large food production industries, such as the milk industry, the meat and meat products industry, the bakery industry, the organized fruit producers, as well as many others of the same type, have conducted extensive health education schemes which have had public health value. These organizations are the first to admit that their primary purpose has been to promote increased sales of their products. Many health officers have been requested to sponsor these various schemes.

The wise health officer will diplomatically decline these requests. The scientific data and authority upon which the commercial companies may base their propaganda may be obtained by them from the scientific literature. The health officer may aid and advise them in selection and preparation of this material, but should not sponsor officially any health educational material, the primary purpose of which is to reap financial gain or secure commercial advantage.

In addition to the unofficial public health agencies that have been organized on a nation-wide basis, one finds in every community, groups of people who have banded themselves together to promote special projects related to public health or public welfare. These organizations are a potent influence in the community and may be of great assistance to the health officer.

The growth of voluntary health organizations has been so rapid and so extensive that these bodies have actually overshadowed the official health organizations in many cities. The White House Conference estimated that in 1930 over $27,500,000 was expended annually in the United States by non-official agencies upon public health or allied matters. This sum is exclusive of any health education activities of commercial organizations. These funds represented at that time nearly one fourth of the total public health expenditures of the nation.

From the above brief description it becomes clear that there exists a great variety of voluntary public health organizations in the United States. Each has its own special field of activity, type of organization and mode of action. The relationship of each organization to the official health service may differ somewhat, but the general principles of co-operative inter-relationship are the same in all.

RELATIONSHIP OF THE OFFICIAL HEALTH AGENCY
TO VOLUNTARY HEALTH ORGANIZATION

**National Public Health Associations.** The great national associations that are interested in the development of public health are all organized in a similar manner. The National Tuberculosis Association, the American Social Hygiene Association, National Committee for Mental Hygiene, American Child Hygiene Association, National Society for Prevention of Blindness, American Society for the Control of Cancer and others are included in this category. The American National Red Cross, and the public health activities of some of the large insurance companies possess many features which make it feasible to include them in the same general grouping.

Each organization has a national headquarters. Most of them are in New York. They have little or no endowment, but depend upon voluntary contributions for their support. State societies are subsidiaries of the parent association, with local affiliated societies in the various communities. Each organization is interested in the advancement of one special phase of public health work, as its name implies. The Nursing Division of the Red Cross is interested primarily in rural nursing service, the insurance companies in health education and morbidity nursing service.

One very important feature of this type of organization is that policies and plans of the organization are determined by the National Society. There is a central responsible body composed of thoughtful, capable people, who are familiar with the general public health problems of the nation. Thus, when any misunderstanding or difficulties are encountered by the local health officer in his relationship with local chapters of national voluntary organizations, it is always easy to rectify the matter through an appeal to the national body.

The local health officer should be familiar with the policies of each of the national organizations, and thus he may make his plans and establish suitable relationship with each local society. This is not always possible when the voluntary health association is organized on a purely local basis. Practically all the national voluntary health organizations have recognized the principle that the local official health organization is directly responsible for the health work of each community. They carry on their special activities in any community in co-operation with the official executive officer of health of the community, and work under his official direction. One major exception is the nursing service of the National Red Cross. The National Red Cross insists that the direction and technical supervision of their full-time nursing field staff shall be the responsibility of the Red Cross and not the local health officer. The policy of the Red Cross is to make the nursing work "a public service, tax supported." It gives authority to its local chapters "to support the nursing service from its own funds or jointly with the public authorities over a considerable period of years until its continuation by public funds on a permanent and adequate basis is definitely assured." But the Red Cross is not willing to affiliate its local nursing activities with those of local official health agencies. They feel that "financial participation should be accompanied by a due measure of control over the work paid for." Administratively, this is an untenable—in fact, an unworkable—situation. It has arisen because many of the Red Cross nurses are located in rural areas where the official health agencies have not been well organized, and often were not familiar with modern public health practice. Any voluntary health organization, however, must recognize the principle that the official health agencies are responsible for the public health program of the community, and cannot surrender their prerogatives or executive functions to any volunteer organization.

The chief functions assumed by the national voluntary health organizations are:

1. Popular health instruction.
2. Advisory and consultation service.
3. Research.
4. Direct service.

*Popular Health Instruction.* The large national health organizations have been very successful in the field of popular health instruction. They are well equipped for this type of activity, and have had an extraordinary influence upon the general public. For the most part this influence has been good. These organizations have a specially trained personnel, are enthusiastically interested in a special subject, and have a wide local chapter membership. Thus, their educational methods have influenced mass opinion to such a degree as to bring about effective activity. At times, their educational policies have not been in accord with the opinions of the official health agencies, and this has led to discord and difficulty. In certain areas, the voluntary organizations have been so active and so influential that some local health departments have developed an unbalanced program, where one or two special activities have consumed the major portion of the personnel and budget, while other equally essential activities have been neglected entirely.

*Advisory and Consultative Service.* The national health organizations have a central group of experts, interested in, and highly trained in, a specific subject. They have had a wide experience and have a national perspective. Some are trained in technical matters; others in administrative detail. Thus the national organization can offer a valuable advisory service along special lines to state and municipal health officers. This advice may relate to legislative procedure, the technic of clinic or hospital organization, specific preventive measures, and many other matters. Health officers may utilize these services to the great advantage of their health activities.

*Research.* Official health organizations seldom have sufficient funds or personnel to carry out research activities. The national voluntary health organizations have an important function to perform in this field. The investigation may be carried out directly by the staff of the voluntary organization, or through grants-in-aid to qualified agencies to make these studies possible. The national organizations have recognized their responsibility in these matters, and have conducted or sponsored some very interesting and valuable studies in administrative practice, epidemiological field work, statistical analysis, and other types of research work.

*Direct Service.* There is a grave question as to whether or not it is the function of a voluntary organization to render a direct health service to the people. When so doing, the voluntary organization is assuming a governmental function. Most of the difficulties between voluntary and official health organizations have occurred in this field. The establishment of public health clinic services, the employment of special nurses, the establishment of tuberculosis hospitals or preventoria under voluntary auspices, and without direct supervision by, or co-operation with, official health agencies, is poor administrative practice, and leads inevitably to difficulty. The voluntary agency may work out a satisfactory public health program in relation to the subject in which it is interested, which will meet the approval of the health officer. It may then supplement the budget or personnel of the official health agency by grants-in-aid or by a co-operative working agreement. It is a sound general principle, however, that voluntary health agencies should not assume responsibility for direct service, but must work through and with the official agencies.

**Social Foundations.** The large social foundations possess a type of organization which is quite different from that of the National Societies, and have somewhat different functions. Their chief usefulness lies in four broad fields:

1. Investigation.
2. Consultative service.
3. Training of personnel.
4. Grants-in-aid for direct service.

*Investigation.* One of the major activities that has been assumed by the large social foundations has been the development of a better public health methodology. There is a great variety of opportunity for this type of work. Experiments may be made in administrative procedure, field studies in epidemiology, studies in the control of communicable disease, public health laboratory studies; in fact, investigation of the whole gamut of established or proposed public health activities. These investigations are not made independently of the official health department, but by direct grant-in-aid to the health department for the study, or by loan of trained personnel and facilities to the health department during a limited period for a special piece of work.

*Consultation Service.* The social foundations all have an expert central staff, which has had wide experience in public health affairs. It is generally conceded that some of the finest talent in the field of public health administration in the United States is centered in the social foundations. Thus these organizations may be of great service to official health agencies through advisory service along public health lines: administrative, epidemiological, sanitary engineering problems, public health nursing technic and organization, etc.

In this general category may be included the activities of the American Public Health Association through its central Committee on Administrative Practice, and also the National Organization for Public Health Nursing. These organizations have determined certain standards of public health practice, and upon request of the local health department will make an appraisal of its health organization and activities. They have also developed standard report forms for health department work and have been of great assistance in many ways to local health officers.

*Training of Personnel.* Aid in the training of public health personnel has been developed by the large social foundations with great success. Official agencies appreciate the importance of trained personnel, but oftentimes have no facilities nor funds for this purpose. Various devices for training of health workers have been established to suit the particular needs of each situation. The best method is the fellowship plan.

The fellowships are given not to individuals, but to the health department for the specific purpose of training one of its staff for a particular position. Training is usually given at one of the Schools of Public Health. A reciprocal agreement is made between the trainee and the health department in order that the Fellow may return to the specified position after the period of training is completed. The Social Security Act, with its liberal grants for training of personnel, greatly augmented the aid that had been given by the social foundations for training of special groups or individuals who were required for specific fields of work.

*Grants-in-Aid for Direct Service.* As a general principle, social foundations should not offer direct health service. A more fundamental and permanent benefit is rendered by the plan of grants-in-aid to the official health departments for development of specific activities. The plan, in essence, consists of a supplement to the health department budget by the voluntary agencies for a temporary period and for a specific purpose. This simple method has been of enormous value in the development of an adequate health service in many parts of the United States.

There is a real peril in relation to these contributions which is not thoroughly appreciated by all health officers. The danger lies in the increasing dependence by official agencies upon funds from voluntary agencies. The guidance of policies may pass out of the hands of the responsible body and into the hands of self-appointed, well-intentioned individuals who are responsible not to government, but only to their boards of directors; and interested only in special subjects, or in special phases of work. These men may have made a special study of certain subjects and have become experts upon the given subject. They have funds to develop their convictions. Official health agencies seldom have sufficient funds to carry out their work. The social foundation has its opinions and also has the money. The experts may not intentionally impose their will upon official organizations, but how can the foundation give the funds unless it feels that the proposed program is satisfactory? The temptation is for the health officer to adjust his program to meet the opinion of the beneficent body.

The risk may not be great and may be counterbalanced by obvious advantages. If the work is not done in this way, it may not be done at all. A health officer may make mistakes, may fall behind in the normal growth of his program, or even, for a time, be unaware or unmindful of his obligations. Granting all this, it must be recognized that the official health executive has the responsibility for the health work of his community and should be perfectly free to determine not only policies, but details of method by which his work is carried out.

Uniformity of health organization for all states and cities is not necessarily beneficial. The health departments may look to the experts for advice and guidance, but must be free to follow many paths and experiment in many directions. Voluntary agencies must realize that just because they are able to give assistance, this fact does not entitle them to dictate the policies of the official organization which they may aid, or to determine exactly how the funds shall be expended. They may suggest definite policies or indicate the names of suitable personnel for a given project. The administrative details and direct responsibility for the activities are the province of the officially selected health organization.

**Visiting Nurse Associations and Other Local Organizations.** Local health organizations having national affiliations have already been discussed. The Visiting Nurse Association is usually organized on a purely local basis, though the general policies are very much the same in all the cities in the United States. The nurses give a morbidity service primarily, though many of their activities include, or are related to, public health affairs. In many cities the official health agencies have a group of nurses that devote themselves exclusively to public health nursing and give no morbidity service. Administrative difficulties that arise in the public health nursing field are due to the fact that there is much overlapping of activities in the two nursing services. The public has difficulty in understanding the exact function of each nurse, official and non-official. This is not surprising, since the health officer himself cannot always draw clear-cut distinctions between preventive and curative activities.

Some socially minded people look forward to the day when local governments will offer hospital service—in and out patient, clinic service and home nursing care, in addition to the preventive services which are offered at the present time. If we accept the complete definition of public health as a "means toward the prolongation of life, and the promotion of physical and mental efficiency through organized community effort," then certainly all the activities given above fall within the scope of the definition. How many of these activities are the direct responsibility of the health department? When do its responsibilities end and other allied activities begin? What is public welfare? When does it begin to be preventive medicine?

Many authorities now believe that generalized nursing service is a most effective plan of organization. This plan includes actual care of the sick in their homes by the nurse, as well as the more clearly defined public health nursing activities. Should bedside nursing be carried out by health department nurses, or should the voluntary nursing associations carry the whole program and receive payment from the city for their public health activities? The borderline activities are the ones which cause administrative difficulty. The system which carries public health nursing and bedside nursing side by side as two separate services is not an efficient plan, but few health officers are willing at present to assume the obligation of complete bedside nursing service.

Most health authorities believe that at some future time health department activities will be centered around community hospitals, with intimate administrative relationship between all community health activities —preventive and curative. Under this plan field nurses will work out from the hospital as a center, and carry on both morbidity work and instructional nursing service. It will be a long time before this type of organization can even be approached, but the alert health officer can shape his program toward the ideal. He may do this by correlation of his activities with those of the voluntary organizations. It is not always necessary for him to draw clear-cut distinctions between official and non-official functions, particularly in the public health nursing field. It is perfectly possible to work out a program whereby the activities of each voluntary organization may be delimited to avoid duplication of effort. It is not necessary, however, to standardize the activities of any one group of workers, or to use the same system in every city. It is even possible for a health department to give good service with no public health nurse on the official staff. The voluntary nursing association may carry the entire field nursing program, and the health department may purchase the public health nursing service by subsidy to the voluntary organization. The health officer should, of course, be on the executive committee of the visiting nurse association and aid in shaping its policies.

### Termination of Voluntary Health Services

One serious difficulty that has been encountered in local communities in relation to voluntary health programs has been the fact that often the voluntary agency does not realize when its work is done. It does not recognize the basic principle that its task is temporary, and that it should gradually terminate its activities and turn them over to the official health agency just as soon as the latter has recognized its obligation, and is willing to undertake the work. If the work of the voluntary organization is well planned and meets a real community need, then this demonstration period should be relatively short. The more important the task, and the better it is done, the sooner will it demonstrate its value. For example, the Visiting Nurse Associations may have been giving the preschool nursing service. This is obviously an official responsibility. A plan should be worked out by the Visiting Nurse Association to turn this work over gradually to the official public health nurses. The voluntary association should not wait until it is sure that the work will be done "just as well" as formerly. It will not be done as well at first, of course. The essential criterion for transfer of the task is that the city health department is ready and willing to undertake the work.

Voluntary tuberculosis associations have conducted extensive tuberculosis programs throughout the nation for many years. Sometimes direct service has been given. The personnel of these associations have sometimes been loath to surrender any of their activities to the official health department. They may be willing to adhere to the principle that they must transfer their responsibilities as rapidly as possible, but the question that remains is: when will their work be finished? Should they set a goal of a specific death rate from tuberculosis for their community of thirty per 100,000? or twenty? or ten? At what stage of the program can all direct service be turned over to the health department? When may the general educational work be curtailed?

The author is of the firm opinion that executive officers of any voluntary health association should make a long-time plan of work, and should contemplate a gradual termination of efforts, along any and all special lines, whenever the demonstration stage of the work has been completed and just as soon as the community has indicated its willingness to incorporate the special procedure as a part of its normal routine.

This principle relates to all special activities of voluntary health associations. There will be a place, for many years to come, for a *general voluntary public health association* in any community. This is quite a different type of organization from the special voluntary health organization which works toward a specific objective.

### THE VOLUNTARY PUBLIC HEALTH ASSOCIATION

As stated above, there is a definite place for this type of enlightened organization in any community. It is a general organization with a representative membership, which is interested in all phases of community health protection and promotion. Its functions are varied:

1. At times pressure may be brought to bear on the local governing body to appoint a health officer or some other key person in the health department for political purposes or other reasons of expediency. A voluntary health organization, sponsored by informed citizens, can have a

powerful influence in securing the appointment of competent, trained and qualified personnel to positions of responsibility.

2. The voluntary health association can use the experimental method in developing new leads and opening up new fields of effective health promotion. The official health department cannot readily do this. Most health officers are loath to expend tax funds for any effort except those that have met the test of time and experience. They feel they cannot use public funds to carry out the experimental method in administrative work. The voluntary health association can do this. In fact, most of the essential and accepted public health activities of today, including dental hygiene, well baby clinic service, pre-natal service, tuberculosis control, public health nursing, venereal disease control, prevention of deafness and blindness, and many more, were inaugurated by voluntary health associations, and later were incorporated as routine official public health tasks.

3. The voluntary health association serves as an outlet of expression of public sentiment in relation to public health affairs. It can interpret the work of the health department to the people. Public sentiment is not yet thoroughly aware of the fact that a health department must be staffed by a competent personnel that has been properly trained in all the technics of the profession. The politician is not yet convinced that appointments to positions in the health department are not his prerogative. Thus, a voluntary public health association, under excellent sponsorship with aggressive and intelligent leadership, can be a most effective organized force for the continued improvement of the health protection activities of a community. It will also serve as a guardian against retrogression, and demoralizing encroachment upon the sincere efforts of a conscientious public health officer and his staff.

**The Public Health Council.** The Public Health Council or Health League is an ingenious administrative device that has solved many of the difficulties in local health departments and has been a tower of strength to the health officer in times of stress. A Health Council is made up of representatives of each and all of the various voluntary organizations in the municipality that are interested in public health. The health officer is a member of the executive committee. The Council meets at regular intervals and discusses the public health needs of the community. The health officer presents his plans to the Council and discusses his difficulties with its members. The Council has no direct operative functions, but simply correlates the activities of all its various member organizations, and integrates their work and their policies with those of the official health organization. The principles of administration of the public health council which were formulated at a special meeting of the American Public Health Association in 1939 are so clear and concise that they are presented herewith.

*"PURPOSE*

"The purpose of a Health Council is to co-ordinate health activities and community health planning.

*"REPRESENTATION*

"A Health Council must be thoroughly representative of the recognized health forces of the community. It should have among its members, lay people and representatives of the official health agency or agencies, of organized medicine, of organized dentistry and of organized nursing, as well as representatives of the unofficial agencies interested primarily in public health work. Liaison with recreational and welfare organizations is essential. It should be without limitation as to race or creed.

*"FUNCTION*

"A Health Council is essentially a conference and co-ordinating body.

"A Health Council shall promote the efficient operation of public health work through the co-ordination of the health activities within the area—local community, state or nation—by means of the elimination of duplication of effort and by the stimulation of new and needed services.

"A Health Council may render common services in such fields as statistics, research, and health education.

"It should not maintain health services except for such demonstration purposes as may meet with the approval of the local health agencies.

"A Health Council should aid in developing public opinion with respect to public health needs, programs, and legislation.

*"ORGANIZATION*

"The form of organization and operation of a local Health Council will vary in details, depending upon local conditions. The larger communities will need to have full time staffs of their own, and reasonable budgets. In other cities, it may be necessary to utilize such part-time service of other staffs as may be available, as for example, the service of a member of the staff of a Council of Social Agencies, Health Department, Medical Society, or other agency.

"In small communities having only a few health activities, such as, for example, health department, school health program, medical society, visiting nurse association, tuberculosis association, and possibly others, there is need for co-ordination of health activities as well as in the larger cities. The Health Council in these smaller communities may utilize such staff resources as may be available from any acceptable source. Some executive service, however, is essential to the most effective Health Council Program. In any community the Secretary of a Health Council should have qualifications appropriate to this field.

"The selection and appointment of the executive should be the responsibility of the agencies which constitute the Health Council with the co-operation of the other local agencies involved.

"A Health Council, to function effectively, must have full scope to determine its own policies consistent with accepted public health principles. Its organic relationship with the Council of Social Agencies may vary in different communities, but the Health Council should always work in co-operation and harmony with both the Council of Social Agencies and the Community Chest or Fund.

"Under proper leadership a rural community (possibly the county) may establish a health council or committee in accordance with the general principles herein set forth even though there may not be available paid executive service or operating budget."

**Summary.** All the activities of voluntary public health organizations are of value. Each has its own particular place in the general scheme of health work. Relationships with official agencies are fraught with difficulty. The chief difficulties have arisen in relation to *direct service*. The reason is that the direct service programs are not always correlated with the work of local health activities. In fact, many times in the past, the voluntary health agencies have made their plans without consulting the health officer and without considering the local health department program.

Difficulties and friction may be avoided easily when one principle is recognized and respected; namely, the official health organization is the body which is responsible for the public health activities of the community. The health department may not be well organized or well staffed. Differences of opinion and clashes of personality may intervene, but the voluntary health organizations in any community must recognize that they have no vested rights. They are the guests of the health department. They must win its sympathy and co-operation, and plan their programs in accordance with the desires and approval of the official agencies. The wise health officer, in turn, will not stand aloof, but will utilize all the potential resources of his community. He will encourage participation by voluntary health agencies in the general program. He should be represented on their administrative boards, be familiar with their plans and in sympathy with their objectives. He should realize that the voluntary health agency is a powerful force and a very helpful one, if properly directed. It often requires a diplomatic talent of no mean order to reconcile the idealism and enthusiasm of the special groups with the general policies and practical everyday working plans of the health department.

The health officer should insist that all the voluntary organizations in the community that are interested in public health should co-ordinate their activities, and he should give the leadership that is required to bring this about. The tendency of each voluntary organization is to become absorbed in its own activities to the exclusion of everything else. There results an overlapping of services, a lack of understanding of community objectives, and a duplication of effort. One agency does not understand what the other is doing or what it desires to do. Often there is no clear-cut allocation of fields or definition of responsibilities. In order that the voluntary agencies may be of greatest service to the community, there must be some systematic plan of cohesion of all their scattered and well-intended, but at times ineffective, activities. The public health council is the simplest device to bring about this co-ordination of service.

In 1945, Selskar Gunn,[2] with the able assistance of Philip S. Platt, published a report of a nation-wide study of voluntary health agencies. It was the last work of a great public health leader who had contributed tremendously to the development of public health, on an international basis. It was one of his best achievements. All public health administrators, as well as all persons interested in the work of voluntary health agencies, should study this report carefully. It recommends, in essence, that local communities should have not multiple, but *one* centralized, unified voluntary health agency, with one board and one executive officer. These general recommendations extend up through the community to the state and national levels.

The report recommends a strong National Health Council, with a pooling of interests of all the various voluntary national health agencies. This Council should have strong executive leadership, and an outstanding board of directors to guide its policies.

The obvious advantages of these recommendations are apparent to all public health administrators.

[2] Gunn, S. M. and Platt, P. S.: *Voluntary Health Agencies. An Interpretive Study.* The Ronald Press Company, New York, 1945.

See also: "Medicine and the Changing Order." Report of a Special Committee of the New York Academy of Medicine. The Commonwealth Fund, New York City, 1947.

Emerson Kendall: "The Role of Voluntary Public Health Agencies." Chap. XLIV of *Preventive Medicine in Modern Practice.* New York Academy of Medicine. Paul B. Hoeber, Inc. New York, 1942.

# CHAPTER XXXIV

## DISASTER RELIEF

THE public health administrative problems relating to disaster relief may seem of little interest to the average health officer. A major disaster is a highly improbable emergency which he may never be called upon to face. But disasters are not so uncommon as one might suppose. Each year, one or more minor disasters occur in some part of the United States. These disasters, though they may be confined within narrow geographic limits, present the same problems for solution on a smaller scale as those which arise in a major disaster.

The major disasters in the United States that have occurred in recent years have been due to a variety of causes, including floods, tornadoes, fire, tidal waves, earthquakes, drought and famine, pestilence, explosions, and, to a lesser degree, train and ship wrecks. Epidemics of disease sometimes assume disaster proportions. The major disasters are always followed by great confusion, untold suffering, and often great loss of life.

Each disaster produces its own peculiar situation so that no plan can be formulated which will exactly fit all conditions and contingencies. In general, however, disaster relief may be divided into three separate activities which follow each other in more or less chronological order. They are:

a. Rescue Work.
b. Emergency Relief.
c. Rehabilitation.

Each activity merges into the next, and no sharp lines may be drawn in a complete disaster relief program.

**Rescue work** is the first thought in any great emergency. No sacrifice is too great to save the lives of the endangered people. Everyone in the community will volunteer for this service and will carry on to the point of physical exhaustion. Natural leaders in the community emerge and take charge of the situation. Every available facility and every available person is drafted to save the lives and prevent further suffering of those endangered.

**Emergency Relief.** Even before the rescue work has been completed, a plan must be formulated, and an organization formed, to meet the emergency needs. Homeless people will be crowded together under un-

514

hygienic conditions, with no shelter, no food, no clothing; their property destroyed, their resources gone. The sick and injured must receive proper care. The dead must be buried. Epidemics of disease may break out to add to the confusion and suffering. It is necessary to understand what needs must be met, what services will be called for, what resources are available, and to have a plan already formulated to meet these needs.

Emergency relief may be divided administratively into two major activities, non-medical and medical.

*The non-medical activities* consist essentially in providing the necessities of life: food, shelter, clothing. In major disasters, refugee camps are usually required. They are set up hurriedly in buildings or tents, and food is provided through community kitchens or canteen service.

*Medical relief* is divided logically into:

a. Medical, surgical, nursing and hospital care of the sick and injured.
b. Protection of the health of those directly affected by the disaster, and protection of the community at large from the unsanitary conditions produced by disruption of normal conditions.

This latter activity (*b*) is an essential function of the official health organization and will be our chief concern in this discussion.

### AGENCIES FOR DISASTER RELIEF

**The rescue work** is carried out by all persons in the community. This work is carried on at a high pitch, amid great confusion, and is accompanied by self-sacrifice and heroism. Everyone aids, every available agency is employed.

*The emergency relief* work which follows can be developed in an orderly way.

**The local Red Cross** is directly responsible for supplying the physical needs of those in distress, including shelter, food and clothing. Local preparedness is one of the tenets of this great organization. When disaster strikes, the local Red Cross chapter is prepared to assume leadership in the emergency relief work. The National Red Cross organization participates only when the emergency is so great as to demand outside assistance.

**The National Red Cross** is the great bulwark in the United States in times of disaster. Thus it is essential that every health authority should understand the plan of organization, the functions and general policies of the National Red Cross in disaster relief.

The Red Cross is a national, semi-official disaster relief agency, chartered as such by the Federal Government. It does not obtain financial support from the Federal Treasury, but from voluntary contributions. The headquarters are in Washington, with approximately three thousand local chapters distributed through all parts of the United States. The National Red Cross in Washington maintains a corps of executives, physicians, and nurses who are trained and experienced in disaster relief, and has necessary supplies and resources available at all times. It is prepared at almost an instant's notice to send relief and aid to any part of the United States.

When disaster occurs, the National Red Cross is frequently requested to come at once and take charge of the situation. This is contrary to its established policy. The National Red Cross insists that administrative responsibility shall rest upon local officials. When it enters a disaster area, it will aid and help in every possible way, but does not supersede the local official agencies.

Furthermore, the local Red Cross chapter is not empowered to call upon the National Red Cross to take charge of the disaster area. The National Red Cross enters the area upon request of the official agencies, usually from the governor of the state.

*The major non-medical functions* of the National Red Cross in disaster relief are to provide shelter, food and clothing for a temporary period for those in distress, to assist these people in rebuilding their homes and to aid in restoring normal living conditions. The local Red Cross chapter has administrative responsibility for these activities in the disaster zone.

*Medical Relief.* The National Red Cross does not sponsor or direct the care of the sick or injured in any disaster area which it has entered. Its function is rather to provide the local medical authorities with supplies, facilities and personnel to meet the emergency. Administrative responsibility for medical, surgical, hospital and nursing care rests upon the local medical society and allied organizations.

In major disasters, the medical facilities usually requested from the National Red Cross are:

1. Provision for additional medical and nursing personnel for the area sufficient to provide for the emergency.

2. Provision for hospitalization, either through expansion of local hospitals or by organization of independent emergency hospitals.

3. The establishment of emergency medical stations at refugee camps and other necessary places.

4. Provision for the necessary surgical and hospital supplies.

5. Provision for complete medical and nursing supervision of refugee centers.

*Public Health and Sanitation.* The National Red Cross does not assume responsibility for sanitation and preventive medicine in any disaster. The local health officials have direct administrative authority in all matters that may arise in disaster relief that pertain to general sanitation or prevention of disease. The National Red Cross may be requested by the constituted authorities to render aid in the emergency. In major disasters the Red Cross usually is called upon to supply:

1. Additional personnel, including physicians trained in public health

administration, sanitary engineers, sanitary inspectors and public health nurses.

2. Aid in sanitation of the area, including establishment of suitable methods to secure a safe water supply, proper sewage and waste disposal, and to safeguard food supplies.

· 3. Aid in control of communicable disease, including immunization of susceptibles against typhoid fever, smallpox, etc.

4. Provision for isolation hospital facilities.

5. Provision for a public health nursing service for the disaster area.

6. Provision for health supplies for use of the health agencies, such as smallpox and typhoid vaccine, diphtheria and tetanus antitoxin, etc.

Although the National Red Cross does not supersede any of the local government authorities in a disaster area, it does insist upon administrative responsibility and authority in two respects:

*a.* Nursing supervision of the Red Cross nursing service.

All the nurses employed by the National Red Cross in disaster relief must serve under the direction and supervision of the National Red Cross nursing service. This includes not only those nurses who are employed in the actual care of the sick and injured, but also the public health nurses assigned to the area.

*b.* Complete administrative responsibility for refugee camps.

The refugee camp is a community organization, a complete unit in itself, for which the Red Cross assumes full charge. This responsibility includes provision for shelter, food, medical and nursing care and sanitary supervision. The Red Cross pays all the expenses of the refugee camps and directs all their activities.

## ORGANIZATION OF THE EMERGENCY RELIEF PROGRAM

It is obvious that there will be some overlapping of functions in the emergency relief in any great disaster. Since everyone is working toward a common purpose, there should be little friction or misunderstanding. It is a poor policy under such circumstances to insist upon the meticulous observance of individual prerogatives. The general tendency is to cut all red tape and to get things done in the most expeditious way. Immediate action is necessary, but it must be remembered that hasty, poorly planned activity is ineffective. An emergency relief program should be so formulated that it is in accordance with established governmental principles, and thus responsibility may be placed where it belongs.

In brief, the administrative responsibilities are threefold: The local Red Cross chapter cares for all non-medical needs; the local medical authorities have charge of medical and hospital care; the local health organization assumes the responsibility for sanitation and public health. The National Red Cross, if asked for assistance, will act as a supplementary organization in furnishing necessary aid to the local agencies that are directly responsible for the relief work.

**Pre-disaster Program.** *An emergency fund* should be set aside in each state government budget which will be available for immediate use in case of disaster. These funds should be expendable at the discretion of the Governor.

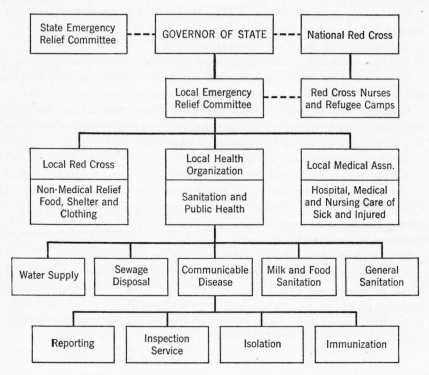

Fig. 41. *Scheme of Organization of Emergency Relief in Disaster.*

*State Disaster Relief Committee.* Each state should have a relief organization committee, at least in skeleton form. It should consist of the Governor, the Adjutant General, the State Health Officer, the Red Cross field representative, the State Commander of the American Legion, and other representatives of the various organizations that are usually called upon in times of disaster relief activities. This committee should have a formulated plan of activity for emergencies, and should possess complete data concerning availability of necessary relief supplies, such as tents, camp equipment, medical supplies, emergency chlorination equipment, etc., with information as to methods whereby these supplies may be obtained with the least delay.

*State Health Organization.* The state health officer should have a plan worked out for the organization of disaster relief, with a personnel trained and prepared to go into immediate action in case of need. These plans need not be elaborate or detailed, but the key personnel should have definite assignments, and the sources of necessary supplies should be known so that when the emergency arises, the relief plan can begin to function immediately.

*Local Emergency Relief Committee.* Since the various local authorities will be directly responsible for administration of disaster relief, there should be a close alliance in every community between the local Red Cross chapter, the medical society, and the local health officials. If a disaster occurs in the community, an immediate organization of responsible authorities can be effected, with proper division of duties. The local committee should be formed immediately. It will be composed of the various representative agencies, and the administration of the major divisions of activity—relief, medical care and sanitation—should be placed in the hands of the responsible local authorities.

**Disaster Program.** *Field Survey.* When disaster strikes, the local authorities should determine as soon as possible:

a. The extent of loss of life and of injury.
b. The extent of destruction of homes and other factors affecting normal life.
c. The destruction of, or damage to, sanitary facilities, such as water supplies, sewage systems, ice plants, milk pasteurization plants, food refrigeration, etc.
d. The extent of other sanitary problems such as disposal of dead bodies, removal of debris, waste and refuse.
e. The prevalence of communicable disease in the area.

As soon as this information is at hand, the local authorities, consisting essentially of the local Red Cross, the medical society representative, and the health officer, should communicate with the Governor of the state, advising him of conditions and requesting the necessary aid. The Governor may then, at his discretion, request aid from the National Red Cross, or from other sources.

*Health Activities.* The state health officer may at his discretion assume entire charge of all matters within the area relating to sanitation and public health. He is empowered to do this in most states, and the ultimate responsibility rests upon him. Usually, this is not done. It is a general principle of administration that, in so far as possible, the state department will delegate the actual rendition of service to the local organization; the state giving supplementary aid and consultant service.

If the state health department assumes charge, due notice must be given to all the local relief workers that all health personnel in the area will become responsible to the state health official who has been placed in administrative charge.

The chief public health activities in the disaster area will be as follows:

*a. Protection of water supplies.* The public water supply should be investigated to determine any damage or interference with its sanitary quality that may have occurred. If necessary, an emergency system of chlorination may be installed and operated under orthotolidin test every three hours. If temporary water supplies are required, the health department must designate and approve them and keep the public informed concerning the quality of the water. Meanwhile, the devastated population must be warned to boil all drinking water until such time as all danger from contamination of public or private supplies has passed. Warning may be given by radio, telegraph, and telephone, by courier and every possible method of rapid transmission of information.

*b. Sewage disposal.* The system should be investigated and, if damaged, should be repaired as soon as possible. If immediate repair is not possible, modern sanitary community latrines should be constructed and maintained in suitable sanitary condition.

*c. Refugee centers.* The health department has general supervision of the sanitation of the refugee centers. If possible, refugees should be housed in available permanent buildings, such as schools, churches, or other public buildings, rather than in tent camps. The state health department standards should constitute the minimum sanitary requirements for refugee camps. (In case the National Red Cross is sponsoring the refugee camp, it assumes direct responsibility for the camp, including sanitation and health supervision.)

*d. Food and milk.* If milk pasteurizing plants have been damaged, they should be repaired at once. If pasteurized milk is not available, the milk should be boiled. Supervision should be maintained over all places where food is stored, refrigerated or prepared. Particular attention should be given to sterilization of eating utensils.

*e. General sanitation.* Sanitation of the area may include disposal of dead bodies, the removal of debris, waste and organic matter. This clean-up work is not the normal function of the health agencies, but the health officials may be called upon to assist in or supervise this work. Burial in sandy soil is the best method of disposal.

*f. Communicable disease.* Special precautions must be taken to prevent the spread of acute communicable disease.

(1) Reporting.

The medical division should report daily by telephone to the health officer in charge of the disaster area in relation to all cases of communicable disease occurring in the disaster area.

(2) Inspection.

There should be a daily inspection for the detection of communicable disease in all the refugee centers.

(3) Immunization.

Tetanus antitoxin should be given to all the wounded. Routine smallpox vaccination is a sound practice, particularly in the refugee camps.

Routine typhoid vaccine should be given if this disease is normally prevalent in the area, or if there is any question about the water or milk supply. Provision should be made for isolation facilities for communicable disease, either in the general temporary hospital or in separate isolation units. The minor contagious diseases of childhood, such as measles and whooping cough, should be isolated, particularly if they occur in the refugee camps.

The health department is not directly responsible for the care of the sick, though it is its obligation to be sure that each case of communicable disease receives proper care. (If an epidemic of disease reaches disaster proportions, it may be necessary for the health authorities to assume a larger measure of responsibility for the care of the sick.)

Measures for the prevention of the spread of diphtheria, malaria, venereal disease, tuberculosis and trachoma, as well as diseases related to improper nutrition, must receive suitable consideration.

The established standards of the state health department should constitute the minimum sanitary regulations in instituting measures for disaster relief. Where measures beyond these standards are required, special local regulations may be instituted by the local health authorities or by the state health officer.

Emergency medical and nursing care is the responsibility of the local medical authority. Usually the county medical society selects an executive committee, and all activities clear through it. Hospitalization of the injured and sick is developed around existing hospital facilities in so far as possible, though temporary emergency field stations may be required. Additional medical and nursing personnel may be needed, as well as additional hospital equipment and medical supplies.

The National Red Cross is the most suitable agency to furnish this aid. The Red Cross has such wide experience in disaster relief that it is prepared to meet almost any emergency on very short notice. The most valuable assistance that it renders is the dispatch to the disaster areas, upon the request of suitable governmental authorities, of trained executives who have had experience in various types of disasters and who are prepared to aid the local authorities in the organization of disaster relief services.

## REHABILITATION

Rehabilitation is a gradual development following emergency relief and is carried forward as rapidly as circumstances will permit. All agencies concerned in emergency relief bend their efforts toward final rehabilitation and the re-establishment of normal conditions.

Sanitary rehabilitation often results in establishment of better conditions than existed before the disaster. Public water supplies may be reconstructed along approved lines, and improved methods of excreta disposal installed.

The beneficial effects of an effective emergency sanitary and public health nursing service when conducted by a competent personnel, are strikingly demonstrated in a well organized relief program. Such demonstration has frequently resulted in the permanent establishment of an effective and comprehensive public health program within the area that has been visited by the disaster.

# CHAPTER XXXV

## THE PRACTICING PHYSICIAN AND THE PUBLIC HEALTH DEPARTMENT

In the early history of the United States practically all public health work was done by practicing physicians as part of their civic duty. Occasionally, when an epidemic occurred, a temporary commission of physicians was appointed by government—state or local—to deal with the immediate situation. When the outbreak ceased, the commission was discharged. This plan was in vogue as late as 1870 in New York, when Stephen Smith was selected as a member of a commission to investigate local health conditions and suggest methods for betterment. The medical profession, individually and as an organized body, was a potent factor, in fact often the only instrumental agency in the community, for protection of the public health.

As community responsibility in these matters grew more and more apparent, it became the general custom of local governments to employ resident physicians on a part-time basis, to carry out certain community health functions, such as isolation and quarantine, fumigation, sanitary inspection, medical examination of school children, etc. In fact, the whole structure of the New York State Health Department as developed by Dr. Biggs was founded on the principle of utilization of a local, part-time physician as the official public health representative in each of the respective communities.

The concept of full-time public health executives, specially trained for their work and with suitable tenure of office, is a relatively recent one. Many of the state health departments were staffed, in their inception, by physicians who gave only part of their time to government work. Even at the present time the public health executives of numerous cities in the United States are local practicing physicians who devote only a portion of their time to the executive duties of their departments.

Only a few farsighted leaders during the past century understood that the nation needed young men and women who would undertake public health as a special profession and make it a life career. Lemuel Shattuck realized this fact in 1850. Charles W. Eliot, the famous President of Harvard University, understood it clearly, and was instrumental in founding the first formal training for public health personnel.

Everyone familiar with the field of public health is now quite cognizant of the fact that public health administration, epidemiology, vital statistics, public health laboratory work, child hygiene activities, sanitary engineering, public health nursing, health education, industrial hygiene, and the like are all special technics that require special training and experience. Young physicians, nurses, engineers and other personnel that are interested in, and have special aptitude for, this type of work now prepare themselves for a life career in their chosen field. They have every assurance that if they possess real ability and prepare themselves properly, they will have the opportunity to obtain interesting and satisfactory employment.

There is still a wide misconception as to just what constitutes proper public health preparation. Many communities have selected their health officer from the group of resident practicing physicians, on the assumption that medical training *per se* will fit a person for the technical duties of public health administration. This assumption is quite wide of the mark. The standard medical training as given in our best medical schools does fit a physician to assume his public health responsibilities as a *practicing physician,* but does not equip him to do public health work.

It is quite true that in the past certain physicians have been chosen from general medical practice and have become excellent public health administrators. They have possessed latent ability and special talents, and have learned their work in the school of experience. It casts no reflection on them to state that this is not the best way to select a competent health officer.

Once the principle was established that public health work was a special career, requiring special training and experience, the pendulum swung too far in the opposite direction, with the result that many health departments tended to exclude all part-time medical personnel, and to carry out all the work of the department with a full-time staff. This is quite proper in state or federal health activities where the very nature of the work is consultative and advisory and where direct service is not rendered. Wherever direct service is rendered, however, as is the case in all local health departments, the resident practicing physician should play a part of greatest importance. No health officer can carry on satisfactory work without the co-operation and whole hearted support of the organized medical profession of his community. No physician can practice modern medicine in an effective way without the aid of a well organized, efficient health department. The dependence of one on the other is mutual, and success is contingent upon mutual understanding and confidence. The health officer should have a real consideration for, and sympathy with, the point of view of the physician; the latter, in turn, should realize that the health department has its difficulties and sometimes makes mistakes.

In the past, a good deal of friction and misunderstanding have arisen between the official health agencies and the practicing physicians. This is entirely unnecessary, but understandable. It has been due in great part to a lack of consideration on the part of the health officer or members of his department for the viewpoint of the physician, and a lack of understanding by the physicians of the purposes and objectives of the health department. One principle must be kept in mind. The fundamental purpose of both the physician and the health department is the same. They are striving for the better health and thus greater happiness of the community. The goal is the same, though it is reached by different paths. These paths cross one another frequently.

The daily work of the physician covers a scope of activities which are related directly or indirectly to almost every part of the health department program. The health department makes many requests of the physicians. These requests are not unreasonable. They represent obligations which the physician assumes when he enters medical practice, and which should be performed as a public duty. The health department makes a fair exchange. It has much to offer to the physicians, so that the final arrangement is one of mutual assistance and mutual advantage.

### THE FUNCTIONS OF THE PRIVATE PHYSICIAN IN HEALTH PROTECTION AND PROMOTION

The physician has two distinct functions in the community in relation to health protection and promotion. First, because of the very nature of his profession, the physician has certain direct obligations to the community. When the state grants him a license to practice medicine, he virtually agrees that he will carry out all his duties and responsibilities in relation to the promotion of the official health services of the community.

The second obligation to the community and to his patients is even more important than the first; namely, the obligation to incorporate the principles of preventive medicine as an essential part of his everyday clinical practice.

Let us consider first the public health functions of the practicing physician.

**Vital Statistics—Birth and Death Reports.** It is an onerous public duty of each physician to report promptly to the health department all births and deaths that occur in his private practice. Busy physicians are often annoyed at the health department for its insistence upon completeness of detail in filling out these records, as well as its requirements for forwarding the forms promptly. For obvious reasons, already given in a previous chapter, it is an important public duty of physicians to fill out the standard forms for registration of births and deaths with greatest care and precision. They are permanent state records, pertaining to the life of the individual and the general welfare of the community. Unless properly filled out, they have little value. This simple procedure is one of the primary obligations to his patients and to the community that a physician assumes when he is granted permission by the state to practice medicine. The health department registrar is only performing his duty when he requires accuracy of the data and prompt filing of the certificates. The health department should make the methods of reporting as simple as possible. For guidance in determining classification of causes of death, all physicians should be furnished copies of the "Physicians' Handbook on Birth and Death Registration," published by the Bureau of the Census.

**Communicable Disease Control.** *Reporting.* One of the chief means of control of communicable disease is the early recognition and immediate isolation of the patient. An epidemic of smallpox, scarlet fever, or other disease may be checked in its incipience, if the first case is controlled. A person with severe sore throat or suspected typhoid fever may be simply an isolated clinical case to the individual practicing physician, but may represent to the health officer a unit of a widespread epidemic. The health department has no satisfactory method of discovering cases of suspected communicable disease, except through physicians. The doctor sees the patient first. A uniform list of communicable diseases that are reportable to the health department has been authorized in practically every state. Each physician should be familiar with this list and should report promptly and faithfully every case of reportable disease that may occur in his practice.

Some of the lists are too inclusive. It is doubtful if the health department should require the reporting of a given disease by the physicians, if the department, in turn, takes no action. Bronchopneumonia is a good example. It is interesting from a statistical point of view to know the number of cases of bronchopneumonia in a community, but we have as yet no effective means of control of the disease, nor is it an index of any other public health problem for which the health department has methods for solution. So why require that it be reported, if nothing is accomplished? Chickenpox is reportable because of its possible confusion with mild smallpox. But there is no logic in requiring that the physician report each and every case of chickenpox unless the reported case is investigated by the health department.

The health department should make the machinery for the reporting of communicable disease by physicians as simple as possible. It should furnish consultative service for communicable disease to physicians. The health department expert should be ready to go at any time on request of a physician to aid in verification of the diagnosis of communicable disease. The physician should institute immediate provisional isolation of a suspected case of communicable disease, but the health department must assume full responsibility for enforcement of the regulations in regard to isolation and quarantine.

*Immunization Programs.* A great deal of misunderstanding and difficulty has arisen between the health department and physicians in regard to immunization programs, particularly those for the prevention of typhoid fever, smallpox and diphtheria. Many physicians feel that the health department should do no clinical work at all, but rather should refer all persons to the private physicians for immunization procedures.

Whenever physicians incorporate standard preventive measures in their private practice, the health department can relinquish immunization programs. It would not be necessary for the health department to carry on immunization against diphtheria and smallpox, if physicians and lying-in hospitals would assume responsibility for each baby delivered in their practice, and guarantee to immunize each child against both small-pox and diphtheria before that child reached one year of age.

The logic of the health department is clear-cut. A given disease is prevalent in the community, or is at least a potential menace, and may occur at any time, causing suffering and loss of life. An effective method of prevention is at hand, namely, mass immunization of the community. Prevention of outbreaks can only be assured when a large proportion of the non-immune population subject to exposure has been properly immunized. Through well recognized channels of mass education and appeal, the community can be advised of the facts. It is the obvious duty of the health department, if the community is not safe against invasion, to offer this mass immunization to the community and thus secure practically complete immunity from invasion. Since the health department is supported by taxation it cannot discriminate between those who can afford to pay for this service and those who cannot. The department should urge that individuals go to their own private physicians, and should furnish biological products for immunization to the doctors, either free, or at cost. But any citizen who brings his child to the health department to be immunized against smallpox, diphtheria or typhoid fever should be given this service free of charge. Experience has shown repeatedly that mass immunization procedures do not rob the physician of his legitimate practice, but rather increase his office visits for the specific procedure five to ten fold.

Some health departments have assumed an educational function in diphtheria prevention campaigns. The health department has used its public health nurses and other personnel in an intensive effort to persuade parents to have their children immunized against diphtheria. The immunizations have been done by practicing physicians. In case the parents could not afford to pay for the work, each physician reported the matter to the health department and was paid a modest sum by the health department for each completed immunization that he gave to an indigent child. It is difficult for the health department to justify this method to the governing body, since the procedure is more expensive than the plan of health department sponsored clinics.

It must be generally conceded as a fundamental principle that the health department should do as little clinical work as possible, compatible with protection of the general health of the community. The health department has undertaken clinical activities because of the obvious immediate necessity. It must allocate these activities to practicing physicians as fast as the medical profession will accept responsibility for them. Whenever mass immunization will prevent outbreaks of disease, however, the health department is under obligation to carry out immunization at public cost by the most effective and least expensive means. The health department considers the community as a whole and not the individual. Mass immunization is done to protect the community. Incidentally, individuals may be safeguarded, but the primary purpose is community protection.

**Tuberculosis and Venereal Disease Clinics.** Tuberculosis and the venereal diseases may be placed in the same category for the purpose of this discussion because both require long continued and expensive treatment. They may be considered together by the health department also because the individual case, for the most part, is the direct source of infection of others and must be rendered non-infectious as soon as possible. Administrative control methods include: search for and control of the infectious person, examination of contacts, and follow-up work of both cases and contacts. Satisfactory results, from both the preventive and the clinical points of view, can be achieved best through early diagnosis and adequate treatment of the individual case. A co-operative relationship between the health department and physicians may be developed in dealing with these diseases. This program should be of mutual advantage to the health department and to physicians. Prompt reporting of all cases is essential to success. The health department should offer the physician all necessary laboratory facilities which serve for early diagnosis and as a check on the effectiveness of treatment. The health department may also offer a purely *diagnostic* clinic service for all who may apply. It may admit patients to the clinic who are referred by their physicians for *consultation,* and may offer facilities for treatment to those individuals who cannot afford to pay a physician, and who are referred, by their own doctors, to the health department clinics for *treatment.*

**Laboratory Service.** One of the major functions of the health department is to offer to physicians free laboratory facilities for the diagnosis of communicable disease. The active extension of this work as part of public health practice has been greatly appreciated by physicians and has been one of the bonds which have drawn the medical profession and health department together. The laboratory results should be accurate, and should be reported to the physicians as promptly as possible. Health departments have not found it feasible or expedient to do urinalysis, microscopic blood work, blood chemistry or any other purely clinical laboratory procedures, but have limited the scope of the laboratory to those diagnostic laboratory procedures which have a public health bearing.

The laboratory has offered an additional service of great value to physicians in many states through furnishing biological products of all types for preventive work of physicians. In some states the health department also furnishes physicians with free therapeutic biological products for their indigent patients.

**Child Hygiene Clinic Service,** including prenatal clinics, well baby clinics, preschool clinics, etc. In many communities health departments, and voluntary health organizations as well, have established various types of maternal and child hygiene clinics, not for the treatment of illness, but for the promotion of good health. The need for this service was so obvious and so urgent that these clinics have been successful from the very beginning.

Many practicing physicians have felt that clinical work of this type is not the normal function of the health department, but represents an encroachment upon the legitimate field of the practice of medicine. Thoughtful public health administrators admit the validity of this contention, and are of the almost universal opinion that all types of clinical activity which are intended to promote the health *of the individual* should be allocated to practicing physicians just as soon as they are willing and ready to undertake this work. Many physicians of the present generation were not taught the principles of preventive medicine in their medical training. Some of the older men find it difficult to adjust themselves to the ever changing conditions of medical practice. The pediatricians have shown the way. Modern practice of pediatrics consists in great part in keeping the child well rather than in seeing the child only when he is sick.

When all physicians and lying-in hospitals give adequate prenatal care, there will be little need for a public prenatal clinic. Well baby service can be given as well or better in the private office than in the public clinic. The health department cannot shirk its responsibility and must furnish facilities for clinic service when it is necessary. But the health department must also clearly understand that clinical work is not its primary function. The poor we shall always have with us. Perhaps no one is better able to judge indigency than the private physician. The logical policy is to admit to public clinics for prenatal work, infant hygiene, preschool hygiene, etc., those mothers and children who are referred to these clinics by private physicians.

In taking this stand we may be charged with inconsistency. If the health department is supported by public funds, why admit only indigent persons to the public clinics? No such distinction was drawn in the immunization programs. The answer is clear. Immunization programs deal with the mass—the community as a whole. They can succeed only if a sufficient number of the non-immune population are immunized in order to prevent any possibility of spread of specific infection. The measures only incidentally protect the individual; their primary purpose is protection of the community. Prenatal work and child hygiene activities relate to the individual and not to the mass. Measures taken for each mother and child affect directly that individual and no other. Protection of the community is essentially a health department function; medical care of the individual is essentially a function of private practice of medicine.

Many health departments have established infant and preschool health conferences to which they admit any and all of the well children of the community. If any defect or illness is discovered in the child, the parent is referred to his private physician for advice. This system has met a real need, and is an educational rather than a remedial or therapeutic activity. Nevertheless, in theory at least, this educational work should be a function of the practicing physician, and if one may venture to be prophetic, it will be done in private practice in the future.

**School Hygiene.** The purpose of the school hygiene program is the protection and promotion of the health of the school child. One of the most important of the various activities of the program is the routine physical examination of all the children by the school medical service for detection of physical defects. Correction of these defects is not a function of the department. The school health service should not maintain a clinic. It should advise the parents and urge them to have their children's defects corrected. It should always recommend that the family physician or dentist be consulted in these matters. In case parents cannot afford to pay for the service of a physician or dentist, the school may aid the parents in utilizing the various available corrective services of the community.

**Adult Hygiene.** There is a growing tendency, on the part of health departments, to take an active interest in the field of adult hygiene. Certain principles that have been worked out successfully in child health promotion and in communicable disease control may be applied almost directly to promotion of the health of adults.

For example, a few health departments and many voluntary health agencies have established cancer prevention clinics, or "cancer detection" clinics. These clinics offer a complete physical examination to presumably well persons, who for one reason or another wish reassurance that they do not have an early undetected cancer.

They are not diagnostic clinics, for if the individual has a definite illness, he is referred to his physician, rather than accepted in the clinic. If any lesion is found by the clinic, the patient is not treated, but is referred to his own physician, or to a suitable hospital.

Perhaps not one person in a hundred will be found to have cancer, in an adult health clinic of this type. But if the examination is complete and properly planned, it is quite possible that other types of degenerative disease may be determined during their early stages of invasion. Furthermore, the skilled clinician may be able to advise the individual who is now well, concerning life habits and hygienic principles, so that future illness and disaster can be avoided.

These clinics for presumably well persons are organized by the health department or by a voluntary agency. The latter may charge for actual costs of the examination, but health departments usually do not. The clinic is staffed by experts who are employed on a *per session* basis, for which they are suitably paid.

Many physicians in private practice offer this type of periodic comprehensive health examination to their clientele. This is a logical step. As group practice is developed, and prepayment for medical care becomes more popular, it seems inevitable that the periodic physical examination of the well adult will become an integral part of adequate medical care.

**Use of Local Physicians for Public Clinic Service.** All clinic activities of the health department, including tuberculosis clinics, venereal disease clinics, prenatal and infant hygiene clinics, immunization programs and school medical service, should be staffed, in so far as possible, by members of the local medical profession. These men should be paid by the health department. A definite item should be included in every public health budget to provide for honoraria to part-time physicians for specified clinical activities. The selection of the personnel for this type of work should be the responsibility of the health officer, but he should make the selections after consultation with the public health committee of the local medical association. This committee, in collaboration with the health officer, should consider the needs of each clinic service and should aid in the selection of suitable personnel for the staffs of the various clinic services.

## THE HEALTH OFFICER AND THE MEDICAL PROFESSION

The health officer should make every effort to win the confidence, friendship and approval of the organized medical body of the community. Misunderstanding will arise between the health officer and practicing physicians concerning health department policies. Mistakes will be made. Feelings will be injured. These conditions are not rectified by hostility and lack of sympathy. The medical society should have a special public health committee. This committee should deal directly with the health officer, should aid and advise him in his programs, and should interpret his policies and activities to the medical profession. The health officer should go out of his way to aid physicians individually and collectively. He should give them every consideration and all the recognition to which they are entitled. Experience has shown that best relations can be established by the health department with the medical profession, if the health officer himself is a physician. He should be abreast of the times clinically, should be a member of the local medical society, and should take an active part in the affairs of that organization. The membership of his Board of Health should always include one or more representative, public spirited physicians. In brief, the relationship between the health department and the medical profession of the community should be one of mutual trust, confidence and respect. Each should have a proper consideration for the point of view of the other. Together they should work out a co-operative program that will be of greatest benefit to the community.

There is at present a definite trend in local health department practice toward greater utilization of the resident practicing physicians as part-time clinical assistants of the health department.

The full-time personnel of the health department are utilized for those activities which require *continuous rendition* of service, such as epidemiological studies, activities aimed toward direct prevention of communicable disease, vital statistics, public health nursing, sanitation services, laboratory activities, etc. The health officials organize, direct and co-ordinate the necessary clinical activities for promotion of the health of individuals in the community. But all the clinical work of the health department—at least in the larger local health departments—should be done by resident practicing physicians.

In order that such a plan be effective, it is necessary that practicing physicians become familiar with the more useful methods and technics that may be utilized in prevention of disease and promotion of health.

### TRAINING IN PREVENTIVE MEDICINE

From the above discussion it becomes clear that the physician who practices in the community must have had suitable training in preventive medicine. He need not receive the technical training required of health officers, but should be prepared to practice preventive medicine. This principle has been understood by the leaders in medical thought of the United States for nearly 100 years,[1] but one must confess that there are still many medical colleges in the United States today where the subject is inadequately taught. It is the firm opinion of the author that the keystone of a sound, well-balanced, intelligent public health program for any state, or any nation, is a well-informed medical profession that has received suitable instruction in the principles of preventive medicine.

The courses of training that have been given in medical colleges have frequently been dull and uninteresting and have emphasized the engineering features of public health. It is true that every educated man should understand the broad general principles of community sanitation, and every physician should know the essential features of water purification, sewage disposal, milk sanitation, the hygiene of food control, and the like. He will seldom be called upon to utilize this knowledge in a direct

[1] *Report of the Sanitary Commission* by Lemuel Shattuck, 1850: "Sanitary professorships should be established in all our Medical Schools, and filled by competent teachers. The science of preserving health and preventing disease should be taught as one of the most important sciences."

way. This is not his field. The essential training of the physician however, should be twofold:

1. Training in matters relating to his public health responsibilities to the community as a practicing physician.

2. Training and experience in the incorporation of preventive principles in dealing with his individual patients in private practice.

The first phase of his training may be given early in his clinical years. He should be given elementary training in medical statistics. This may be followed by a brief course in environmental sanitation. The epidemiological features of the major diseases that will be encountered in practice should be considered, as well as methods dealing with their control. He should be taught the principles of health administration and should study the social and economic factors that may influence health and disease. He should learn the part that a private physician will play in the promotion of community health. All these matters are taught in a separate department of preventive medicine.

The incorporation of the principles of preventive medicine *in clinical practice* should be presented to the student by the clinicians. This training can often be planned as a co-ordinated exercise of the Departments of Preventive Medicine and of Curative Medicine. The essential thing is that the medical student be imbued with the idea that preventive medicine is an integral part of medical practice.

## REFERENCES

1. *Medical Care of the American People.* Final Report of the Committee on the Costs of Medical Care. University of Chicago Press, Chicago. 1932.
2. Warbasse, J. P. *The Doctor and the Public.* Paul B. Hoeber, Inc., New York. 1935.
3. Galdston, Iago. *Progress in Medicine.* Alfred A. Knopf, New York. 1940.
4. *Preventive Medicine in Modern Practice.* New York Academy of Medicine. Paul B. Hoeber, Inc., New York. 1942.
5. Smillie, W. G. *Preventive Medicine and Public Health.* The Macmillan Company, New York. 1946.
6. *Medicine and the Changing Order.* Report of the Committee on Medicine and the Changing Order, New York Academy of Medicine. The Commonwealth Fund, New York City. 1947.
7. Stieglitz, E. J. *A Future for Preventive Medicine.* The Commonwealth Fund, New York City. 1945.
8. *Proceedings of the Conference on Preventive Medicine and Public Health.* Published by the School of Public Health, University of Michigan, Ann Arbor, Michigan. 1947.

# CHAPTER XXXVI

## TRAINING OF PUBLIC HEALTH PERSONNEL

It is a truism to state that good health work cannot be accomplished without stimulating leadership and a competent, enthusiastic personnel. How shall this leadership and competence be obtained? What qualities are required for leadership? What factors produce competence? What preparation and training are desirable?

There are two main classifications of activity in health work:

    *a.* The administrative duties of the department.
    *b.* The technical activities.

Some members of the staff are occupied primarily with administrative work: for example, the health officer himself and most of the clerical staff. Others have almost no administrative work, but are primarily engaged in technical work. The principal special technics include vital statistics, epidemiology, the diagnosis and control of communicable disease, laboratory service, public health nursing, child hygiene in all its phases, health education, industrial hygiene, mental hygiene, dental hygiene, and sanitation in its various divisions.

It is obvious that some members of the department must have special training in these various highly specialized technics; others must have administrative ability and experience.

**Training of the Health Officer.** The health officer is the key man in any health organization, large or small. The position is essentially an administrative one. Thus, executive ability is required. Is executive ability an inherited or an acquired trait? If inherent, may not the talent be developed by suitable training? The health officer has the responsibility for a large number of diverse activities, some of which have a clinical significance, others bearing no relationship to clinical medicine. In smaller organizations he will carry out many of these activities himself; in larger organizations he will have charge of a group of highly trained technical people and be responsible to the government for their activities. How much should he know about the details of the work of his technicians? He must recognize that he cannot master the specialized technics of the whole department, and be at the same time a vital statistician, epidemiologist, sanitary engineer, laboratorian, industrial hygienist and pediatrician. How much should he know in order to carry out his program efficiently, and how should this knowledge be acquired?

One of the greatest defects in our system of public health administration in America has been our inability to provide properly trained personnel for positions of responsibility. Public health has not been generally recognized as a definite specialty of medicine—few of the young medical school graduates have thought of public health as a suitable outlet for a life of responsibility and interest. When an administrative position in public health becomes vacant, it is still a common practice in many parts of the United States to select for the position a resident physician whose only real qualification for the work is that he has graduated from a medical school.

In fact, the only primary requisite that has been generally accepted as essential for the position of health officer is that he shall possess a medical degree. This fact is clearly brought out, if we check the qualifications of a list of full-time health officers in the United States. The list represents a group of men who may be considered as seriously interested in public health as a career. With few exceptions they are physicians. A few municipalities and one or two states have recognized that administrative ability and special training in public health methods are as important qualifications as medical training, and have selected non-medical health officers. There is no gainsaying, however, that a medical degree represents a very valuable *basic* training for any health officer. He must deal constantly with physicians and must hold their respect and win their esteem. A well balanced medical curriculum gives not only a general knowledge of disease processes, but special training also in bacteriology, communicable disease diagnosis and control methods; training in obstetrics, pediatrics, nutrition; knowledge of physical defects of school children and the methods for their correction, psychiatry, and many other clinical data that are of primary importance to the work of the health department. Furthermore, many medical schools now give all their students a formal training in preventive medicine, and instil in them a sense of responsibility to their community for all matters relating to public health. This basic medical training is invaluable to a health officer, but the intelligent physician is the first to admit that it does not prepare him to assume the responsibility for the direction of a department of public health.

How shall the prospective health officer obtain the proper preparation? In the past, a great many successful health officers in the United States acquired their training in the school of experience, often under the apprentice system. Less than a century ago the great proportion of physicians in the United States got their medical training in this same way. It is a good system, if the preceptor is an able man and a capable teacher. A much more comprehensive and less expensive method is a formal academic course of training in a school of public health. There are now several schools of public health in the United States and Canada that are equipped primarily to train medical health officers for positions of responsibility, and several other universities give special training in the various public health technics.

The ideal training for a health officer includes collegiate training, a medical degree and at least one year's hospital internship. The hospital internship should include, if possible, special work in communicable disease and in pediatrics. This basic training should be followed by an academic year of formal training in a school of public health. Many men have found it advantageous to spend two or three years in the field in some phase of public health activity after they have finished the hospital internship, before taking formal public health training. When they enter the school of public health these men are already well oriented; they appreciate the practical difficulties that arise in any health department, and absorb the formal public health training much more rapidly than the men who enter the school of public health directly from the hospital internship.

The chief difficulty with the above plan of ideal training is that it is too prolonged and too expensive.

The large social foundations and other voluntary organizations have been most liberal in granting scholarships to state and local governments for the training of their personnel. The results were so satisfactory that in 1935, when the Social Security Act was passed, a large appropriation was made by the Federal Government for the specific purpose of training public health personnel.

The United States Public Health Service does not offer the training, but gives grants to the states whereby suitable candidates who are selected by the State Health Officer may receive appropriate training. The trainee is usually granted tuition and a stipend for maintenance for one academic year at an accredited university. Customarily the State sending the candidate for training agrees to give him at least one year's trial employment on completion of his theoretical training, and the trainee in turn agrees to return to his State Health Department for at least one year of service.

Practically all medical specialties have developed "specialty boards," which provide accreditation in the given specialty. A specialty board for health officers as well as other types of medical health personnel is a logical step in the development of this profession.

**Academic Training in Public Health Administration.** The average physician does not possess the qualities that are required of a good administrator. If he did have these innate talents, the chances are that he would have chosen some other profession than that of medicine. Men who lack the qualities that are required to handle administrative problems will not become good public health administrators by taking a theoretical course in a school of public health. Theoretical and practical training will develop qualities when an individual possesses native ability, but it cannot be expected to supply administrative capacity.

Administration in any field is concerned with (*a*) formulation of policies, and (*b*) the carrying into effect of these policies. Formulation of policy involves the study of present conditions and the weighing of past experience. One is then able to obtain a trend, and plan for the future with reasonable foresight. But conditions may change, or judgment may be faulty. Thus, the good administrator in formulating his policies must maintain a flexibility such that he can readjust his program when necessary to meet unexpected conditions.

The execution of policies requires:

1. A comprehensive knowledge of the task at hand.

2. An aptitude for marshalling resources.

3. Qualities of leadership, and particularly the ability to select, train, and assign men according to their talents, and in relation to the task to be done.

4. The development of a plan of supervision, whereby the administrator may be sure that all assignments are faithfully carried out.

5. A talent for the careful timing of action, so that most efficient results will be obtained from the energy expended.

6. A system of constant appraisal of results, so that policies may be changed if necessary, because of changed conditions or because the methods that have been adopted are not effective. This requires a system of careful record-keeping which will rapidly make available all data concerning activities and achievements.

State health officers who assign trainees to a school of public health cannot expect that all the above technics will be acquired in one year of training. As we have already said, academic training in public health administration will never generate new qualities in an individual. All that can be anticipated is that the trainee will develop wisdom and skill in forming judgments and in organizing his work. It is true that the trainee would gain the same knowledge by direct experience, but experience is a slow and costly teacher. The academic training is intended to give the student the experience of others, and to lead him in an orderly and comprehensive way to develop theory and to make generalizations. Its chief purpose is that it aids the trainee in substituting logical thought for an intuitive action, which is often based on an unconscious reaction to past experience.

**Field Training in Public Health.** The American Public Health Association has sponsored the accreditation of schools of public health and has developed minimum standards for academic training in this field. The theoretical training will assemble a large amount of information for the trainee, but this in itself will be of little value unless the student is given an opportunity to carry out his theoretical concepts in practice under supervision. Thus, the work in theory should be supplemented by a period of apprenticeship, or externship.

Many state health officers have followed the apprenticeship plan.

They have selected the trainee, provided for a period of academic training—usually a year—and then have given him a period of orientation in the field in which he is to be assigned, where he works under the direction of an experienced health administrator. New York State has reversed the process, and has given the candidate a preliminary apprenticeship before the theoretical training is acquired.

In a few areas, public health "residencies" have been given. This type of training is almost exactly parallel to the hospital internship. The trainee, on completion of his theoretical training, obtains an appointment of one year in a health department. He rotates from one type of service to another in regular sequence, and takes part in all the various health department activities, always working under supervision. These residencies bear a remuneration which is equivalent to maintenance, and the health department is under no obligation to employ the resident on termination of his externship.

The apprenticeship plan and the residency plan are quite similar, except that in the one the trainee usually works in one field and under one director, and there is a definite commitment on the part of both trainee and health department that the candidate will be continued in service on salary if his apprenticeship has been satisfactory; the resident has a definite and varied program, and thus gains experience in all types of service. The latter plan is particularly valuable if it can be correlated with university work.

The Committee on Professional Education of the American Public Health Association, under the guidance of Dr. Gaylord Anderson, has attempted to define [1] the various types of field training that may be planned for public health personnel. These plans are particularly designed for training medical health officers, but are quite inclusive and may be utilized for the training of all types of public health personnel. The major categories of training may be defined as:

A. **Observation.**

**Definition.** A planned visit to a health agency to observe the public health program without active participation therein.

**Objective.** To see the functioning of an efficient community health program. The duration of the visit is usually brief (one to a few days). The planning is individualized on the basis of past experience and special interests. Observation may be of value to the uninitiated as well as to the highly skilled.

B. **Orientation.**

**Definition.** Preparation of a person for a specific job under the auspices of the employing agency.

**Objective.** To acquaint the prospective employee with administrative details and policies of the employing and related agencies and the

[1] *Standards for Field Training* (in press). Committee on Professional Education, American Public Health Assn., 1790 Broadway, New York 19, N. Y.

conditions under which he is to work; for example, background, laws, regulations, records, personnel, and health problems of the area. The duration of a planned period for orientation is usually a matter of a few weeks.

C. **Supervised Field Experience.**

**Definition.** Planned instruction, observation, and active participation in a comprehensive organized public health program as an integral part of or a sequel to formal academic training in public health.

**Objective.** To learn to apply the basic principles and skills studied in a university course to an actual field situation. It may or may not be a requirement for an academic degree. The duration of a planned period of field experience is usually from two to four months.

D. **Apprenticeship.**

**Definition.** An extended period of active service under supervision in a public health program, but without prior academic training in public health.

**Objective.** To select personnel best suited for formal academic training, to prepare them to receive the maximum benefit from such training and to develop certain elementary skills which may enable them to participate in the public health program as assistants to qualified workers in their professional field. The period of apprenticeship is usually for a period not to exceed one year.

E. **Residency.**

**Definition.** An extended period of active service under supervision in a public health program following a period of formal academic training in public health.

**Objective.** To develop through supervised practice a high degree of technical skill and confidence in a person who has had broad basic academic training in public health. This is usually accomplished through occupancy of a first level staff position in an organized health agency already employing competent supervisory personnel. It corresponds to the year of supervised experience required in public health nursing and is comparable to the residence required for certification in medical specialties. It may or may not be a requirement for an academic degree.

The Committee has set forth the minimum standards that should be required for established field training areas that are organized to give this service.

It is obvious that each of the various states should finance their own orientation training, but grants-in-aid from Federal or other sources will probably be required to finance adequately the field training stations that will be needed for supervised field experience and for apprenticeship training. The universities that give the theoretical academic training in public health will maintain a vital interest in field training, but they should not have the direct administrative responsibility for these field training centers.

STANDARD QUALIFICATIONS FOR PUBLIC HEALTH PERSONNEL

Standard minimum qualifications for public health personnel are highly advantageous to public health administrators.

The Committee on Professional Education of the American Public Health Association has made recommendations in regard to the educational qualifications of health officers, public health nurses, public health engineers, sanitarians, sub-professional field personnel in sanitation, public health statisticians, school health educators, and for other types of professional personnel. The minimum qualifications for public health nurses are practically identical with the recommendations of the National Organization for Public Health Nursing. These recommendations have been officially adopted by the Governing Council of the American Public Health Association. These standards are all given in the Appendix, and therefore they require no further discussion in this chapter. Suffice it to say that the author served on the Committee on Professional Education for years, and is in full accord with the recommendations that have been made relating to the training of all types of public health personnel.

**Training of Physicians in Public Health.** Satisfactory community programs in public health are dependent in the end upon the co-operation and support of the private practitioners of medicine. The physician is not only the health adviser to the individual and the family, but is looked up to as an authority in community health matters. In any governmental unit, be it city, county, or state, the physicians should be the leaders in the promotion of community programs for the betterment of public health. The average physician is public spirited and sincerely interested in community affairs. In many parts of the United States, the practicing physicians have realized the importance of their public duty, and have been largely responsible for the advances that have been made in public health practice. One serious difficulty has been encountered, in that many physicians have not had the opportunity for basic training in preventive medicine. Medical schools are beginning to realize this hiatus in their curricula, and the better schools have introduced formal courses in preventive medicine. But the curriculum is always crowded. Courses in preventive medicine and hygiene have been added as an appendage—perhaps as a separate department—often as a part of some other division of teaching, such as bacteriology. It is clear that preventive medicine is not a separate entity, but an integral part of the practice of medicine. The pediatricians are well aware of the facts, and are far in advance of other departments of medical teaching. They are rapidly incorporating the teaching of preventive medicine with curative medicine, with little or no distinction between the two subjects. Other departments have been slow to follow.

The lack of appreciation of the preventive viewpoint on the part of many physicians has compelled the official health department to assume essential clinical functions for protection of the health of the individual and the community. These activities are not primarily community functions, but a responsibility of every practicing physician and every parent.

## PUBLIC HEALTH INSTITUTES

Public health institutes, if properly conducted, are continuation courses in public health. They are very valuable. Each state may hold an annual conference for each type of personnel employed—health officers, nurses, sanitary inspectors, etc. These institutes familiarize the personnel with the recent advance in public health technic, and encourage free discussion of the general health policies of the state.

Correspondence courses in public health have been organized in a few states for the health personnel in the field. They have a limited value, and the best that can be said for them is that they are better than no instruction at all.

The chief purpose of the annual meeting of the American Public Health Association is that it serves as a continuation course, giving opportunity for instruction, exchange of viewpoint and discussion of problems. The annual Surgeon General's Conference for the State Health Officers has been a powerful agency in advancing public health procedures in the United States through the information and counsel given to the state health leaders.

## IN-SERVICE TRAINING

A plan of continuous training of personnel is essential to good health administration. This principle has been recognized by departments of education for years, in that teachers in the public schools have been required to continue their education, and keep abreast of modern methods of teaching. The field of preventive medicine has grown even more rapidly than that of education. New technics are continuously being developed, so that it is essential that all members of the health department shall be encouraged to continue their professional education.

Courses may be offered by the health department, using departmental personnel for teaching in so far as possible, with assistance from community leaders and from state health department resources. In the large cities, teaching centers may be developed, perhaps by utilizing the facilities of a university or medical college in planning the courses.

An effort should be made to instruct the personnel of each division in the perfection of its own technics. In addition, instruction may be given which will broaden the horizon of the personnel and teach them what the other divisions of the department are doing. Thus, they may learn how their own work fits into the activities of others in the department.

Rural health departments may not have local facilities to enable them to organize their own in-service training courses. One of the important functions of the state health department is to aid these smaller organizations in the planning and conduct of in-service training.

**Library Facilities.** Every health department, no matter how small, should maintain a library. The rural health unit with limited budget can spend no more, perhaps, than $30 to $50 a year for books and periodicals, but if care is used in selection, a very satisfactory reference library can be built up.

The library should be built around the periodicals, particularly the American Journal of Public Health, the Journal of the American Medical Association, the Journal of Public Health Nursing, and the publications of the United States Public Health Service. Excellent health educational materials may be obtained at cost from the Children's Bureau, the various national public health organizations such as the National Tuberculosis Association, and from the large insurance companies. The American Medical Association and the Surgeon General's Library in Washington have extensive loan services.

The larger municipal health departments should develop their own libraries for all employees. The State Health Department can be of great assistance to the smaller local health departments through the organization of a loan library system. The State Health Department libraries may aid the local health departments in selection of a small reference library for local permanent use, and may supplement the local libraries through loan of a wide selection of special texts and monographs. The Book Service of the American Public Health Association publishes an excellent list of books on public health subjects, from which selections may be made.

## REFERENCES

The reader who is interested in the whole field of training of public health personnel is referred to the various current publications of the:

Committee on Professional Education, American Public Health Association, 1790 Broadway, New York City.

The Education Committee of the National Organization of Public Health Nursing, 1790 Broadway, New York City, maintains current educational standards of training for public health nurses. (See Appendix.)

The training qualifications for public health personnel of the United States Public Health Service and the Children's Bureau, Washington, D. C., are also of interest.

# CHAPTER XXXVII

## BUDGETS AND BUDGET MAKING [1]

GLADSTONE: "Budgets are not merely affairs of arithmetic, but in a thousand ways go to the root of prosperity of individuals, the relation of classes, and the strength of kingdoms."

Apparently, it is the fate of all scientists and most medical men to have difficulty with finances. The bacteriologist may be able to make careful observations and keep minute and exact records concerning the details of his experiments, but the details of his monthly bank statement drive him to distraction. The practicing physician is a notoriously poor business man, and is a prey to every get-rich-quick promoter who may secure his momentary attention.

The medical student absorbs these traditions from his first medical contacts. He soon encounters the notorious feud that exists between the clinical staff of the hospital and the administrative staff. The hospital intern is encouraged by the clinician to despise and to consider as beneath his contempt all matters which relate to business management. Osler used to tell his students, "The practice of medicine is an art, and not a trade."

It is true that medicine may be and has been successfully and splendidly practiced without giving any concern to the ordinary simple principles of business management. It must be recognized, however, that one great difference between the practice of Public Health and the practice of Medicine is that the former *must be conducted on business principles.*

The tradition of poor financial administrative methods has been carried into public health work. It must be confessed that medical health officers should bear a large part of the responsibility for this state of affairs. This condition cannot continue. The medical health officer must learn that public health activities cannot be conducted in the same haphazard financial manner as private practice. Public health brings an added responsibility. Not only must it be conducted on sound scientific principles, but, since the cost of the work is met from taxation, the expenditure of the funds becomes a public trust.

Scientific training and sound judgment are required in public health work to determine just which procedures will probably be most effective

[1] The textbook of Mark Carter Mills and Geo. W. Starr on *Readings in Public Finance and Taxation* (1932, The Macmillan Co.) has been referred to freely in preparation of this chapter.

in preventing disease and promoting the health of the public. Business judgment is required to determine just how the available funds can be expended to yield the maximum return. Scientific knowledge determines what should be done and which activities are most important; business judgment determines what can be accomplished with the resources at hand.

## THE BUDGET

The budget is a useful business invention which enables the administrator to utilize his resources to greatest advantage. There is nothing mysterious about it, nor is it a panacea which will solve all financial difficulty. In fact, the budget plan has distinct limitations. For example, the budget is always made for a limited time, usually one year. It presupposes that the resources for a given project are known and fixed. This is not always the case. Unless very carefully drawn, it may defeat its own purpose and serve as a hindrance rather than an aid to the administrator. The administrator may discover in the middle of his budgetary period that he has not allotted enough funds to a given item to carry the work through to a successful conclusion. He is then in the embarrassing position of being required either to give up the work or ask for a revision of his budget.

**Essentials of the Budget System.** The budget should be prepared and submitted to the legislative body by the executive who will have the responsibility for expenditures after enactment of the budget. Thus the essentials of the budget system are:

1. Responsible executive leadership.
2. Broad and accurate information concerning the given project.
3. A complete budgetary plan.

The health department budget represents only a part of governmental activity. The whole governmental budget represents a plan for all governmental activities for a definite period. Segregation of the funds assigned to the various departmental budgets into individual budget items is seldom necessary. Once proper executive leadership and suitable arrangements have been established to administer and control expenditures, it becomes a wise policy to make appropriations for the activities of a given department in a lump sum, rather than in detail.

The budget is made for a definite period—usually one year—sometimes two years. This limitation does not make it necessary for the executive to limit his administrative plans to one budgetary period. It does require the establishment of a financial calendar. Most states adopt the federal fiscal year of July 1 to June 30. The calendar year is most frequently adopted by municipalities and counties.

*General Principles in Relation to the Budget.* Certain general principles should be observed in developing a budget system:

1. The budget should not exceed the probable source of income. This most obvious principle is frequently violated.

2. The budget must be adhered to strictly. If this is not done, the whole purpose of the budget system is nullified.

3. There should be some effective method of controlling the execution of the budget. A constant check should be made of expenditures. This routine check of disbursements should be under the direct supervision of the executive, who, in the end, is responsible for the proper expenditure of the available funds. This method enables the executive to know where the department stands financially at any given time, and also renders it possible to make a more satisfactory budget for the next fiscal period.

4. A small contingent fund is essential. It gives some elasticity to the budget, as it may be used at the discretion of the executive, and may be expended for any budget item (except to augment salaries). The contingent fund should seldom exceed 5 per cent of the total budget. A large contingent fund is a confession by the executive of failure in the exact estimation of his needs.

*Purposes of the Budget.* The chief purposes of the budget are that it assists the administrator:

1. To clarify his own mind as to his objectives.

2. To plan his work for a definite period.

3. To balance his program so that he is not placing too great emphasis on unessentials and neglecting some important activities.

In an organization as large as a state health department or a large city health department, with several bureaus of activity, the budget is an invaluable administrative aid to the chief executive. The budget is arranged so that each division head knows just what his resources will be for the current year. Salaries are fixed, thus minimizing the danger of internal dissension and friction. When any question arises as to over-expenditure of items, such as for supplies, for travel, etc., there is always the court of last appeal—the budget.

The budget is the most important document in the department. It is kept in a special place, carefully guarded and frequently consulted. It is sacred, and must not be violated. The tradition is built up in a well-organized health department that the greatest crime of administrative practice is over-expenditure of a budget item.

Like all despots and tyrants, the budget has its disadvantages. It is inflexible, unwieldy and cumbersome. When emergencies arise, or when mistakes in judgment have been made in drawing up the budget, the executive may find it impossible to modify expenditures to meet the needs of the situation until the budgetary period has elapsed. Despite these and other disadvantages, however, the carefully prepared budget is essential in health department practice.

Most state health departments have adopted the budget system only within recent years. Many of the smaller health departments have not yet adopted the budget plan. In these latter organizations, financial disbursements are made on more or less the same plan that most men follow in managing their own personal expenditures. A certain sum is allotted for the work of the whole department and the money is doled out to the various bureau heads as they ask for it. The one who is most insistent gets the greatest share, with all hands suffering privation as the end of the fiscal period draws near.

**Budget Making.** There are certain broad principles in regard to making up a budget that are more or less applicable to any organization, large or small. A budget is an estimate of expenditures for various items of activity carried out by the organization during a certain limited time. There should be a proper classification of items, and this classification may be made in various ways. The common methods that are useful for health department practice are: [2]

1. Classification by Unit of Organization.
2. Classification by Function.
3. Classification by Character.
4. Classification by Source of Funds.

Each of these classifications will be discussed in relation to its application to health department practice.

*Classification by Unit of Organization.* Classification of the budget by unit of organization is made for the purpose of locating responsibility. When a budget is prepared, the chief executive is responsible:

    *a.* For each estimate that is made.
    *b.* For seeing that the money granted is expended by departmental executives with proper economy and in accordance with the law.

The chief executive officer of the health department is directly responsible for all the estimates and expenditures of the various units under his supervision. It is his duty to execute contracts, to approve purchase orders, vouchers, payrolls, and to control all expenditures.

The actual responsibility for detailed expenditures usually rests upon each one of the division directors in charge of the different units of organization. Thus, the health officer may delegate his authority to a division chief, but, nevertheless, the chief executive is, himself, ultimately responsible for all budget items. In order to locate responsibility, therefore, it is necessary to arrange the budget, at least for large organizations, by classification according to organization unit.

Let us select, for example, a State Health Department with eight divisions. The state health officer has direct personal supervision over the division of administration only; each of the other seven divisions is in the charge of a full-time divisional director. Each of these divisional directors is allotted a specified sum in the budget for a year's activity. A

[2] Adapted from Francis Oakey's *Principles of Government Accounting and Reporting.*

suitable classification of the budget by unit of organization is shown in Budget A.

BUDGET A

*Budget Summary for a State Health Department with Eight Divisions, Each with a Division Director*

The budget is classified according to unit of organization.
Period of the Budget: 1 year.

| Item No. | Title | Amount |
|---|---|---|
| 1. | Administration | $ 40,100 |
| 2. | Vital Statistics | 26,600 |
| 3. | Public Health Laboratories | 46,300 |
| 4. | Sanitation | 36,200 |
| 5. | Communicable Disease Control | 41,300 |
| 6. | Child Hygiene and Public Health Nursing | 42,200 |
| 7. | Public Health Education | 17,300 |
| 8. | Local Health Organization, including subsidy to local health departments | 130,000 |
| 9. | Contingent Fund | 20,000 |
| | | $400,000 |

This budget classification gives a general idea of the distribution of activities of the department through the *titles* of the various items. It is not, however, a classification by function. It gives no idea as to cost of detailed activities, since there may be overlapping of functions in the various organization units.

*Classification by Function.* A function of government is "a service that is rendered or purpose accomplished by an organ or agent through performing a complement of related processes." Each function of government represents a service rendered directly to the people, or service performed as a means of controlling or directing services that may be directly rendered. For example, the control of tuberculosis and the supervision of public water supplies are official public health functions.

A distinction should be made between function and activity. Function indicates the *end sought,* rather than the specific work done. Thus, the health department performs the governmental function of promotion of the general sanitation of the community. In performing this function, many activities are engaged in, such as inspection of dairies, supervision of food handlers, bacteriological examination of water supplies, etc.

*Standardization of the Title of Items.* The value of this type of classification depends upon the extent to which the nomenclature of the various functions and activities of a health department have been standardized. The scope and definition of every budget item must be exactly specified and clearly understood. Every title of each item must be the standard which is generally accepted by health officials throughout the nation. Statements of expenditures for various types of activity may then be prepared that convey exact information as to the cost of each type of work.

BUDGET B

*Example of Budget Classification by Function*

Annual Expenditures for Maternal and Child Health Protection ...... $100,000

 Item 1. Prenatal Clinics .......................... $ 4,000
 Item 2. Well Baby Clinics ........................ 12,000
 Item 3. Preschool Health Service ................. 7,000
 Item 4. Dental Hygiene .......................... 8,000
 Item 5. Home Nursing Service for Mothers and Babies.. 18,000
 Item 6. School Health Program
    *a.* School Medical Service $ 6,000
    *b.* School Nursing Service 24,000
    *c.* School Health Education 12,000

    TOTAL ......................... 42,000
 Item 7. Care of Crippled and Defective Children ...... 5,000
 Item 8. Nutrition Service ......................... 4,000

    GRAND TOTAL .............. $100,000

*Purpose of Classification by Function.* A classification of expenditures by function is essential in order that the executive may:

 *a.* Determine the cost of carrying on some special type of work.
 *b.* Be aided in determining policies in regard to future procedures concerning expansion or contraction of specific services.
 *c.* Compare the cost of a given activity with the cost of the same type of work in a prior period.
 *d.* Compare the cost of similar functions performed by other health departments.
 *e.* Give an account of stewardship to the legislative body and to the public.

Thus, a classification of the budget by function enables the executive to develop a properly balanced program, and aids him in securing intelligent legislative action.

From the standpoint of the chief executive—as for example, the governor of the state or mayor of the city—as well as the legislature and the public, budget classification by function has three main purposes:

 *a.* It gives exact knowledge of the cost of a given public service which has been performed.
 *b.* It gives definite information as to efficiency of departmental executives.
 *c.* It furnishes information as to the classes of work that are carried out by the various organization units.

This third purpose aids in the elimination of duplication in governmental service. A classification by function shows the extent to which other bureaus and departments are carrying on work in the same or similar fields. For example, classification by function of the Federal Governmental Budget revealed that at least five major Federal departments were engaged in public health activities to a greater or lesser extent.

*Classification by Character.* For general governmental purposes, it is important to classify budget items by character. Segregation of expenditures is made into three main groups.

    *a.* Expense for administration, operation and current repairs.
    *b.* Capital outlays.
        This item includes expenditures which increase capital assets or reduce capital liabilities. The cost of construction of a health center, a tuberculosis hospital, or a public health laboratory would be included under this item. The title includes, also, expenditures for acquisition, betterment or replacement of permanent property, as well as redemption of outstanding long-term bonded indebtedness.
    *c.* Fixed charges.
        "Fixed charges are non-asset producing expenditures for existing obligations that were created by previous administrators and over which the present administration has no control. An example is expenditures for interest on bonded indebtedness."

It is obvious that the two latter classes will seldom apply to ordinary health department practice unless the department has the responsibility for hospitalization. If the health department actually maintains and operates institutions, such as tuberculosis hospitals, contagious disease hospitals, etc., this classification is essential. The increasing tendency for the development of health centers in municipal health department practice, with the required outlay for capital construction, necessitates more and more consideration of this type of budget classification.

The first group of expenditures under classification by character may be subdivided into three groups: (1) Administration, (2) Operation, (3) Upkeep.

1. The budget item for cost of administration represents the efforts of the executive and his immediate staff. Expenditures under this item include administrative salaries and all expenses related to the application of administrative effort.

2. The budget item for cost of operation includes all efforts directly applied to the rendition of actual public service, such as:

    *a.* Salaries and wages of all those engaged in a specific activity.
    *b.* Supplies and materials required for a given activity. Rent, heat and light are included in this item of operation.

It is often difficult to distinguish between administration and operation. In certain instances the decision must be arbitrary, since some items may be chargeable to either administration or operation. The only important thing is to determine some rule of distinction and adhere to it. For example, the deputy health officer of a city health department may aid in general administration, but his major activities are concerned with communicable disease control. It is quite appropriate to allocate his salary to the latter under *operation,* and not divided between the two classifications.

3. Upkeep. This item represents partial and continuous restorations of property that are necessary to keep the property in fit and serviceable condition. Depreciation charges on automobiles owned by the health department might be classified under this item.

*Classification by Source of Funds.* The funds for given health functions or activities may come from various sources. Most of the funds will be derived from taxation and will be allocated to the health department by legislative action, usually in a lump sum. In many instances special funds may be allotted to the health department for special or for general purposes. For example, a local, city, or county health department may receive a subsidy from the state for a venereal disease clinic. The Federal Government may make a grant to the state for the development of rural health work. Unofficial sources, such as the local tuberculosis association, may aid the municipal health department in some special activity. The expenditures from special funds for these several operations should be clearly shown in the consolidated budget statement.

When considering the costs of various health department activities, the actual resources from which the various funds have been secured must be stated in the budget. These funds must be properly allocated to the activities and to the personnel for which they are intended. In other words, the items of the budget are arranged so that a detailed statement of expenditures may be definitely related to the actual cost of given standard activities and may be analyzed also as to the various sources of the funds.

From the above discussion we note that the budget for the health department may be prepared so that a ready analysis can be made on the basis of the various classifications.

*a. Expenditures by unit organization.* This analysis will show the expenditures of each bureau or division, without reference to the purpose of the expenditures except as the title of the division might explain.

*b. Expenditures for various functions and activities* may be determined, as, for example, the cost of control of tuberculosis, the cost of vital statistics activities, of milk sanitation, etc.

*c. Classification by character* will separate the costs of administration and of operation. Since most local health departments are operating units, this classification is seldom applicable in its entirety to health department practice. It may be a very useful classification in the larger organizations. Even in the small units, the subdivision of operation into: (*a*) Salaries, (*b*) Supplies, and (*c*) Travel, is an essential procedure.

*d. Classification by source of funds* will determine the source of revenue for each and all of the activities of the health department.

In health department practice the primary classification of the budget is usually by *unit of organization.* If this method is used, the items should be subdivided so that the budget may be analyzed on the basis of classification by function, character and source of funds.

An example of a simple county health unit budget which brings out the principal feature of classification is given below.

BUDGET C

*Simple Budget to Bring Out Various Classifications* [3]

County Health Unit
Period: January 1 to December 31

| Item | | | Source of Funds | | |
|---|---|---|---|---|---|
| Salaries | Total | County Court | County Dept. of Education | State Subsidy | Federal Aid |
| 1. Health Officer | $ 4,500 | $ 2,500 | | $2,000 | |
| 2. Secretary | 1,500 | 1,500 | | | |
| 3. Sanitary Officer | 3,000 | 1,000 | | 2,000 | |
| 4. Public Health Nurse-Supervisor | 2,400 | 1,200 | | | $1,200 |
| 5. School Nurses (2) | 3,600 | | $3,600 | | |
| 6. Nurse—Maternal and Infant Welfare | 1,800 | | | | 1,800 |
| 7. Medical and Dental Assistance (part time) | 2,000 | 1,000 | | 1,000 | |
| 8. Travel | 4,500 | 2,500 | | 1,000 | 1,000 |
| 6 automobiles for health officer, sanitary officer and each nurse | | | | | |
| Running expenses $2,500 | | | | | |
| Depreciation 2,000 | | | | | |
| 9. Supplies | 3,000 | 2,000 | | | 1,000 |
| Administration $1,500 | | | | | |
| School Health 750 | | | | | |
| Infant Health 750 | | | | | |
| 10. Contingent Fund | 700 | 700 | | | |
| | $27,000 | $12,400 | $3,600 | $6,000 | $5,000 |

Population: 35,000      Per capita annual cost: 77 cents

**Analysis of Budget C.** *By Unit of Organization.* The organization is a complete unit in itself and is a part of county government. Thus the portion of the budget presented represents only a part of a complete

[3] The student is asked to consider this budget as illustrative of the principles of budget making, and not as a declaration of the author's ideas of suitable salary ranges. Fluctuations in the cost of living, in time, and in various parts of the nation, make it impossible to prepare an "ideal" budget.

budget that has already been classified on the basis of unit of organization. The county appropriation body can determine from the budget exactly what the health services cost per capita.

*By Function and Activity.* It is not possible to analyze the cost of all health functions completely in this small unit of organization, as the health officer performs so many functions. His major activities are: Administration, Communicable Disease Control, Child and School Hygiene, etc. Activities may be classified as follows:

*Item*
1. Medical Activities. Health Officer, salary and travel, and Medical Assistance .......... $ 7,250
2. Office Costs. Salary of secretary and office supplies ...... 3,000
3. Sanitation. Salary of Sanitary Officer and his travel ...... 3,750
4. School Hygiene. Salary of 2 nurses, travel and supplies ...... 5,850
5. Infant and Preschool Hygiene. Supervising nurse, salary of one nurse, travel and supplies ...... 6,450
6. Contingent ...... 700
     $27,000

*By Character.* The county health department is an operating unit. Thus, all costs of the work may be allocated to operation, with no separate division for administration. Operation is subdivided into salaries, travel and supplies. The approximate allocation according to this classification, therefore, is:

*Operation*
Salaries ............................. $18,000
Travel ............................. 2,500
Supplies .......................... 3,000
*Upkeep,* depreciation on cars ............. 2,000
*Contingent* .......................... 700
     $27,000

*By Source of Funds.* This budget clearly states the source of funds, namely,

County Court ............... $12,400
Dept. of Education .......... 3,600
State Subsidy ............... 6,000
Federal Aid ............... 5,000
     $27,000

It also indicates the allocation of each of these funds to the various items of activity. Thus each agency that has contributed to the budget may determine exactly how its funds have been allocated. By analysis of the annual report of activities it will be possible to determine the cost of each major activity and thus determine whether or not the results achieved are commensurate with expenditures.

**Steps in Drawing a Budget.** In planning the budget for his department, the health officer must consider first the relative importance of the various activities that he wishes to carry out during the coming fiscal period and the emphasis he wishes to place on each. He must determine approximately the available total funds that will be at his disposal, from both official and unofficial sources. He will use his present organization and personnel as a basis and give due consideration to the budgetary experiences of the previous fiscal periods. He may then make a tentative draft of the budget, classifying the items according to *function,* and allotting proportionate amounts to each item. This is done in order to obtain a balanced program.

Using this tentative budget as a basis, he can then take the second step. He should draw a budget, classified according to *character,* and should allow suitable amounts to individual items, such as travel, salaries, etc. In this way he can plan the allocation of suitable personnel for each project. If new work is to be undertaken, the budget can be arranged so as to meet probable needs. When the health officer has determined what activities he wishes to emphasize and has also determined what personnel and proportionate expenditures he can devote to each activity, he can then take the third and final step in drawing his budget. The final (consolidated) budget will probably be drawn on the primary basis of *unit* of organization, but so classified that it may be analyzed, in the final draft, on the basis of either character or function. The sources of funds must also be stated, so that there can be no question that the revenue granted for a specific purpose will be expended for any purpose other than that for which it was intended.

It is not feasible, nor is it necessary, to give in this text a complete type budget of a large organization. The general principles are the same for all. In making up any budget certain rules must be remembered:

1. The budget shall be held inviolate; otherwise, its very purpose is defeated. If it becomes obvious during the fiscal period that the budget is unworkable, a revision may be obtained. This should not be customary practice.

2. The budget is at best inflexible and unwieldy. For this reason the executive should have certain discretion, within budgetary limits, in allocation of funds. For example, in the County Health Unit given above, he may apply portions of contingent items to supplement any of the other budget items, *except salaries.* He may even use the whole contingent fund for an emergency.

3. Budget items should not be too detailed. For example, it is unwise to allocate a definite budget item for postage, another for telephone, another item for stationery, etc. This is particularly true in small operating units. Operating costs may be estimated in a lump sum, thus giving to the executive the power to allocate funds within the item as necessity demands. Under the travel item, for example, it may be found that the

health officer and sanitary inspector will travel much more than the nurses. In order that the work shall not be curtailed, a lump sum is estimated for travel for the whole unit rather than allocated in equal parts to each employee. For example, under Budget C the health officer would first allocate $25 a month for depreciation on each car, and then permit some variation of travel expenditures for each of the staff. The total of the budget item, however, must not be over expended, nor should it be expended for other purposes than travel.

4. Budget items for salaries should not be violated during the budgetary period. If some of the other budget items are unexpended during the fiscal period, they cannot be applied toward the salaries of personnel, but should be accumulated to the end of the fiscal period. Each unexpended item is then returned to the original source of funds.

5. Detailed records must be kept of all actual expenditures. These records should be itemized in accordance with the budgetary classification. Thus, at any and all periods during the fiscal year, the executive will know whether or not current expenditures are exceeding the allocation of any single budgetary item.

**Revision of the Budget.** Because of unforeseen circumstances, it may be necessary to ask for revision of the budget. This should not be undertaken unless a real emergency arises. As already stated, it is bad budgetary practice to transfer funds from one item to another during the fiscal year. The executive should never, because of decrease in an activity or through unexpected savings, use the unexpended funds of these items toward augmentation of salaries.

Some organizations permit unexpended balances to be carried over to the next fiscal period. This may be justified, if development along specific lines of activity has been delayed temporarily for some obvious reason. Otherwise, unexpended funds should be returned to the general treasury.

Any fees or other sources of revenue from health department activities should not go into departmental funds to be expended as occasion arises, but should be turned into the general treasury and not included in the budget.

It may seem to the average reader that too great emphasis has been placed in this text upon budgets and their importance to good health department practice. Certain reiterations and repetitions will be noted in the text. These have been included intentionally in order to emphasize certain points. It is the author's opinion that no single instrument is of greater value to the health executive than a properly drawn and frequently consulted budget. The New York Bureau of Municipal Research, 1907, in "Making a Municipal Budget" states succinctly, "No document can tell in such condensed form so many significant facts about community needs and governmental efforts to meet those needs as the municipal budget."

## REFERENCES

1. Buck, A. E. *The Development of the Budget Idea in the United States.* Annals of the American Academy of Political and Social Science. 1924, Vol. CXIII, pp. 31–39.
2. Mills, M. C. and Starr, G. W. *Readings in Public Finance and Taxation.* 1932. The Macmillan Company.
3. Oakey, Francis. *Principles of Government Accounting and Reporting.* 1921 D. Appleton and Co., New York City.

# CHAPTER XXXVIII

## THE NATIONAL HEALTH PROGRAM

PUBLIC health protection in the United States has developed on a community basis. First, the community met each individual situation as it arose; then, gradually, permanent local health organizations were formed. The state did not consider health protection to be an essential state-wide governmental function, and no state health work was organized until the nation was nearly 100 years old. An abortive attempt was made to establish a National Board of Health in 1879, but it failed; no nation-wide responsibility was assumed for health protection until a good many years later.

The importance of good health to the national economy was brought to the attention of the nation by the "Report on National Vitality: Its Waste and Conservation," in 1909.[1] The National Conservation Commission, at the instigation of President Theodore Roosevelt, surveyed the whole problem of health protection as an essential part of the conservation of the national resources, and made this excellent report, which met with little response.

The White House Conference on Child Health and Protection,[2] which was called by President Hoover in 1930, was the next important study of our national needs for health protection. This study had a broad and lasting effect in the determination of public health procedures and policies in the United States, but the nation was not yet ready for a definite national health program, guided by national leadership, and supported by federal appropriation.

The Committee on Economic Security,[3] which made its report to President Franklin D. Roosevelt in 1935, brought home to this country the failures that we had made in the application of our knowledge in relation to the prevention of illness and the promotion of health. This committee estimated the loss in wages caused by sickness in families with modest income to be nearly a billion dollars annually, and stated that the actual

[1] *Bulletin 30, Committee of One Hundred on National Health*, National Conservation Commission. U. S. Government Printing Office, 1909.

[2] See *Reports of the White House Conference on Child Health and Protection*, published by The Century Company in 1930, 1932, and 1933.

[3] *Report of the Committee on Economic Security*, January 15, 1935. Government Printing Office, Washington, D. C.

cost to these income groups for medical, nursing, and hospital care was over one and one-half billion dollars. The committee found that every million persons living in the United States during a given year would suffer from 800,000 cases of illness. Over half would be sick at least once; 70,000 would suffer three or more illnesses. Many of these cases of illness are not preventable, of course—at least with our present knowledge. But it must be granted that, in view of our great advances in medical science and knowledge of methods of protecting the public health, "the American people are not as healthy as they have a right to be."

It is true that the infant death rate was cut in half following the first 25 years of active child health promotion, but it must be recognized that it can easily be cut in half again. The mortality rate from tuberculosis has been reduced by half in half a century; the next 25 years should see a similar reduction. Two thirds of the annual maternal deaths could be prevented. The ravages of typhoid fever, diphtheria, and smallpox have been greatly reduced, but they have by no means been eliminated.

The expectation of life at 50 years of age is little greater now than it was in 1900—or, in fact, in 1850. The most important age group from a productive point of view is that from 20 to 45 years, yet in this age group tuberculosis is still one of the principal causes of death. To this group accidents and industrial illness are highly destructive, and organic heart disease is the third most important cause of death. Studies of causes of illness and of physical disability have revealed, more clearly than mortality statistics, the extent of impairment of bodily vigor and vitality in this most efficient period of human life. These matters were all clearly brought out by the Committee on Economic Security.

In view of the need for nation-wide development of means for public health promotion, the Committee attempted to establish a basic national concept concerning the responsibility of the Federal Government for a national public health program. The Committee stated:

"It has long been recognized that the Federal, State, and local Governments all have responsibilities for the protection of all the population against disease. The Federal Government has recognized its responsibility in this respect in the public-health activities of several of its departments. There also are well-established precedents for Federal aid for State health administration and for local public health facilities, and for the loan of technical personnel to States and localities. What we recommend involves no departure from previous practices, but an extension of policies that have long been followed and are of proven worth. What is contemplated is a Nation-wide public-health program, financially and technically aided by the Federal Government, but supported and administered by the State and local health departments."

On the basis of this general recommendation, the Committee proposed that appropriations be made to the United States Public Health Service and to the Children's Bureau for:

*a.* Increase of public health activity by the Federal Government itself.

*b.* Provision for grants-in-aid to states for

(1) The development of state health department activities;

(2) Development of local health services in communities that were unable to finance adequate health protection programs.

The essentials of these recommendations were embodied by Congress in the Social Security Act of August 14, 1935.

### THE SOCIAL SECURITY ACT OF 1935

"The Social Security Act presents the public health profession of this country with the greatest opportunity to establish constructive programs of health service that has been given to any group in our history." (E. L. Bishop)

The purpose of the Social Security Act adopted by Congress and approved by the President on August 14, 1935, is stated in the general title of the Act to be the following:

"To provide for the general welfare by establishing a system of Federal old-age benefits, and by enabling the several States to make more adequate provision for aged persons, blind persons, dependent and crippled children, maternal and child welfare, public health, and the administration of their unemployment-compensation laws; to establish a Social Security Board; to raise revenue; and for other purposes."

The Act has eleven titles, as follows:

I. Grants to States for old-age assistance.
II. Federal old-age benefits.
III. Grants to States for unemployment-compensation administration.
IV. Grants to States for aid to dependent children.
V. Grants to States for maternal and child welfare.
VI. Public-health work.
VII. Social Security Board.
VIII. Taxes with respect to employment.
IX. Tax on employers of eight or more persons.
X. Grants to States for aid to the blind.
XI. General provisions.

The Act provided for the organization of the Social Security Board, which was given the responsibility for all the grants-in-aid features of the Act.

Two titles of the act are of major public health import, as follows:

Title V: Those parts of the Act relating to maternal and child health, and to child welfare, were allocated to the Children's Bureau.

Title VI: Public health work was assigned to the United States Public Health Service.

The provisions of the Act that relate to health protection and promotion are administered as follows:

**Title V** (except for part 4) is administered by the Children's Bureau. The primary purposes of this section were to extend health protection services for women and children:

1. In rural areas.
2. In areas suffering from severe economic distress.
3. Among groups in special need.

The initial appropriations were:

1. Maternal and child health services .......... $3,800,000
2. Service for crippled children .............. 2,850,000
3. Child welfare services ..................... 1,500,000

*1. Maternal and Child Health Services.* The purpose of this appropriation was to give grants-in-aid to the various states in order to extend and improve services for the promotion of the health of mothers and children, particularly in rural areas and areas that suffer from severe economic stress. Apportionment to each state was made on the following basis:

1. A uniform apportionment of $20,000.
2. An allotment on the basis of live births.
3. Additional aid "to certain States on the basis of financial need."

*2. Services for Crippled Children.* Grants were made to each state for the purpose of finding crippled children and for providing for medical, surgical, and corrective care with facilities for diagnosis, hospitalization, and after-care of children who may be crippled or who suffer from conditions that may lead to crippling.

*3. Child Welfare Services.* The purpose of this part of Title V was to co-operate with state public welfare agencies in establishing, extending, and strengthening, especially in the rural areas, welfare services for the protection and care of homeless, dependent, and neglected children, and children who may be in danger of becoming delinquent.

Grants to each of the states for each of the above purposes were contingent upon:

1. Financial participation by the state.
2. Provision by each state for proper administrative procedures, and properly qualified personnel to insure efficient operation of the plan.
3. Provision for regular reports to the Children's Bureau regarding the accomplishments and activities in the various fields of work, as well as an accounting of expenditure of funds.

**Title VI.** Administered by the United States Public Health Service. The initial appropriation was $8,000,000. This appropriation was for the purpose of assisting states, counties, health districts, and other political subdivisions of the states in establishing and maintaining adequate public

health services, including the training of personnel for state and local
health work. The allotment to each state was determined on the basis of:

1. Population.
2. Special health problems.
3. Financial need.

Funds were made available to each state for two major purposes:

1. To strengthen the service division of the state health department.
2. To aid the state health department in the promotion and administrative
   guidance of full time city, county, and district health organizations.

Allotments to each state were contingent upon the establishment by it
of a properly organized state health department on a full-time basis. The
essential services required were:

1. A qualified full time state health officer.
2. Adequate provision for administrative guidance of local health services.
3. An acceptable vital statistics service.
4. A suitable state public health laboratory service.
5. Special services for the control of preventable disease and for health promotion.
6. Services for the study, promotion, and supervision of environmental sanitation.

Grants-in-aid to states for the development of local health services were
contingent upon:

1. Co-ordinate financial assistance to the local health departments from state
   funds.
2. The local health services should be under the direction of a full time health
   officer.
3. Each health department must have as a minimum: a full time health officer,
   two nurses, one sanitation officer, and one clerk. This basic personnel must
   be on a full time basis, and must meet the standard qualifications established
   by the Conference of State and Territorial Health Officers.

The original funds allotted to the Public Health Service were allocated
in five major classes:

1. A flat grant of $7,843 to each state and territory ...... $   400,000
2. Grants on a per capita basis ........................      4,000,000
3. An equalizing fund to meet economic needs in certain
   states  ................................................   1,200,000
4. Grants made on the basis of special health problems
   (for example, malaria) ...........................        1,200,000
5. A special fund for the training of personnel ...........   1,200,000
                                                             _____
                                                             $8,000,000

The administration of the titles of the Social Security Act relating to
public health and to maternal and child care was successful from the very
beginning. The Act followed established lines of action and did not

require the uprooting of traditions or the development of new social philosophies.

Activities were developed by an enthusiastic, capable personnel, and large funds were expended with conspicuous absence of waste and inefficiency. Some of the states felt at first that the Federal Government was usurping state prerogatives and invading state sovereignty, but it soon became clear that the restrictions of allotments to states were on a sound basis and represented real assistance to each state in building up its public health program. The great hiatus at the outset was the lack of trained personnel to carry out the provisions of the Act. But wise forethought had made suitable provision for funds to provide for training of personnel. Short courses of training for all types of personnel were set up at strategic places throughout the nation to meet the emergency. It was understood from the beginning that these short courses were makeshifts. They did serve a valuable purpose as a "screening test." Often the short course of training served as a guide to the trainee concerning his capability and fitness for a career in public health.

The initiation of the Social Security Act of 1935 has been given in detail because it represents a very important milestone in the social development of our nation. No one can deny that Federal Government subsidy represents a certain degree of Federal supervision and control. It represents also uniformity of program, standardization of personnel training, and fiscalization of state and of local expenditures.

If the leadership that is furnished by the Public Health Service and the Children's Bureau continues to be intelligent, tactful, imaginative, dynamic, and broad in its understanding and interpretation of the functions of the Federal Government in the promotion of national public health, then the Social Security Act must represent a great advance in our national economy and conservation of our social resources.

The plan contains the seeds of a bureaucratic centralization of national affairs that is entirely foreign to all our established traditions; but if it is wisely administered, its potentialities for national benefit are enormous. Success is dependent upon the principle that the administration and operation of health services should be left to the local communities and to the states, and that the Federal Government should not control or dictate to the local communities or states in the management of these functions. It is obvious that the Federal Government cannot be indifferent to remediable deficiencies or inadequacies in the provision of services that are necessary to health. It should take steps to aid the states and, through them, the local communities, in the provision of necessary health services to their inhabitants. The primary opportunity for the Federal Government is to give financial and technical aid to the states, so that the state, in turn, may use Federal funds to aid in the development of local health services.

The development of health services under the Social Security Act led directly to the concept that the community functions of medical care are, basically, public health functions.

## MEDICAL CARE AS A PUBLIC HEALTH RESPONSIBILITY

Public health in the United States has been developed from a social concept that it is the function of the community to protect its people against the hazards of community life. Thus public health—*i.e.*, the prevention of disease, the prolongation of life, and the promotion of physical and mental health by organized community effort—has not included, as a rule, the organization of a community-wide plan for medical care. (It should be noted that in all our discussion, medical care includes all those services that are performed for care of the sick, and is not limited to physician care.)

One exception to the above rule is that health departments often give medical care in communicable disease. Many communities have established hospitals for contagious disease, as an integral part of health department organization. This procedure is an outgrowth of the "pest houses" which were temporary structures that were erected outside the community, in an isolated place, and were used only in emergencies.

The original purpose of the contagious disease hospital was:

First, to protect the community from further spread of infection; second, to be of benefit to the patient.

We have now learned that these institutions are of great benefit to the patient who is ill with an infection, but that they have very little protective value to the community. The reasons are clear: Isolation of the patient is usually ineffective in preventing spread of infection because

1. Most infections are transmissible during the incubation period.

2. Unrecognized cases of a contagious disease are important sources of infection.

3. Carriers are also important "silent" sources of infection.

For these and other reasons, an excellent system of hospitalization for infectious disease will have little influence upon checking the spread of these diseases in the community.

There are important exceptions to this rule. Persons with typhoid fever, with open pulmonary tuberculosis, and those individuals in the infectious stages of syphilis, should always be hospitalized. A few other rare diseases may be hospitalized for the purpose of community benefit. Included in this list are: leprosy, smallpox, cholera, plague, and yellow fever.

In most instances, however, hospitalization of infectious disease is of primary benefit to the individual. Furthermore, we now believe that most of these cases can be cared for adequately in a special ward of a general hospital, rather than in a special institution.

**Medical Care as a Welfare Function.** Traditionally, in the United States, community programs for medical care have been developed as a welfare function. They were organized first as voluntary benevolent institutions. The earliest organizations were the dispensaries for the sick poor. These were followed by the establishment of hospitals which were little more than alms houses, and which provided, for the most part, for the care of chronic illness of the destitute.

The third step was the development by the community of institutions for custodial care of chronic illness. Care of mental disease initiated this activity, and was the first medical care facility developed on a state-wide basis and paid for from state funds. Later, the state and local communities assumed responsibility for the hospitalization of tuberculosis, for crippled children, for poliomyelitis, arthritis, and other types of special hospitalization.

Still later, a few states, and many cities, undertook the establishment of a *general hospital* service for the care of acute illness. Always these were benevolent functions of the community—a welfare activity for the sick poor. They were never organized as a public health function, and their administration was seldom assigned to the health officer.

Nursing care of the sick poor in their homes was established as a benevolent enterprise in the early eighties. The nurses soon realized that economic and social factors played an overwhelming part in the problems encountered by them. This led them to begin a true preventive service, as an integral part of nursing care. This service led directly to the establishment of a public health nursing service, sponsored and paid for by local tax funds. Miss Lillian Wald of the Henry Street Visiting Nurse Service in New York, which was a voluntary philanthropic organization, was responsible for this transition. She loaned one of her nurses to the Bureau of Child Hygiene of the New York City Health Department in 1902, to conduct school nursing, and later loaned a nurse, as an experiment, for infant hygiene work.

This action represents the birth of public health nursing in the United States. It was planned as a separate service, and did not represent a co-ordinated bedside nursing and public health nursing program. The two types of community nursing were kept separate down through the years,—the one a philanthropic plan for home nursing care of the sick poor, and the other a separate system of public health nursing conducted by public health department personnel. The distinction was sometimes quite artificial, and the people were often confused concerning the function of the two different types of nursing, as well as by the overlapping of activities.

The next concept that invaded our social consciousness was that the community had greater responsibility to its individual members than the simple older concept of the public health function as a protection against the hazards of community life.

This new concept was that an individual is a community asset, to be valued and conserved as any other asset. Under this theory, the health and welfare of each and every person in the community become a direct community responsibility.

As noted above, our whole philosophy of community responsibility in health promotion that had been developed over the years had been that the community was responsible for certain mass health protection measures, which the individual could not, from his own resources, provide for himself. The community protected the individual from those menaces to individual health that grew out of community activity. Thus, public health administration in the United States has been developed almost exclusively as an organization that was concerned with the health protection and promotion of the community *as a unit,* rather than health promotion for the individual or his family. Procedures directed toward an individual might be of value to him, but the primary purpose of each activity was *community welfare.* It was agreed that the promotion of the health of the individual was highly desirable from each individual's point of view. It was generally conceded that a sound, healthy body is one of life's richest possessions, to be safeguarded as carefully as any other prized personal or family possession. But this was an individual matter, requiring participation and interest on the part of each person. A man's health, in last analysis, was his own very personal responsibility.

Gradually it began to be understood that health promotion of the individual was of wide importance from a community point of view, in that ill health of individuals is a direct menace to the economic security of the community as a whole.

The principal risks to economic security that arise from ill health are:

1. The danger of impairment of individual capacity for productive work.

2. Loss of earnings that results from disabling illness among employable age groups.

3. The cost to the community of medical, nursing, and hospital care for preventable illness.

The community has sought in a great many ways to meet the menace of ill health to economic security. Some have believed that if sound provision is made by the community for economic security, then the individual will solve his own problems of ill health. Suggested methods are:

   *a.* Unemployment compensation.
   *b.* Wage increases.
   *c.* Old-age pensions and annuities.
   *d.* Stabilization of employment.
   *e.* Direct relief to the unfortunate.

These methods of meeting the risk to economic security due to ill health can have but an indirect effect on health promotion, since they do not strike at the basic causes of illness.

Certain general technics have been developed by community effort, and whenever they have been systematically applied, they have had some influence on the prevention of disease, and have influenced community-wide health in a favorable manner. Examples of the methods of approach are:

1. Slum clearance and housing programs.
2. Popular education in the general principles of personal hygiene.
3. Provision for an adequate food supply.
4. Education of all the people concerning the nutritional requirements of the body.
5. Development of community facilities for healthful recreation and physical training.
6. Suitable methods of "population control."

These methods are all valuable, and each has its particular importance, but here again the community efforts represent an indirect attack upon the basic problem of ill health and its relationship to the economic security of the community.

Three major methods have been employed by the community in a *direct attack* upon ill health and its attendant economic and social consequences:

*1. Standard Public Health Procedures.* Here are included all those measures of proved effectiveness which may be undertaken by organized community effort, which will reduce disease and promote mental and physical health *on a community-wide basis.*

*2. Medical, nursing, and hospital care of the indigent* and other groups in the community who, for some reason, are unable to obtain these benefits from their own resources.

*3. Sickness Insurance.* This method is essentially a comprehensive plan for the distribution of the costs of illness for any given individual or family over a period of time and among large groups of individuals in the community.

These three methods have not developed simultaneously throughout the United States. The first method—namely, organized public health work—has had the longest period of systematic development and has met with a reasonable measure of success.

The second social method—*i.e.,* medical care of the indigent—as we have already noted, has developed independently of public health, and has been carried out as a function of government which is more or less parallel to the public health function. In many instances, there has been an overlapping of activity, as well as a great deal of co-ordination of activities; but in the main they have been parallel, rather than inter-related services.

The third plan of *sickness insurance* is a recent development in our social thinking. It has had a stormy career. For the most part, it has not been developed as a co-ordinated service with public health and medical care of the indigent, but as a completely separate community activity.

## SICKNESS INSURANCE

In 1932 a representative committee that had made an extensive study of the costs of medical care published a report on this subject.[4] The essential fact brought out by this report was that medical care, including nursing and hospitalization, was abundantly supplied in the larger centers, but these facilities were not always available to the scattered rural populations. The report drove home the fact that some communities provided amply for the medical care of the sick poor, while others had not met this responsibility. In a few states, a state-wide system for medical care of the sick poor was in force, with subsidy by the state to the local communities. The report emphasized the fact that there was no nation-wide plan of medical care of the indigent, nor was there any Federal Government subsidy for the care of the sick poor.

This report caused unprecedented discussion, much of which did not bear directly upon the points at issue. The members of the committee did not agree among themselves. Both the majority and the minority groups, in their final report, agreed upon the following recommendations:

1. That the promotion of public health facilities should be undertaken on a nation-wide basis.
2. That government should assume control of measures relating to medical, nursing, and hospital care of the indigent.

There were some minor differences of opinion relating to administration of these governmental activities.

The Committee's investigation emphasized one fact that had long been tacitly conceded: the report demonstrated that the well-to-do in the United States received excellent medical care, and also that community responsibility for the medical care of the indigent had been rather generally assumed throughout the land, though the service was not always organized effectively. But *the average man of low income* was unable to provide for the medical and surgical emergencies that might arise in his family. Some of the Committee thought that he was unable to obtain adequate medical care at all, at least in most communities.

The majority of the Committee recommended as a solution of this problem:

*a.* A system of group practice centering around a community hospital.
*b.* Some system of sickness insurance under Government sponsorship.

This latter suggestion introduced an entirely new element into the social structure of the nation and caused a great deal of discussion and

---

[4] *Medical Care for the American People.* Final Report of the Committee on the Cost of Medical Care. University of Chicago Press, 1932.

opposition. During the five years following this report, and possibly in response to it, there grew up rather extensive experiments in *hospitalization insurance* with limited benefits. Group medical practice did not expand to any appreciable degree, and sickness insurance, though widely discussed, was not initiated, except in a few scattered instances.

The Division of Public Health Methods in the National Institute of Health made an extensive national health survey in 1935 and 1936. This report [5] gave an estimate of the amount of disabling illness in the nation, and studied the relationship of illness and medical care to economic and social status. Following this report, President Roosevelt called a national health conference in July, 1938. It was called The Interdepartmental Committee to Co-ordinate Health and Welfare Activities. The report of this conference set forth that it had determined that:

"1. Preventive health services for the Nation as a whole are grossly insufficient.
"2. Hospital and other institutional facilities are inadequate in many communities, especially in rural areas, and financial support for hospital care and for professional services in hospitals is both insufficient and precarious, especially for services to people who cannot pay the costs of the care they need.
"3. One third of the population, including persons with or without income, is receiving inadequate or no medical service.
"4. An even larger fraction of the population suffers from economic burdens created by illness."

The Conference made recommendations [6] for:

1. Expansion of the public health and maternal and child health services.
2. Expansion of national hospital facilities.
3. A national program for the medical care of the indigent, with one half the total annual costs to be met by the Federal Government.
4. A suggestion that Federal Government aid be granted to states to study their own problems and develop their own plans in regard to sickness insurance.
5. A plan for insurance against loss of wages during sickness.

The annual cost of this program, or at least of Recommendations 1, 2, and 3, to Federal, state, and local governments was estimated to be about $80,000,000 annually.

The President [7] embodied the essentials of this report and the recommendations of the Interdepartmental Committee to Co-ordinate Health and Welfare Activities in his message to Congress on January 23, 1939.

The elements of this message were included in Bill S. 1620, which was

[5] *National Health Survey of Sickness and Medical Care.* Bulletins 1 to 6, published by the National Institute of Health, Washington, D. C., 1938.
[6] *Proceedings of the National Health Conference, July 18–20, 1938.* Government Printing Office, Washington, D. C., 1938.
[7] *Health Security:* President's Message, Document 120, House of Representatives, 76th Congress, 1939.

presented to the 76th Congress by Senator Wagner in February, 1939.

The American Medical Association strongly opposed certain features of the report of the Interdepartmental Committee, of the President's Message, and of Bill S. 1620, and formulated a platform, as follows:

"1. The establishment of an agency of the Federal Government under which shall be co-ordinated and administered all medical and health functions of the Federal Government exclusive of those of the Army and Navy.

"2. The allotment of such funds as the Congress may make available to any state in actual need, for the prevention of disease, the promotion of health and the care of the sick on proof of such need.

"3. The principle that the care of the public health and the provision of medical service to the sick is primarily a local responsibility.

"4. The development of a mechanism for meeting the needs of expansion of preventive medical services with local determination of needs and local control of administration.

"5. The extension of medical care for the indigent and the medically indigent with local determination of needs and local control of administration.

"6. In the extension of medical services to all the people, the utmost utilization of qualified medical and hospital facilities already established.

"7. The continued development of the private practice of medicine, subject to such changes as may be necessary to maintain the quality of medical services and to increase their availability.

"8. Expansion of public health and medical services consistent with the American system of democracy."

It will be noted that the basic contention of the American Medical Association was that the promotion of public health and the medical care of the sick are primarily local responsibilities. Thus, the determination of need and the administration of affairs should be in the hands of local authorities. Grants-in-aid and technical assistance may be received from state and Federal Government sources, but the determination of policy should be a matter of local autonomy.

**Hospitalization Insurance** was widely introduced following the Report on the Cost of Medical Care. In some communities the plan worked very well, and proved to be a boon to hospital administrators; in other cities the plan encountered serious difficulties because of poor planning and faulty actuarial information. Gradually it became clear that insurance against serious medical emergencies, including hospitalization, is a satisfactory solution of medical emergency problems for the average family.

The "Blue Cross" plan became the most successful of the hospitalization insurance plans. It was organized as a non-profit association under the following general principles:

1. Limited hospital benefits. The risks covered were, basically, for an acute illness which requires a short period of hospitalization, in a general hospital.

2. Physician and surgeon care were excluded from most contracts. Most of the essential hospitalization expenses were covered in the agreement.

3. Groups of persons were insured, and not individuals.

4. The cost of insurance was moderate, varying with the hospitalization costs in different parts of the nation. The average initial cost of insurance was about $10 per person per year.

5. The primary purpose was to buffer hospitalization costs of acute illness for the middle income group. The Blue Cross contract did not meet the requirements of the persons in the lowest income brackets, and made no provision for hospitalization for chronic diseases nor for hospitalization of indigent persons.

The Blue Cross plan spread to all parts of the nation, but was particularly successful in industrial communities. (By January 1, 1947, over 24 million persons were enrolled in the Blue Cross or in similar hospital insurance plans.) It met an obvious community need, since hospitalization is a family catastrophe against which the breadwinner has made no provision. The average person feels quite capable of meeting the usual costs of illness from current resources, but hospitalization is a disaster which falls in the class of a prepaid insurable risk. It is an episode which strikes a family perhaps only once in a decade, and thus is comparable to accident insurance, fire insurance, and the like.

**Voluntary Sickness Insurance.** The success of hospitalization insurance suggested the possibility of including the surgeon's fee in the coverage for other hospitalization expenses. This plan was attempted in some sickness insurance contracts, with limited success. The next logical development was the suggestion of a plan for comprehensive medical care coverage, through a system of prepayment insurance against all the costs of all types of illness. There has been a great deal of discussion of this subject, with much violent argument. Most of the opposition has come from physicians.

The development of prepayment plans for coverage of costs of illness is in its initial stages in the United States. Actuarial data upon the extent of illness, and the actual facilities that would be required to provide for adequate medical care, are not fully available. The report on medical care by Pastore [8] and "Planning for the Care of the Chronically Ill" by the New York State Health Preparedness Commission [9] are steps in the right direction, in that they furnish information concerning the

[8] Pastore, John B.: *Medical Care Program: Report to the Committee on Future Plans of The New York Hospital and Cornell University Medical College*, New York City, October 1945.

[9] New York State Legislative Document No. 78A: "Planning for the Care of the Chronically Ill in New York State—Regional Aspects." New York State Commission to Formulate a Long Range Health Program, also known as New York State Health Preparedness Commission. Williams Press, Inc., Albany, 1946.

community facilities that would be needed to provide any community with well-rounded facilities for comprehensive medical care.

Various voluntary associations have attempted to formulate a satisfactory plan for community-wide sickness insurance. Some of these programs have been organized by large industries, some by labor unions, or by farmers' co-operative groups. In a few instances, the organized medical society of a community has developed a plan for prepaid comprehensive medical care.[10]

The proposals of the "Health Insurance Plan of Greater New York" may be taken as a type of sickness insurance contract. The general principles of this plan are:

The medical services that are provided will be comprehensive. They include preventive, diagnostic, and therapeutic medical and nursing services in the home, in the physician's office, and in the hospital.

Hospitalization will be furnished through a joint arrangement with the Blue Cross plan, and thus the hospitalization coverage has certain limitations.

Long-time institutional care is not provided for. Dental care is not included in the contract.

Groups will be insured—not individuals. For example, a single contract may be drawn for all city employees that have a low to moderate salary range. Individuals in the group of employees who have high salaries are not included in the contract. (An annual income of $5,000 or more is considered a high salary.)

Medical care is provided through a contract with a group of physicians. Each group shall be approved by a Medical Control Board. This board is appointed by officers of the Plan, and consists of representative physicians selected by the County Medical Society. This board acts as adviser in the determination of general medical policies, and also provides professional standards for the participating medical groups.

The association is a non-profit membership corporation, and the annual cost of the compulsory coverage is consistent with sound actuarial practice.

**Compulsory Sickness Insurance Plans.** A program for nation-wide compulsory sickness insurance was advocated by President Truman in his address to Congress in 1946, and a plan of this scope was incorporated in the Wagner-Murray-Dingell Bill, S. 1606, which was presented to Congress and discussed in committee in 1946. These matters will doubtless be considered further in subsequent deliberations of Congress.

Our text is not a suitable place for discussing the details of plans for

[10] The Council on Medical Service of the American Medical Association had approved 52 plans of voluntary medical service associations by December 1, 1946. "Each plan has gone its individual way in setting up what locally has seemed best. Soon will come the time to strive for some semblance of standardization."—*News Letter*, Council on Medical Service, American Medical Association, Chicago, Dec. 16, 1946, Vol. III, No. 12.

sickness insurance, either on a voluntary or compulsory basis. Suffice it to say that the author is of the opinion:

1. That the philosophy of prepayment plans for meeting the costs of comprehensive medical care is a logical social development. It is the only feasible method, in his opinion, which will make it possible to incorporate an adequate system of preventive medicine in a community-wide comprehensive system for medical care.

2. That the establishment of a nation-wide system of compulsory sickness insurance for the whole of the United States at the present stage in our social development is an unwise procedure, which is quite contrary to the principles of local self-government, and antagonistic to the historical developmental policies of our nation.

The author has expressed his opinion on this matter in some detail in a previous publication,[11] and will not repeat these ideas at this point. He believes that a series of local evolutionary community-wide social experiments in sickness insurance, planned to meet the special needs of each local community, is a forward-looking and very wise procedure. He believes that nation-wide compulsory sickness insurance would not meet with ready acceptance, either by the people who receive the service, or by the physicians, who are the key persons in rendering this service, and in the end, largely responsible for its success.

**Federal Aid in the Development of Local Programs for Medical Care.** A plan of nation-wide Federal assistance in the development of hospital facilities for local communities was realized through the passage by Congress in 1946 of Bill S. 191, called the Hill-Burton Bill.

**Hill-Burton Bill.** A Federal appropriation was made of $3,000,000, which was allotted to the various states to make careful surveys of local needs for hospitals and for health centers.

A sum of $75,000,000 annually was appropriated for aid in hospital construction in areas that were found to be in need of this facility; the Federal contribution to be matched in the ratio of 2:1 by local funds. The program was projected over a period of 5 years. Administration of the funds was centered in the Surgeon General of the U. S. Public Health Service, advised by a Federal Hospital Council. This council was appointed by the Federal Security Administrator and had veto powers, including the right to disapprove a state plan which did not conform to Federal regulations.

Each state had wide latitude in the development of its own hospital program. Sponsors of hospital or health center construction might be the state itself, cities, counties, other governmental agencies, or, within certain limits, private non-profit hospitals.

**Hospital and Health Center Needs.** The U. S. Public Health Service made an estimate for an adequate community hospital program as follows:

[11] Smillie, W. G.: *Preventive Medicine and Public Health*. New York, The Macmillan Company, 1946, p. 573.

## HOSPITAL REQUIREMENTS FOR THE UNITED STATES AS A WHOLE

Estimated by the U. S. Public Health Service,[12] 1946

| Service | Bed Ratio | New Beds | Replacements |
|---|---|---|---|
| 1. General hospital beds | 4.5 per 1,000 pop. | 170,000 | 84,000 |
| 2. Tuberculosis | 2.5 per annual death | 65,000 | 17,000 |
| 3. Nervous and mental diseases | 5.0 per 1,000 pop. | 200,000 | 100,000 |
| 4. Chronic disease | no ratio | 270,000 | —— |
| 5. Public health centers | —— | 4,500 | —— |

It has been estimated that the five-year plan which was encompassed by the Hill-Burton Bill would cover nearly 25 per cent of the estimated total needs for hospital and health center construction in the nation.

**Prevention of Disease an Integral Part of Comprehensive Medical Care.** A new concept appeared in the course of discussion of plans for adequate medical care. This concept is that the prevention of illness and the promotion of health are integral parts of the community program for comprehensive medical care. If this thesis is correct, then any plan for community-wide health care which provides only for the care of those who have already become ill, is meeting only half of its obligation. The point of view emerges that there is no real separation of preventive from curative medicine. In this case, the community obligation to provide facilities for health protection and also to provide for adequate care of those who are ill, are not separate functions, nor are they joint and closely correlated activities, but are actually a unified function of government.

If this thesis is accepted, then the entire community program for health protection, including plans for care of the sick, should logically be administered as a unit, since it represents closely related functions of government.

This concept has been vigorously opposed by many community leaders, who have felt that prevention of disease as a community responsibility is a distinct and separate community function—a function quite apart from the care of those who become ill. Furthermore, they insist that in a co-ordinated health promotion and sickness care plan, the preventive aspects of medical care would be overwhelmed and completely submerged by the large costs and great administrative details of a sickness care program.

### THE PLACE OF THE HEALTH OFFICER IN THE NATIONAL HEALTH PROGRAM

The National Health Program has been discussed in some detail in this text, because of the fact that the health officer is considered by

[12] National Health Act of 1945, and Hospital Survey and Construction Bill, reported to the Committee on Education and Labor, Senate Committee Print No. 3, 79th Congress, 2d Session, March 1946, pp. 158 ff.

many to be the logical person in the community to administer all the official medical aspects of the plan. It is obvious that the health officer must be vitally concerned in all matters that may affect an extension of his administrative activities. He should also give thought to all developments that relate to improvement in medical and nursing care of the people of his community.

Leading health authorities have taken diametrically opposing positions as to the future responsibility of the health department in these matters. Dr. Haven Emerson, for example, believes that "logic and practice have distinctly separated the functions of public health from those of the care of the sick"; and he states that "the usual health officer, whether state or local, should not be charged with the care of the sick among the poor of the population." [13]

Dr. Edward Godfrey, on the other hand, in his presidential address to the American Public Health Association in 1939, stated:

"The only safeguard that would seem to insure continuance of a dynamic public health movement, and to insure that any government expansion of medical services has the improvement of health as its primary objective, is to place the administration of any such expansion squarely upon the shoulders of departments of health—national, state, city, and county."

Later in this same address, he said:

"There are those who believe that public health work should be limited to sanitation of the environment and to control of communicable disease. . . . They profess to see a sharp distinction between curative and preventive medicine, between functions which may properly be operated by health departments and those which belong either to another department of government, or are the exclusive reserve of private medical practice and medical philanthropy. Events tend constantly to disprove the accuracy of their vision. Experimental effort disproves the accuracy of their prophecies."

Agencies other than the health department are vitally interested in these matters. Departments of Public Welfare in most local communities and many states have long administered the medical relief of the sick poor, under the same logic that permits them to provide other necessities of life, such as shelter, food, and clothing. They believe that the administration of community medical care of the indigent and medically indigent is a *welfare* responsibility.

The organized medical societies are quite firm in their contention that they shall have a determining voice in any modification in the "American system" of medical practice. They insist that sickness insurance programs, programs for the care of the medically indigent, expansion of public health services, and developments of group practice require full debate and general acceptance by the medical profession. Practically every one

[13] Emerson, Haven. "The Physician's Part in Organized Medical Care." *Amer. J. Public Health*, 1940, Vol. 30, p. 9.

concedes that the organized medical societies must have a strong representation in the determination of policies relating to administration of these plans, whether they are developed on a local, state, or national basis.

The issue is clear. A national health program will be formulated. It will require strong Federal support and assistance, both financial and technical. Time and experiment will determine whether or not the program will include sickness insurance, and also whether the plans can best be administered by the health departments—national, state, and local—more or less as at present constituted, or under some other and completely different administrative device.

It is the author's opinion that different systems will be developed to meet the needs of different communities. In the rural areas, such as county health units, the health officer and his associates will probably be the most logical and effective persons to administer the whole program of public health and medical assistance. The program will develop around the community hospital. The hospital will be much more than a center for surgical operations and the diagnosis of difficult cases. It will be the medical and nursing center of the community. Its facilities will be extended to the homes. Nursing service will ramify through the community. The administrator of the hospital will also be the administrator of the preventive services of the community.

In large cities, it seems quite probable that the work will be organized on a different basis. One agency might continue the present functions of a health department, and a separate "Bureau of Hospitals and Medical Care" might be required to administer all problems relating to public medicine.

**Co-ordinated Health and Hospital Service.** The United States Public Health Service has proposed an administrative unit of co-ordinated health and hospital facilities which is illustrated in Figure 42.

Under such a plan, the health centers would become the foundation stones upon which all medical care is constructed.

The core of the organization is a base hospital which has three major functions: (1) teaching, (2) research, and (3) consultation. District hospitals are located radially from the base hospital, with suitable interspersion of institutions for convalescent care, and for care of chronic illness. The health centers are at the periphery, and are the part of the organization that has direct and intimate contact with the people. Practically all *direct services* will be initiated here.

More than 90 per cent of all health protection measures, including diagnosis of disease and actual medical care, will be rendered at or through the health center and the local practicing physicians.

The district hospital will care for those persons who are referred from the health center. Less than 10 per cent of those referred to the district hospital will prove to be of such a nature that they must be sent to the base or consultation hospital.

A free interchange of trained medical personnel should flow from

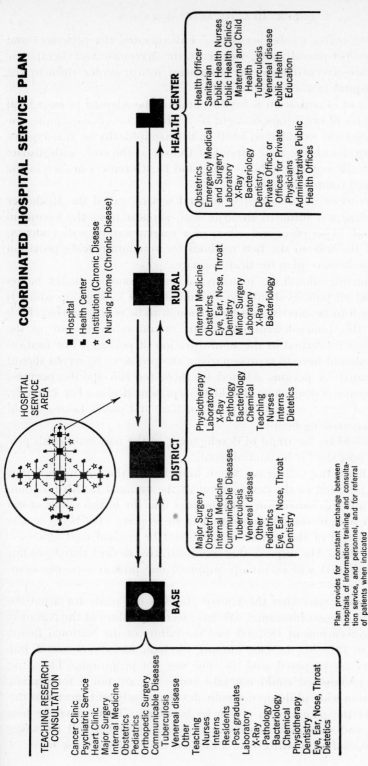

# COORDINATED HOSPITAL SERVICE PLAN

**HOSPITAL SERVICE AREA**

■ Hospital
■ Health Center
★ Institution (Chronic Disease)
△ Nursing Home (Chronic Disease)

**BASE**

**TEACHING RESEARCH CONSULTATION**

Cancer Clinic
Psychiatric Service
Heart Clinic
Major Surgery
Internal Medicine
Obstetrics
Pediatrics
Orthopedic Surgery
Communicable Diseases
Tuberculosis
Venereal disease
Other
Teaching
Nurses
Interns
Residents
Post graduates
Laboratory
X-Ray
Pathology
Bacteriology
Chemical
Physiotherapy
Dentistry
Eye, Ear, Nose, Throat
Dietetics

**DISTRICT**

Major Surgery
Obstetrics
Internal Medicine
Cummunicable Diseases
Tuberculosis
Venereal disease
Other
Pediatrics
Eye, Ear, Nose, Throat
Dentistry
Physiotherapy
Laboratory
X-Ray
Pathology
Bacteriology
Chemical
Teaching
Nurses
Interns
Dietetics

**RURAL**

Internal Medicine
Obstetrics
Eye, Ear, Nose, Throat
Dentistry
Minor Surgery
Laboratory
X-Ray
Bacteriology

**HEALTH CENTER**

Obstetrics
Emergency Medical and Surgery
Laboratory
X-Ray
Bacteriology
Dentistry
Private Office or Offices for Private Physicians
Administrative Public Health Offices

Health Officer
Sanitarian
Public Health Nurses
Public Health Clinics
Maternal and Child Health
Tuberculosis
Venereal disease
Public Health Education

Plan provides for constant exchange between hospitals of information training and consultation service, and personnel, and for referral of patients when indicated

Fig. 42. *A Diagram Showing Relationships among Base, District, and Rural Hospitals and Health Centers in a Coordinated Service Plan.* From Mountin, J. W., Pennell, E. H., and Hope, V. M.: "Health Service Areas: Requirements for General Hospitals and Health Centers," *Public Health Bulletin No. 292,* Gov't Print. Off., Washington, 1945.

the teaching center to the periphery. Functionally, the personnel and services flow peripherally and, vice versa, the diagnostic and therapeutic problems are screened from the peripheral health center through the district hospital to the base hospital.

This unit of organization is flexible, and can be adapted to meet local needs. A unit of organization might be a whole state. For example, the state of Colorado would lend itself well geographically to this type of health service, with the state capital of Denver as the core, with district hospitals in the major peripheral cities, and health centers in each of the various small communities.

An experiment in co-ordinated hospital service, called the Rochester (N. Y.) plan, was initiated in 1946, with support from the Commonwealth Fund. This plan, and others of a similar nature, will undoubtedly point the way to the best methods for community-wide provision for a comprehensive plan for health service.

One principle should be inviolate. Local autonomy should be respected, and all policies should be determined by a local group which is small enough to be effective, yet large enough to be representative. Each person in this policy-determining board should represent one of the agencies most concerned in the administration of policies. The medical profession should have its representatives; the people to be served should be represented by persons selected by them for this specific purpose. Local governmental agencies should be represented also. For example, executives of the departments of public welfare and public health should be on the controlling board.

What should be the trend of development in the national health program, and how shall it be administered?

The author is not willing to commit himself as to the best method that should be followed in the development of the national health program, nor to indicate his conviction as to the part that the health officer of the future will play in the administration of these plans. He believes that the development of the national plan should be gradual, and along experimental lines. He suspects that administrative devices that have not yet been initiated will eventually supplant our present type of organization.

He feels quite sure that the United States is not ready for a nationwide plan of sickness insurance. We have seen the failure of the National Sanitary Conventions of 1857–60, and the failure of the National Board of Health in 1879–82. In each instance the basic ideas were sound, but the soil was not prepared, and the time was not propitious. Thus, the seeds that germinated could not take root. We are not a totalitarian nation; nation-wide philosophies must develop slowly and must win the approval of the people who are to be benefited. There must be free discussion, and stumbling experiments. Foolish mistakes will be made. Out of this confusion will evolve a method that will meet the needs of the people and satisfy their requirements. When the American people want a nation-wide plan of universal sickness insurance, it certainly will evolve.

Dr. Abel Wolman, while president of the American Public Health Association, made a prediction as to the probable plan of administration of

FIG. 43. *Health Center with 10-Bed Nursing Unit.* Plan suggsted by Hospital Facilities Section, U. S. Public Health Service.

This hospital service plan is intended only for rural communities which cannot support even a "rural hospital." Its primary function is to bring public health facilities to the small community; its secondary one to provide nursing service mainly for obstetrical care, plus facilities for emergency or minor surgical work. A noteworthy feature is the provision of offices and examination room for private physicians; it is anticipated that local doctors will want to avail themselves of the diagnostic facilities now so generally lacking.

The nursing unit, though small, is complete. The isolation suite should be especially appreciated in places where this unit would be built. Rooms are designed for south orientation, on a one-sided corridor for good natural ventilation. Nurses' station is located for control of entrance at night.

The health center wing provides facilities for complete public health work. Since health education is one of the more important phases of this work, there is a lecture or demonstration room opposite the entrance. Examination room would serve for various clinics, scheduled on days and hours to coordinate with its use by private physicians. Laboratory facilities also would serve for multiple use by clinician, epidemiologist, nurse, and sanitary engineer.

Such a unit as this would operate as an outpost in the coordinated health service scheme, bringing either resident or visiting technicians to the locality, handling minor cases, referring others to "rural," "district," or "base" hospital as required.

Source: *Architectural Record,* August 1945.

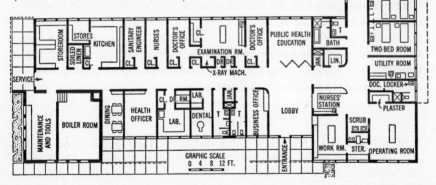

a community health protection service, which we present as an indication of the trend of the leading opinion in these matters.

"1. Within 10 years the major elements of the national health program will be in effect, because the people want it, can pay for it and are entitled to it.

"2. The public health officer will play a major role in the evolution of the program, not always because he wants it, but because the forces of logic normally place the responsibility upon him.

"3. Medical care will be universalized for the medically needy and for the lower income groups. It is probable that this universalization will proceed through the channels of tax-supported subsidies and voluntary insurance programs and ultimately toward a compulsory insurance scheme. This approach through experimental operations to compulsory health insurance will probably consume several decades, because in this as in all other efforts toward social amelioration, we must experience the same mistakes made elsewhere, before we learn to avoid them. These mistakes, contrary to the views of many, have considerable constructive value since they result in processes adjusted to the peculiarities of our own people and institutions.

"4. In the fields of medical care and public health, equalization or levelling of necessary service independent of geography or economic status will occur as it has in universal education, postal service, transportation, public welfare, and other basic necessities for a safe and healthy society of people. Resistance to universalizing these services is doomed to fail as long as we preserve a true faith in democratic institutions." [14]

Ten years is a short time. Let us imagine that the next twenty-five years will bring about some of these changes. If this is the case, then the health officer who is just entering the field should prepare himself to meet these changing conditions. Since he will deal so intimately with physicians and with problems relative to illness, it is obvious that he should be a well trained physician. But he must have suitable training in sociology, in economics, and in hospital administration. He should have a knowledge of the principles of public administration and of the functions of government. He should be familiar with business methods and serve an apprenticeship in administrative affairs.

The health officer of the future must be an exceptional man, with special talents and special training, for he will be called upon to assume the responsibility for matters of great importance and value to the nation. Public health administration will be a dignified and respected profession, which should attract young men and women of superior ability, and offer them a full and satisfactory life career.

## REFERENCES

1. *Medicine and the Changing Order.* Report of the Committee on Medicine and the Changing Order, New York Academy of Medicine. The Commonwealth Fund, New York City. 1947. See also supplementary publications of the Committee.

2. Mountin, J. W. *Content and Administration of a Medical Care Program. A Brief of the Report on Medical Care in a National Health Program.* Am. Jour. Pub. Health. 1944, Vol. 34, p. 1217.

3. Goldmann, Franz. *Public Medical Care.* Columbia University Press, New York. 1945.

[14] Wolman, A.: "The National Health Program: How Far? How Fast?" *Amer. Journal of Pub. Health,* 1939, Vol. 29, p. 628.

4. Davis, Michael M. *America Organizes Medicine*. Harper and Brothers, New York. 1941.
5. *Medical Care for the People of New York State*. Report of the New York State Legislative Commission on Medical Care. Feb. 15, 1946.
6. *Principles of a Nation-Wide Health Program*. Committee on Research in Medical Economics, 1790 Broadway, New York City. Nov. 1944.

The reprints and reports of the Hospital Facilities Section, Division of States Relations, U. S. Public Health Service, are particularly recommended.

See also current publications of the American Medical Association, the American Hospital Association, the American Public Health Association, and other discussions of these matters.

# APPENDIX

## EDUCATIONAL QUALIFICATIONS OF HEALTH OFFICERS [1]

### I. GENERAL SCOPE OF THE FIELD

**A.** *Specific Contribution to Public Health by Workers in This Field*

IT has long been established that public health is a concern of government and the necessity for an official designated by law as health officer is universally recognized. Past accomplishment of the health officer and his associates as measured by the prevention of sickness and death and the prolongation of life is a matter of common knowledge. As progress has been made in certain fields of preventive medicine, other and more complex problems have come into prominence, such as accident prevention, the prevention or amelioration of the chronic and degenerative diseases, and the maintenance of optimum health. Scientific discoveries of wide practical application have been rapid in the past few decades and the demand for public services for the prevention and cure of disease has become greater and in all probability will so continue. Opportunities for challenging and constructive service in the field of public health have developed rapidly and the needs for specific education and training have increased accordingly.

The health officer's responsibilities vary considerably in different public health organizations, but in general he has administrative responsibility for all activities of the official health agency operating in the area and directs the staff promoting those activities.

The provision of medical care, or the administration of a medical care program in certain special fields or as an emergency activity, has with increasing frequency been accepted as a responsibility of official health agencies. The medical treatment of a large proportion of persons suffering from the venereal diseases, tuberculosis, and certain of the acute infectious diseases has for some time been directly or indirectly the responsibility of health departments, as has a medical and surgical treatment program for the physically handicapped in many communities. Partial responsibility for the treatment of cancer and other chronic diseases is sometimes assumed by the health department, and during recent years as an "emergency" measure, the administration of medical services for the wives of certain members of the armed forces, and general pediatric care for this segment of the population, have been undertaken by the official health agencies. There are indications that the health officer's responsibilities in the field of medical care may be increased rather than decreased in the future.

**B.** *Future Outlook*

It is generally recognized that there should be coverage of every population and area unit of our nation with competent, full-time local health service. Both

---

[1] "Report of the Committee on Professional Education." Reprinted from *The American Journal of Public Health*, August 1946, vol. 36.

the American Public Health Association and the American Medical Association have declared in official pronouncements their interest in the complete coverage of the United States by local units of health jurisdiction, and continued efforts in this direction are to be expected in the future. Between 1915 and 1935, the number of counties in the United States with full-time local health services increased from 14 to 762. Passage of the Social Security Act in 1935 stimulated and accelerated this development, so that there are now over 1,800 counties that receive full-time health service. A third of the population, however, is still without the services of a full-time local health officer.

Local communities in the United States are now being served by approximately 1,100 full-time health officers and 1,800 other full-time administrators. Of this number over 90 per cent hold the degree of Doctor of Medicine and 20 per cent hold this degree and in addition have a postgraduate degree in public health. The majority of full-time local health officers are employed by cities, counties, and combinations thereof. In some states, district health officers on the staffs of state departments of health are assigned to local areas and render direct service. A large number of individuals qualified as health officers are employed by federal and state agencies and by voluntary organizations. The establishment of new subdivisions within health departments to provide service in the fields previously neglected by the official agencies, such as accident prevention, cancer control, general nutrition, and industrial hygiene, gives reason to believe that the future will show expansion into new fields as well as an intensification of the existing activities of the health agency.

## II. FUNCTIONS OF HEALTH OFFICERS

Many functions of the health officer are defined by statute, such as his power to enforce sanitary laws and regulations, his responsibility for the preparation of budgets and the proper expenditure of funds. He has also the important functions of interpreting public health activities to governing bodies, co-ordinating the activities of official and voluntary agencies, performing the duties of a public office and of assuming a position of leadership in the community in all matters pertaining to health. Besides administrative duties and exercising leadership in his field, the health officer takes part in specific activities for disease prevention and control, using technical procedures that call for a high degree of medical and sanitary knowledge. In larger organizations the health officer may not personally render direct service but directs and evaluates the work of his subordinates and must be able to exercise both technical skill and professional judgment in so doing. The health officer's position is such that he may have broad opportunity for special studies and research in public health. In smaller localities he may perform all or numerous medical and other professional functions himself. In general, the health officer must have some training and assume some responsibility for the proper development of the official agency's activities in the following fields:

1. Environmental sanitation including water, milk, and food sanitation, insect and rodent control, and nuisance abatement.
2. Acute communicable disease control.
3. Tuberculosis control.
4. Venereal disease control.
5. Child hygiene.

6. School hygiene.
7. Dental hygiene.
8. Maternal hygiene.
9. Public health laboratory service.
10. Vital statistics.
11. Public health nursing.
12. Public health education.
13. Industrial hygiene.
14. Nutrition.
15. The chronic or degenerative diseases.
16. Mental hygiene.
17. Accident prevention.
18. Medical care administration.
19. Audit and Accounts.
20. Personnel management and training.
21. Hospital administration.

A. *Lines of promotion*

In large local jurisdictions and in federal and state agencies there are numerous subordinate positions, such as those of deputy and assistant health officer. Several grades of positions with administrative duties are provided, and there are definite lines of promotion. The health officer showing ability may progress from the administration of small official health units to positions of responsibility in larger organizations or larger areas, or he may advance from a subordinate position such as an assistant health officer to full responsibility for the direction of a department, agency, or district. In general, a classification of health officers includes the following titles descriptive of the area of jurisdiction or degree of responsibility: state, city, district or county health officer or commissioner; deputy commissioner, assistant commissioner or deputy health officer; assistant and senior public health officer or physician. Occasionally, an official health agency offers training positions to which a special title is given, such as apprentice health officer.

III. THE EDUCATIONAL BACKGROUND OF HEALTH OFFICERS

The basic educational background for the position of health officer should be as follows:

1. Fundamental training in the sciences and the humanities at least equivalent to that required for a college degree in the Arts or Sciences.

2. Completion of a course leading to the degree of Doctor of Medicine [2] in a medical school approved by the Council on Medical Education and Hospitals of the American Medical Association, or graduation from a medical school of recognized standing.

3. Internship of at least one year in an approved general hospital, preferably including communicable disease service.

[2] Because of the trend upon the part of governmental bodies to insist upon the medical degree as a prerequisite to appointment as health officer, it is inadvisable to encourage the candidate for a public health degree to look forward to a career as health officer unless he is also the possessor of a medical degree. In making this recommendation, the American Public Health Association expressly recognizes the professional standing of non-medical persons now performing creditable service as health officers.

4. Eligibility to examination for medical licensure in the state where service is to be rendered.

## IV. GRADUATE EDUCATION AND TRAINING

Graduate education and training for the position of health officer should include the following:

1. Preliminary supervised field training in a well organized health department for a period sufficient to give acquaintance with the general aspects of public health and to give the candidate an opportunity to determine his own liking and fitness for such work.

2. Completion of a program of study leading to a degree in public health of not less than one full academic year in a university approved by the American Public Health Association. The university in which such a program of study is pursued should have a well organized school or department of public health with a corps of full-time instructors recognized as leaders in their respective fields, ample laboratory, library, and other facilities, and access to official and voluntary health agencies willing to provide facilities for field training and experience.[3] The program of study should cover the general field of public health administration, biostatistics, environmental sanitation, epidemiology, health education, laboratory methods, public health nursing, physiological hygiene, the socio-economic aspects of health and disease, and should be accompanied by special instruction in the application of basic principles to the functions and duties of a public health administrator.

3. An additional year of practical experience in a subordinate position is highly desirable before the graduate in public health assumes full direction of even a small health unit.

4. Full-time practical experience is an essential part of the education of the health officer, and it is recognized that great achievement can usually be attained only after an adequate period of experience. Physicians otherwise qualified who have achieved notable success and who have had many years of full-time experience in a well-organized health agency should be considered as qualified to serve as health officers even though lacking formal academic training. However, it is to be emphasized that an exception to the requirements of a postgraduate course and supervised field training should be made only if the candidate, in addition to years of experience, has actually demonstrated unusual ability as a public health administrator.

5. If the health officer is vested with the administration of a medical care program, efficient performance of these functions requires knowledge and skills of a special nature. Courses of instruction in this field should be included in the postgraduate course in public health, at least as electives in the program of training of potential health officers. Instruction should include courses in the socio-economic aspects of health and disease and in methods of establishing standards of quality of medical care, budgeting requirements and special administrative technics, including hospital administration.

---

[3] See Criteria for Accreditation of Schools of Public Health Granting the Master of Public Health Degree, prepared as a basis for accreditation by the Committee on Professional Education of the American Public Health Association and published in the *American Journal of Public Health* for March, 1946.

## V. Personal Qualities

The health officer should possess the qualities of personality and character necessary to insure the successful prosecution of the scientific and administrative duties. These include such qualities as leadership, the ability to establish and maintain favorable relations with the public and his own personnel, creative ability, far-sighted sound judgment and common sense, and the will to serve honestly and industriously at all times, subordinating his own desires to the best interests of the community.

ERNEST L. STEBBINS, M.D., *Referee*

### Committee on Professional Education

W. P. SHEPARD, M.D., *Chairman*          GEORGE H. RAMSEY, M.D.
REGINALD M. ATWATER, M.D., *Secretary*   LOWELL J. REED, PH.D.
GAYLORD W. ANDERSON, M.D.                WILSON G. SMILLIE, M.D.
W. W. BAUER, M.D.                        ERNEST L. STEBBINS, M.D.
ROBERT D. DEFRIES, M.D.                  RALPH E. TARBETT, C.E.
EDWARD S. GODFREY, JR., M.D.             CLAIR E. TURNER, DR.P.H.
PEARL McIVER, R.N.

## RECOMMENDED QUALIFICATIONS FOR PUBLIC HEALTH NURSING PERSONNEL [4]

### 1940-1945

SINCE the publication of *Minimum Qualifications for Those Appointed to Positions in Public Health Nursing* in 1936, far-reaching developments have taken place that need to be considered in setting new goals for the next five years. The years 1935–1940 have seen the greatest expansion of public health nursing in its history, due in large part to the health provisions of the Social Security Act. Despite the pressing need for nurses to fill available public health nursing positions, there has been an increasing appreciation by administrators of the importance of appointing nurses specifically prepared for the public health nursing field. The Social Security Act has assisted in this trend by making provision for many nurses to get the needed preparation as well as requiring through a later amendment that appointments be made under a merit system of personnel administration.

The completion of the revised *Curriculum Guide for Schools of Nursing* by the National League of Nursing Education in 1937 has given impetus to the enrichment of the undergraduate curriculum so that the nurse may be more adequately prepared to make her contribution to the health and social welfare of the community in whatever field she enters. However, since this requires a faculty prepared to assist in the integration of the health and social aspects of nursing throughout the curriculum, emphasis has been placed increasingly on the importance of faculty preparation in these areas by many schools. Also, it is apparent that the graduates from the schools which offer such an enriched curriculum, with a wide range of clinical experience including communicable and mental

[4] "Report of the Committee on Professional Education." Reprinted from *The American Journal of Public Health,* July 1942, vol. 32.

diseases, will be considered potentially the most promising for public health nursing service. The membership list of the Association of Collegiate Schools of Nursing and the National League of Nursing Education's list of accredited schools will be helpful in furnishing another basis for the selection of graduate nurses for public health nursing.

The growth of merit systems as a method of selecting personnel both in official and nonofficial agencies has made for greater understanding by agencies and by citizens of the need for specific requirements for the various positions in the field of public health nursing. The qualifications recommended here have been formulated in the light of these present trends in qualifications for public health nurses wherever they may be employed.

Determined effort to reduce further certain existing health problems, such as crippling in children, maternal and neonatal hazards, tuberculosis, and the venereal diseases, has made emphasis on special services in these areas necessary. Each of these is recognized as one part of the whole family health service, and, as such, is most adequately carried on by the field nurse who is responsible for all phases of the public health nursing program. The nurse, however, needs help from consultants who in addition to the necessary equipment as supervisors have had preparation in the special field in which they are engaged.

Mindful of these trends and realizing that the first principle underlying the improvement of service is the appointment of qualified personnel, the Education Committee of the National Organization for Public Health Nursing and the American Public Health Association recommend these qualifications for those appointed to public health nursing positions as the goal for 1945. They are based on the principles: (1) that one of the most essential requisites in public health nursing is the ability to work effectively with people, (2) that the public health nurse must be a competent nurse with sound basic theoretical and clinical preparation in nursing and with an understanding of its social and health aspects, (3) that additional study, including supervised field experience, is essential to prepare the graduate nurse for the specific functions of public health nursing, (4) that continued in-service education including qualified supervision (see II, A of outline) is necessary to further the development of the nurse's potentialities for improved service to the individual family and community, which is the goal of all public health nursing.

### PERSONAL FACTORS IMPORTANT

While the following qualifications may seem to stress academic preparation and professional experience, personality remains a major factor in successful public health nursing service, and therefore must always be given due consideration. Also, good physical health as determined by a pre-employment examination should be considered essential because without it the other qualifications are rendered less effective.

Improvement in the technic of personal interviews and the collection of credentials, through study of personnel methods in other fields, will help in developing more accurate methods for the selection of applicants with fundamental requisites. Tests and other measurements need to be studied as a means of determining individual abilities and capacities.

On the other hand, it is important for both the nurse and the employer to understand the purpose and value of theoretical preparation for public health nursing. University study should be an economical means to the end of greater competency in daily work and not an end in itself. It is a means for the nurse to review under guidance past and present practice in this field in order to become familiar with sound, workable principles and thereby avoid some of the trial-and-error learning common to all new workers. It is an opportunity to gain additional tools, both in content and method, which will make work in the field more pertinent and more productive.

Unusual competence in the work to which the nurse is assigned is the only sound basis for promotion to greater responsibility, and the one most frequently used. Well utilized graduate study should assist in the development of such competence. The amount of study suggested in these recommended qualifications is believed to represent the minimum needed for each type of worker described.

While these qualifications apply specifically to new appointees, the importance of corresponding additional preparation for those already appointed should receive careful consideration in relation to each nurse. Under certain conditions, it might be desirable for agencies to adopt a policy urging those appointed within the last few years to meet within a specified period of time the recommended theoretical preparation for the respective positions.

## I. STAFF NURSES [5]

A. *For the nurse working on the staff of an official or private agency under the direct supervision of a nurse supervisor who meets the qualifications herein set forth—*

Duties: To carry on the direct nursing service of the agency in the home, clinic, conference, school, or industry.

Preparation:

1. General education—High school graduation or its educational equivalent which meets college entrance requirements. Education on a college level is desirable.

2. Basic nursing education—Graduation from an accredited [6] school of nursing connected with a hospital having a daily average of 100 patients, with the necessary affiliation, which gives the nurse a broad clinical experience in medical nursing, including acute communicable disease, tuberculosis, and the venereal diseases; psychiatric and pediatric nursing (including the care of children with orthopedic and cardiac conditions); and an understanding of the social and health aspects of nursing, both physical and mental, through an integrated program of instruction in classroom, ward, outpatient department, with appropriate use of community facilities.

3. State registration.

4. Postgraduate study—Completion of the year's program of study in public health nursing in a university program approved by the National Organization for Public Health Nursing, previous to or within five years after appointment.

---

[5] See "Minimum Qualifications for Nurses Appointed to School Nursing Positions." *Pub. Health Nurs.*, Feb., 1938, p. 108. Also "Desirable Qualifications of Nurses Appointed to Public Health Nursing Positions in Industry." *Pub. Health Nurs.*, July, 1939, p. 410 and *A.J.P.H.*, 29, 7:789 (July), 1939.

[6] Accredited by the state board of nurse examiners.

B. *For the nurse in an official or private agency not working under direct supervision—*

Duties: In addition to carrying on the direct nursing service of the agency as in A, to assist in organizing the service; to work with lay and professional groups; to carry on the activities in special situations such as the school and industry.

Preparation:

1. General education—Same as listed for staff nurse under A.
2. Basic nursing education—Same as listed for staff nurse under A.
3. State registration.
4. Postgraduate study—Completion of the year's program of study in public health nursing in a university program approved by National Organization for Public Health Nursing, before appointment.
5. Experience—At least one year's experience under qualified nursing supervision in a public health nursing agency in which family health is emphasized.

## II. SUPERVISORS AND EXECUTIVES

A. *For the supervisor—*

Duties: To supervise the staff nurses in an official or private agency and to assist in their growth and development; to plan and develop the nursing program for which she is responsible in relation to the total program of the agency; to correlate it with that of other agencies in the educational, social, and health fields; to study and evaluate the program within her own area.

Preparation:

1. General education—College degree.
2. Basic nursing education—Same as listed for staff nurse under I, A.
3. State registration.
4. Postgraduate study—Same as listed for staff nurse under I, B., and in addition, a course in principles of supervision.
5. Experience—At least two years' experience, one of which was under direct, qualified nursing supervision in a public health nursing service in which family health is emphasized.

B. *For the consultant—*

Duties: To assist in analyzing the needs and developing the service in the special field; to correlate this service with other services offered by the agency and with the programs of other agencies; to advise regarding policies, technics, and procedures in the special field; to participate in the supervisory and staff-education program of the agency in co-operation with the other supervisory personnel.

Preparation:

1. General education—College degree.
2. Basic nursing education—Same as listed for staff nurse under I, A.
3. State registration.
4. Postgraduate study—Same as listed for staff nurse under I, B., and in addition a course in principles of supervision and advanced preparation in the special field, including content in that field, courses in general education, and methods of making and using studies.
5. Experience—At least two years' experience, one of which was under direct,

qualified nursing supervision in a public health nursing service in which family health is emphasized, and at least one year's experience as a generalized supervisor.

**C.** *For the educational director or instructor in public health nursing—*
Duties:

In public health nursing agencies—To plan and to direct the educational program for the new nurse, for the student, and for the staff as a whole, and to correlate and develop the resources of the agency and of related community services for teaching purposes.

In schools of nursing—To assist in directing, to correlate, and to participate in the efforts to give the undergraduate student the concept of the social and health aspects of nursing, both physical and mental, through an integrated program of instruction in classroom, ward, and outpatient department, with appropriate use of community facilities.

Preparation:

1. General education—College degree.
2. Basic nursing education—Same as listed for staff nurse under I, A.
3. State registration.
4. Postgraduate study—Same as listed for staff nurse under I, B., and in addition, courses in principles of supervision and in the philosophy and principles of education.
5. Experience—At least two years' experience, one of which was under direct, qualified nursing supervision in a public health nursing service in which family health was emphasized, and at least one year's experience as a supervisor in a public health nursing service.

**D.** *For the director—*

Duties: To administer the nursing service of the official or private agency; to determine with the administrative official or the board the policies and program to be followed; to interpret the needs of the nursing service to the administrative officials, to the board, to committees, and to the community; to participate in community planning and action in health and social welfare.

Preparation:

1. General education—College degree.
2. Basic nursing education—Same as listed for staff nurse under I, A.
3. State registration.
4. Postgraduate study—Same as listed for staff nurse under I, B., and in addition, courses in supervision and in principles of administration.
5. Experience—At least three years' experience, preferably in more than one type of agency—*i.e.,* official and private—including experience in supervision.

**E.** *For the director of a university program of study—*

Duties: To assume direct responsibility for the planning and administration of the program.

Preparation:

1. General education—Graduate degree.
2. Basic nursing education—Same as listed for staff nurse under I, A.
3. State registration.

4. Postgraduate study—Completion of the year's postgraduate program of study in public health nursing in one of the university programs approved by the National Organization for Public Health Nursing, before appointment, and advanced university courses in general education and in supervision and administration in public health nursing.

5. Experience—A minimum of five years' public health nursing experience, preferably in more than one agency, one year of which should have been in a general public health nursing agency with direct, qualified supervision, emphasizing family health. This experience should include experience as a staff nurse and experience as a supervisor, executive, or educational director.

## PROPOSED REPORT ON THE EDUCATIONAL QUALIFICATIONS OF PUBLIC HEALTH ENGINEERS [7]

THE term "public health engineer" as used in this report refers to the sanitary engineer, employed by a public health agency, who is trained in methods for the control and proper use of factors of the environment to the end that the public health is improved or protected.

The term "public health engineering" as used in this report includes the public health aspects of all types of environmental conditions whose control is based upon engineering principles. All procedures of public health agencies that depend upon engineering materials or methods for environmental conditions should be considered as public health engineering activities.

### I. GENERAL SCOPE OF ENGINEERS IN PUBLIC HEALTH PROGRAMS

Sanitary engineers with basic training in civil engineering early developed competence in water supply, sewage, and waste disposal. In order adequately to meet the problems of design and operation of such sanitary work, a knowledge of the chemistry and biology of these services became essential. This enlarged their sphere of interest, and in the course of time caused them to take an active part in all those problems concerned with the promotion and preservation of the public health to which engineers are able to contribute a significant solution.

The practice of public health engineering includes not only the activities of engineers in official health agencies in their investigations, review of plans, and supervision of the operation of sanitary works, but also the functions of engineers in private practice or in government organizations other than health agencies in the design, operation, and control of sanitary works. In order to be qualified to review plans and supervise operations, therefore, the public health engineer must be trained and qualified not only to advise on problems of sanitation, but also to design and construct sanitary works.

Public health activities may be divided into two distinct but closely interrelated fields, one having to do with the human element and the other with the environment. The first is normally the field of the physician and the nurse, while the second is that of the engineer and other sanitation personnel. There is no distinct separation between these activities, but there is a middle ground in which the activities of the physician and engineer merge. Therefore, success-

[7] "Report of the Committee on Professional Education." Reprinted from *The American Journal of Public Health*, January 1947, vol. 37.

ful operation of a public health program demands administrative participation and careful planning by both physician and engineer.

A complete public health program must include adequate provision for both the human element and the environment. The health officer aided by an adequate and competent engineering staff can assure the needed administrative assistance and technical advice necessary to provide a complete program. Not only is the public health engineer responsible for the engineering aspects of strictly public health phases of community life but he must also participate and assist in planning, designing, building, and operating of other engineering facilities, which are the primary responsibility of other branches of government, in order to promote and protect public health.

It is evident then that the department of health, through its engineering division or bureau, does not operate as an isolated unit, but that it contributes to the maintenance of an orderly and properly functioning society in co-operation with many other departments of government having engineering functions. A broad concept of the social, political, and economic forces that operate in the community is essential to the recognition and development of such a program.

There is a considerable expansion of health programs taking place both at state and local levels as well as in industry. The number of engineers in public health work must be increased enormously if the needs are to be met. Expansion of related programs of public works construction, slum clearance, and urban redevelopment, industrial activity and stream pollution control will require additional numbers of similarly trained men. Conservative estimates place the number of public health engineers needed, in addition to those on the job now, at more than 1,000 to meet only the minimum needs for local health services. It is recommended that a population unit of 50,000 or more requires the services of at least one public health engineer plus an adequate number of assistants. Only by the establishment of high professional standards, with a corresponding increase in salaries, can the required number of competent persons be obtained and their services retained.

## II. The Activities and Functions of Engineers in Public Health

One of the major activities of public health engineers is that of supervising the development and operation of sanitary works in order to control properly those aspects that may affect the public health. The engineering procedures involved and the place of the public health engineer in the supervision, development and operation of such works are:

a. Investigating and planning.
b. Designing and preparing specifications.
c. Construction.
d. Maintenance and operation.

Except as discussed later, the design and construction of sanitary works is commonly assigned to engineers in private or consulting practice, public engineering organizations developed for this specific purpose, such as the New York Board of Water Supply or the Chicago Sanitary District, and the personnel of existing governmental agencies, such as the Department of Public Works. The maintenance and operation of the structures is then generally taken over by existing or specially organized departments or appropriate political subdivisions.

The proper development and operation of sanitary works are matters of public concern in general and of public health in particular. Since profit or other economic motives are often associated with the development and operation of sanitary works, and since there may be a conflict of interest between different regions, communities, or industries and their sanitary needs, supervision and regulation is placed in governmental agencies including the engineering subdivision of health departments. Briefly, those organizations are entrusted with the following activities:

e. Investigation of sanitary needs, and stimulation to provide necessary remedial measures.
f. Advice relative to and approval of proposed works and approval of completed works.
g. Supervision of operation and maintenance of existing works.
h. Development and enforcement of rules and regulations.

Procedures (e) to (h) are complementary to the fundamental engineering procedures involved in the development and operation of sanitary works procedures (a) to (d) and have been interpolated for the purpose of establishing a reasonable system of checks and balances in the interest of health and welfare. Competently to fulfill procedures (e) to (h) the responsible engineer must possess the fundamental qualifications required by procedures (a) to (d) as well as additional qualifications related to the public health and welfare aspects of these activities. In the Federal Government and in some states and their subdivisions, the design, construction, and operation of sanitary works connected with governmental institutions and the design, construction, and operation of mosquito-control and rodent-control projects are assigned to the engineering organizations of their respective health agencies.

Public health engineering includes not only supervision of the development and operation of sanitary works as outlined above, but also participation in the planning, design, construction, operation, and maintenance of other physical elements that contribute to the support of community life so that the protection and promotion of public health can be assured. Some of these other physical elements are: dwellings; structures, and equipment used to produce, process, and distribute the food supply; environmental conditions which support disease-bearing insects and rodent life, and the growth of noxious weeds; industrial structures and equipment with especial reference to the effect on the air breathed in such industries as well as the other physical hazards therein.

The following are listed as public health engineering activities, as now carried on:

1. Water supply and treatment; design and installation of sewers, sewage and industrial waste disposal; stream pollution control; bathing place control; and mosquito control measures.
2. Municipal and rural waste disposal and insect, rodent, vermin and weed control.
3. Food sanitation, including the production and pasteurization of milk and the manufacture of ice cream and other dairy products; the sanitary production of shellfish, and the production, storage, and distribution of meat, poultry, pastry, bakery goods, fish, and other foods as well as the sanitation of eating and drinking establishments.

4. The sanitation of schools, camps, public places, swimming pools, and recreational areas.

5. Programs to promote healthful housing for all people.

6. Industrial hygiene and sanitation. This involves those special engineering problems incident to industrial processes and includes the many features of environmental sanitation. Industrial sanitation should, therefore, be under the direction of a public health engineer.

7. In cities particularly, proper city planning, heating, lighting, and ventilation of buildings, plumbing, aerial pollution, and noise. These problems are largely engineering in character. Any program to influence them for the benefit of public health must be based on engineering investigations and solutions.

### III. The Educational Background of Public Health Engineers

Public health engineers must possess two distinct and essential educational qualifications: (a) basic education and training in engineering, and (b) specialized knowledge and ability in sanitary science, sanitary engineering, and public health.

#### a. *Basic Engineering Education*

The public health engineer should be a graduate of a full four-year or longer course leading to a bachelor's or higher degree [8] at a college or university of recognized standing [9] with the major study and the basis of the degree in a course such as sanitary or public health engineering, or the sanitary option in civil engineering. In the case of public health engineers entering industrial sanitation, mechanical or chemical engineering is preferred.

In so far as the academic requirements are concerned, the basic education of the engineer should make him eligible for admission to examination for licensure to practise professional engineering in the state of his employment.

#### b. *Specialized Education and Training*

The varied functions of a public health engineer necessitate additional education beyond that ordinarily acquired by basic training in engineering. Successful performance in his field requires: (a) an intimate and working knowledge of the physical, chemical, biological, and engineering sciences upon which the sanitary control of the environment is based, and (b) the ability to identify, evaluate, and explain in terms of their public health implications those environmental factors that will promote and protect health or those that are capable of injuring health.

This specialized knowledge lies mainly in three fields: (1) sanitary science, (2) sanitary engineering, and (3) public health. The elements of these are indicated in the outline of graduate education, Section IV. In the rigorous under-

[8] In making this recommendation the American Public Health Association expressly recognizes that there are many persons now actively engaged in public health work who are lacking in formal education but whose training or experience should be accepted as fully equivalent to the basic engineering education defined above. The basis of substitution shall be at least two years of appropriate training or experience equivalent to one year of formal engineering education. Such persons who have sufficient equivalent training or experience to substitute for the accredited engineering education they lack shall be considered professional engineers for the purpose of this report.

[9] A college or university of recognized standing is defined as one which is accredited by a national or regional accrediting association such as the Association of American Universities, or the New England, Middle State, North Central, Southern, or Northwest Association of Secondary or Higher Schools, or one whose engineering curricula have been accredited by the Engineers' Council for Professional Development.

graduate engineering curriculum the amount of time that can be allotted to specialized study in these three fields without impairing the basic engineering education is quite limited—generally not more than about 15 per cent of the total scheduled instruction. Adequate preparation of an engineer for a career in public health requires one or more years of specialized study as outlined in Section IV and a period of supervised experience in addition to the minimum of four years required for graduation in engineering. However, to enable the graduate in engineering to begin work and gain experience and to prepare him for graduate study it is desirable that his undergraduate program should include as much instruction as possible in the fundamental sanitary sciences—especially bacteriology and chemistry—and in the principles of sanitary engineering and public health.

The program of study, preparing for a career in public health engineering, falls into three categories:

1. Sanitary Options in Four-year Undergraduate Curricula of Civil Engineering—In 1944 twenty-three such curricula remained accredited by the Engineers' Council for Professional Development.[10] The accredited options, for which information is available, allotted from 8 to 20 per cent of the period of study to the subjects of primary importance to sanitary engineers; namely, chemistry (beyond freshman chemistry), biology (including bacteriology), hydrology or hydraulic engineering, sanitary engineering, and public health. There are no sanitary options in chemical and mechanical engineering, those most closely allied to industrial hygiene.

2. Four-year Undergraduate Curricula in Sanitary Engineering—In 1944 three such curricula remained accredited by the Engineers' Council for Professional Development. One of these three accredited curricula had been discontinued by its institution. Registration for programs of this type has long been very low and the outlook for a continuation of these programs is uncertain. The accredited curricula allotted from 13 to 25 per cent of the period of study to the subjects of primary importance to sanitary engineers (see "1" above). None of these curricula is oriented particularly toward the practice of industrial hygiene.

3. Graduate Curricula in Sanitary Engineering and Public Health—These include two general types of programs, those in which the major study and graduate degrees are in sanitary engineering and those in which the major study and degree are in public health. Such programs provide opportunities for engineers with little or no training in public health engineering to develop a sufficient background to begin work in public health. They also provide advanced graduate instruction for those who have completed undergraduate programs in sanitary options or sanitary engineering. Either of the two types of programs should be accepted as satisfactory for these purposes if they include adequate instruction in each of the three essential fields of knowledge previously outlined and enough choice of electives to meet the needs of students with varying backgrounds of previous training and experience. As yet there are no accrediting agencies that examine and accredit graduate curricula in sanitary or public health engineering.

As a minimum for initial employment as a public health engineer the graduate engineer should have completed an approved undergraduate sanitary option or sanitary engineering program; or, in addition to graduation in engineering, should have received an equivalent amount and similar character of approved

[10] At the present time the Engineers' Council for Professional Development is the only accrediting agency of national scope which examines and accredits curricula in sanitary engineering and sanitary option of civil engineering.

postgraduate education or in-service training. Such postgraduate training can best be obtained through study in an approved educational institution but may be provided by postgraduate self-education or in-service training during a period of probationary employment under competent public health engineering supervision. A young engineer, at first occupied in a subordinate position, should work under close public health engineering supervision until he has prepared himself by experience or graduate study for positions of major responsibility. Graduate education affords the greatest assurance that the public health engineer will become both broadly competent and well grounded in the subjects that are fundamental to sanitary progress.

## IV. Graduate Education

The true value of the public health engineer rests squarely on his ability within his professional field.

Because of the wide difference in the technical knowledge required in the various fields of public health engineering activity, opportunity should be afforded for some specialization. Depending upon the student's preparation, a suitable program of graduate study should be developed from the following elements of sanitary science, engineering technology, and public health practice.

a. Sanitary sciences including (but not limited to): bacteriology, chemistry, parasitology, planktology, entomology and human physiology as related to problems of public health engineering interest.

b. The principles and practices of engineering analysis, design and operation as applied to works and projects for the protection and promotion of the public health including (but not limited to) the following: water supply and purification, sewerage and sewage treatment, the collection and disposal of municipal, rural and industrial wastes; projects for the control of insect, rodent, and other vectors of disease transmission; the engineering and administrative phases of food and milk sanitation; the sanitation of buildings including ventilation, air conditioning, heating, plumbing, and illumination; housing; industrial sanitation with particular reference to those industrial health hazards the correction of which is largely an engineering problem.

c. The principles of public health including (but not limited to) the following: public health administration sufficient to give the student a clear understanding of the purposes, functions, and legal bases of the general public health program and the responsibilities of the engineer within that program; epidemiology and communicable disease control; statistical methods in sanitary engineering and public health practice.

Emphasis should be placed upon the fundamental scientific engineering and public health content of the subject matter presented—the student being supervised and guided in his development of possible technics and practices based upon sound fundamental concepts.

The type of institution best fitted to give the instruction is a university which includes both a faculty of engineering and a faculty of public health, and in which close co-operation is maintained between the members of the two faculties who are responsible for instruction in public health engineering.

## V. Classification of Public Health Engineers

In any organization having a staff of engineers, classification is necessary. In general such classification automatically occurs and it is a general requirement under usual civil service procedures. However, lack of uniformity in classification exists among the various health agencies employing engineers. The following classification with educational and experience requirements is suggested. It is based on the requirements of several states, federal Civil Service, the United States Public Health Service for Commissioned Officers, and the classification of engineers as adopted by the American Society of Civil Engineers.

The education, training, and experience stated in the classification should be regarded as the minimum that is normally acceptable. It is not intended that the qualifications should be retroactive but rather that they should apply to the selection of new employees and serve as a guide in the future advancement of sanitary engineering personnel.

Because of the present limited supply of qualified public health engineers, it is proposed that in any grade, three years of acceptable experience in public health engineering under competent supervision may be substituted for the one year of graduate study set forth in this report. However, the advantages of specialized graduate study in the sound and early development of public health engineers for positions of responsibility are recognized. Therefore, as soon as practicable, at least one academic year of approved graduate study as described in Section IV should be made a basic requirement for appointment or promotion to Grade III or to higher grades in this classification.

*Education and Experience*

The minimum educational requirements for all grades are: (1) graduation in engineering from a college or university of recognized standing; (2) satisfaction of academic requirements for admission to examination for licensure to practice engineering in the particular state; and (3) completion of an approved undergraduate sanitary option or sanitary engineering program or, lacking such training, an equivalent amount of postgraduate orientation. Such postgraduate training may consist of at least three months of approved university guidance; or a like period of well rounded and systematic in-service orientation and supervised practice. Tentative or provisional appointments may be authorized for graduate engineers without public health engineering training or experience to allow a sufficient period for graduate study or in-service training to qualify them for permanent classification.

With the exception of Grades I and II, specialized education should include, in addition to the minimum educational requirements, at least one academic year of graduate study in a recognized institution of learning leading to a graduate degree and with major study in sanitary science, sanitary engineering, and public health. In lieu of a year of graduate study, three years of suitable practice under the supervision of a competent public health engineer in public health work may be substituted *provided* that, (1) such substitutions of experience for graduate study normally should not be allowed for grades higher than Grade III, and (2) a sanitary engineer who later completes a year or more of graduate study should receive equivalent credit in his classification for the years of experience previously substituted in lieu of graduate study.

Attainment of the doctor's degree in sanitary engineering or in public health if based on special studies in the field of public health engineering in a school of recognized standing should be considered as the equivalent of and may be substituted for a part of the experience requirements of the classification below as follows: Grade III—one year; Grade IV—two years; and Grade V—three years.

*Classification*

The qualifications for each grade should conform with the educational requirements or equivalent experience as described above in addition to the experience indicated below:

Grade I—No experience required.

Grade II—At least one year of suitable experience in sanitary engineering work under competent supervision.

Grade III—At least two years of suitable experience in sanitary engineering work in a grade comparable to Grade II, of which at least one year of the total experience must be in public health work. (Total 3 years sanitary engineering, 1 of them in a public health agency.)

Grade IV—At least two years of sanitary engineering experience in a grade comparable to Grade III, of which at least two years of the total experience must be in a responsible position in public health work. (Total 5 years sanitary engineering, 3 of them in a public health agency.)

Grade V—At least five years of engineering experience in a grade comparable to Grade IV, of which at least five years of the total experience must be in a responsible position in public health work. (Total 10 years sanitary engineering, 5 of them in a public health agency.)

*Personal Qualities*

To attain success in full measure, public health engineers should not only be competent in their field of learning and practice but should also be able to establish and maintain favorable relations in their own department and with the public on the basis of creative ability, far-sighted leadership, sound engineering judgment, common sense, honesty, and industry.

VI. QUALIFICATIONS FOR DIRECTING PERSONNEL

*Director*

The qualifications for the position of Director of a Division of Sanitation (however designated) in a health department will vary depending upon the size of the division and the responsibilities of the position. He should have the educational requirements set forth for all public health engineers, a general knowledge of all phases of public health engineering, and an intimate knowledge of those problems which are of importance in the particular area or community in which he is to be employed. He should have the ability to organize and direct the work of his division.

In small health units where only one employee is engaged in environmental sanitation activities, this employee should meet the qualifications of one of the public health engineering grades unless he is working under the technical direction of a public health engineer of the staff of an overlying governmental health agency.

*Assistant Director*

An Assistant Director should have the qualifications for the next grade below that in which the director is classified.

## THE EDUCATIONAL QUALIFICATIONS OF HEALTH EDUCATORS [11]

### I. The General Scope of Health Education

THE health educator assists in helping people to become intelligently aware of individual and community health problems and to share the responsibility for their solution. He interprets health needs, desirable health behavior, and the services of professional health agencies. Successful health education can rarely be accomplished by the use of publicity technics alone. It almost always includes the development of satisfactory learning experiences within organized groups and the training of other public health personnel to aid them in improving the educational opportunities presented by their contacts with individuals.

Health education is rapidly becoming recognized as one of the important fields of service in the modern public health movement. The emphasis upon health education and the demand for professionally trained health educators are increasing. We are without accurate data on the number of health educators now employed in the United States. It is estimated that there are probably four hundred to five hundred, exclusive of teachers of health in public schools and institutions of higher learning. Increasing consideration is being given to the organization of unified, community-wide programs. Thus, promotional progress may be anticipated by the beginning health educator, both through the expansion of his program and through transfer to the service of larger population groups, as his ability is demonstrated.

The health educator in the health department works under the administrative leadership and direction of the health officer. The health educator working in the school system as a teacher, supervisor, or consultant, is a member of the staff of the school and will, of course, meet whatever professional educational standards are set by the school for the type of work involved. Health educators may be employed jointly by health departments and school systems. They are also employed by voluntary agencies. The educational qualifications of a health educator, whether employed by a governmental or by a voluntary agency, should meet generally accepted standards.

This report proposes desirable areas of competence for the health educator, based upon the functions which he is expected to perform. The recommendations are made for the guidance both of officials responsible for the appointment of health educators and of individuals looking forward to careers in health education. The professional standing of persons now performing creditable service as health educators has been established. Successful experience and demonstrated ability should be recognized at the present time as evidence of professional qualification.

### II. The Functions in Health Education

The following functions are believed to be essential for carrying out complete community-wide programs in health education. Such programs include health education in the schools and health education with the general public. It is recognized that there is an increasingly close relationship between these two

[11] "Report of the Committee on Professional Education." Reprinted from *The American Journal of Public Health*, August 1933, vol. 33.

phases of health education. Health educators in various positions will be expected to undertake some or all of the following functions or activities which involve the formulation of plans and methods, the application of specific technics and skills, the supervision of the work of others, and the maintenance of group relations. A job analysis of existing positions reveals wide variations in their scope.

The functions of health educators in community-wide programs of health education are:

In accordance with the administrative policy of the health department or other employing agency:

1. To be responsible for assistance in planning and organizing a program of health education of suitable scope and activities to meet adequately the needs of the community, state, or area to be served. This includes at the outset a study or survey of the needs, the determination of health problems which may be solved, at least in part, by the educational process, and an appraisal of resources.
2. To assist the community in organizing itself to find and solve its health problems.
3. To assist in establishing and maintaining close co-operative working relationships between all agencies (official and nonofficial) which may contribute to health education.
4. To aid in the planning, development, and conduct of training programs for employed personnel, in accordance with the policy of the agency involved, for (a) health agency personnel, (b) school personnel, and (c) personnel of other agencies.

   Nearly all public health personnel have important educational opportunities. To increase the effective use of these opportunities is an important function of health education leadership.
5. To give aid in accordance with the policy of the institution concerned, in planning the health education aspects of pre-service training programs for professional personnel, including (a) public health personnel, (b) school personnel, and (c) others.
6. To provide consultation and guidance to various individuals and groups (such as Parent Teacher Associations, service clubs, and others) in developing and improving their health education activities.
7. To assist in promoting, organizing, and guiding study programs in the field of health for adult and group-work agencies, such as divisions of adult education, Young Men's Christian Associations, and similar groups.
8. To contribute to the improvement of the quality of the health education of the school child in accordance with the standards and policies of the school system.
   a. Through aid in planning school health programs and curricula of health instruction
   b. Through conferences with teachers, supervisors, and school administrators
   c. Through such other activities as the school may desire
9. To organize and operate an informational service to provide answers to inquiries and to supply source materials and source references in answer to requests.
10. To be responsible for the preparation, selection, assembly, and distribution of health education materials, using the services of special technicians and health experts as necessary. Such materials include:
    a. Reports and other printed materials

   b. Visual aids, such as motion pictures, photographs, graphic materials, ex-
      hibits, and posters
   c. News releases
11. To organize and assist in conducting a speakers' bureau, conferences, meet-
    ings, and radio programs.
12. To see that there is established a program of continuing appraisal of health
    education methods and materials in order to evaluate the effectiveness of
    health education procedures.

### III. Broad Educational Background

The procedure used in determining the educational qualifications here listed,
was to analyze each of the above functions in terms of needed professional qualifications and to group these qualifications in suitable areas.

Certain facts should be borne in mind in approaching this discussion. Not all
positions in health education, as indicated above, are of the same scope. The
health officer or other appointing authority may not deem it necessary to require
all the qualifications listed below for every position. They are the qualifications
believed desirable for the director of a large and complete program. Nevertheless it is believed that the continuing improvement in the training of health
educators will provide more and more workers who have this training, and that
such a person will eventually prove most useful.

Experts in various technics who are not health educators are commonly needed
to assist in editorial work and in the development of films, exhibits, and other
graphic materials. The health educator concerned with the production of such
material will know the nature, limitations, and possibilities of the processes involved. He will know how to work effectively with printers, motion picture
producers, and other specialists. This report does not consider the qualifications
of these technical experts.

It is clear that the health educator will be helped by broad cultural background and by a knowledge of (a) the structure, functions, and care of the body,
elements of the commoner pathologic processes and elements of epidemiology in
its broadest sense; (b) motivation and behavior in human life; (c) society as it
is constituted—social forces and their control; (d) forces which affect living—
environment and economics; (e) the scientific method in approaching the process of living, distinguishing science from pseudo-science; and (f) the processes
of education—why we learn and how we learn.

There is also need for knowledge and skills which are more specifically professional in nature. The division between essentially basic preparation and
strictly professional training cannot be readily drawn. Neither is it feasible to
indicate here a specific training program in terms of institutions to be attended,
degree secured, years of study or specific courses taken.

Some health educators have begun training for this field immediately upon
reaching the university level. More will do so in the future. At the same time
it is recognized that many of the professional fields in the health and social sciences, including education, contain many of the elements of training which are
desirable for the health educator. Many successful health educators have acquired their training through supplementing the training in one of these professional fields by study in those previously omitted areas of knowledge which are
required for health education. It is not feasible to discuss here the entrance
into health education from various professional fields. We shall not attempt

to define optimal training. We shall attempt to state the essential qualifications.

Present requirements in the training of health educators should be sufficiently flexible to be adapted to the scope of work required from the individual in question. Without attempting to indicate subjects of instruction or the division between fundamental and professional study, and based upon the duties to be performed in a complete program of health education, there is listed below the areas of knowledge and skill considered desirable for professional competence in health education. Well known areas of knowledge are listed in brief, general terms, while some of the specific skills needed are listed in more detail.

Desirable qualifications are:

1. Basic cultural education, including the development of appreciations and skills in the use of the English language
2. Basic science education, including physics, chemistry, biology, anatomy, physiology and bacteriology
3. Training in education and educational psychology to provide a knowledge of and functional experiences with
   a. The nature of the learning process, involving individual psychology, interests and reactions, and indirect as well as direct learnings
   b. The principles and practices of education
   c. Methods and possibilities of adult education
   d. The nature of the school health program, including health services, physical education, and other activities.
   e. Methods of educational evaluation and their possibilities and limitations in respect to the evaluation of health education programs
   f. Curricula and curriculum development in public schools and in schools of higher learning
   g. Educational supervision and administration
   h. Existing practices and viewpoints of professional groups for which in-service training is provided, and recent trends in their education
   i. How to organize and conduct field training for students at the pre-service level (in the case of a field station for professional training)
4. Social science education to provide an appreciation of the importance of respect for human personality and a knowledge of
   a. Racial, social and cultural characteristics of the people and their mores
   b. The significance of the economic status of population groups
5. Education in the field of hygiene and public health to provide a knowledge of
   a. Physiologic hygiene, including personal hygiene, nutrition and mental hygiene
   b. Environmental sanitation
   c. Basic principles in the organization and administration of public health
   d. Methods of communicable disease control, including the nature of the causative organisms and methods of transmission
   e. Public health statistics and principles of statistical reliability
   f. Survey methods
   g. Relative importance of health problems and mode of attack
6. Training in the area of public administration to provide a knowledge of
   a. Governmental and community organization
   b. Community agencies, their functions, aims and interests
   c. Technics for the successful interview and consultative conference (particularly in public school work)
   d. The qualities of leadership, how to discover leaders and how to work with them

    e. Group-work methods
    f. Principles of planning
7. Training in special skills required in health education to include ability in public speaking and the conduct of public meetings and knowledge of
    a. Methods and materials in health education, their possibilities, and limitations
    b. The evaluation of sources of material and information
    c. How to write informative and friendly letters
    d. How to compile bibliographies
    e. Filing and clipping methods
    f. How to write and edit material for publication
    g. The nature of the printing and duplicating processes and their use
    h. How to distribute educational material effectively
    i. The nature, preparation, and use of visual aids
    j. Possibilities of community participation in the development of educational material
    k. Press relations and technics
    l. Radio methods and technics
    m. Conference technics
    n. How to organize, advertise, and conduct meetings

Carefully planned and supervised field experience and "internship" should be regarded as an important element in the training of the health educator and in the development of skill and ability in the field of health education.

*Personal Qualities*

A candidate for a position as health educator should possess such personal characteristics as creative ability, leadership, good personal health, good judgment, pleasing personal appearance, common sense, and adaptability. Such important characteristics, along with the ability to work with people, the ability to size up and meet situations, and the ability to present pertinent facts simply and effectively, are not guaranteed by academic records in formal courses of instruction. The health practices of the health educator himself are also important.

*Length of the Training Period*

If one were to enter upon a program of planned study in the first year of university life, this essential training could not be secured, we believe, in less than 5 years. Study beyond this point would probably be desirable, especially for those aiming for positions of larger responsibility.

If such a 5 year program were followed, the essential basic preparation could be obtained by a 4 years' course leading to a Bachelor's degree with major emphasis upon: (1) the basic health sciences, (2) education, with emphasis upon educational psychology, and (3) the social sciences.

In such a case, the graduate work would include supplementary courses in the above and allied fields, courses to give a working knowledge of the public health program and its operation, and courses in health education, plus supervised field training wherever possible. The content and extent of the graduate work required would vary according to the amount of undergraduate preparation and the interval between undergraduate and graduate study and the quality and type of experience the individual has had.

*The Place for Graduate Training*

It is recommended that programs of professional study in health education be offered in those institutions which are providing professional education in other fields of public health, and which have available the required instructional facilities. Field training stations are desirable.

## THE EDUCATIONAL QUALIFICATIONS OF SCHOOL PHYSICIANS [12]

### I. GENERAL SCOPE OF THE FIELD

A. *Specific Contributions to Public Health*

SCHOOL physicians have always had unique opportunities to improve the health of children and communities. For many years, however, the most important function of the school physician was regarded as the physical examination of pupils. Today he has responsibilities of a much broader nature. Although not responsible for medical care of individual children, his responsibilities do include a thorough knowledge of:

1. The growth and development of normal children
2. Diseases of children
3. The values, methods and limitations of advisory service to parents, teachers, school administrators, and pupils concerning the promotion of optimum growth and development
4. The over-all school program and the types of adjustment which are possible and necessary for health reasons for some children
5. Methods of co-ordinating the medical and nursing services and other school health work with classroom instruction, physical education and recreation, lunchroom and nutrition services so that he may assist all school personnel to make their most effective contribution to optimum pupil health
6. The facilities available for treatment in the community (chief of which is the private physician)
7. The technics of explaining to the parents, child, and teacher the reasons why good health practices are desirable and why treatment is necessary
8. Individual and community health problems which may be attacked through education
9. The place of the school as an integral part of the community's health resources

These modern functions of the school physician enable him to contribute much more to the health and welfare of children and of the community than did the medical examiner or inspector of past years. They necessitate, however, special educational qualifications over and above the M.D. degree. The purpose of this report is to describe this broadened concept of the school physician's functions and suggest the training and experience necessary.

B. *Future Outlook*

With the increased public attention being given child health, public health and education authorities face greater demands for further development of

[12] Report of the Committee on Professional Education." Reprinted from *The American Journal of Public Health*, September 1944, vol. 34.

school health programs. Well qualified medical leadership is essential to sound school health work in both private and public schools.

## C. Number Engaged in This Field

There are probably well over 5,000 physicians in the United States who give either part-time or full-time service to schools. During the past 25 years the number of full-time physicians in schools has increased considerably.

## D. By Whom Employed

School physicians may be employed either by the board of health or the board of education, or jointly by both. In some states the law requires that boards of education employ school physicians. In other places the board of health is legally responsible for school medical work. In some localities the board of education contracts with the local health department for school health work, including the employment of physicians, nurses, and sanitary inspectors. In other localities the school medical director is employed jointly by the board of education and the health department. He may be the director of the bureau of maternal and child health in the health department. In smaller communities the full-time health officer is sometimes designated school medical director.

## E. Promotional Progress

Opportunities for advancement in this field occur through promotion from subordinate to administrative positions, by moving from smaller to larger school systems, by promotional progress through the health department, and through the growth and expansion of local, state, and national programs.

## II. Functions of School Physicians

### A. The Duties and Functions of the School Physician Include:

1. *Periodic medical examination of children*—This is to demonstrate the value of health examinations, to give children the educational experience of learning how well they are, to evaluate growth and development, to reveal conditions which might adversely affect the health or educational progress of children, and to furnish recommendations for the care and alleviation of these conditions. Teachers and even parents are often unaware of abnormalities in the child and are frequently unfamiliar with the sources of, and necessity for, treatment. This function necessarily includes mass-testing procedures such as for vision and hearing.

2. *Professional consultation in health education*—Actually, the pupil's medical examination in the presence of the parents [13] can be made one of the most potent health education influences in the child's life. These examinations offer the school physician opportunities of presenting health information to pupils and parents, and to confer with teachers regarding individual findings, thus enabling him to influence their ideas on health. Correcting misconceptions, dispelling superstitions, and instilling a desire for accurate, scientific facts are fundamental contributions of physicians to health education.
   As a consultant in the preparation of health courses he can check the medical accuracy of study and source materials, suggest timely topics for inclu-

---

[13] Elementary school children are usually best examined in the presence of one or both parents. High school students are often seen individually, and a consultation with parents arranged at a later time.

sion, and advise on the selection of health facts important for pupils as distinguished from those of less importance. The *1942 Year Book* of the American Association of School Administrators states: "The functions of the modern school physician are educational. The school requires a medical inventory of the health status of its children, both for their general welfare and to indicate necessary variations in school procedures. The health examination, ideally made in the presence of the parents, serves to screen out children where conditions require diagnosis and those whose obvious ill health indicates a need for immediate attention. To the family physician and to available clinics or other approved medical agencies, belongs the responsibility of diagnosis and appropriate treatment. To the school physician and other members of the school staff belongs the responsibility of result-producing health guidance in cases where action is indicated."

3. *Responsibility for the prevention and control of communicable diseases in the school*—Procedures established by the school physician and health officer for preventing the spread of such diseases must be carefully explained to administrators, teachers, custodians, parents, and pupils. Smallpox re-vaccination, diphtheria reimmunization and such other specific preventive measures as are supplementary to the earlier protection given infants and pre-school children and are approved by the local medical profession are systematically organized by the school physician, bearing in mind that these too are potent and beneficial educational experiences. The carrying out of measures in the school for the control of epidemics is often a responsibility delegated to him by the health officer. Guidance in the use of tuberculin testing and other methods of tuberculosis case finding are also the province of the school physician.

4. *School safety and safety education*—This is another part of the school physician's educational function. One of his first responsibilities is the establishment of well understood policies and procedures for the care of school emergencies. The smooth functioning of these procedures when a child is hurt is a valuable piece of safety education for all concerned. His advisory responsibility for the safety of school buildings and grounds, together with his professional knowledge of the results and underlying physical and emotional causes of accidents, make him an invaluable consultant in teaching safety.

5. *Directing teachers and school nurses in systematic and continuous observation of the health of pupils*—so that they may identify those who are normal and so that deviations from normal will be discovered early and investigated by experts. This may include programs for weighing and measuring, for testing vision and hearing, and for securing health histories.

6. *Selecting pupils for special educational programs*—such as lip reading instruction, speech correction, sight conservation, visiting teacher service, modified physical education, shortened school day, rest periods, advising with teachers in constructing educational programs for the physically handicapped. This includes guidance of physical education and corrective physical education teachers in providing modified and suitable exercises for those suffering from postural defects, nervous and crippling disorders and the like.

7. *General supervision of sanitation and other environmental health factors within the school buildings and grounds*—This includes the safety of water, safety of food and milk supplies in the lunchroom and their safe treatment by food handlers, the proper disposal of sewage and wastes, sanitation of drinking fountains and wash rooms, proper eating, lighting, heating and ventilation, safety of gymnasium and playground.

8. *Medical advice to school authorities on mental and emotional health influences*—such as the length of the school day, extracurricular activities, the frequency of recess periods, type of examinations, methods of marking, and technic of handling individual children.

9. *Professional guidance in the field of teacher's health*—The teacher's mental as well as her physical health is of direct concern to her employer because of its effect on the quality of her work. In this area the school physician is comparable to the medical director of an industry who is given broad responsibility for employees' health maintenance, while actual diagnosis and treatment are usually done by the employee's private physician, the school physician often conducts periodic health examinations and offers consultation to employees with health problems.

10. *Administrative functions*—such as the skilled supervision of personnel within his department, preparation of budgets and reports, the development of health and medical records, and the statistical analysis of records and results.

11. *Responsibility to the school system and the community for integrating the school health program into the public health program of the community* [14]— Health maintenance and protection are of equal importance to infants, children, adults, and aged. The school health program has too often been considered a separate entity, apart from the community health program as a whole. It is a co-operative enterprise both inside and outside the school. Outside the school it involves co-operative effort with health departments, voluntary health agencies, welfare agencies, clinics and hospitals, individual physicians, and organized medicine. Inside the school it involves co-operation between physicians, dentists, nurses, principals, psychologists, cafeteria directors, custodians, classroom teachers, supervisor, and superintendents. The school physician interprets his job to agencies and individuals outside the school. He elicits and fosters the assistance of departments and individuals within the school. He recognizes the interrelationships of all individuals and groups who can help attain the goal of healthier, happier people.

12. *Incidental functions and duties*—which are important but need not be detailed—include co-operation in the development of an effective physical education program on the basis of sound health standards including the health supervision and guidance of athletes; advice to those responsible for the school cafeteria to insure the sanitary safety of food and its nutritional adequacy; assistance with the in-service training of teachers in health subjects; continued search for and elimination of outmoded procedures and policies which impede the securing of medical care and other remedial work; assistance with the vocational guidance of the physically handicapped.

B. *Two Classifications of School Physicians*

There are variations in the responsibilities and duties of school physicians depending in part on the size of the schools served, the number of physicians employed, and the completeness of the school health program. In a large school system there may be many physicians working under the general supervision and direction of a chief physician. In still larger school systems the chief physician may have one or more deputies, some of whom may have special titles, descriptive of their specialized duties. In smaller communities one physician

---

[14] The school administrator is responsible for integrating the activities of the entire school system with the work of many agencies in the community. In his work with community health agencies the school physician is guided by the administrator's general policies and keeps him currently informed.

may be employed to serve several school systems. In many areas a part-time physician is used.

To differentiate between the qualifications needed by a physician who administers, or assists with the administration, of a school health program, devoting his full time thereto, and one who works under the supervision of another, two classifications of school physicians are designated for the purpose of this report. They will be referred to here as "Director, Deputy, or Assistant Director of School Health" and "School Medical Adviser." These titles are not necessarily recommended to school systems, but are used here to differentiate between the qualifications needed for the duties performed by two classes of medical personnel.

1. *Director, Deputy, or Assistant Director of School Health*—Regardless of whether this is his actual title, this type of school physician will ordinarily be a full-time employee of the board of education or the health department, with a rank of, or equivalent to, an assistant superintendent for those employed by schools or assistant health officer or deputy for those employed by health departments. He establishes policies, selects other medical personnel, is responsible to the school superintendent or health officer, or both, supervises, guides, and evaluates all medical phases of the school health program. Ideally, such a physician with the special qualifications set forth below should be obtained to administer and supervise the medical aspects of the school health program in all schools. This is almost an essential in large communities. In smaller communities a practical solution is for several schools in one or more counties or districts to join in the employment of such a person. In other small communities it is often practical to employ the health officer in this capacity especially if he has the basic qualifications set forth below and has the ability to administer the two positions. This has the advantage of assuring the integration emphasized above.

2. *School Medical Advisers*—Regardless of whether this is his actual title, this type of school physician will be a staff member working under the direction of a "Director of School Health." While good administration will require that the director consult his staff members regarding policies and procedures, "School Medical Advisers" will be concerned primarily with carrying out established procedures. They will ordinarily be part-time physicians. They will be recruited from competent physicians in the community, who wish to devote part of their time to public health, and whose qualifications meet those listed below. The selection of "School Medical Advisers" should rest with the "Director of School Health" or the health officer if he is acting in that capacity, subject to such Civil Service or Merit System regulations as may exist. Selections of medical personnel usually calls for careful scrutiny of personal and professional qualifications which is best done by one who is himself well trained in medicine and public health.

### III. BROAD EDUCATIONAL BACKGROUND OF SCHOOL PHYSICIANS

Both "Directors of School Health" and "School Medical Advisers" should above all be good doctors. They should have the M.D. degree from a Class A medical school, so designated by the Council on Medical Education and Hospitals of the American Medical Association, plus an internship in a hospital approved by that Council.

## IV. Graduate Education

**Note:** This section proposes desirable areas of competence for physicians engaged in school health work. The recommendations are made for the guidance of (1) officials responsible for the appointment of school physicians, (2) individuals looking forward to careers in school health work, (3) universities contemplating the offering of special courses in this field.

The professional competence of persons now performing creditable service as school physicians is recognized. It is realized that many have not had the opportunity to acquire the formal education or graduate degrees suggested herein. However, it is to be emphasized that an exception to the requirements for a postgraduate course and the other qualifications listed should be made only if the candidate in addition to years of experience has actually demonstrated unusual ability as a school physician.

### A. *"School Medical Adviser"*

A beginning policy of limiting recommendations to those workers who are devoting themselves to a career in full-time public health work has been adopted. The "School Medical Adviser" is not ordinarily a full-time career worker. Recognizing his value to the school health program, however, and the dilemma sometimes confronting school superintendents when local physicians are recommended for school appointments by influential people, the following suggestions are submitted:

Preference should be given to physicians who have had special training and experience in the fields of pediatrics or internal medicine. Physicians who, in addition to a sound background of clinical experience in pediatrics or internal medicine, have had special training and experience in the field of public health, should receive additional consideration for appointment.

Special training in pediatrics may be judged by possession of one or more of the following qualifications, which are named in the order of their importance: (1) Certification as a pediatrician by the American Board of Pediatrics; [15] (2) Eligibility for certification by the American Board of Pediatrics, or qualifications meeting Board requirements; (3) Completion of one year as a Resident in Pediatrics in a hospital approved for such residency by the Council on Medical Education and Hospitals of the American Medical Association; (4) Completion of one year on the pediatrics staff of a hospital which has a Resident in Pediatrics and which has been approved for such residency by the Council on Medical Education and Hospitals, American Medical Association; (5) Completion of 18 months' internship, including an appointment in pediatrics in a hospital approved by the Council on Medical Education and Hospitals, American Medical Association; (6) Specializing part-time in pediatrics with an appointment in pediatrics in a hospital approved by the Council on Medical Education and Hospitals, American Medical Association.

In larger school systems it is assumed that "School Medical Advisers" will be working under the administrative and supervisory direction of a "Director of School Health." Their training and experience will be augmented by in-service

[15] The American Board of Pediatrics is an independent board of pediatricians established to provide a uniform standard of competency in the field of pediatrics. For information regarding these standards, address the Board at 707 Fullerton Avenue, Chicago, Ill.

training provided by the director through individual conferences, special studies, group projects, and other supervisory technics.

## B. *Director, Deputy, or Assistant Director of School Health*

1. *Specific Knowledge, Skill and Experience*—The scope of modern school health activities requires that the "Director of School Health" be a career man with special training both in education and in public health. In addition to being a well-trained physician with some of the qualifications listed above for the "School Medical Adviser" he will need the following special training and experience:

   a. Basic principles of public health including general philosophy of mass health protection, epidemiology, vital statistics, record systems and record keeping, environmental sanitation, and the principles of public health administration.

   b. Principles of growth and development of the child, the philosophy of modern education and its relationship to other community endeavors, an understanding of school procedures and organization, the principles of educational supervision and administration, educational psychology, the administration of school health programs, including development of health education curricula, the organization and conduct of special classes such as speech correction, lip reading, and sight saving, and the development of school mental hygiene programs including mental testing. Ideally, the "Director of School Health" should be qualified as a "School Medical Adviser" and should have had two or more years' experience in that capacity. Those who do not have the suggested public health and educational background should obtain it as soon as possible after appointment. This should be stipulated at the time of appointment.

   c. Upon completion of the "in residence" training listed above, the trainee should have an opportunity for observation and practice in well selected field training centers where outstanding work is being done. This may require a few weeks to three months depending on the amount of previous practical experience.

   These are essentially the requirements for the Master of Public Health degree in most schools.

2. *Personal Qualities*—The need for co-operative effort with many diverse groups and individuals emphasizes the importance of personal qualities of leadership, such as understanding of others, ability to select and help develop subordinates, ability to evaluate and improve accepted procedures, a friendly but dignified manner, a liking for children, and for preventive medicine.

3. *Approximate Time Required for Special Training*—The physician interested in this field presents an educational status somewhat different from the undergraduate or the non-professional student. For this reason, it is believed that one calendar year of specialized, concentrated work, which would include his field work, is sufficient.

4. *Type of Institution Best Fitted for Such Training*—It is important, however, that this work be undertaken in a school where his individual needs are carefully assayed and courses offered to fulfil these needs, where his time is well planned, and where there are rich opportunities for professional association and discussion as well as practice and observation in the field. It is essential that there be close association between the school of public health and the school of education. Neither school alone can complete the training of a potential director of school health. The leading schools of public health in this country and Canada, which have close association with the school of

education, particularly those meeting the "minimum facilities needed for graduate instruction in public health" [16] as listed by the Committee on Professional Education, American Public Health Association, are usually well suited to offer this type of training in the time suggested.

## V. EDUCATIONAL QUALIFICATIONS, OTHER TYPES OF PUBLIC HEALTH PERSONNEL

The educational qualifications for public health laboratory workers, nutritionists in health agencies, executives of voluntary health associations, public health statisticians, public health dentists, industrial hygienists, and administrators of other specialized health activities, may be obtained by writing directly to the Committee on Professional Education, American Public Health Association, 1790 Broadway, New York 19, New York.

[16] See "Memorandum Regarding Minimum Educational Facilities for the Postgraduate Education of Those Seeking Careers in Public Health," prepared by the Committee on Professional Education, American Public Health Association and published in the *American Journal of Public Health*, May, 1942.

# INDEX

Abramson, H., 273

Accidents: accidental deaths, 191; health officer's interest in, 5, 399; home, 386; industrial, 330, 331, 333, 335, 338, 386; in mines, 331; school-age children, 282; traffic, 386

Adenoids, diseased, 357

Adult hygiene, 371–387; accident prevention, 386; cancer, 377–381; diabetes, 375–376; general health education, 386; heart disease, 381–383; industrial hygiene, 330–346; mental disease, 381; periodic examinations, 372, 383–385; practicing physicians, 530–531; rheumatism, 373–375. For a more detailed index, *see* the specific subjects mentioned

Aedes mosquitoes, 177

Aestivo-autumnal fever, 141–142

Agustsson, H., 69

Air-borne disease, theory of, 241. *See also* Communicable disease control, Respiratory infections

Air sanitation and sterilization, 50, 121, 256–257

Airsols, 121

Alabama: ascariasis in, 170; board of health, 15; county health organization, 444; hookworm disease in, 206; malaria control in (Fig. 19), 199; malaria control: regulations governing impounding of waters, 147; malaria epidemic in, 209, 210 (Fig. 21); maternity care demonstration, 266; syphilis prevalence in Jefferson County, 103–108; typhus fever in, 179

Alaska, 485, 487, 488

Albany, N. Y., 198

Alcoholism, 318, 320

Alexandria, Va., 15

Altman, I., 251

Altmann, F., 59

Amatruda, C. S., 295

Amberson, J. B., Jr., 101

American Academy of Pediatrics, 276

American Association of Industrial Physicians, 332

American Association of School Administration, 295

American Child Health Association, 313, 501, 503

American College of Dentists, 291

American Epidemiological Society, 202

American Heart Association, 387

American Hospital Association, 579

American Legion, 518

American Medical Association: Council on Medical Education and Hospitals, 585; Council on Medical Service, 570; Journal of, 542; physical examination forms, 383, 387; platform of, for national health program, 568, 579; public health education material, 314; survey of state health departments, 419, 420

American National Red Cross: county health work, 440; disaster relief, 501, 515–521; entry into field of public health, 19; nursing service in rural areas, 237, 426–427, 501, 503–504; nutritional services, 369; type of organization, 503

American Public Health Association: Book Service, 542; Committee on Administrative Practice, 420, 445, 447, 506; Committee on Hygiene of Housing, 252; Committee on Professional Education, 227, 229, 236, 260, 311, 538, 542, 581–611; history of formation, 6, 13, 16, 17, 18; Journal of, 542; and National Board of Health, 18; national health program, publications concerning, 579; Presidents of: Dr. Godfrey, 573; Dr. Wolman, 576; proceedings of, 15, 16, 20, 209, 481; qualifications for public health personnel, 581–611; Subcommittee on Communicable Disease Control, 30

American Red Cross, *see* American National Red Cross

American Social Hygiene Association, 118, 314, 501, 503

American Society for the Control of Cancer, 387, 501, 503

Analyses, *see* Laboratory

Andalusia, Ala., 199

Anderson, G. W., 34, 42, 83, 538, 585

Andrewes, C. H., 131

Anopheles crucians, 142, 209

Anopheles gambeii, 495

Anopheles maculipennis, 142

Anopheles punctipennis, 142

Anopheles pseudopunctipennis, 142

munity program, 35, 38, 39–42; in individual case, 35, 38–39; decline in, 18, 35, 36; disinfection, 39; epidemiologic investigations, 27–29, 40; epidemiology, 35–38, 214; etiology, 35, 37; hospitalization, 29, 38, 39; immunity, 207; immunization, 35, 38, 39, 40–41 (Fig. 5), 434–435; incubation period, 37; isolation, 38; laboratory diagnosis of, 40, 221–222; mode of spread, 37; morbidity rate, 36 (Fig. 4); prevalence, 37; quarantine, 30, 38–39, 494; reporting, 26, 38; Schick test, 35, 39, 40, 41, 42, 223; symptomatology, 37; therapy, 38; toxoid, 35, 38, 40, 41, 42, 218, 434–435; treatment with penicillin, 43

Disaster relief, 514–522: agencies for, 515–517, 519; communicable disease, 520–521; emergency relief, 514; field survey in, 519; food and milk, 520; organization of emergency program, 517; predisaster program, 518; Red Cross, 501, 515–521; refugee centers, 517, 520; rehabilitation following, 521; rescue work, 514; sewage disposal, 520; state disaster relief committee, 518; water supplies, 520

Disease: air-borne theory, 241; germ theory, 17, 21; prevention of the function of health department, 19, 32, 371, 475, 500, see also Health promotion and protection; propagation of by decaying animal and vegetable matter, 4, 11, 241, 303–304, 439; social, 84, 114, see also Social and economic factors; study of, see Epidemiology; visitation of Providence, 11; zymotic, 13. See also Chronic disease, Communicable disease, Degenerative disease, Epidemics, Industrial disease, Resistance, Sickness, and the various specific diseases

Disinfection: in Colonial times, 12, 17; concurrent, 31; terminal, 31, 241, 399, see also Fumigation

Dispensary: industrial, 335, 339; for sick poor, 563. See also Clinics, Hospitals

District health centers, see Health centers

District health officer, see Health officer

District health unit, 425–426, 441–446: plan of organization, 442, 443 (Fig. 36); state subsidy, 444

District nursing associations, 501. See also Public health nursing, Visiting Nurse Associations

District of Columbia, 15, 189, 485, 487, 488

District plan of state health organization, 460

Dochez, A. R., 125, 130

Dog bites, 151. See also Rabies

Dogs: registration of, 151; vaccination clinics for, 152

Donald, A. B., 68

Donnally, H. H., 137, 138

Dorn, H. F., 387

Douglas, B. H., 101

Doull, J. A., 130

Dowling, J. D., 153, 154

Drainage: Act of 1709, 11; of marshes, 12, 16, 140. See also Sewage disposal

Draize, J. H., 148

Drill, V. A., 182

Drinker, P., 346

Drug addiction, 493

Drugs, see Food and drugs

Dublin, L. I., 382, 387

DuBois, C., 183

Dubos, R. J., 90

Dudley, S. F., 202

Duerschner, D. R., 50

Duncan, J. T., 80, 83

Dungal, N., 68, 69

Dust: ascariasis transmission, 170; dispersion of, 256; industrial law for removal, 331, 333; prevention of function of health department, 4; silica, 93, 330; streptococcus infection, 50

Dusty trades, 332, 343

Dyer, R. E., 132, 179

Dysentery, amebic, 26, 71, 81–82: control of, 82; epidemic at World's Fair, 81, 245

Dysentery, bacillary, 26, 71, 79–81: cause of, 80; control of, 80–81; control of carriers, 81; detection of, 80, 221; epidemiology, 80; treatment, 81

E. histolytica, 82, 400

Eberthella typhi, 71

Echinococcus infection, 247, 248

Economic and social factors in illness, see Social and economic factors

Eddie, B., 183

Education, included in "Census of Boston," 13. See also Public health education, Public health personnel, educational qualifications, Schools

Edwards, H. R., 99, 101

Ehlers, V. M., 261

Ekas, M. P., 201

Eklund, C. N., 183

Eldering, G., 63, 68

Eliot, C. W., 523

Ellingson, H. V., 176

Ellis, R., 137, 138

Elmsford, N. Y., 28 (Fig. 3)

Elvove, Elias, 357

Emergency Maternity and Infant Care Program, 237, 265, 470, 477, 487–488

Emergency relief program: in Colonial days, 12, 13; committees in, 518–519; scheme of organization, 517–518. See also Disaster relief

cer, municipal; Municipal health department

Municipal health department, 391–424: adult hygiene, 401–402; budget, 411–412, 421 (Fig. 33); cancer clinics, 401–402; child hygiene, 397–399, 408–409; combined city-county health department; communicable disease control, 393, 396, 407–408; epidemiological activities, 215; functions of, 391–402; industrial hygiene, 401; infectious disease control, 408; laboratories, 400–401, 410; popular health instruction, 401; preschool hygiene, 398; public health nursing, 409–410; public welfare, 416–418; relationship to state health department, 419, 457; sanitation of milk, food and water, 399–400, 406; school hygiene, 398, 409; tuberculosis, 408; venereal disease, 408; vital statistics, 392–393, 407

Municipal health department organization, 402–410: board of health, 404; city manager plan, 403–404; divisions of, 406; divisional organization, 406–410; health officer, 405; mayor and city council, 403; plan for small city, 403 (Fig. 30); public health council, 405–406; San Francisco, 417 (Fig. 32); staff meetings, 406. *See also* Boards of health, Health officer

Munro, T. A., 319
Munson, W. L., 114, 117, 208
Murphy, W. J., 182, 204
Mustard, H. S., 424, 446, 481
Mycobacterium tuberculosis, 87

Narcotic addiction, 493. *See also* Food and drugs
Nasopharyngitis, *see* Colds
Nassau County, N. Y., 152
National Advisory Health Council, 490
National Association of Manufacturers, 340
National Board of Health, 18, 21, 556, 576
National Cancer Institute, 489, 491
National Committee for Mental Hygiene, 326, 329, 501, 503
National Conference on Local Health Units, 447
National Conservation Commission, Report on National Vitality, 556
National Dental Hygiene Association, 296
National Foundation for Infantile Paralysis, 501
National Health Act of 1945, 572
National Health Conference, 1938, 567
National Health Council, 513
National health program, 9, 556–579: concept of need for, 557, 566; development of, trend in, 576–578; health officer in,

9, 572–573, 578; Hill-Burton Bill, 571; "Principles of a National Health Program," 579; surveys of national health, 556, 567. *See also* Federal health administration, Medical care, Social Security Act
National Health Survey, 1935–36, 373, 375, 567
National Institute of Health, 491–492: Biologics Control Laboratory, 491–492; Chemistry Laboratory, 492; Division of Infectious Diseases, 491; Division of Physiology, 491; Division of Public Health Methods, 567; Division of Research Grants, 492; Functional Chart, 499; Industrial Hygiene Research Laboratory, 492; and National Advisory Health Council, 490; National Cancer Institute, 491; Pathology Laboratory, 491; Zoology Laboratory, 492
N.I.H. swab, 171
National League of Nursing Education, 587, 588
National Leprosarium, 489, 493
National Organization for Public Health Nursing, 237: appraisal form, 423, 506; definition of public health nursing, 228; Educational Committee, 540, 542, 586; Manual of, 229, 240; and state nursing programs, 471
National Red Cross, *see* American National Red Cross
National Registration Area, 189
National Research Council, 349, 350, 370
National Sanitary Conventions, 16, 576
National Society for the Prevention of Blindness, 401, 503
National Tuberculosis Association, 100, 101, 238, 314, 401, 426, 440, 501, 503
Nebraska, 85, 342, 473
Necator americanus, 166–167, 206
Neefe, J. R., 182
Negri bodies, 150, 151, 154
Neisseria gonorrhea, 109
Neisseria intracellularis, 161
Nelson, A. A., 148
Nelson, K. R., 132
Nelson, N. B., 160
Nelson's Loose-Leaf Medicine, 170
Neonatal mortality, 272–273: birth injury, 272; epidemic diarrhea, 273; malformation, 272; premature infants, care of, 272; Rh factor in, 273; syphilis, 273
Neonatal mortality rate, definition of, 189
Nevada, 342, 448, 461, 473
New England, 139, 225, 425, 428, 440, 443, 456
New Jersey, 85, 152, 189, 225
New Mexico, 342, 452, 473
New Orleans, La., 15